Medical Insurance

An Integrated Claims Process Approach
Third Edition

JoanneValerius, RHIA, MPH
Chair, Information Management Department
Associate Professor, College of Saint Catherine

Nenna L.Bayes, B.A., M.Ed.
Associate Professor, Ashland Community and Technical College

Cynthia Newby, CPC

Janet I. B. Seggern, M.Ed., M.S., CCA
Professor of Business, Lehigh Carbon Community College

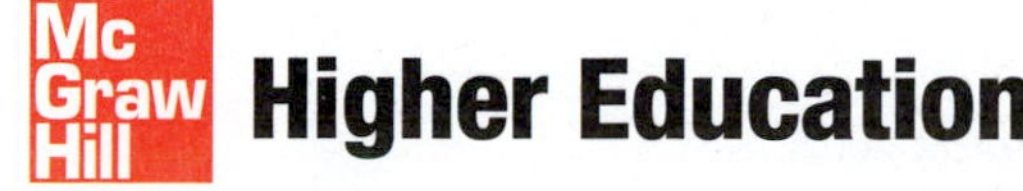

Boston Burr Ridge, IL Dubuque, IA New York San Francisco St. Louis
Bangkok Bogotá Caracas Kuala Lumpur Lisbon London Madrid Mexico City
Milan Montreal New Delhi Santiago Seoul Singapore Sydney Taipei Toronto

The McGraw·Hill Companies

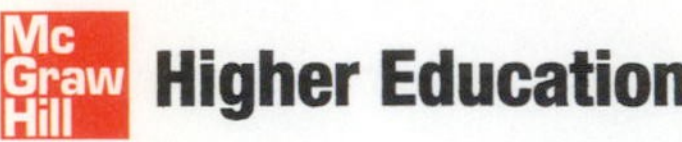

MEDICAL INSURANCE: AN INTEGRATED CLAIMS PROCESS APPROACH, THIRD EDITION

Published by McGraw-Hill, a business unit of The McGraw-Hill Companies, Inc., 1221 Avenue of the Americas, New York, NY 10020.

Some ancillaries, including electronic and print components, may not be available to customers outside the United States.

This book is printed on recycled, acid-free paper containing 10% postconsumer waste.

3 4 5 6 7 8 9 0 QPD/QPD 0 9 8

ISBN 978-0-07-352191-6
MHID 0-07-352191-4

Publisher: *Michelle Watnick/David T. Culverwell*
Senior Sponsoring Editor: *Roxan Kinsey*
Managing Developmental Editor: *Patricia Hesse*
Senior Marketing Manager: *Nancy Bradshaw*
Senior Project Manager: *Kay J. Brimeyer*
Senior Production Supervisor: *Sherry L. Kane*
Lead Media Project Manager: *Audrey A. Reiter*
Senior Coordinator of Freelance Design: *Michelle D. Whitaker*
Cover/Interior Designer: *Studio Montage*
(USE) Cover Image: *Computer monitor: ©Photodisc/Vol. OS52*
Compositor: Carlisle Publishing Services
Typeface: 11/13 *Berkeley*
Printer: *Quebecor World Dubuque, IA*

The Student Data Template CD-ROM, illustrations, instructions, and exercises in MEDICAL INSURANCE: AN INTEGRATED CLAIMS PROCESS APPROACH are compatible with the Medisoft™ Advanced Version 11 Patient Accounting software available at the time of publication. Adaptations may be necessary for use with subsequent versions of the software. Text changes will be made in reprints when possible. Medisoft Advanced Version 11 software must be available to access the data on The Student Data Template CD-ROM. It can be obtained by contacting your McGraw-Hill sales representative.

CPT codes are based on CPT 2007.
ICD-9-CM codes are based on ICD-9-CM 2007.

All names, situations, and anecdotes are fictitious. They do not represent any person, event, or medical record.

www.mhhe.com

Brief Contents

PREFACE XI

PART 1 WORKING WITH MEDICAL INSURANCE AND BILLING 1

Chapter 1 Introduction to the Medical Billing Process 2

Chapter 2 HIPAA and Medical Records 35

Chapter 3 Patient Encounters and Billing Information 73

PART 2 CLAIM CODING 109

Chapter 4 Diagnostic Coding: Introduction to ICD-9-CM 110

Chapter 5 Procedural Coding: Introduction to CPT 143

Chapter 6 Procedural Coding: Introduction to HCPCS 188

PART 3 CLAIM PREPARATION 203

Chapter 7 Visit Charges and Compliant Billing .204

Chapter 8 Health Care Claim Preparation and Transmission 237

PART 4 PAYERS 285

Chapter 9 Private Payers/Blue Cross and Blue Shield 286

Chapter 10 Medicare 332
Chapter 11 Medicaid 373
Chapter 12 TRICARE and CHAMPVA 398
Chapter 13 Workers' Compensation and Disability 422

PART 5 PAYMENT PROCESSING 447
Chapter 14 Payments (RAs/EOBs), Appeals, and Secondary Claims 448
Chapter 15 Patient Billing and Collections 484

PART 6 HOSPITAL SERVICES 511
Chapter 16 Hospital Billing and Reimbursement 512

PART 7 CLAIM CASE STUDIES 543
Chapter 17 Primary Case Studies 544
Chapter 18 RA/EOB/Secondary Case Studies 580

GUIDE TO MEDISOFT 593
APPENDIX A MEDICAL SPECIALTIES AND TAXONOMY CODES 617
APPENDIX B PLACE OF SERVICE CODES 623
APPENDIX C PROFESSIONAL WEBSITES 625
APPENDIX D FORMS 631

ABBREVIATIONS 633
GLOSSARY 637
INDEX 654

Contents

Preface xi
What Every Instructor Needs To Know xv
What Every Student Needs to Know xviii
Acknowledgments xx
How Can I Succeed in This Class? xxii

PART 1 WORKING WITH MEDICAL INSURANCE AND BILLING 1

Chapter 1 Introduction to the Medical Billing Process 2

Insurance Basics 3
Health Care Plans 6
Medical Insurance Payers 14
Duties of the Medical Insurance Specialist: The Medical Billing Process 16
Procedures, Communication, and Information Technology in the Medical Billing Process 21
Employment as a Medical Insurance Specialist 22
Chapter Review 29

Chapter 2 HIPAA and Medical Records 35

Medical Record Documentation 36
Health Care Regulation 45
HIPAA Privacy Rule 48
HIPAA Security Rule 56
HIPAA Electronic Health Care Transactions and Code Sets 57
Fraud and Abuse Regulations 59
Enforcement and Penalties 62

Compliance Plans 63
Chapter Review 66

Chapter 3 Patient Encounters and Billing Information 73

Gathering Patient Information 74
Establishing Financial Responsibility 86
Updating Patient Diagnoses, Procedures, and Charges 92
Collecting Time-of-Service Payments and Checking Out Patients 95
Chapter Review 102

PART 2 CLAIM CODING 109

Chapter 4 Diagnostic Coding: Introduction to ICD-9-CM 110

The ICD-9-CM 111
Organization of the ICD-9-CM 112
New Version: ICD-10-CM 113
The Alphabetic Index 114
The Tabular List 117
V Codes and E Codes 122
Coding Steps 124
Official Coding Guidelines 125
Overview of ICD-9-CM Chapters 130
Chapter Review 137

Chapter 5 Procedural Coding: Introduction to CPT 143

Current Procedural Terminology, Fourth Edition (CPT) 144
The Index 147
The Main Text 149
CPT Modifiers 152
The Appendixes 155
Coding Steps 156
Evaluation and Management Codes 157
Anesthesia Codes 169
Surgery Codes 171
Radiology Codes 176
Pathology and Laboratory Codes 177
Medicine Codes 179
Category II and III Codes 180

Chapter Review . . . 181

Chapter 6 Procedural Coding: Introduction to HCPCS . . . 188

Overview of HCPCS . . . 189
Level II Codes . . . 189
HCPCS Coding Procedures . . . 193
HCPCS Billing Procedures . . . 194
Chapter Review . . . 197

PART 3 CLAIM PREPARATION 203

Chapter 7 Visit Charges and Compliant Billing . . . 204

Compliant Billing . . . 205
Knowledge of Billing Rules . . . 205
Compliance Errors . . . 210
Strategies for Compliance . . . 212
Audits . . . 215
Comparing Physician Fees and Payer Fees . . . 220
Payer Fee Schedules . . . 222
Payment Methods . . . 225
Chapter Review . . . 230

Chapter 8 Health Care Claim Preparation and Transmission . . . 237

Introduction to Health Care Claims . . . 238
Completing the CMS-1500 Claim . . . 239
Completing the HIPAA 837 Claim . . . 260
Clearinghouses and Claim Transmission . . . 267
Chapter Review . . . 274

PART 4 PAYERS 285

Chapter 9 Private Payers/Blue Cross and Blue Shield . . . 286

Private Insurance . . . 287
Features of Group Health Plans . . . 290
Types of Private Payer Plans . . . 292
Consumer-Driven Health Plans . . . 296

Major Private Payers and the Blue Cross and Blue Shield Association . . . 299
Participation Contracts . . . 304
Interpreting Compensation and Billing Guidelines . . . 307
Private Payer Billing Management and Claim Completion . . . 312
Capitation Management . . . 320
Chapter Review . . . 323

Chapter 10 Medicare . . . 332

The Medicare Program . . . 333
Medicare Coverage and Benefits . . . 335
Medicare Participating Providers . . . 340
Nonparticipating Providers . . . 344
Original Medicare Plan and Medicare Advantage Plans . . . 346
Medigap Insurance . . . 349
Medicare Billing and Compliance . . . 351
Preparing Primary Medicare Claims . . . 355
Chapter Review . . . 363

Chapter 11 Medicaid . . . 373

The Medicaid Program . . . 374
Federal Eligibility . . . 375
State Programs . . . 377
Medicaid Enrollment Verification . . . 380
Covered and Excluded Services . . . 384
Types of Plans . . . 385
Payment For Services . . . 385
Third-Party Liability . . . 386
Claim Filing Guidelines . . . 387
Medicaid Claim Completion . . . 388
Chapter Review . . . 391

Chapter 12 Tricare and Champva . . . 398

The TRICARE Program . . . 399
TRICARE Standard . . . 401
TRICARE Prime . . . 403
TRICARE Extra . . . 404
TRICARE Reserve Select . . . 404
TRICARE and Other Insurance Plans . . . 404

Filing Claims 405
Fraud and Abuse 406
CHAMPVA 409
Chapter Review 413

Chapter 13 Workers' Compensation and Disability 422
Occupational Safety and Health Administration 423
Federal Workers' Compensation Plans 423
State Workers' Compensation Plans 424
Classification of Injuries 426
Workers' Compensation Terminology 427
Workers' Compensation and the HIPAA Privacy Rule 428
Claim Process 429
Billing and Claim Management 433
Disability Compensation Programs 434
Government Programs 434
Preparing Disability Reports 436
Chapter Review 438

PART 5 PAYMENT PROCESSING 447

Chapter 14 Payments (RAs/EOBs), Appeals, and Secondary Claims 448
Claim Adjudication 449
Monitoring Claim Status 453
The Remittance Advice/Explanation of Benefits (RA/EOB) 456
Reviewing and Processing RAs/EOBs 462
Appeals, Postpayment Audits, Overpayments, and Grievances 464
Billing Secondary Payers 468
Chapter Review 478

Chapter 15 Patient Billing and Collections 484
Patient Billing 485
Organizing For Effective Collections 492
Collection Regulations and Procedures 494
Credit Arrangements and Payment Plans 499
Collection Agencies and Credit Reporting 500
Skip Tracing 502
Writing Off Uncollectible Accounts 503

Record Retention. 505
Chapter Review 506

PART 6 HOSPITAL SERVICES 511

Chapter 16 Hospital Billing and Reimbursement 512

Health Care Facilities: Inpatient Versus Outpatient 513
Hospital Claim Processing 514
Inpatient (Hospital) Coding 523
Payers and Payment Methods 526
Claims and Follow-Up 529
Chapter Review 537

PART 7 CLAIM CASE STUDIES 543

Chapter 17 Primary Case Studies 544

Chapter 18 RA/EOB/ Secondary Case Studies 580

GUIDE TO MEDISOFT™ 593

Part 1: *Getting Started with Medisoft* 593
Part 2: *Overview and Practice*. 597

APPENDIX A MEDICAL SPECIALTIES AND TAXONOMY CODES 617
APPENDIX B PLACE OF SERVICE CODES 623
APPENDIX C PROFESSIONAL WEBSITES 625
APPENDIX D FORMS 631
ABBREVIATIONS 633
GLOSSARY 637
INDEX 654

Preface

Welcome to the third edition of *Medical Insurance*. This program introduces you to the concepts, knowledge, and skills you will need for a successful career in medical insurance. Medical billing is one of the 10 fastest-growing allied health occupations. This employment growth is the result of the increased medical needs of an aging population, advances in technology, and the growing number of health practitioners.

Your Career in Medical Insurance, Billing, and Reimbursement

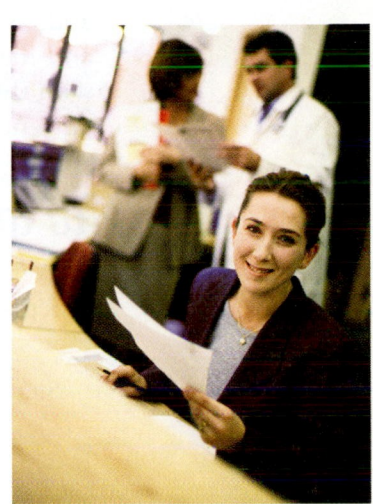

Medical insurance specialists play important roles in the financial wellbeing of every health care business. Billing for services in health care is more complicated than in other industries. Government and private payers vary in payment for the same services, and health care providers deliver services to beneficiaries of several insurance companies at any one time. Medical insurance specialists must be familiar with the rules and guidelines of each health care plan in order to submit the proper documentation so that the office receives maximum appropriate reimbursement for services provided. Without an effective administrative staff, a medical office would have no cash flow!

Medical billing is a challenging, interesting career, where you are compensated according to your level of skills and how effectively you put them to use. Those with the right combination of skills and abilities may have the opportunity to advance to management positions, such as patient account managers, physician office supervisors, and medical office managers. The more education the individual has, the more employment options and advancement opportunities are available. Individuals who have a firm understanding of the medical billing process will find themselves well prepared to enter this ever-changing field.

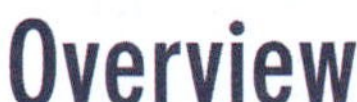

Overview

Whether your course of study is medical assisting, medical insurance, or health information technology, this text/workbook gives you the background, knowledge and skills needed to successfully perform insurance-related duties. It focuses on three components required to handle the medical billing process:

1. Knowledge of procedures–including the administrative duties important in medical practices and an understanding of how to bill both payers and patients.

2. Communication skills–effectively working with physicians, patients, other members of the health care team, and payers using written and oral communications.
3. Health information management skills–using computer technology to manage patients' records and the billing/collections process, electronically transmit claims, conduct research, and for communications.

Medical insurance specialists must also understand medical coding guidelines and principles in order to verify diagnosis and procedure codes and use them to report patients' conditions on health care claims and encounter forms. For this reason, the text/workbook provides a fundamental understanding of diagnostic and procedural coding, preparing you to effectively and efficiently submit claims in accordance with payers' requirements.

Of special importance is the coverage of HIPAA. In today's health care environment, claims cannot be simply correct. Claims, as well as the process used to create them, must also comply with the rules imposed by federal and state law and by government and private payer health care program requirements. Medical insurance specialists help ensure that physician practices receive maximum appropriate reimbursement for reported services by submitting correct and compliant claims, reducing the chance of an investigation of the practice and the risk of liability if an audit occurs. *Medical Insurance 3e* provides you with the concepts and facts needed to understand applicable rules and to stay current with the changing regulatory environment.

To the Student

The third edition of *Medical Insurance* follows a ten-step medical billing process, illustrated on the inside front cover of your text, that organizes the topics for you. This sequence includes:

Step 1 Preregister patients

Step 2 Establish financial responsibility for visits

Step 3 Check in patients

Step 4 Check out patients

Step 5 Review coding compliance

Step 6 Check billing compliance

Step 7 Prepare and transmit claims

Step 8 Monitor payer adjudication

Step 9 Generate patient statements

Step 10 Follow up patient payments and handle collections

The seven instructional parts of the text/workbook follow this sequence:

- Part 1, *Working with Medical Insurance and Billing,* introduces the major types of medical insurance, payers, and regulators; the medical insurance specialist's functions, ethical responsibilities, and certification; the medical billing process; and HIPAA Privacy, Security, and Electronic Health Care Transactions/Code Sets rules.
- Part 2, *Claim Coding,* builds skills in correct coding procedures, use of coding references, and compliance with proper linkage guidelines.
- Part 3, *Claim Preparation,* covers the general procedures for calculating reimbursement, how to bill compliantly, and preparing and transmitting

claims using the CMS-1500 (08/05) paper claim and the HIPAA electronic claim.

- Part 4, *Payers*, provides descriptions of the major third-party private and government-sponsored payers' procedures and regulations. Each chapter contains specific filing guidelines.
- Part 5, *Payment Processing*, explains how to handle payments from payers, follow up and appeal claims, file secondary claims, and correctly bill and collect from patients.
- Part 6, *Hospital Services*, provides necessary background in hospital billing, coding, and payment methods.
- Part 7, *Claim Case Studies*, provides exercises to reinforce your knowledge of completing primary/secondary claims, processing payments from payers, and handling patients' accounts.

After completing *Medical Insurance: An Integrated Claims Process Approach*, students can enhance their qualifications for employment by studying *Computers in the Medical Office*, which develops skills in the use of Medisoft™, a popular medical billing and accounting software program, that can easily be transferred to any software program on the job. These skills can then be cemented through *Case Studies for the Medical Office: Capstone Billing Simulation*, an excellent "internship in a box." *Case Studies for the Medical Office: Capstone Billing Simulation* contains a simulation covering two weeks of work in a medical office using Medisoft.

What Every Instructor Needs to Know

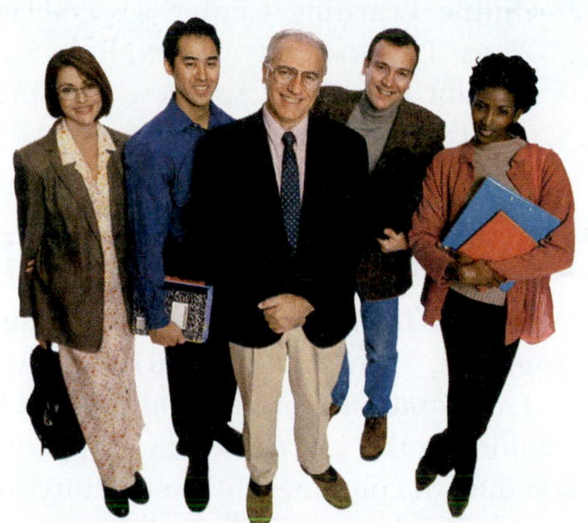

What's New in the Third Edition?

- **NEW text subtitle, *An Integrated Claims Process Approach*, and the medical billing process illustration** printed on the inside front cover for easy reference, together reflect the emphasis on the ten-step billing cycle that organizes the text presentation. Chapter 1 previews this medical billing process so that students understand the medical insurance specialist's role in the logical flow from patient encounter, claim coding and preparation, to patient billing and collections that ensures maximum appropriate payment for the physician's services. The process is then integrated into each subsequent chapter to enhance comprehension of the related tasks.
- NEW ***Workbook to Accompany Medical Insurance: An Integrated Claims Process Approach*** has been created to reinforce, apply, and extend student knowledge of essential concepts. Each workbook chapter contains assisted outlining, objective questions covering key terms, critical thinking questions, guided web activities, and an Applying Concepts section to reinforce and extend abstracting insurance information, calculating insurance math, and using insurance terms.
- **NEW worked-out examples and case studies** in every chapter that build the basic skills of abstracting insurance information, calculating insurance math, and insurance communications.
- **NEW chapters** "Payments (RAs/ROBs), Appeals, and Secondary Claims" and "Patient Billing and Collections" include handling payers' remittance advices, preparing secondary claims, laws regulating patient collections, the role of collection agencies, and handling uncollectible accounts in the medical office. Students understand the entire collections process of identifying overdue accounts, planning for follow-up, correctly communicating with patients over the telephone, creating collections letters, and monitoring the collections process.
- **NEW case studies** in Chapters 17 and 18 provide over fifty primary/secondary claims, RA/EOBs, and patient account exercises.

- **NEW Customizable Lesson Plans** integrate the text pedagogy, the supplied lecture and testing tools, and the new *Workbook to Accompany Medical Insurance: An Integrated Claims Process Approach* as well as the updated 2007–2008 *Medical Insurance Coding Workbook.* An Instructor Productivity CD-ROM contains chapter-by-chapter PowerPoint® presentations and EZTest test generator. Questions from EZTest can be used with eInstruction's Classroom Performance System.
- **Online Learning Center** *www.mhhe.com/medinsurance3e* includes Lesson Plans, Power Point® Slides, links to professional organizations, and PDF files for teaching resources. Also provided for student review are games, flashcards, and additional questions.

Learning and Teaching Supplements

***Workbook to Accompany Medical Insurance: An Integrated Claims Process Approach*, Third Edition (0-07-340210-9)**

The *Workbook to Accompany Medical Insurance* has excellent material for (1) reinforcing the text content, (2) applying concepts, and (3) extending understanding. It combines the best features of a workbook and a study guide. Each workbook chapter enhances the text's strong pedagogy through:

- Assisted Outlining—reinforce the chapter's key points
- Key Terms—objective questions and crossword puzzles/word finds
- Critical Thinking—questions that stimulate process understanding
- Guided Web Activities—build skill in locating and then evaluating information on the Internet
- Applying Concepts—reinforce and extend abstracting insurance information, calculating insurance math, and using insurance terms

Matching the text chapter-by-chapter, the workbook reinforces, applies, and extends the text to enhance the learning process.

***Medical Insurance Coding Workbook for Physician Practices*, 2007–2008 Edition (0-07-352205-8)**

The *Medical Insurance Coding Workbook* provides practice and instruction in coding and compliance skills. Since medical insurance specialists verify diagnosis and procedure codes and use them to report physicians' services, a fundamental understanding of coding principles and guidelines is the baseline for correct claims. The coding workbook reinforces and enhances skill development by applying the coding principles introduced in *Medical Insurance 3e* and extending knowledge through additional coding guidelines, examples, and compliance tips. More than 75 NEW case studies have been added to simulate more real-world application.

For the Instructor

Instructor's Medisoft™ Advanced Version 11 Software

This full working version allows a school to place the live software on the laboratory or classroom computers (only one copy needs to be sent per campus location).

Instructor's Manual (0-07-352195-7) includes:

- course overview.
- information on ordering and installing Medisoft™ Advanced Version 11 software.

- software troubleshooting tips
- answers to the text's Thinking It Through and end-of-chapter questions
- workbook answers
- answer key for *Medical Insurance Coding Workbook*
- correlation tables: SCANS, AAMA Role Delineation Study Areas of Competence (2003), and AMT Registered Medical Assistant Certification Exam Topics

If you elect to use Medisoft™ Advanced Version 11 program for the claim case studies, you can rely on the manual for important information that you can use to help your students work through the exercises in the book.

Instructor Productivity Center CD-ROM (packaged with the Instructor's Manual) includes:

- instructor's PowerPoint® presentation of Chapters 1–16.
- electronic testing program featuring McGraw-Hill's EZ Test. This flexible and easy-to-use program allows instructors to create tests from book specific items. It accommodates a wide range of question types and instructors may add their own questions. Multiple versions of the test can be created and any test can be exported for use with course management systems such as WebCT, Blackboard, or PageOut.
- Instructor's Manual.
- Medisoft backup file (VAPCclaims.mbk) for instructor use.

Online Learning Center (OLC), *www.mhhe.com/medinsurance3e,* Instructor Resources include:

- Instructor's Manual in Word and PDF format
- Customizable Lesson Plans
- PowerPoint® files for each chapter
- links to professional associations
- Medisoft™ tips and frequently asked questions
- Medisoft™ Advanced Version 11 installation instructions
- PageOut link
- PDF files for teaching resources
- Medisoft backup file (VAPCclaims.mbk) for instructor use.

For the Student

Student-at-Home Medisoft™ Advanced Version 11 Software

This version is an option for distance education or students who want to practice with the software at home.

Student Data Template CD-ROM is packaged with every copy of the text. The data template provides the patient database to complete Medisoft™ Advanced, Version 11 claim case studies.

Online Learning Center (OLC), *www.mhhe.com/medinsurance3e* includes additional chapter quizzes and other review activities.

What Every Student Needs to Know

Many tools to help you learn have been integrated into your text.

Chapter Features

Chapter Outline—gives you an overview of the key concepts and organization.

Learning Outcomes—present a list of the most important points you should focus on in the chapter.

Key Terms—list the important vocabulary words alphabetically to build your insurance terminology. Key terms are highlighted and defined when introduced in the text.

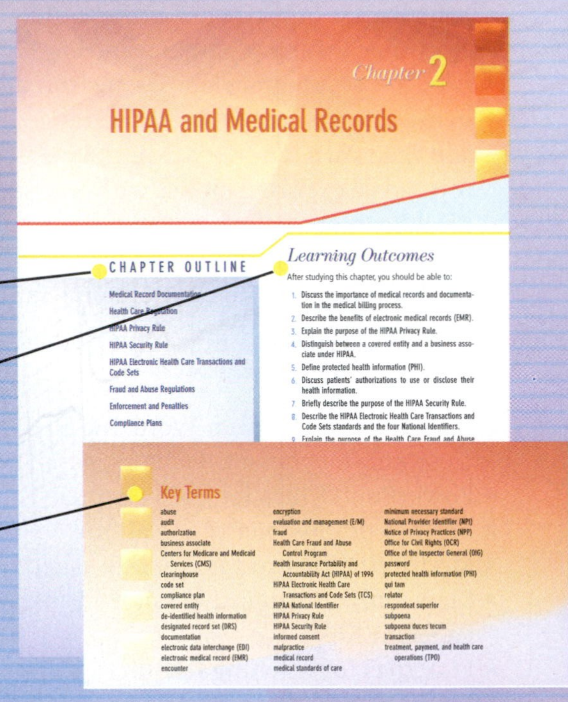

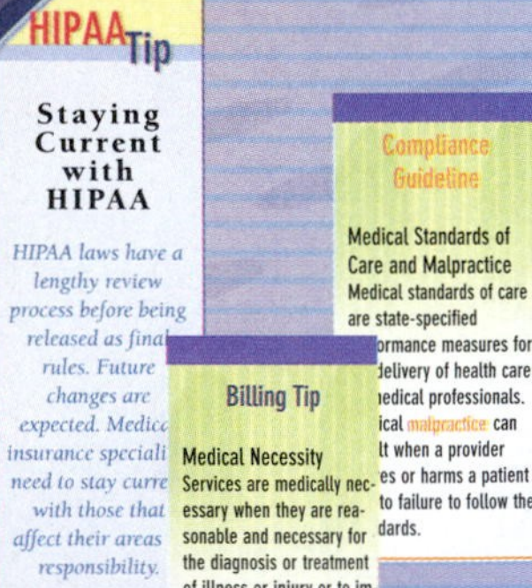

HIPAA, Billing, and Compliance Tips—connect you to the real world of insurance billing. These tips on HIPAA rules, billing points, and ensuring compliance with correct billing and coding practices are located in the margins near the related chapter topics.

Figures, Forms, and Screen Captures—illustrate the key concepts in the chapter visually.

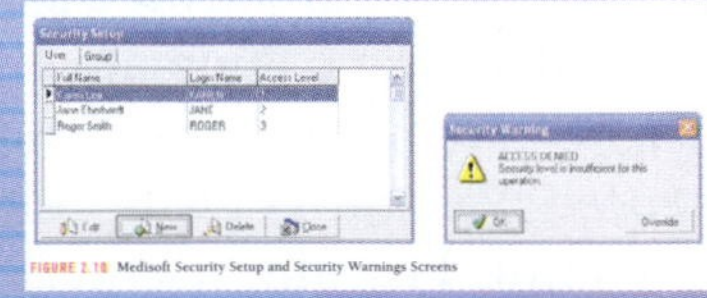

Thinking It Through—challenges you to stop and think through the questions that are posed at major points in the chapter.

Thinking It Through — 2.2

Based on the information in Figure 2.7:

1. What document is required when a patient asks Valley Associates to transfer a record to another person or organization?
2. Is written authorization from a patient needed to use or disclose health information in an emergency?
3. What is the purpose of an "accounting of disclosures"?

I found all of the Applying Your Knowledge exercises to be right on track and beneficial to student success.

Carol Putkamer,
Alpena Community College

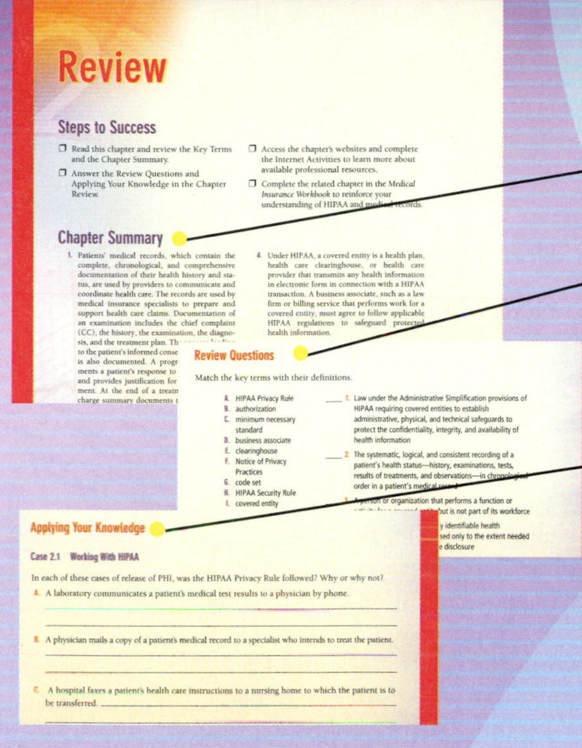

Chapter Review

Chapter Summary—provides a helpful review of the chapter's key concepts.

Review Questions—reinforce the important facts and points made in the chapter. Question formats include matching, true-false, completion, and short answer.

Applying Your Knowledge—utilizes cases that ask you to apply the knowledge gained by studying the chapter for correct answers.

Icons point you to the *Medical Insurance Coding Workbook* to reinforce your understanding of major coding points.

Internet Resources and Activities
describe relevant websites and direct you to use the Internet to research and report your findings. The goal of the activities is to extend your knowledge of the selected topics and to learn to use the Internet as a research tool.

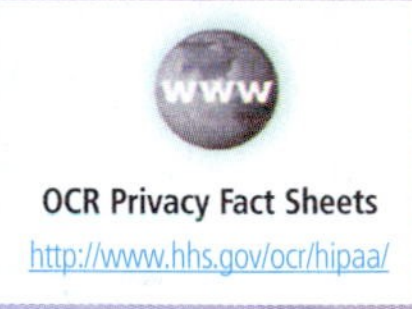

Claim Case Studies

The claim case studies in Chapters 8 through 13 and in Chapters 17–18 let you practice your knowledge of correctly preparing primary and secondary claims.

Abbreviations and Glossary

The most important insurance, billing, and coding abbreviations and definitions are found at the back of the text for easy reference.

Online Learning Center (OLC)

www.mhhe.com/medinsurance3e
The OLC offers additional learning and teaching tools.

> *Chapter 13 presents extensive information in a concise and organized manner. This chapter is a definite strength of the textbook. The material is well organized and offers insights to job responsibilities.*
>
> Patricia Stich,
> Waubonsee Community College

Acknowledgments

For insightful reviews and helpful suggestions, we would like to acknowledge the following individuals.

Contributors

Chapter 6, Procedural Coding: Introduction to HCPCS:

Wilsetta L. McClain, BBA, RMA, CMB, NCICS, NR-CMA, EMT-B

For technical review of coding instruction in Chapters 4 and 5:

Daphne Balacos, CPC, approved AAPC PMCC instructor

Third Edition Reviewers:

LaBera A. Ard, B.A., M.A., CPC
Bluegrass Community and Technical College
Lexington, KY

Elaine Bellcourt, M.S.
ECPI College of Technology
Greenville, SC

Gerry A. Brasin, C.M.A., A.S., CPC
Premier Education Group
Springfield, MA

BethAnn Clouser, B.A.
formerly Thompson Institute
Harrisburg, PA

Marianne Durling, Medical Coding Program Coordinator/Instructor
Vance Granville Community College
Henderson, NC

Deborah S. Gilbert, Ed.S., MBA
Dalton State College
Dalton, GA

Kelley Fazzone, B.A.
Blair College
Colorado Springs, CO

Nina Gookin-Peterson, M.S.
Blackhawk Technical College
Janesville, WI

Carol Hinricher, M.A.
University of Montana College of Technology
Missoula, MT

Gerald J. Levy, M.S., C.H.I.
International Development Institute
New York, NY

Wilsetta L. McClain, BBA, RMA, CMB, NCICS, NR-CMA
Baker College of Auburn Hills
Auburn Hills, MI

Janice Manning, M.A., CPC
Baker College, Jackson Campus
Jackson, MI

Michael A. Meyer, D.O., CCS, CPC
FMU South Orlando, DeVry Online, South University Online
Orlando, FL

Angela Parmley, AABA
Sanford Brown Institute
Trevose, PA

Carol Putkamer, M.S., RHIA
Alpena Community College
Alpena, MI

Patricia A. Stich, M.A.
Waubonsee Community College
Sugar Grove, IL

Stacy L. Taylor, B.S.
formerly Florida Career College
West Palm Beach, FL

Nina Thierer, CMA
Ivy Tech State College
Fort Wayne, IN

Sandra A. Thomas, NCICS, NCMA, Academic Director, Medical Billing & Coding Instructor
Professional Careers Institute
Houston, TX

Jim Wallace, MHSA
Maric College—Los Angeles
Los Angeles, CA

Stacey F. Wilson, B.S., CMA, MT
Cabarrus College of Health Sciences
Concord, NC

Second Edition Reviewers:

Lisa Ann Cook, B.S.H.S.

Mercedes A. Fisher
Indian River Community College

Linda Iavarone, B.X., R.T.
National Institute of Technology

Margaret McCoy
Ivy Tech State College
Fort Wayne, IN

Dr. Linda F. Samson
Governors State University

Ann Marti-Segrini, RHIA
Santa Fe Community College
Gainesville, FL

Kristi Sopp
MTI College

Valeria D. Truitt
Craven Community College
New Bern, NC

How Can I Succeed in this Class?

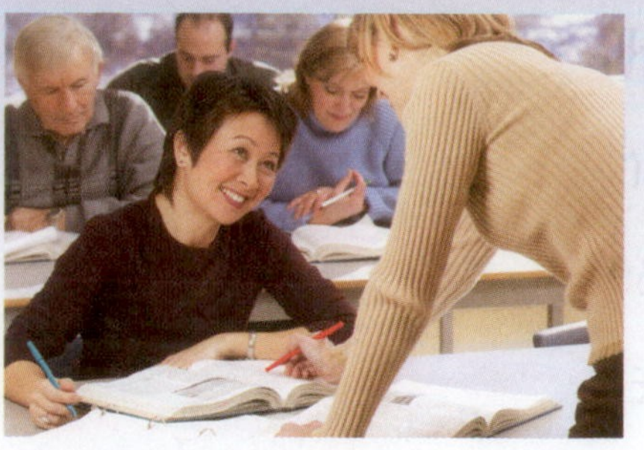

An important step in effective learning begins with a solid study strategy. Many students feel overwhelmed when learning new concepts and a new software program at the same time. The following study tips will help ensure your success in this course.

"You are the same today that you are going to be five years from now except for two things: the people with whom you associate and the books you read."

Charles Jones

Right now, you're probably leafing through this book feeling just a little overwhelmed. You're trying to juggle several other classes (which probably are equally as intimidating), possibly a job, and on top of it all, a life.

It's true—you are what you put into your studies. You have a lot of time and money invested in your education. Don't blow it now by only putting in half of the effort this class requires. Succeeding in this class (and life) requires:

A commitment—of time and perseverance

- **Knowing and motivating yourself**
- **Getting organized**
- **Managing your time**

This special introduction has been designed specifically to help you learn how to be effective in these areas, as well as offer guidance in:

- **Getting the most out of your lecture**
- **Thinking through—and applying—the material**
- **Getting the most out of your textbook**
- **Finding extra help when you need it**

Making a commitment—of time and perseverance

Learning—and mastering—takes time. And patience. Nothing worthwhile comes easily. Be committed to your studies and you will reap the benefits in the long run.

Consider this: your accounting courses are building the foundation for your future—a future in your chosen profession. Sloppy and hurried craftsmanship now will only lead to ruins later.

Knowing and motivating yourself

What type of a learner are you? When are you most productive? Know yourself and your limits and work within them. Know how to motivate yourself to give your all to your studies and achieve your goals. Quite bluntly, you are the one who benefits most from your success. If you lack self-motivation and drive, you are the first person who suffers.

Know yourself—There are many types of learners, and no right or wrong way of learning. Which category do you fall into?

- **Visual learner**—You respond best to "seeing" processes and information. Particularly focus on the text's figures and tables.
- **Auditory learner**—You work best by listening to—and possibly tape recording—the lecture and by talking information through with a study partner. Be sure not to miss any lectures.
- **Tactile/kinesthetic learner**—You learn best by being "hands on." You'll benefit by applying what you've learned during lab time. Think of ways to apply your critical thinking skills in application ways. Be sure to complete all the computer exercises in the textbook.

Identify your own personal preferences for learning and seek out the resources that will best help you with your studies. Also, learn by recognizing your weaknesses and try to compensate/work to improve them.

Getting organized

It's simple, yet it's fundamental. It seems the more organized you are, the easier things come. Take the time before your course begins to look around and analyze your life and your study habits. Get organized now and you'll find you have a little more time—and a lot less stress.

- **Find a calendar system that works for you.** The best kind is one that you can take with you everywhere. To be truly organized, you should integrate all aspects of your life into this one calendar—school, work, leisure. Some people also find it helpful to have an additional monthly calendar posted by their desk for "at a glance" dates and to have a visual of what's to come. If you do this, be sure you are consistently synchronizing both calendars so as not to miss anything. *More tips for organizing your calendar can be found in the time management discussion on the next page.*
- **Keep everything for your course or courses in one place**—and at your fingertips. A three-ring binder works well because it allows you to add or organize handouts and notes from class in any order you prefer. Incorporating your own custom tabs helps you flip to exactly what you need at a moment's notice.
- **Find your space.** Find a place that helps you be organized and focused. If it's your desk in your dorm room or in your home, keep it clean. Clutter adds confusion, stress, and wastes time. Or perhaps your "space" is at the library. If that's the case, keep a backpack or bag that's fully stocked with what you might need—your text, binder or notes, pens, highlighters, Post-its®, phone numbers of study partners

(hint: a good place to keep phone numbers is in your "one place for everything calendar").

*A **Helpful Hint**—add extra "padding" into your deadlines to yourself. If you have an assignment due on Friday, set a goal for yourself to have it done on Wednesday. Then, take time on Thursday to look over your work again, with a fresh eye. Make any corrections or enhancements and have it ready to turn in on Friday.*

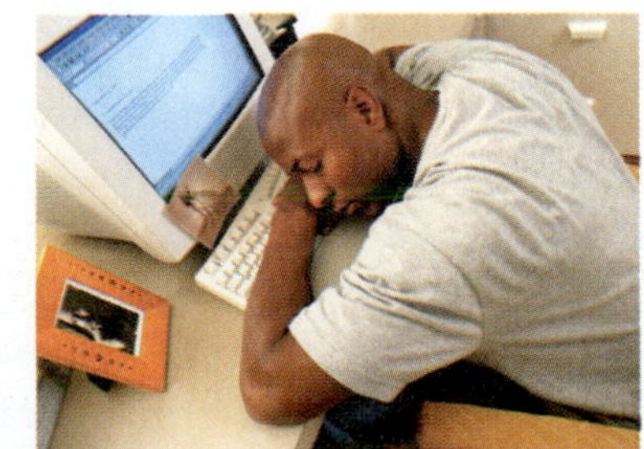

Managing your time

Managing your time is the single most important thing you can do to help yourself. And, it's probably one of the most difficult tasks to successfully master.

You are taking this course because you want to succeed in life. You are preparing for a career. You are expected to work much harder and to learn much more than you ever have before. To be successful you need to invest in your education with a commitment of time.

How time slips away

People tend to let an enormous amount of time slip away from them, mainly in three ways:

1. **procrastination**, putting off chores simply because we don't feel in the mood to do them right away
2. **distraction**, getting sidetracked by the endless variety of other things that seem easier or more fun to do, often not realizing how much time they eat up
3. **underestimating the value of small bits of time**, thinking it's not worth doing any work because we have something else to do or somewhere else to be in 20 minutes or so.

We all lead busy lives. But we all make choices as to how we spend our time. Choose wisely and make the most of every minute you have by implementing these tips.

Know yourself and when you'll be able to study most efficiently

When are you most productive? Are you a late nighter? Or an early bird? Plan to study when you are most alert and can have uninterrupted segments. This could include a quick 5-minute review before class or a one-hour problem solving study session with a friend.

Create a set study time for yourself daily

Having a set schedule for yourself helps you commit to studying, and helps you plan instead of cram. Find—and use—a planner that is small enough that you can take with you—everywhere. This can be a $2.50 paper calendar or a more expensive electronic version. They all work on the same premise—**organize *all* of your activities in one place.**

Less is more. Schedule study time using shorter, focused blocks with small breaks. Doing this offers two benefits:

1. You will be less fatigued and gain more from your effort, and
2. Studying will seem less overwhelming and you will be less likely to procrastinate.

Plan time for leisure, friends, family, exercise, and sleep

Studying should be your main focus, but you need to balance your time—and your life.

Try to complete tasks ahead of schedule. This will give you a chance to carefully review your work before you hand it in (instead of at 1 a.m. when you are half awake). You'll feel less stressed in the end.

Prioritize!

In your calendar or planner, highlight or number key projects; do them first, and then cross them off when you've completed them. Give yourself a pat on the back for getting them done!

Try to resist distractions by setting and sticking to a designated study time (remember your commitment and perseverance!) Distractions may include friends and surfing the Internet. . .

Multitask when possible

You may find a lot of extra time you didn't think you had. Review material or organize your term paper in your head while walking to class, doing laundry, or during "mental down time." (Note—mental down time does NOT mean in the middle of lecture.)

Getting the most out of lectures

Believe it or not, instructors want you to succeed. They put a lot of effort into helping you learn and preparing their lectures. Attending class is one of the simplest, most valuable things you can do to help yourself. But it doesn't end there. . . . getting the most out of your lectures means being organized. Here's how:

Prepare Before You Go To Class

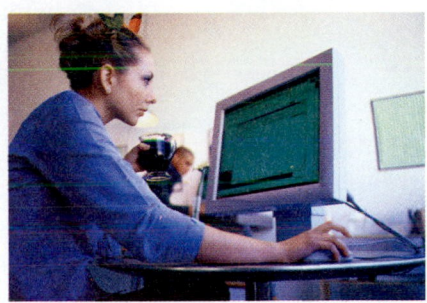

Really! You'll be amazed at how much more comprehensible the material will be when you preview the chapter before you go to class. Don't feel overwhelmed by this already. One tip that may help you—plan to arrive to class 5-15 minutes before lecture. Bring your text with you and skim the chapter before lecture begins. This will at the very least give you an overview of what may be discussed.

Be a Good Listener

Most people think they are good listeners, but few really are. Are you?

Obvious, but important points to remember:

1. You can't listen if you are talking.
2. You aren't listening if you are daydreaming.
3. Listening and comprehending are two different things. If you don't understand something your instructor is saying, ask a question or jot a note and visit the instructor after hours. Don't feel dumb or intimidated; you probably aren't the only person who "doesn't get it."

Take Good Notes

1. Use a standard size notebook, and better yet, a three-ring binder with loose leaf notepaper. The binder will allow you to organize and integrate your notes and handouts, integrate easy-to-reference tabs, etc.
2. Use a standard black or blue ink pen to take your initial notes. You can annotate later using a pencil, which can be erased if need be.
3. Start a new page with each lecture or note-taking session (yes—you can and should also take notes from your textbook).
4. Label each page with the date and a heading for each day.
5. Focus on main points and try to use an outline format to take notes to capture key ideas and organize sub-points.

6. Review and edit your notes shortly after class—at least within 24 hours—to make sure they make sense and that you've recorded core thoughts. You may also want to compare your notes with a study partner later to make sure neither of you have missed anything.

Get a Study Partner

Having a study partner has so many benefits. First, he/she can help you keep your commitment to this class. By having set study dates, you can combine study and social time, and maybe even make it fun! In addition, you now have two sets of eyes and ears and two minds to help digest the information from lecture and from the text. Talk through concepts, compare notes, and quiz each other.

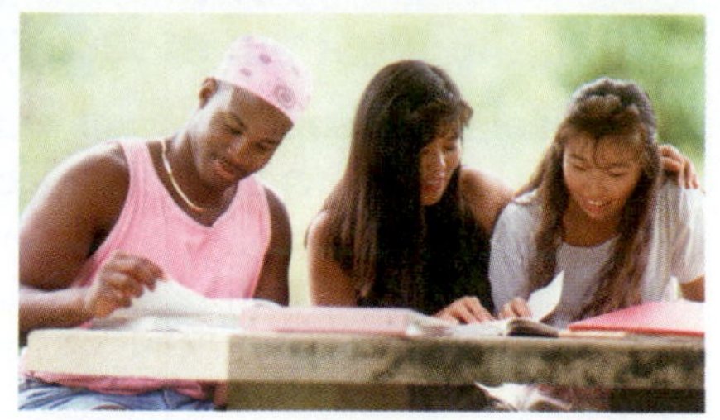

An obvious note: Don't take advantage of your study partner by skipping class or skipping study dates. You obviously won't have a study partner—or a friend—much longer if it's not a mutually beneficial arrangement!

Part 1 Working with Medical Insurance and Billing

Chapter 1
Introduction to the Medical Billing Process

Chapter 2
HIPAA and Medical Records

Chapter 3
Patient Encounters and Billing Information

Chapter 1

Introduction to the Medical Billing Process

CHAPTER OUTLINE

Insurance Basics

Health Care Plans

Medical Insurance Payers

Duties of the Medical Insurance Specialist: The Medicalbilling Process

Procedures, Communication, and Information Technology in the Medical Billing Process

Employment as a Medical Insurance Specialist

Learning Outcomes

After studying this chapter, you should be able to:

1. Describe the basic features of medical insurance policies.
2. Compare indemnity and managed care plans.
3. Discuss the fee-for-service and the capitation methods of payment for medical services.
4. Compare health maintenance organizations, point-of-service plans, and preferred provider organizations.
5. Describe the key features of a consumer-driven health plan.
6. Describe the major types of payers for medical insurance.
7. List the ten steps in the medical billing process.
8. Identify the most important skills of medical insurance specialists.
9. Discuss the types of health care organizations that employ medical insurance specialists.
10. Compare medical ethics and etiquette.

Key Terms

accounts receivable (A/R)
benefits
capitation
coinsurance
compliance
consumer-driven health plan (CDHP)
copayment
covered services
deductible
diagnosis code
ethics
etiquette
excluded services
fee-for-service
health care claim
health maintenance organization (HMO)
health plan
indemnity plan
managed care
managed care organization (MCO)
medical coder
medical insurance
medical insurance specialist
medical necessity
network
noncovered services
open-access plans
out-of-network
out-of-pocket
participation
patient ledger
payer
per member per month (PMPM)
point-of-service (POS) option
policyholder
practice management program (PMP)
preauthorization
preexisting condition
preferred provider organization (PPO)
premium
preventive medical services
primary care physician (PCP)
procedure code
provider
referral
schedule of benefits
self-funded health plan
third-party payer

Patients who come to physicians' practices for medical care are obligated to pay for the services they receive. Some patients pay these costs themselves, while others have medical insurance to help them cover medical expenses. Administrative staff members help collect the maximum appropriate payments by handling patients' financial arrangements, billing insurance companies, and processing payments to ensure both top-quality service and profitable operation.

Insurance Basics

The trillion-dollar health care industry—including pharmaceutical companies, hospitals, doctors, medical equipment makers, nursing homes, assisted-living centers, and insurance companies—is a fast-growing and dynamic sector of the American economy.

Rising Spending

Spending on health care in the United States continues to rise, for two reasons. The first factor is the cost of advances in medical technology. An X-ray machine that cost less than $200,000 ten years ago is upgraded to a more powerful CT scan device that costs over $1 million. The second factor is an aging American population that requires more health care services. Average life expectancy is increasing, and by 2030 people over the age of sixty-five will make up 20 percent of the population. More than half of the patients receiving care from physicians are older than forty-five. Older people need more health care services than do younger people; more than half of the money spent on health care goes to managing chronic diseases, such as diabetes, hypertension, osteoporosis, and arthritis, which are more common in people older than sixty-five.

Who Pays for Health Care?

Since medical costs are rising faster than the overall economy is growing, more of everyone's dollars are spent on health care. Federal and state government budgets

U.S Department of Labor
Bureau of Labor Statistics

Occupational Outlook Handbook

Health Information Technicians

- Health Information technicians are projected to be one of the 20 fastest growing occupations.
- Job prospects for formally trained technicians should be very good. Employment of health information technicians is expected to grow much faster than the average for all occupations through 2010, due to rapid growth in the number of medical tests, treatments, and procedures which will be increasingly scrutinized by third-party payers, regulators, courts, and consumers.
- Most technicians will be employed in hospitals, but job growth will be faster in offices and clinics of physicians, nursing homes, and home health agencies.

Medical Assistants

- Employment of medical assistants is expected to grow much faster than the average for all occupations through 2010 as the health services industry expands due to technological advances in medicine and a growing and aging population. It is one of the fastest growing occupations.
- Employment growth will be driven by the increase in the number of group practices, clinics, and other health care facilities that need a high proportion of support personnel, particularly the flexible medical assistant who can handle both administrative and clinical duties. Medical assistants work primarily in outpatient settings, where much faster than average growth is expected.
- Job prospects should be best for medical assistants with formal training or experience, particularly those with certification.

Medical Administrative Support

- Growth in the health services industry will spur faster than average employment growth for medical support staff.
- Medical administrative support employees may transcribe dictation, prepare correspondence, and assist physicians or medical scientists with reports, speeches, articles, and conference proceedings. They also record simple medical histories, arrange for patients to be hospitalized, and order supplies. Most medical administrative support staff need to be familiar with insurance rules, billing practices, and hospital or laboratory procedures.

Figure 1.1 Employment Opportunities

increase to pay for medical services, employers pay more each year for medical services for their employees, and patients also pay higher costs. These rising costs increase the financial pressure on physicians' practices. To remain profitable, physicians must carefully manage the business side of their practices. Knowledgeable medical office employees are in demand to help. Figure 1.1 describes the rapidly growing employment possibilities in the health care administrative area.

Medical Insurance Terms

Understanding how to work with the medical billing process begins with medical insurance basics. **Medical insurance**, which is also known as health insurance, is a written policy that states the terms of an agreement between a **policyholder**—an individual—and a **health plan**—an insurance company. The policyholder (also called the insured, the member, or the subscriber) makes payments of a specified amount of money. In exchange, the health plan provides **benefits**—defined by the Health Insurance Association of America as payments for medical services—for a specific period of time. Because they pay for medical expenses, then, health plans are often referred to as **payers.**

Health plans create a variety of insurance products that offer different levels of coverage for various prices. In each product, they must manage the risk that some individuals they insure will need very expensive medical services. They do that by spreading that risk among many policyholders.

Health Care Benefits

The medical insurance policy contains a **schedule of benefits** that summarizes the payments that may be made for medically necessary medical services which policyholders receive. The payer's definition of **medical necessity** is the key to coverage and payment. A medically necessary service is reasonable and is consistent with generally accepted professional medical standards for the diagnosis or treatment of illness or injury.

Payers scrutinize the need for medical procedures, examining each bill to make sure it meets their medical necessity guidelines. The **provider** of the service must also meet the payer's professional standards. Providers include physicians, nurse-practitioners, physicians' assistants, therapists, hospitals, laboratories, long-term care facilities, and suppliers such as pharmacies and medical supply companies.

Covered Services

Covered services are listed on the schedule of benefits. These services may include primary care, emergency care, medical specialists' services, and surgery. Coverage of some services is mandated by state or federal law; others are optional. Some policies provide benefits only for loss resulting from illnesses or diseases, while others also cover accidents or injuries. Many health plans also cover **preventive medical services,** such as annual physical examinations, pediatric and adolescent immunizations, prenatal care, and routine screening procedures such as mammograms.

Not all services that are covered have the same benefits. A policy may pay less of the charges for psychiatric care or treatment for alcohol and drug abuse than for physically related treatments. Many services are also limited in frequency. A payer may cover just three physical therapy treatments for a condition, or a certain screening test every five years, not every year.

Noncovered Services

The medical insurance policy also describes **noncovered services**—those for which it does not pay. Such **excluded services** or exclusions may include all or some of the following:

- Most medical policies do not cover dental services, eye examinations or eyeglasses, employment-related injuries, cosmetic procedures, or experimental procedures.
- Policies may exclude specific items such as vocational rehabilitation or surgical treatment of obesity.
- Many policies do not have prescription drug benefits.
- If a new policyholder has a medical condition that was diagnosed before the policy took effect—known as a **preexisting condition**—medical services to treat it are often not covered.

Billing Tip

Third-Party Payers
There are actually three participants in the medical insurance relationship. The patient (policyholder) is the first party, and the physician is the second party. Legally, a patient-physician contract is created when a physician agrees to treat a patient who is seeking medical services. Through this unwritten contract, the patient is legally responsible for paying for services. The patient may have a policy with a health plan, the third party, which agrees to carry some of the risk of paying for those services and therefore is called a third-party payer.

Thinking It Through — 1.1

Describe the type of medical insurance coverage you have. If you are not insured, describe the policy held by someone you know, or select a plan to research by accessing the website of America's Health Insurance Plans (AHIP) at http://www.ahip.org, searching on "health plans," and selecting the most recent Chartbook of Findings. According to the plan's policy information (often printed in a pamphlet that accompanies the policy itself or available online at the plan's website), what benefits does the policy cover? Are some services excluded from coverage? Are any preventive medical services included?

Group or Individual Medical Insurance Policies

Either groups or individuals may be insured. In general, policies that are written for groups cost policyholders less than those written for individuals. Group plans are bought by employers or organizations. The employer or the organization agrees to the contract and then offers the coverage to its group members. People who are not eligible for group insurance from employers—for example, independent contractors, temporary or part-time employees, or unemployed people—may purchase individual policies directly from health plans. In either a group or an individual plan, the policyholder's dependents, customarily the spouse and children, may also be covered for an additional cost.

Disability Insurance and Workers' Compensation

Other types of health-related insurance are available. A patient may have disability insurance that provides reimbursement for income lost because of the person's inability to work. Disability insurance is discussed in Chapter 13.

Workers' compensation insurance is purchased by employers to pay benefits and provide medical care for employees who are injured in job-related accidents and to pay benefits to employees' dependents in the event of work-related death. State laws determine the coverage that is required. Chapter 13 also covers workers' compensation insurance.

Health Care Plans

Although there are many variations, all insurance plans are based on one of the two essential types of plans, indemnity and managed care.

> **Billing Tip**
>
> **Filing Claims for Patients**
> The practice usually handles the process of billing the insurance company for patients; patients are generally more satisfied with their office visits when this is done for them, and the practice receives payment more quickly.

Indemnity

An indemnity is protection against loss. Under an **indemnity plan**, the payer indemnifies the policyholder against costs of medical services and procedures as listed on the benefits schedule. Patients choose the providers they wish to see. The physician usually sends the **health care claim**—a formal insurance claim in either electronic or hard copy format that reports data about the patient and the services provided by the physician—to the payer on behalf of the patient.

Conditions for Payment

For each claim, four conditions must be met before the insurance company makes a payment:

1. The medical charge must be for medically necessary services and covered by the insured's health plan.

2. The patient's payment of the **premium**—the periodic payment the patient is required to make to keep the policy in effect—must be up to date. Unless the premium is current, the patient is not eligible for benefits and the insurance company will not make any payment.
3. If part of the policy, a **deductible**—the amount that the insured pays on covered services before benefits begin—must have been met (paid). Deductibles range widely, usually from $200 to thousands of dollars annually. Higher deductibles generally mean lower premiums.
4. Any **coinsurance**—the percentage of each claim that the insured pays—must be taken into account. The coinsurance rate states the health plan's percentage of the charge, followed by the insured's percentage, such as 80-20. This means that the payer pays 80 percent of the covered amount and the patient pays 20 percent after the premiums and deductibles are paid.

The formula is as follows:
Charge − Deductible − Patient Coinsurance = Health Plan Payment

Example

An indemnity policy states that the deductible is the first $200 in covered annual medical fees and that the coinsurance rate is 80-20. A patient whose first medical charge of the year was $2,000 would owe $560:

Charge	$2,000
Patient owes the deductible	$ 200
Balance	$1,800
Patient also owes coinsurance (20% of the balance)	$ 360
Total balance due from patient	$ 200 + $360 = $560

In this case, the patient must pay an **out-of-pocket** expense of $560 this year before benefits begin. The health plan will pay $1,440, or 80 percent of the balance:

Charge	$2,000
Patient payment	–$560
Health plan payment	$1,440

If the patient has already met the annual deductible, the patient's benefits apply to the charge, as in this example:

Charge	$2,000
Patient coinsurance (20%)	$ 400
Health plan payment (80%)	$1,600

Fee-For-Service Payment Approach

Indemnity plans usually reimburse medical costs on a fee-for-service basis. The **fee-for-service** payment method is retroactive: The fee is paid after the patient receives services from the physician (see Figure 1.2 on page 8).

Managed Care

Managed care offers a more restricted choice of (and access to) providers and treatments in exchange for lower premiums, deductibles, and other charges than traditional indemnity insurance. This approach to insurance combines the financing and management of health care with the delivery of services.

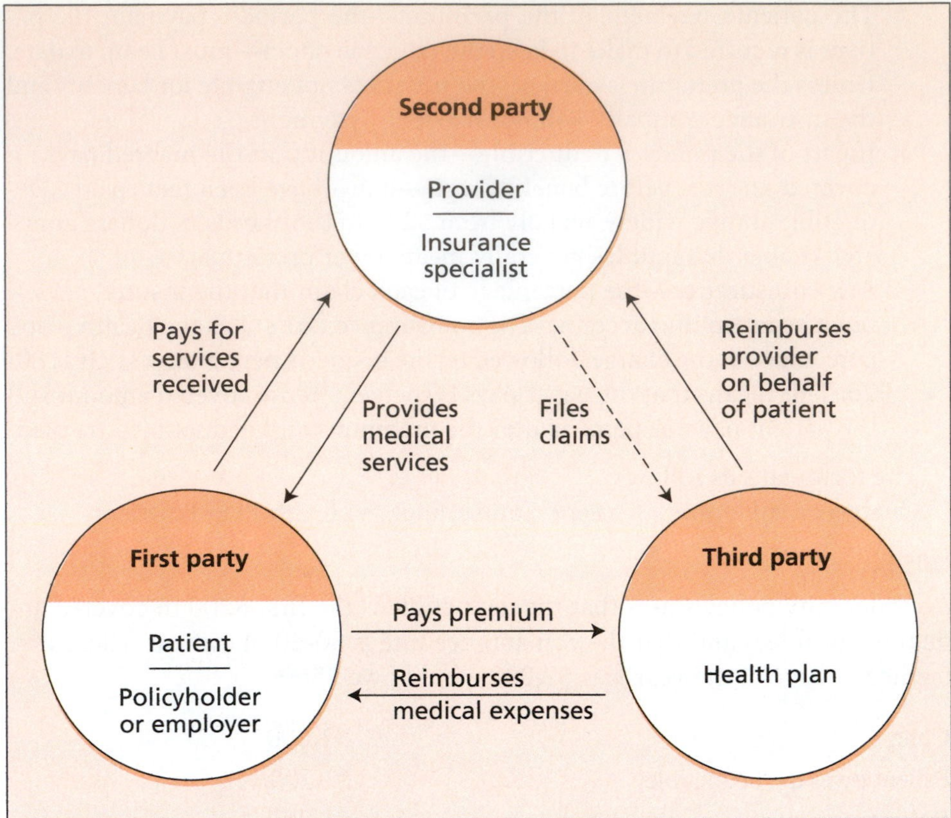

Figure 1.2 Payment Under Fee-for-Service

Managed care organizations (MCOs) establish links between provider, patient, and payer. Instead of only the patient having a policy with the health plan, both the patient and the provider have agreements with the MCO. This arrangement gives the MCO more control over what services the provider performs and the fees for the services.

Managed care plans, first introduced in California in 1929, are now the predominant type of insurance. Over 90 percent of all insured employees are enrolled in some type of managed care plan, and thousands of different plans are offered. The basic types are:

- Health maintenance organizations
- Point-of-service plans
- Preferred provider organizations
- Consumer-directed health plans

> **Billing Tip**
>
> **Participation as a Provider**
> **Participation** means that a provider has contracted with a health plan to provide services to the plan's beneficiaries. Participation brings benefits, such as more patients, as well as contractual duties and, usually, reduced fees.

Health Maintenance Organizations

A **health maintenance organization (HMO)** combines coverage of medical costs and delivery of health care for a prepaid premium. Over 20 percent of insured employees are enrolled in HMOs.

The HMO creates a network of physicians, hospitals, and other providers by employing or negotiating contracts with them. The HMO then enrolls members in a health plan under which they use the services of those network providers. In most states, HMOs are licensed and are legally required to provide certain services to members and their dependents. Preventive care is often required as appropriate for each age group, such as immunizations and well-baby checkups for infants and screening mammograms for women.

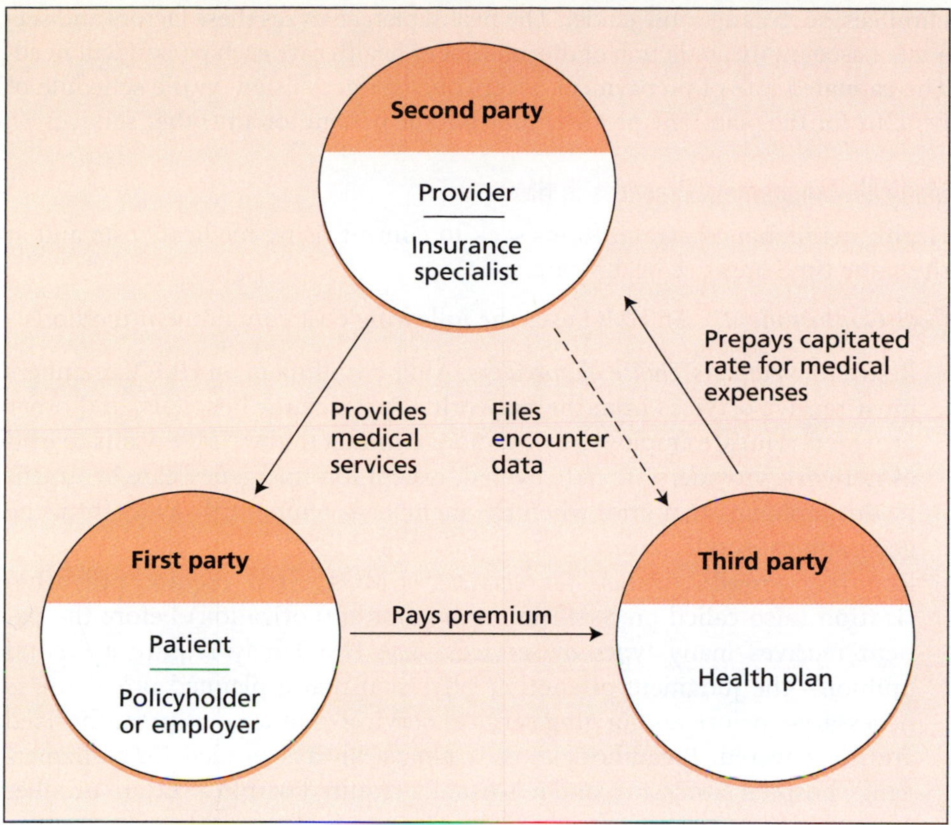

Figure 1.3 Payment Under Capitation

Capitation in HMOs

Capitation (from *capit*, Latin for *head*) is a fixed prepayment to a medical provider for all necessary contracted services provided to each patient who is a plan member (see Figure 1.3). The capitated rate is a prospective payment—it is paid *before* the patient visit. It covers a specific period of time. The health plan makes the payment whether the patient receives many or no medical services during that specified period.

In capitation, the physician agrees to share the risk that an insured person will use more services than the fee covers. The physician also shares in the prospect that an insured person will use fewer services. In fee-for-service, the more patients the provider sees, the more charges the health plan reimburses. In capitation, the payment remains the same, and the provider risks receiving lower per-visit revenue.

Example

A family physician has a contract for a capitated payment of $30 a month for each of a hundred patients in a plan. This $3,000 monthly fee ($30 × 100 patients = $3,000) covers all office visits from all the patients. If half of the patients see the physician once during a given month, the provider in effect receives $60 for each visit ($3,000 divided by 50 visits). If, however, half of the patients see the physician four times in a month, the average fee is $3,000 divided by 200 visits, or $15 for each visit.

A patient is enrolled in a capitated health plan for a specific time period, such as a month, a quarter, or a year. The capitated rate, which is called **per member per month (PMPM)**, is usually based on the health-related characteristics of the enrollees, such as age and gender. The health plan analyzes these factors and sets a rate based on its prediction of the amount of health care each person will need. The capitated rate of prepayment covers only services listed on the schedule of benefits for the plan. The provider may bill the patient for any other services.

Medical Management Practices in HMOs

Health maintenance organizations seek to control rising medical costs and at the same time improve health care.

Cost Containment An HMO uses the following cost containment methods:

- *Restricting patients' choice of providers:* After enrolling in an HMO, members must receive services from the **network** of physicians, hospitals, and other providers who are employed by or under contract to the HMO. Visits to **out-of-network** providers are not covered, except for emergency care or urgent health problems that arise when the member is temporarily away from the geographical service area.
- *Requiring preauthorization for services:* HMOs often require **preauthorization** (also called precertification or prior authorization) before the patient receives many types of services. The HMO may require a second opinion—the judgment of another physician that a planned procedure is necessary—before authorizing service. Services that are not preauthorized are not covered. Preauthorization is almost always needed for nonemergency hospital admission, and it is usually required within a certain number of days after an emergency admission.
- *Controlling the use of services:* HMOs develop medical necessity guidelines for the use of medical services. The HMO holds the provider accountable for any questionable service and may deny a patient's or provider's request for preauthorization.

  For example, a patient who has a rotator cuff shoulder injury repair can receive a specific number of physical therapy sessions. More sessions will not be covered unless additional approval is obtained. Emergency care is particularly tightly controlled because it is generally the most costly way to deliver services. These guidelines are also applied to hospitals in the network, which, for instance, limit the number of days patients can remain in the hospital following particular surgeries.
- *Controlling drug costs:* Providers must prescribe drugs for patients only from the HMO's list of selected pharmaceuticals and approved dosages, called a formulary. Drugs that are not on the list require preauthorization, which is often denied.
- *Cost-sharing:* At the time an HMO member sees a provider, he or she pays a specified charge called a **copayment** (or copay). A lower copayment may be charged for an office visit to the primary care physician, and a higher copayment may be required for a visit to the office of a specialist or for the use of emergency-department services.

One other cost-control method is now used less frequently but was a major feature of initial HMOs. This required a patient to select a **primary care physician (PCP)**—also called a "gatekeeper"—from the HMO's list of general or family practitioners, internists, and pediatricians. A PCP coordinates patients' overall care to ensure that all services are, in the PCP's judgment, necessary. In gatekeeper plans, an HMO member needs a medical **referral** from the PCP before seeing a specialist or a consultant and for hospital admission. Members who visit providers without a referral are directly responsible for the total cost of the service.

Historically, the first HMOs used all of these cost-containment methods and reduced operating costs. However, both physicians and patients became dissatisfied with the policies. Physicians working under managed-care contracts complained that they were not allowed to order needed treatments and tests. Patients often reported that needed referrals were denied. In response, the medical management practices of HMOs increasingly emphasize the quality of health care as well as the cost of its delivery. Just as providers must demonstrate that their services are both effective and efficient, HMOs must demonstrate that they can offer these services at competitive prices while improving the quality of health care.

Health Care Quality Improvements The quality improvements made by HMOs are illustrated by these features, which most plans contain:

- *Disease/case management:* Some patients face difficult treatments, such as for high-risk pregnancies, and others need chronic care for conditions such as congestive heart failure, diabetes, and asthma. HMOs often assign case managers to work with these patients. Some conditions require case managers who are health care professionals. Others are assigned to people who are familiar with the health care system, such as social workers. The goal of case managers is to make sure that patients have access to all needed treatments. For example, physician case managers coordinate appropriate referrals to consultants, specialists, hospitals, and other services. Other types of case managers provide patient education, special equipment like a blood glucose meter for a diabetic, and ongoing contact to monitor a patient's condition.
- *Preventive care:* Preventive care, which seeks to prevent the occurrence of conditions through early detection of disease, is emphasized through provisions for annual checkups, screening procedures, and inoculations.
- *Pay-for-performance (P4P):* HMOs collect and analyze large amounts of data about patients' clinical treatments and their responses to treatment. In this way, the HMOs can establish the most effective protocols—detailed, precise treatment regimens that work best. HMOs use financial incentives to encourage their providers to follow these protocols.

Billing Tip

Open-Access Plans
Many HMOs have switched from "gatekeeper" plans that require referrals to all specialists to open-access plans, in which members can visit any specialists in the network without referrals. Even if referrals are required for specialists, patients can usually see ob-gyn specialists without referrals.

Point-of-Service Plans

Many patients dislike HMO rules that restrict their access to physicians. In order to better compete for membership, a **point-of-service (POS) plan**, also called an open HMO, reduces restrictions and allows members to choose providers who are not in the HMO's network. Over 20 percent of employees covered by employers' health care plans are enrolled in this type of plan.

Members must pay additional fees that are set by the plan when they use out-of-network providers. Typically, 20 to 30 percent of the charge for out-of-network service must be paid by the patient, and the deductible can be very high. The HMO pays out-of-network providers on a fee-for-service basis.

Preferred Provider Organizations

A **preferred provider organization (PPO)** is another health care delivery system that manages care. PPOs are the most popular type of insurance plan. They create a network of physicians, hospitals, and other providers with whom they have negotiated discounts from the usual fees. For example, a PPO might sign a contract with a practice stating that the fee for a brief appointment will be $60, although the practice's physicians usually charge $80. In exchange for

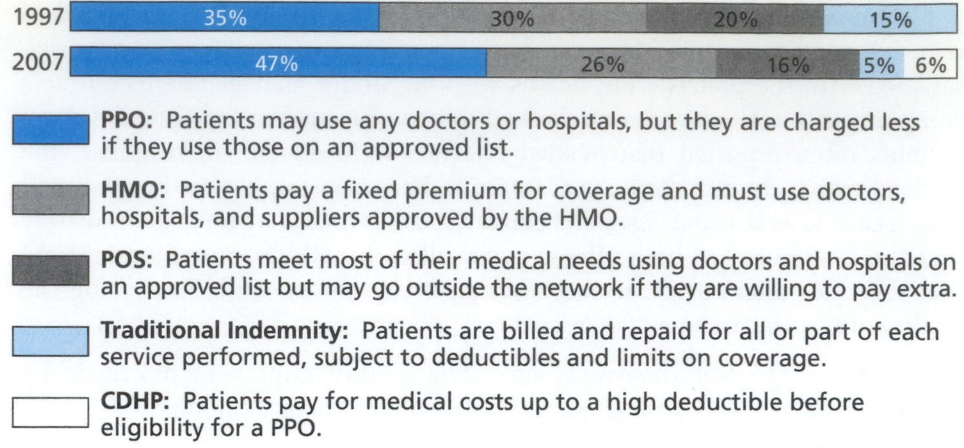

1997
35%
30%
20%
15%
2007
47%
26%
16%
5%
6%
PPO: Patients may use any doctors or hospitals, but they are charged less if they use those on an approved list.
HMO: Patients pay a fixed premium for coverage and must use doctors, hospitals, and suppliers approved by the HMO.
POS: Patients meet most of their medical needs using doctors and hospitals on an approved list but may go outside the network if they are willing to pay extra.
Traditional Indemnity: Patients are billed and repaid for all or part of each service performed, subject to deductibles and limits on coverage.
CDHP: Patients pay for medical costs up to a high deductible before eligibility for a PPO.

Figure 1.4 Employer-Sponsored Health Plans

accepting lower fees, providers—in theory, at least—see more patients, thus making up the revenue that is lost through the reduced fees. As shown in Figure 1.4, PPOs enroll almost 50 percent of the Americans workers who are insured through their employers.

A PPO requires payment of a premium and often of a copayment for visits. It does not require a primary care physician to oversee patients' care. Referrals to specialists are also not required. Premiums and copayments, however, are higher than in HMO or POS plans. Members choose from many in-network generalists and specialists. PPO members also can use out-of-network providers, usually for higher copayments, increased deductibles, or both.

Example

A PPO member using an in-network provider pays a $20 copayment at the time of service (the visit), and the PPO pays the full balance of the visit charge. A member who sees an out-of-network provider pays a $40 copayment and is also responsible for part of the visit charge.

As managed care organizations, PPOs also control the cost of health care by:

- *Directing patients' choices of providers:* PPO members have financial incentives to receive services from the PPO's network of providers.
- *Controlling use of services:* PPOs have guidelines for appropriate and necessary medical care.
- *Requiring preauthorization for services:* PPOs may require preauthorization for nonemergency hospital admission and for some outpatient procedures.
- *Requiring cost-sharing:* PPO members are also required to pay copayments for general or specialist services.

Consumer-Driven Health Plans

Consumer-driven health plans (CDHP) combine two elements. The first element is a health plan, usually a PPO, that has a high deductible (such as $1,000) and low premiums. The second element is a special "savings account" that is used to pay medical bills before the deductible has been met.

TABLE 1.1 Comparison of Health Plan Options

Plan Type	Provider Options	Cost Containment Methods	Features
Indemnity Plan	Any provider	• Little or none • Preauthorization required for some procedures	• Higher costs • Deductibles • Coinsurance • Preventive care not usually covered
Health Maintenance Organization (HMO)	Only HMO network providers	• Primary care physician manages care; referral required • No payment for out-of-network nonemergency services • Preauthorization required	• Low copayment • Limited provider network • Covers preventive care
Point-of-Service (POS)	Network providers or out-of-network providers	• Within network, primary care physician manages care	• Lower copayments for network providers • Higher costs for out-of-network providers • Covers preventive care
Preferred Provider Organization (PPO)	Network or out-of-network providers	• Referral not required for specialists • Fees are discounted • Preauthorization for some procedures	• Higher cost for out-of-network providers • Preventive care coverage varies
Consumer-Driven Health Plan	Usually similar to PPO	• Increases patient awareness of health care costs • Patient pays directly until high deductible is met	• High deductible/low premium • Savings account

The savings account, similar to an individual retirement account (IRA), lets people put aside untaxed wages that they may use to cover their out-of-pocket medical expenses. Some employers contribute to employees' accounts as a benefit.

Cost containment in consumer-driven health plans begins with consumerism—the idea that patients who themselves pay for health care services become more careful consumers. Both insurance companies and employers believe that asking patients to pay a larger portion of medical expenses reduces costs. To this are added the other controls typical to a PPO, such as in-network savings and higher costs for out-of-network visits.

The major types of plans are summarized in Table 1.1.

Thinking It Through — 1.2

Managed care organizations often require different payments for different services. Table 1.2 below shows the copayments for a HMO health plan. Study this schedule and answer these questions:

- **Does this health plan cover diabetic supplies? Dental exams? Emergency services?**
- **Is the copayment amount for a PCP visit higher or lower than the charge for specialty care?**

TABLE 1.2 Example of Benefits under an HMO

	Copayments
Primary Care Physician Visits	
Office Hours	$20 copay
After Hours/Home Visits	$20 copay
Specialty Care	
Office Visits	$30 copay
Diagnostic Outpatient Testing	$20 copay
Phys, Occ, Speech Therapy	$20 copay
SPU Surgery	$250 copay
Hospitalization	$250 copay
Emergency Room (copay waived if admitted)	$35 copay
Maternity	
First OB Visit	$30 copay
Hospital	$250 copay
Mental Health	
Inpatient	$250 copay, 60 days
Outpatient	30% copay
Substance Abuse	
Detoxification	$250 copay
Inpatient Rehab (combined w$MH)	$250 copay
Outpatient Rehabilitation	30% copay
Preventive Care	
Routine Eye Exam	Not covered
Routine GYN Exam	$30 copay
Pediatric Preventive Dental Exam	Not covered
Chiropractic Care (20 visits/condition)	$20 copay
Prescriptions	$15/$20/$20 copay $150 deductible/calendar year
Contraceptives	Covered
Diabetic Supplies	Covered
31–90 Day Supply (Retail & Mod)	$30/40/60 copay
Durable Medical Equipment	No copay

Compliance Guideline

Unpaid Health Care
Under the federal Emergency Medical Treatment and Active Labor Act, or EMTALA, hospital emergency departments must provide care for all patients in need of medical services, regardless of their ability to pay. More than $100 billion in unpaid health care is provided annually for uninsured and underinsured patients.

Medical Insurance Payers

Nearly 250 million people in the United States have medical coverage through either private payers or government programs (see Figure 1.5). Another 45 million people—about 16 percent of the population—have no insurance. Many of the uninsured people work for employers that either do not offer health benefits or do not cover certain employees, such as temporary workers or part-time employees.

Private Payers

A small number of large insurance companies dominate the national market and offer all types of health plans. The three largest are WellPoint, United-Health Group, and Aetna. There are also a number of nonprofit organizations, such as Kaiser Permanente, which is the largest nonprofit HMO. Some organizations, such as the Blue Cross and Blue Shield Association, have both for-profit and nonprofit parts.

Private payers have contracts with businesses to provide benefits for their employees. These may be large-group or small-group health care plans. Payers may also offer individual insurance coverage.

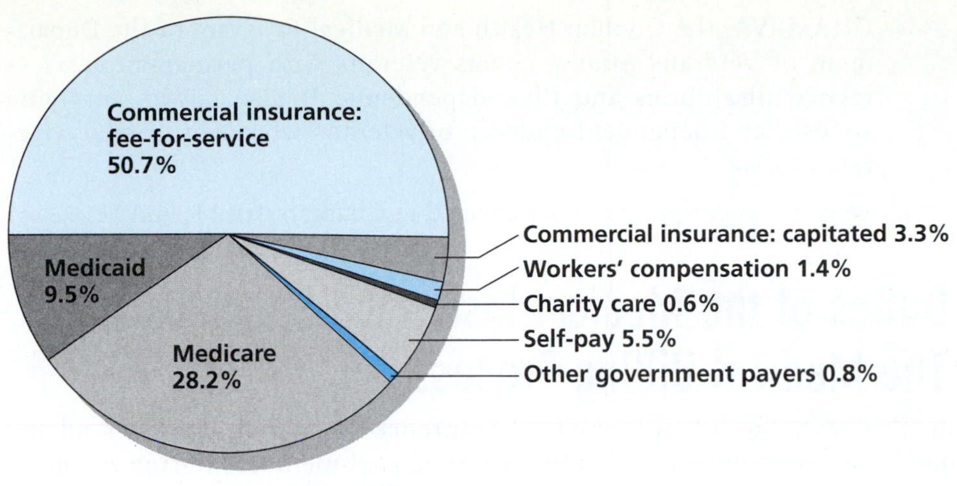

Figure 1.5 Types of Insurance Held

Source: Reprinted with permission from the Medical Group Management Association, 104 Inverness Terrace East, Englewood, Colorado 80112-5306; 877.ASK.MGMA. www.mgma.com. Copyright 2006.

Self-Funded Health Plans

Some 50 million employees have health insurance through employers that have established themselves as **self-funded (self-insured) health plans.** Examples are General Motors, UPS (United Parcel Service), and DaimlerChrysler. Rather than paying premiums to an insurance carrier, the organization "insures itself." It assumes the risk of paying directly for medical services and sets up a fund from which it pays for claims. The organization establishes the benefit levels and the plan types it will offer. Self-funded health plans may set up their own provider networks or, more often, buy the use of existing networks from managed care organizations.

Most self-funded health plans are set up as PPOs; fewer than 10 percent are set up as HMOs. As discussed in Chapter 9, being self-insured changes the regulations under which a plan works, giving the employer some financial advantages over paying for coverage through a typical insurance company.

Government-Sponsored Health Care Programs

The four major government-sponsored health care programs offer benefits for which various groups in the population are eligible:

1. Medicare is a 100 percent federally funded health plan that covers people who are sixty-five and over, are disabled, or have permanent kidney failure (end-stage renal disease, or ESRD).
2. Medicaid, a federal program that is jointly funded by federal and state governments, covers low-income people who cannot afford medical care. Each state administers its own Medicaid program, determining the program's qualifications and benefits under broad federal guidelines.
3. TRICARE, a Department of Defense program, covers medical expenses for active-duty members of the uniformed services and their spouses, children, and other dependents; retired military personnel and their dependents; and family members of deceased active-duty personnel. (This program replaced CHAMPUS, the Civilian Health and Medical Program of the Uniformed Services, in 1998.)

4. CHAMPVA, the Civilian Health and Medical Program of the Department of Veterans Affairs, covers veterans with permanent service-related disabilities and their dependents. It also covers surviving spouses and dependent children of veterans who died from service-related disabilities.

These government programs are covered in Chapters 10, 11, and 12.

Duties of the Medical Insurance Specialist: The Medical Billing Process

In this text, the job title **medical insurance specialist** addresses all the tasks that are completed by administrative staff members during the medical billing process. Typically, *front office* staff members handle duties such as reception (registration) and scheduling. *Back office* staff duties are related to billing, insurance, and collections. Job titles in common use are billing clerk, insurance specialist, reimbursement specialist, and claims specialist. The broad picture of the medical insurance specialist is presented in *Medical Insurance*, Third Edition, to provide the widest background for future employment.

The main job functions of medical insurance specialists are:

- To understand patients' responsibilities for paying for medical services
- To analyze charges and insurance coverage to prepare accurate, timely claims
- To collect payment for medical services from health plans and from patients

These functions entail:

- Verifying patient insurance information and eligibility before medical services are provided
- Collecting payments that are due, such as copayments, at the time of service
- Maintaining up-to-date information about health plans' billing guidelines
- Following federal, state, and local regulations on maintaining the confidentiality of information about patients
- Abstracting information from patients' records for accurate billing
- Billing health plans and patients, maintaining effective communication to avoid problems or delayed payments
- Assisting patients with insurance information and required documents
- Processing payments and requests for further information about claims and bills
- Maintaining financial records
- Updating the forms and computer systems the practice uses for patient information and health care claims processing

To complete their duties, medical insurance specialists follow a medical billing process. This process is a series of steps that lead to maximum, appropriate, timely payment for patients' medical services (see Figure 1.6).

> **Billing Tip**
>
> **The Medical Billing Process**
> Study the medical billing process in Figure 1.6 as you read the steps below. The process is also printed on the inside front cover of your text for your convenience. Refer to the process as you read the text's chapters; it serves as your path toward expertise in medical insurance.

Step 1 Preregister Patients

The first step in the medical billing process is to preregister patients. There are two main tasks involved:

- Schedule and update appointments
- Collect preregistration demographic and insurance information

VISIT	Step 1	Preregister patients
	Step 2	Establish financial responsibility for visits
	Step 3	Check in patients
	Step 4	Check out patients
CLAIM	Step 5	Review coding compliance
	Step 6	Check billing compliance
	Step 7	Prepare and transmit claims
POST-CLAIM	Step 8	Monitor payer adjudication
	Step 9	Generate patient statements
	Step 10	Follow up patient payments and handle collections

Figure 1.6 The Medical Billing Process

New patients who call for appointments provide basic personal and insurance information to the scheduler. Both new and returning patients are asked about the medical reason for the visit, so appropriate visits can be scheduled for them.

Step 2 Establish Financial Responsibility for the Visit

The second step is very important: determine financial responsibility for the visit. For insured patients, these questions must be answered:

- What services are covered under the plan? What medical conditions establish medical necessity for these services?
- What services are not covered?
- What are the billing rules of the plan?
- What is the patient responsible for paying?

Knowing the answers to these questions is essential to correctly bill payers for patients' covered services. This knowledge also helps medical insurance specialists ensure that patients will pay their bills when benefits do not apply.

To determine financial responsibility, these procedures are followed:

- Verify patients' eligibility for their health plan
- Check the health plan's coverage
- Determine the first payer if more than one health plan covers the patient, the first payer is determined (this is the payer to whom the first claim will be sent)
- Meet payers' conditions for payment, such as preauthorization, the correct procedures are followed to meet them

The practice's financial policy—when bills have to be paid—is explained so that patients understand the medical billing process. Patients are told that they are responsible for paying charges that are not covered under their health plans. Uninsured patients are informed of their responsibility for the entire charge. Payment options are presented if the bill will be substantial.

Step 3 Check in Patients

The third step is to check in individuals as patients of the practice. When new patients arrive for their appointments, detailed and complete demographic and medical information are collected at the front desk. Returning patients are asked to review the information that is on file for them, making sure that demographics and medical data are accurate and up-to-date. Their financial records are also checked to see if balances are due from previous visits.

Both the front and back of insurance cards and other identification cards such as drivers' licenses are scanned or photocopied and filed in the patient's record. If the health plan requires a copayment, the correct amount is noted for the patient. Copayments should always be collected at the time of service. Some practices collect copayments before the patient's encounter with the physician; others after the encounter.

A number of other important forms may need to be completed by patients. These forms are part of the process of recording administrative and clinical facts about patients. Often they involve authorizing planned procedures and payments to the practice from the health plan.

Step 4 Check Out Patients

Check-out procedures follow patients' encounters (visits) with providers. The first task is to record the medical codes for the visit.

When physicians or other licensed health care professionals examine or treat patients, they document patients' diagnoses and procedures in medical records. To bill for the visit, the medical diagnoses and procedures must be assigned medical codes. In some practices, physicians assign these codes; in others, a **medical coder** or a medical insurance specialist handles this task. The medical insurance specialist may verify the codes with data in the patient's medical record.

The patient's primary illness is assigned a **diagnosis code** from the *International Classification of Diseases*, Ninth Revision, *Clinical Modification* (ICD-9-CM) (see Chapter 4).

Example

The ICD-9-CM code for Alzheimer disease is 331.0.

The ICD-9-CM code for influenza with bronchitis or with a cold is 487.1.

Similarly, each procedure the physician performs is assigned a **procedure code** that stands for the particular service, treatment, or test. This code is selected from the *Current Procedural Terminology* (CPT) (see Chapters 5 and 6). A large group of codes cover the physician's evaluation and management of a patient's condition during office visits or visits at other locations, such as nursing homes. Other codes cover groups of specific procedures, such as surgery, pathology, and radiology. Another group of codes covers supplies and other services.

Example

99431 is the CPT code for the physician's examination of a newborn infant.

27130 is the CPT code for a total hip replacement operation.

The physician identifies the patient's diagnoses and procedures. This information is used by the medical insurance specialist after the encounter to update the patient's account. The transactions for the visit, which include both the charges and any payment the patient made, are entered in the **patient ledger** (the record of a patient's financial transactions; also called the patient account record), and the patient's balance is updated. Following is an example of the account for one patient's recent series of visits:

Date/Procedure		Charge	Payment		Balance
7/2/08	OV	200.00		200.00	—
7/3/08	OV	150.00			
7/4/08	INS	—		—	150.00
7/13/08	PMT		Insurance	120.00	30.00
7/25/08	STM	—		—	30.00
7/30/08	PMT		Patient	30.00	0.00

This formula is followed to calculate the current balance:

Previous Balance + Charge – Payment = Current Balance

In this example, on 7/2/08 the patient's office visit (OV) resulted in a $200 charge. The patient paid this bill, so there is no current balance. The patient's next office visit, 7/3/08, resulted in a charge of $150. The medical insurance specialist sent a health care claim to the health plan (INS for insurance) the next day, and the payer paid $120 (PMT) on 7/13. This payment is subtracted from the charge to equal the current balance of $30.

As noted on the account, then a statement (STM) (a bill) was sent to the patient on 7/25 showing the current balance now owed. The patient sent a payment of $30 (PMT) received on 7/30, which reduced the patient's current balance to zero.

At the time of the visit, patients may owe a previous balance, coinsurance, deductibles, and/or fees for noncovered services. Payments may be made by cash, check, or credit/debit card. When a payment is made, a receipt is given to the patient. Patients' follow-up visits are also scheduled.

Steps 1 through 4 are covered in Chapters 3 through 6 of this text.

Step 5 Review Coding Compliance

Compliance means actions that satisfy official requirements. In the area of coding, compliance involves following official guidelines when codes are assigned. Also, after diagnosis and procedure codes are selected, they must be checked for errors. The diagnosis and the medical services that are documented in the patient's medical record should be logically connected (linked), so that the payer understands the medical necessity of the charges.

Step 6 Check Billing Compliance

Each charge, or fee, for a visit is related to a specific procedure code. The provider's fees for services are listed on the medical practice's fee schedule. Most medical practices have standard fee schedules listing their usual fees.

Although there is a separate fee associated with each code, each code is not necessarily billable. Whether a code can be billed depends on the payer's rules. Following these rules when preparing claims results in billing compliance. Some payers include particular codes in the payment for another code. Medical insurance specialists apply their knowledge of payer guidelines to analyze what can be billed on health care claims.

Steps 5 and 6 are covered in Chapter 7.

Step 7 Prepare and Transmit Claims

A major step in the medical billing process is the preparation of accurate, timely health care claims. Most practices prepare claims for their patients and send them electronically. A claim communicates information about the diagnosis, procedures, and charges to a payer. A claim may be for reimbursement for services rendered or to report an encounter to an HMO. The practice has a schedule for transmitting claims, such as daily or every other day, which is followed.

General information on claims is found in Chapter 8. Chapters 9 through 13 explain how to prepare correct claims for each major payer group:

Private payers/Blue Cross and Blue Shield

Medicare

Medicaid

TRICARE and CHAMPVA

Workers' compensation and disability

A related topic, hospital billing, is covered in Chapter 16.

Step 8 Monitor Payer Adjudication

Once health care claims have been sent to health plans, it is important to collect payments as soon as possible. The money due from the plans, as well as payments due from patients, add up to the practice's **accounts receivable (A/R)**—the money that is needed to run the practice.

Payers review claims by following a process known as *adjudication*. This term means that the payer puts the claim through a series of steps designed to judge whether it should be paid. What the payer decides about the claim—to pay it in full, to pay some of it, or to deny it—is explained on a report sent back to the provider with the payment. When patients are covered by more than one health plan, the additional plans are then sent claims based on the amounts still due.

The amount of the payment depends on the practice's contract with the payer. Seldom do the practice's fee and the payer's fee match exactly. Most payers have their own fee schedules for providers with whom they have contractual arrangements. The medical insurance specialist compares each payment with the claim to check that:

- All procedures that were listed on the claim also appear on the payment transaction
- Any unpaid charges are explained
- The codes on the payment transactions match those on the claim
- The payment listed for each procedure is correct according to the contract with the payer

If discrepancies are found, an appeal process may be started. In this process, the medical insurance specialist follows payers' or state rules to seek full appropriate reimbursement for a claim.

When a patient is covered by more than one health plan, the second and any other plans must be sent claims.

Step 8 is covered in Chapter 14.

Step 9 Generate Patient Statements

Payers' payments are applied to the appropriate patients' accounts. In most cases, these payments do not fully pay the bills, and patients will be billed for the rest. The amount paid by all payers (the primary insurance and any other insurance) plus the amount to be billed to the patient should equal the expected fee. Bills that are mailed to patients list the dates and services provided, any payments made by the patient and the payer, and the balances now due.

Step 10 Follow Up Patient Payments and Handle Collections

Patient payments are regularly analyzed for overdue bills. A collection process is often started when patient payments are later than permitted under the practice's financial policy.

Patient medical records and financial records are filed and retained according to the medical practice's policy. Federal and state regulations govern what documents are kept and for how long.

Steps 9 and 10 are covered in Chapter 15.

Procedures, Communication, and Information Technology in the Medical Billing Process

Each step of the medical billing process has three parts: (1) following procedures, (2) communicating effectively, and (3) using information technology.

Following Procedures

Each step in medical billing has procedures. Some procedures involve administrative duties, such as entering data and updating patients' records. Other procedures are done to comply with government regulations, such as keeping computer files secure from unauthorized viewing. In most offices, policy and procedure manuals are available that describe how to perform major duties.

For most procedures, medical insurance specialists work in teams with both licensed medical professionals and other administrative staff members. Providers include physicians and nurses as well as physician's assistants (PA), nurse-practitioners (NP), clinical social workers, physical therapists, occupational therapists, audiologists, and clinical psychologists. Administrative staff may be headed by an office manager, practice manager, or practice administrator to whom medical assistants, patient services representatives or receptionists, and billing, insurance, and collections specialists report.

Communicating Effectively

Communication skills are as important as knowing about specific forms, codes, and regulations. Using a pleasant tone, a friendly attitude, and a helpful manner when gathering information increases patient satisfaction. Having interpersonal skills enhances the billing and reimbursement process by establishing professional, courteous relationships with people of different backgrounds and communication styles. Effective communicators have the skill of empathy; their actions convey that they understand the feelings of others.

Equally important are effective communications with physicians and other professional staff members. Conversations must be brief and to the point, showing that the speaker values the provider's time. People are more likely to listen when the speaker is smiling and has an interested expression, so speakers should be aware of their facial expressions and should maintain moderate eye contact. In addition, good listening skills are important.

> **Billing Tip**
>
> **Practice Management Programs: Medisoft**
> In this text, Medisoft Advanced Patient Accounting from Per-Se Technologies is the program used to illustrate typical PMP data entry screens and printed reports.

Using Practice Management Programs

Medical insurance specialists use information technology (IT)—computer hardware and software information systems—in almost all physician practices. **Practice management programs (PMP)**, which are used in over 70 percent of medical offices for scheduling appointments, billing, and financial record keeping, are a good example of IT. They streamline the process of creating and following up on health care claims sent to payers and on bills sent to patients.

Expertise in the use of practice management programs is an important skill in the medical practice. Medical insurance specialists use them to:

Schedule patients

Organize patient and payer information

Collect data on patients' diagnoses and services

Generate, transmit, and report on the status of health care claims

Record payments from payers

Generate patients' statements, post payments, and update accounts

Create financial and productivity reports

Electronic Medical Records

Very gradually, another IT application is being introduced in physician practices: electronic medical records, or EMR. EMR systems are set up to gather patients' clinical information using the computer rather than paper. Most EMR systems are designed to exchange information with—to "talk" to—the PMP and to cut out the need for many paper forms. Electronic medical record systems are discussed further in Chapter 2.

A Note of Caution: What Information Technology Cannot Do

Although computers increase efficiency and reduce errors, they are not more accurate than the individual who is entering the data. If people make mistakes while entering data, the information the computer produces will be incorrect. Computers are very precise and also very unforgiving. While the human brain knows that *flu* is short for *influenza*, the computer regards them as two distinct conditions. If a computer user accidentally enters a name as *ORourke* instead of *O'Rourke*, a human might know what is meant; the computer does not. It would probably respond with a message such as "No such patient exists in the database."

Employment as a Medical Insurance Specialist

The health care industry offers many rewarding career paths for well-qualified employees. Providers must compete in a complex environment of various health plans, managed care contracts, and federal and state regulations. Employment in positions that help providers handle these demands is growing, as are opportunities for career development. According to *The Physician's Advisory*, a health care journal:

> good, experienced billing/coding specialists are in short supply; to retain good workers in these very important positions, going up in salary is a bargain compared to risking their going to another employer . . . the work of insurance specialists is an increasingly complex job.

Thinking It Through — 1.3

In your opinion, is each of the following procedures likely to be considered medically necessary by a payer's health care claims examiner? Why?

A. Diagnosis: deviated septum

_____ Procedure: nasal surgery

B. Diagnosis: mole on a female patient's cheek, questionable nature

_____ Procedure: surgical removal and biopsy

C. Diagnosis: male syndrome hair loss

_____ Procedure: implant hair plugs on scalp

D. Diagnosis: probable broken wrist

_____ Procedure: comprehensive full-body examination, with complete set of lab tests, chest X-ray, and ECG

Medical insurance specialists' effective and efficient work is critical for the satisfaction of the patients—the physician's customers—and for the financial success of the practice.

Roles and Responsibilities

In addition to working in physicians' practices, medical insurance specialists work in clinics, for hospitals or nursing homes, and in other health care settings such as in insurance companies as claims examiners, provider relations representatives, or benefits analysts. Positions are also available in government and public health agencies. Employment with companies that offer billing or consulting services to health care providers is an option, as is self-employment as a claims assistance professional who helps consumers with medical insurance problems or as a billing service for providers.

In small physician practices, medical insurance specialists handle a variety of billing and collections tasks. In larger medical practices, duties may be more specialized. Billing, insurance, and collections duties may be separated, or a medical insurance specialist may work exclusively with claims sent to just one of many payers, such as Medicare or workers' compensation. Practice size varies by specialty. Seventy-five percent of physicians provide care in small settings, usually in practices with from one to three physicians. Specialties that require a lot of technology, such as radiology, tend to have large single-specialty medical groups.

Requirements for Success

A number of skills and attributes are required for successful mastery of the tasks of a medical insurance specialist.

Skills

Knowledge of medical terminology, anatomy, physiology, and medical coding: Medical insurance specialists must analyze physicians' descriptions of patients' conditions and treatments and relate these descriptions to the systems of diagnosis and procedure codes used in the health care industry.

Communication skills: The job of a medical insurance specialist requires excellent oral and written communications skills. For example, patients often need explanations of insurance benefits or clarification of instructions such as referrals. Courteous, helpful answers to questions strongly influence patients' willingness to continue to use the practices' services. Memos, letters, telephone calls, and e-mail are used to research and follow up on changes in health plans' billing rules. Communication skills also are needed to create and send collection letters that are effective and claim attachments that explain special conditions or treatments so as to obtain maximum reimbursement.

Attention to detail: Many aspects of the job involve paying close attention to detail, such as correctly completing health care claims, filing patients' medical records, recording preauthorization numbers, calculating the correct payments, and posting payments for services.

Flexibility: Working in a changing environment requires the ability to adapt to new procedures, handle varying kinds of problems and interactions during a busy day, and work successfully with different types of people with various cultural backgrounds.

Billing Tip

Keeping Up to Date: The Internet
The Internet is frequently used for research about government regulations, payer billing updates, and code updates. Ignorance of new instructions, rules, or codes is not an excuse for incorrect billing. Experienced medical insurance specialists make it a habit to regularly check the websites that are most important for their billing environment. Many are provided throughout this text and summarized in Appendix C.

Information technology (IT) skills: Most medical practices use computers to handle billing and to process claims. Many also use or plan to use computers to keep patients' medical records. General computer literacy is essential, including working knowledge of the Microsoft Windows operating system, a word-processing program, a medical billing program, and Internet-based research. Data-entry skills are also necessary. Many human errors occur during data entry, such as pressing the wrong key on the keyboard. Other errors are a result of a lack of computer literacy—not knowing how to use a program to accomplish tasks. For this reason, proper training in data-entry techniques and in using computer programs are essential for medical insurance specialists.

Honesty and integrity: Medical insurance specialists work with patients' medical records and with finances. It is essential to maintain the confidentiality of patient information and communications as well as to act with integrity when handling these tasks.

Ability to work as a team member: Patient service is a team effort. To do their part, medical insurance specialists must be cooperative and must focus on the best interests of the patients and the practice.

Attributes

A number of attributes are also very important for success as a medical insurance specialist. Most have to do with the quality of professionalism, which is key to getting and keeping employment. These factors include the following:

Appearance: A neat, clean, professional appearance increases other people's confidence in your skills and abilities. When you are well-groomed, with clean hair, nails, and clothing, patients and other staff members see your demeanor as businesslike.

Attendance: Being on time for work demonstrates that you are reliable and dependable.

Initiative: Being able to start a course of action and stay on task is an important quality to demonstrate.

Courtesy: Treating patients and fellow workers with dignity and respect helps build solid professional relationships at work.

Medical Ethics and Etiquette in the Practice

Licensed medical staff and other employees working in physicians' practices share responsibility for observing a code of ethics and for following correct etiquette.

Ethics

Medical **ethics** are standards of behavior requiring truthfulness, honesty, and integrity. Ethics guide the behavior of physicians, who have the training, the primary responsibility, and the legal right to diagnose and treat human illness and injury. All medical office employees and those working in health-related professions share responsibility for observing the ethical code.

Each professional organization has a code of ethics that is to be followed by its membership. In general, this code states that information about patients and other employees and confidential business matters should not be discussed with anyone not directly concerned with them. Behavior should be consistent with the values of the profession. For example, it is unethical for an employee to take money or gifts from a company in exchange for giving the company business. Study Figures 1.7 and 1.8 on pages 26 and 27, which are examples of codes of ethics that relate to the role of medical insurance specialists.

Etiquette

Professional **etiquette** is also important for medical insurance specialists. Correct behavior in a medical practice is generally covered in the practice's employee policy and procedure manual. For example, guidelines establish which types of incoming calls must go immediately to a physician or to a nurse or assistant and which require a message to be taken. Of particular importance are guidelines about the respectful and courteous treatment of patients and all others who interact with the practice's staff.

Securing and Advancing on a Job

Completion of a medical insurance specialist program, coding specialist program, or medical assisting or health information technology program at a postsecondary institution provides an excellent background for many types of positions in the medical insurance field. Another possibility is to earn an associate degree or a certificate of proficiency by completing a program in a curriculum area such as health care business services. Further baccalaureate and graduate study enables advancement to managerial positions.

Moving ahead in a career is often aided by membership in professional organizations that offer certification in various areas. Certification by a professional organization provides evidence to prospective employers that the applicant has demonstrated a superior level of skill on a national test.

Medical Assisting Certification

Two organizations offer tests in the professional area of medical assisting. After earning a diploma in medical assisting from an accredited school (or having a year's work experience), medical assistants may sit for the Certified Medical Assistant (CMA) titles from the American Association of Medical Assistants or the Registered Medical Assistant (RMA) designation from the American Medical Technologists.

CMA

American Association of Medical Assistants (AAMA)
20 N. Wacker Drive,
Suite 1575
Chicago, IL 60606-2903
312-899-1500
http://www.aama-ntl.org

RMA

American Medical Technologists (AMT)
710 Higgins Road
Park Ridge, IL 60068-5765
847-823-5169
http://www.amt1.com

AHIMA Code of Ethics 2004

Ethical Principles: The following ethical principles are based on the core values of the American Health Information Management Association and apply to all health information management professionals.

HIM professionals:

I. Advocate, uphold, and defend the individual's right to privacy and the doctrine of confidentiality in the use and disclosure of information.
II. Put service and the health and welfare of persons before self-interest and conduct themselves in the practice of the profession so as to bring honor to themselves, their peers, and to the health information management profession.
III. Preserve, protect, and secure personal health information in any form or medium and hold in the highest regard the contents of the records and other information of a confidential nature, taking into account the applicable statues and regulations.
IV. Refuse to participate in or conceal unethical practices or procedures.
V. Advance health information management knowledge and practice through continuing education, research, publications, and presentations.
VI. Recruit and mentor students, peers, and colleagues to develop and strengthen professional work force.
VII. Represent the profession accurately to the public.
VIII. Perform honorably health information management association responsibilities, either appointed or elected, and preserve the confidentiality of any privileged information made known in any official capacity.
IX. State truthfully and accurately their credentials, professional education, and experiences.
X. Facilitate interdisciplinary collaboration in situations supporting health information practice.
XI. Respect the inherent dignity and worth of every person.

Figure 1.7 AHIMA Code of Ethics

Health Information Certification

Students who are interested in the professional area of health information (also known as medical records) may complete an associate degree from an accredited college program and pass a credentialing test to be certified as a Registered Health Information Technology, or RHIT. An RHIT examines medical records for accuracy, reports patient data for reimbursement, and helps with information for medical research and statistical data.

Also offered is the Registered Health Information Administration (RHIA), requiring a baccalaureate degree and national certification. RHIAs are skilled in the collection, interpretation, and analysis of patient data. Additionally, they receive the training necessary to assume managerial positions related to these functions. RHIAs interact with all levels of an organization—clinical, financial, and administrative—that employ patient data in decision making and everyday operations.

RHIAs enjoy job placements in a broad range of settings that span the continuum of health care, including office-based physician practices, nursing homes, home health agencies, mental health facilities, and public health agencies. The growth of managed care has created additional job opportunities in HMOs, PPOs, and insurance companies. Prospects are especially strong in these settings for RHIAs who possess advanced degrees in business or health administration.

RHIT, RHIA, CCS, CCS-P, CCS-A

American Health Information Management Association (AHIMA)
233 N. Michigan Ave., Suite 2150
Chicago, IL 60601-5800
800-335-5535
http://www.ahima.org

American Academy of Professional Coders

Code of Ethical Standards

- Members of the American Academy of Professional Coders shall be dedicated to providing the highest standard of professional coding and billing services to employers, clients and patients. Behavior of AAPC members must be exemplary.
- AAPC members shall maintain the highest standard of personal and professional conduct. Members shall respect the rights of patients, clients, employers and all other colleagues.
- Members shall use only legal and ethical means in all professional dealings, and shall refuse to cooperate with or condone by silence, the actions of those who engage in fraudulent, deceptive or illegal acts.
- Members shall respect the laws and regulations of the land, and uphold the mission statement of the AAPC.

AAPC Mission Statement

Establish and maintain ethical and educational standards for professional coders.

Provide a national certification and credentialing process.

Support the national and local membership by providing educational products and opportunities to network.

Increase and promote national recognition and awareness of procedural and diagnostic coding.

- Members shall pursue excellence through continuing education in all areas applicable to their profession.
- Members shall strive to maintain and enhance the dignity, status, competence and standards of coding for professional services.
- Members shall not exploit professional relationships with patients, employees, clients or employers for personal gain.
- Above all else, we will commit to recognizing the intrinsic worth of each member.

This code of Ethical Standards for members of the American Academy of Professional Coders strives to promote and maintain the highest standard of professional service and conduct among its members. Adherence to these standards assures public confidence in the integrity and service of professional coders who are members of the American Academy of Professional Coders.

Figure 1.8 Code of Ethical Standards, American Academy of Professional Coders

Coding Certification

Medical coders are expert in classifying medical data. They assign codes to physicians' descriptions of patients' conditions and treatments. For employment as a medical coder, employers typically prefer—or may require—certification. AHIMA offers three coding certifications: the Certified Coding Associate (CCA),

CPC, CPC-H, CPC-P, CPC-A

American Academy of Professional Coders
2480 South 3850 West, Suite B
Salt Lake City, Utah 84120
800-626-2633
http://www.aapc.com

Thinking It Through — 1.4

*Dorita McCallister, the office manager of Clark Clinic, ordered medical office supplies from her cousin, Gregory Hand. When the supplies arrived, Gregory came to the office to check on them and to take Dorita out to lunch. Is Dorita's purchase of supplies from her cousin ethical? Why?

*George McGrew is a medical insurance specialist in the practice of Dr. Sylvia Grets. Over the last few weeks, Dr. Grets has consistently written down codes that stand for one-hour appointments, but George knows that these visits were all very short, no longer than fifteen minutes each. Is it ethical for George to report these codes on health care claims?

Billing Tip

Moving Ahead in Your Career
Professional certification, additional study, and work experience contribute to advancement to positions such as medical billing manager and medical office manager. Billers may also advance through specialization in a field, such as radiology billing management. Some become medical coders or coding managers.

intended as a starting point for entering a new career as a coder; the Certified Coding Specialist (CCS); and the Certified Coding Specialist-Physician-based (CCS-P). The American Academy of Professional Coders (AAPC) grants the Certified Professional Coder (CPC) and the Certified Professional Coder-Hospital (CPC-H) certifications. The AAPC also offers the CPC-P, a payer certification; the CPC-A, an associate level for those who do not yet have medical coding work experience; and a number of advanced specialty coding certifications.

Continuing Education

Most professional organizations require certified members to keep up to date by taking annual training courses to refresh or extend their knowledge. Continuing education sessions are assigned course credits by the credentialing organizations, and satisfactory completion of a test on the material is often required for credit. Employers often approve attendance at seminars that apply to the practice's goals and ask the person who attends to update other staff members.

Review

Steps to Success

- ❐ Read this chapter and review the Key Terms and the Chapter Summary.
- ❐ Answer the Review Questions and Applying Your Knowledge in the Chapter Review.
- ❐ Access the chapter's websites and complete the Internet Activities to learn more about available professional resources.
- ❐ Complete the related chapter in the *Medical Insurance Workbook* to reinforce your understanding of medical insurance, billing, and reimbursement.

Chapter Summary

1. Group and individual policies provide medical insurance coverage. The policy defines the payments that are required, such as premiums, coinsurance, and copayments. It also describes the services that are covered and those that are not. In addition to medical insurance, two other policy types are important for medical insurance specialists: disability insurance that covers loss of income due to a person's inability to work and workers' compensation that provides benefits for job-related claims.
2. An indemnity health plan reimburses beneficiaries according to the contract's schedule of benefits in exchange for payment of a specified premium, deductibles, and coinsurance. Patients with indemnity plans receive care from the providers of their choice. Managed care plans, in contrast, contract with both beneficiaries and providers to control the delivery and cost of health care services. In exchange for lower premiums and other cost reductions, plan members agree to a reduced choice of health care providers and tighter regulation of access to services.
3. Fee-for-service reimbursement is a retroactive payment method in which payment is made after services are provided. In capitation, a fixed prospective payment is made for services to be provided during a specified period of time.
4. An HMO locks patients into receiving services from providers with whom it has contracts; sometimes a primary care physician coordinates care and makes required referrals to specialists. A POS offers more flexibility to choose providers, but at an increased cost to the patient. A PPO offers patients lower fees in exchange for receiving services from plan providers but does not usually require care coordination or referrals.
5. A consumer-driven health plan combines a high-deductible, low-premium PPO with a pretax savings account to cover out-of-pocket medical expenses up to the deductible point.
6. Private payers of health benefits are either insurance companies or self-insured employers. Most private health insurance is employer-sponsored. Government-sponsored health care programs include Medicare, Medicaid, TRICARE, and CHAMPVA.
7. The ten steps in the medical billing process are: (1) preregister patients, (2) establish financial responsibility for the visit, (3) check in patients, (4) check out patients, (5) review coding compliance, (6) check billing compliance, (7) prepare and transmit claims, (8) monitor payer adjudication, (9) generate patient statements, and (10) follow up patient payments and handle collections.
8. Medical insurance specialists must know medical terminology, anatomy, physiology, and medical coding, have communication and information technology skills, pay attention to detail, be flexible and honest, and be able to work as team members.

9. Medical insurance specialists work in a variety of environments ranging from small to very large medical practices and for insurance companies, government-sponsored programs, and billing services.

10. Ethical conduct in medical practices means being honest and truthful and acting with integrity. Professional etiquette sets standards for good manners in dealing with others.

Review Questions

Match the key terms with their definitions.

A. health maintenance organization (HMO)
B. capitation
C. schedule of benefits
D. fee-for-service
E. coinsurance
F. deductible
G. copayment
H. premium
I. preferred provider organization (PPO)
J. indemnity

____ 1. A list of the medical services covered by an insurance policy
____ 2. The amount of money paid to a health plan to buy an insurance policy
____ 3. A managed care network of providers under contract to provide services at discounted fees
____ 4. An amount that an insured person pays at the time of a visit to a provider
____ 5. The percentage of each claim that an insured person must pay
____ 6. A prospective payment to a provider made for each plan member
____ 7. A health plan that reimburses policyholders based on the fees charged
____ 8. An organization that contracts with a network of providers for the delivery of health care for a prepaid premium
____ 9. The amount that an insured person must pay before reimbursement for medical expenses begins
____10. A retroactive reimbursement method based on providers' charges

Decide whether each statement is true or false.

____ 1. Employment opportunities for medical insurance specialists are increasing because providers need trained, knowledgeable staff members to maximize revenue and ensure patient satisfaction.
____ 2. The third party to a medical insurance contract is the policyholder.
____ 3. A discounted fee-for-service schedule provides for prospective payment.
____ 4. In order to receive prospective payments for enrollees in a capitated managed care plan, a provider must have given medical services to each member at least once a month.
____ 5. Under an indemnity plan, the premium, deductible, and coinsurance are taken into account before the insured is reimbursed.
____ 6. Members of a POS plan must use network providers to be covered.
____ 7. Both HMOs and PPOs use capitation as their main reimbursement method.
____ 8. PPOs are the most popular type of health plan.
____ 9. A consumer-directed health plan is a type of HMO.
____ 10. Everyone who works in a medical practice, whether a physician, a nonphysician practitioner, or an administrative staff member, has ethical responsibilities.

Select the letter that best completes the statement or answers the question

1. In an HMO with a gatekeeper system, a _____ coordinates the patient's care and provides referrals.
   A. PPO
   B. EPO
   C. PCP
   D. NPP
2. Which of the following permits members to see out-of-network providers?
   A. POS
   B. PCP
   C. URO
   D. EOC
3. Health plans pay for _____ services.
   A. indemnity
   B. covered
   C. coded
   D. out-of-network
4. In an HMO, securing _____ may be required before services are provided.
   A. preauthorization
   B. utilization
   C. gatekeeper
   D. formulary
5. A self-insured health plan may use its own
   A. physician-employees
   B. funds
   C. gatekeepers
   D. primary care physicians
6. Unlike an HMO, a PPO permits its members to use _____ providers, but at a higher cost.
   A. subcapitated
   B. out-of-network
   C. nonphysician practitioner
   D. primary care
7. The major government-sponsored health programs are
   A. TRICARE, CHAMPVA, Medicare, and Medicaid
   B. HEDIS, Medicare, Medicaid, and CHAMPUS
   C. Medicare and Medicaid
   D. Medicare and TRICARE
8. Coinsurance is calculated based on
   A. the number of policyholders in a plan
   B. a fixed charge for each visit
   C. a capitation rate
   D. a percentage of a charge
9. When a patient has insurance coverage for which the practice will create a claim, the patient bill is usually done
   A. before the encounter
   B. during the encounter
   C. after the encounter when the health care claim is transmitted
   D. after the encounter and after the payer's payment is posted
10. If a patient's payment is later than permitted under the financial policy of the practice, the _____ may be started.
    A. copayment process
    B. appeal process
    C. coding process
    D. collection process

Answer the following questions.

1. List the ten steps in the medical billing process.

   Step 1 ______________________________

   Step 2 ______________________________

   Step 3 ______________________________

   Step 4 ______________________________

   Step 5 ______________________________

Step 6 ______________________________

Step 7 ______________________________

Step 8 ______________________________

Step 9 ______________________________

Step 10 ______________________________

2. List at least four important skills of medical insurance specialists.
   A. ______________________________
   B. ______________________________
   C. ______________________________
   D. ______________________________

Applying Your Knowledge

Case 1.1 Abstracting Insurance Information

A patient shows the following insurance identification card to the medical insurance specialist:

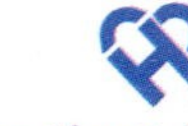

Connecticut HealthPlan

I.D.#:	1002.9713
Employee:	DANIEL ANTHONY
Group #:	A0000323
Eff. date:	03/01/2008
Status:	Dependent Coverage? F
In-network:	$10 Co-Pay
Out-of-network:	$250 Ded; 80%/20%

Front of card

IMPORTANT INFORMATION
Notice to Members and Providers of Care

To avoid a reduction in your hospital benefits, you are responsible for obtaining certification for hospitalization and emergency admissions. The review is required regardless of the reason for hospital admission. For specified procedures, Second Surgical Opinions may be mandatory.
For certification, call Utilization Management Services at 800-837-8808:
- At least 7 days in advance of Scheduled Surgery of Hospital Admissions.
- Within 48 hours after Emergency Admissions or on the first business day following weekend or holiday Emergency Admissions.

CONNECTICUT HEALTHPLAN C/O
WEISS
Robert S. Weiss
& Company
Silver Hill Business Center
500 S. Broad Street
P.O. Box 1034
Meriden, CT 06450
(800) 466-7900

THIS CARD IS FOR IDENTIFICATION ONLY AND DOES NOT ESTABLISH ELIGIBILITY FOR COVERAGE BY CONNECTICUT HEALTH PLAN. Please refer to your insurance booklet for further details.

Back of card

A. What copayment is due when the patient sees a network physician?

B. What payment rules apply when the patient sees an out-of-network physician?

C. What rules apply when the patient needs to be admitted to the hospital?

Case 1.2 Calculating Insurance Math

Calculate the payment(s) billed in each of the following situations.

A. The patient's health plan has a $100 annual deductible. At the first visit of the year, the charges are $95. What does the patient owes?

B. The patient's coinsurance percentage is stated as 75-25 in the insurance policy. The deductible for the year has been met. If the visit charges are $1,000, what payment should the medical insurance specialist expect from the payer? What amount will the patient be billed?

C. The patient's coinsurance percentage is stated as 80-20 in the insurance policy. The deductible for the year has been met. If the visit charges are $420, what payment should the medical insurance specialist expect from the payer? What amount will the patient be billed?

D. The patient is enrolled in a capitated HMO with a $10 copayment for primary care physician visits and no coinsurance requirements. After collecting $10 from the patient, what amount can the medical insurance specialist bill the payer for an office visit?

E. The patient has a policy that requires a $20 copayment for an in-network visit, due at the time of service. The policy also requires 30 percent coinsurance from the patient. Today's visit charges total $785. After subtracting the copayment collected from the patient, the medical insurance specialist expects a payment of what amount from the payer? What amount will the patient be billed?

F. A patient's total surgery charges are $1,278. The patient must pay the annual deductible of $1,000, and the policy states a 80-20 coinsurance. What does the patient owe?

G. A patient has a high-deductible consumer-driven health plan. The annual deductible is $2,500, of which $300 has been paid. After a surgical procedure costing $1,890, what does the patient owe? Can any amount be collected from a payer? Why?

H. A patient with a high-deductible consumer-driven health plan has met half of the $1,000 annual deductible before requiring surgery to repair a broken ankle while visiting a neighboring state. The out-of-network physician's bill is $4,500. The PPO that takes effect after the deductible has been met is an 80-20 in-network plan and a 60-40 out-of-network plan. How much does the patient owe? How much should the PPO be billed?

Case 1.3 Using Insurance Terms

Read the following information from a medical insurance policy.

> Policy Number 054351278
> Insured Jane Hellman Brandeis
> Premium Due Quarterly $1,414.98
>
> AMOUNT PAYABLE
> Maximum Benefit Limit, per *covered person*. $2,000,000
> Stated Deductible per *covered person*, per *calendar year*. $2,500
> EMERGENCY ROOM DEDUCTIBLE (for each visit for *illness* to an emergency room when not directly admitted to the *hospital)* $50
> Note: After satisfaction of the emergency room deductible, *covered expenses* are subject to any applicable *deductible amounts* and coinsurance provisions.
>
> PREFERRED PROVIDER COINSURANCE PERCENTAGE, per *calendar year*
> For *covered expenses* in excess of the applicable stated deductible, payer pays. 10%

A. What type of health plan is described: HMO, PPO, or indemnity?

B. What is the *annual* premium? ____________________________

C. What is the annual deductible? ____________________________

D. What percentage of preferred provider charges does the patient owe after meeting the deductible each year? ____________________________

E. If the insured incurs a $6,000 in-network medical bill after the annual deductible has been paid, how much will the health plan pay? ____________________________

Internet Activities

1. The Internet is a valuable source of information about many topics of interest to medical insurance specialists. For example, to explore career opportunities, study the job statistics gathered by the *Occupational Outlook Handbook* of the Bureau of Labor Statistics at http://stats.bls.gov/oco. Using the site map at that home page, choose Keyword Search of BLS Web Pages, and enter a job title of interest, such as medical assistants or health information technicians. In particular, review the job outlook information.
2. Using a search engine (such as Google or Yahoo!), investigate the following organizations, studying their membership, career ladders, and certification or credentials offered:
   ACA International (formerly American Collectors Association)
   American Academy of Professional Coders
   American Association of Healthcare Administrative Management
   American Health Information Management Association
   Association of Medical Billers
   Healthcare Billing and Management Association
   Healthcare Financial Management Association
   Medical Group Management Association
   Professional Association of Health Care Office Management

Chapter 2

HIPAA and Medical Records

CHAPTER OUTLINE

Medical Record Documentation

Health Care Regulation

HIPAA Privacy Rule

HIPAA Security Rule

HIPAA Electronic Health Care Transactions and Code Sets

Fraud and Abuse Regulations

Enforcement and Penalties

Compliance Plans

Learning Outcomes

After studying this chapter, you should be able to:

1. **Discuss the importance of medical records and documentation in the medical billing process.**
2. **Describe the benefits of electronic medical records (EMR).**
3. **Explain the purpose of the HIPAA Privacy Rule.**
4. **Distinguish between a covered entity and a business associate under HIPAA.**
5. **Define protected health information (PHI).**
6. **Discuss patients' authorizations to use or disclose their health information.**
7. **Briefly describe the purpose of the HIPAA Security Rule.**
8. **Describe the HIPAA Electronic Health Care Transactions and Code Sets standards and the four National Identifiers.**
9. **Explain the purpose of the Health Care Fraud and Abuse Control Program and related laws.**
10. **Discuss the ways in which compliance plans help medical practices avoid fraud and abuse.**

Key Terms

abuse
audit
authorization
business associate
Centers for Medicare and Medicaid Services (CMS)
clearinghouse
code set
compliance plan
covered entity
de-identified health information
designated record set (DRS)
documentation
electronic data interchange (EDI)
electronic medical record (EMR)
encounter
encryption
evaluation and management (E/M)
fraud
Health Care Fraud and Abuse Control Program
Health Insurance Portability and Accountability Act (HIPAA) of 1996
HIPAA Electronic Health Care Transactions and Code Sets (TCS)
HIPAA National Identifier
HIPAA Privacy Rule
HIPAA Security Rule
informed consent
malpractice
medical record
medical standards of care
minimum necessary standard
National Provider Identifier (NPI)
Notice of Privacy Practices (NPP)
Office for Civil Rights (OCR)
Office of the Inspector General (OIG)
password
protected health information (PHI)
qui tam
relator
respondeat superior
subpoena
subpoena duces tecum
transaction
treatment, payment, and health care operations (TPO)

Medical Record Documentation

A patient's **medical record** contains facts, findings, and observations about that patient's health history. The record also contains communications with and about the patient. In a physician practice, the medical record begins with a patient's first contact and continues through all treatments and services. The record provides continuity and communication among physicians and other health care professionals who are involved in the patient's care. Patients' medical records are also used in research and for education.

Medical Records

Medical records, or charts, are created by physicians and other providers. These records are stored—on paper or electronically—by physician practices, hospitals, surgery centers, clinics, and other health care facilities. Records are created and shared to help make accurate diagnoses of patients' conditions and to trace the course of care.

Compliance Guideline

Medical Standards of Care and Malpractice
Medical standards of care are state-specified performance measures for the delivery of health care by medical professionals. Medical malpractice can result when a provider injures or harms a patient due to failure to follow the standards.

Example

A patient's medical record contains the results of all tests a primary care physician (PCP) ordered during a comprehensive physical examination. To follow up on a problem, the PCP refers the patient to a cardiologist, also sending the pertinent data for that doctor's review. By studying the medical record, the specialist treating a referred patient learns the outcome of previous tests and avoids repeating them unnecessarily.

Documentation means organizing a patient's health record in chronological order using a systematic, logical, and consistent method. A patient's health history, examinations, tests, and results of treatments are all documented. Complete and comprehensive documentation is important to show that physicians have followed the **medical standards of care** that apply in their state. Health care providers are liable (that is, legally responsible) for providing this level of care to their patients. The term *medical professional liability* describes this responsibility of licensed health care professionals.

Patient medical records are legal documents. Good medical records are a part of the physician's defense against accusations that patients were not treated correctly. They clearly state who performed what service and describe why, where, when, and how it was done. Physicians document the rationale behind their treatment decisions. This rationale is the basis for medical necessity—the clinically logical link between a patient's condition and a treatment or procedure.

> **Billing Tip**
>
> **Medical Necessity**
> Services are medically necessary when they are reasonable and necessary for the diagnosis or treatment of illness or injury or to improve the functioning of a malformed body member. Such services must also be consistent with generally accepted standards of care.

Documenting Encounters with Providers

Every patient **encounter**—the face-to-face meeting between a patient and a provider in a medical office, clinic, hospital, or other location—should be documented with the following information:

- Patient's name
- Encounter date and reason
- Appropriate history and physical examination
- Review of all tests that were ordered
- Diagnosis
- Plan of care, or notes on procedures or treatments that were given
- Instructions or recommendations that were given to the patient
- Signature of the provider who saw the patient

In addition, a patient's medical record must contain:

- Biographical and personal information, including the patient's full name, Social Security number, date of birth, full address, marital status, home and work telephone numbers, and employer information as applicable
- Copies of all communications with the patient, including letters, telephone calls, faxes, and e-mail messages; the patient's responses; and a note of the time, date, topic, and physician's response to each communication
- Copies of prescriptions and instructions given to the patient, including refills
- Original documents that the patient has signed, such as an authorization to release information and an advance directive
- Medical allergies and reactions, or their absence
- Up-to-date immunization record and history if appropriate, such as for a child
- Previous and current diagnoses, test results, health risks, and progress
- Copies of referral or consultation letters
- Hospital admissions and release documents
- Records of any missed or canceled appointments
- Requests for information about the patient (from a health plan or an attorney, for example), and a detailed log of to whom information was released

Medicare's general documentation standards are shown in Table 2.1 on page 38.

> **Billing Tip**
>
> **Working with Medical Records**
> Medical insurance specialists abstract billing information from the medical record, including the date of service, the diagnoses and procedures, and the provider.

SOAP Format

Medical insurance specialists work with a number of methods that are used to organize patient medical records. The most common format is called a *problem-oriented medical record* (POMR). The problem-oriented medical record has a

TABLE 2.1 Documentation Pointers

1.	Medicare expects the documentation to be generated at the time of service or shortly thereafter.
2.	Delayed entries within a reasonable time frame (twenty-four to forty-eight hour) are acceptable for purposes of clarification, error correction, and addition of information not initially available, and if certain unusual circumstances prevented the generation of the note at the time of service.
3.	The medical record cannot be altered. Errors must be legibly corrected so that the reviewer can draw an inference about their origin. Corrections or additions must be dated, preferably timed, and legibly signed or initialed.
4.	Every note stands alone—that is, the performed services must be documented at the outset.
5.	Delayed written explanations will be considered for purposes of clarification only. They cannot be used to add and authenticate services billed and not documented at the time of service or to retrospectively substantiate medical necessity. For that, the medical record must stand on its own, with the original entry corroborating that the service was rendered and was medically necessary.
6.	All entries must be legible to another reader to a degree that a meaningful review can be conducted.
7.	All notes should be dated, preferably timed, and signed by the author.
8.	In the office setting, initials are acceptable as long as they clearly identify the author.
9.	If the signature is not legible and does not identify the author, a printed version should be also recorded.

general section with data from the initial patient examination and assessment. When the patient makes subsequent visits, the reasons for those encounters are listed separately and have their own notes. A problem-oriented medical record contains SOAP notes, as shown in Figure 2.1. In the SOAP format, a patient's encounter documentation has four parts: Subjective, Objective, Assessment, and Plan:

S: The *subjective* information is what the patient names as the problems or complaints.

O: The *objective* information is what the physician finds during the examination of the patient; it may include data from laboratory tests and other procedures.

A: The *assessment*, also called the impression or conclusion, is the physician's diagnosis.

P: The *plan*, also called advice or recommendations, is the course of treatment for the patient, such as surgery, medications, or other tests, including necessary patient monitoring, follow-up, and instructions to the patient.

Evaluation and Management Services Reports

When providers evaluate a patient's condition and decide on a course of treatment to manage it, the service is called **evaluation and management (E/M)**. Evaluation and management services may include a complete interview and physical examination for a new patient or for a new problem presented by a person who is already a patient. There are many other types of E/M encounters, such as a visit to decide whether surgery is needed or to follow up on a patient's problem. An E/M service is usually documented with chart notes.

History and Physical Examination A complete history and physical (H&P) is documented with four types of information: (1) the chief complaint, (2) the

Rayelle Smith-Jones

SUBJECTIVE: The mother brought in this 1-month-old female. The patient is doing very well. They have been using the phototherapy blanket. She is thirsty, has good yellow stooling, and continues on formula. Her alertness is normal. Other pertinent ROS is noncontributory.

OBJECTIVE: Afebrile. Comfortable. Jaundice is only minimal at this time. No scleral icterus. Good activity level. Normal fontanel. TMs, nose, mouth, pharynx, neck, heart, lungs, abdomen, liver, spleen, and groins are normal. Normal cord care. Good extremities.

ASSESSMENT: Resolving physiologic jaundice on phototherapy.

PLAN: Will stop phototherapy and do a bilirubin level a couple of days to make sure there is no rebound. The patient is to be seen in one week. Push fluids. Routine care was discussed.

FIGURE 2.1 Example of a SOAP Note

history and physical examination, (3) the diagnosis, and (4) the treatment plan (see Figure 2.2 on page 40).

The physician documents the patient's reason for the visit, often using the patient's own words to describe the symptom, problem, condition, diagnosis, or other factor. For clarity, the physician may restate the reason as a "presenting problem," using medical terminology.

The physician also documents the patient's relevant medical history. The extent of the history is based on what the physician considers appropriate. It may include the history of the present illness (HPI), past medical history (PMH), and family/social history. There is usually also a review of systems (ROS), in which the doctor asks questions about the function of each body system considered appropriate to the problem.

The physician performs a physical examination and documents the diagnosis—the interpretation of the information that has been gathered—or the suspected problem if more tests or procedures are needed for a diagnosis. The treatment plan, or plan of care, is described. It includes the treatments and medications that the physician has ordered, specifying dosage and frequency of use.

Other Chart Notes Many other types of chart notes appear in patients' medical records. Progress reports, as shown in Figure 2.3 on page 41, document a patient's progress and response to a treatment plan. They explain whether the plan should be continued or changed. Progress reports include:

- Comparisons of objective data with the patient's statements
- Goals and progress toward the goals
- The patient's current condition and prognosis
- Type of treatment still needed and for how long

Compliance Guideline

Informed Consent
If the plan of care involves significant risk, such as surgery, state laws require the physician to have the patient's informed consent in advance. The physician discusses the assessment, risks, and recommendations with the patient and documents this conversation in the patient's record. Usually, the patient signs either a chart entry or a consent form to indicate agreement.

James E. Ribielli
5/19/2006

CHIEF COMPLAINT: This 79-year-old male presents with sudden and extreme weakness. He got up from a seated position and became light-headed.

PAST MEDICAL HISTORY: History of congestive heart failure. On multiple medications, including Cardizem, Enalapril 5 mg qd, and Lasix 40 mg qd.

PHYSICAL EXAMINATION: No postural change in blood pressure. BP, 114/61 with a pulse of 49, sitting; BP, 111/56 with a pulse 50, standing. Patient denies being light-headed at this time.

HEENT: Unremarkable.

NECK: Supple without jugular or venous distension.

LUNGS: Clear to auscultation and percussion.

HEART: S1 and S2 normal; no systolic or diastolic murmurs; no S3, S4. No dysrhythmia.

ABDOMEN: Soft without organomegaly, mass, or bruit.

EXTREMITIES: Unremarkable. Pulses strong and equal.

LABORATORY DATA: Hemoglobin, 12.3. White count, 10.800. Normal electrolytes. ECG shows sinus bradycardia.

DIAGNOSIS: Weakness on the basis of sinus bradycardia, probably Cardizem induced.

TREATMENT: Patient told to change positions slowly when moving from sitting to standing, and from lying to standing.

John R. Ramirez, MD

FIGURE 2.2 Example of History and Physical Examination Documentation

Discharge summaries, as shown in Figure 2.4, are prepared during a patient's final visit for a particular treatment plan or hospitalization. Discharge summaries include:

- The final diagnosis
- Comparisons of objective data with the patient's statements
- Whether goals were achieved
- Reason for and date of discharge
- The patient's current condition, status, and final prognosis
- Instructions given to the patient at discharge, noting any special needs such as restrictions on activities and medications.

Jennifer Delgado
8/14/2006

SUBJECTIVE: The patient has had epilepsy since she was 10. She takes her medication as prescribed; denies side effects. She reports no convulsions or new symptoms. She is a full-time student at Riverside Community College.

OBJECTIVE: Phenobarbital 90 mg twice a day as prescribed since 1994. The motor and sensory examination results are normal.

ASSESSMENT: Well-controlled epilepsy.

PLAN: Patient advised to continue medication regimen. Schedule for follow-up in 6 months.

Jared R. Wandaowsky, MD

FIGURE 2.3 Example of a Progress Report

Myrna W. Pearl
8/20/2006

SUBJECTIVE: Myrna came in for suture removal from a right-knee wound. She reports that she is healing well.

OBJECTIVE: The wound appears dry and clean, with no signs of infection.

ASSESSMENT: Uncomplicated suture removal.

PLAN: All six sutures were removed and a bandage applied. Patient was advised to continue to keep the wound clean. No further treatment is required.

Grady Longuier, MD

FIGURE 2.4 Example of a Discharge Summary

Procedural Services Documentation

Other common types of documentation are for specific procedures done either in the office or elsewhere:

- Procedure or operative reports for simple or complex surgery
- Laboratory reports for laboratory tests

Angela Di Giorono
April 5, 2005

CC: Two days ago, patient saw a red swollen lump on her medial thigh. Today it is reddened and painful. She wonders if this is an ingrown hair.

OBJECTIVE: There is an indurated area measuring 3 cm in diameter in the proximal medial right thigh. In the center is a darker area of erythema with a small pustule. There is a wider area of erythema surrounding this, consistent with a cellulitis. There are no red streaks going up toward the groin.

Explanation of the process was given to the patient, and she agreed to having the procedure performed.

The abscessed area was cleansed with Betadine and anesthetized with 1% Xylocaine. An incision and drainage were done with a #11 blade. Scant pus was obtained. A pocket was curetted out and then packed with Iodoform gauze.

DIAGNOSIS: Abscess with cellulitis.

PLAN: Patient was given Ancef I gm 1M. Tomorrow, she is to start Keflex 500 mg q.i.d. #40 capsules. She was given Tylenol #3 for pain, 10 tablets. She is to remove the packing tomorrow and start warm soaks 3 times a day, 10 minutes each time. Signs of infection were discussed with her. She was told to return immediately if she notices any of these signs; otherwise, recheck in about 5 days.

Carol Rice, MD

FIGURE 2.5 Example of an Office Procedure Note

- Radiology reports for the results of X-rays
- Forms for a specific purpose, such as immunization records, pre-employment physicals, and disability reports

An office procedure report is shown in Figure 2.5.

Termination of the Provider-Patient Relationship

At times, either the patient or the provider terminates the relationship. In such cases, the provider must still maintain the patient's medical record according to the provisions of federal and state law. The provider also sends the patient a letter that documents the situation and provides for continuity of care with the next provider. For example, if a patient wishes to be released from a physician's care, the provider documents this fact and any part of the treatment plan that was still underway at the time of termination. On the other hand, a patient's actions, such as refusing to observe a treatment plan, take required medication, or keep appointments, may cause the provider to decide to terminate the relationship. In this event, the patient is informed in writing. A copy of this letter, as shown in Figure 2.6, becomes part of the patient's medical record.

Dear __________:

I find it necessary to inform you that I am discharging you as a patient for the reason that you have continually refused to follow my medical advice and treatment. Because your condition requires medical attention, I suggest that you find another physician to provide you with care promptly. If you wish, I will provide care for a period of up to five days after you receive this letter. This should give you enough time to select a physician from the many competent providers in this area. With your authorization, I will make your medical record available to the physician you select.

Sincerely,

_______________, MD

FIGURE 2.6 Example of a Termination Letter

Electronic Medical Records

Because of the advantages, health care leaders in business and government are pressing for laws to require the switch to **electronic medical records (EMR)**. An electronic medical record is a collection of health information that provides immediate electronic access by authorized users.

The federal government, in President George W. Bush's Executive Order 13335, has set the goal of using electronic records for all patients by 2014. However, it is estimated that fewer than one in five group physician practice currently has electronic patient records. Some of these in fact have hybrid systems that combine paper and electronic records. Cost, technical support, and privacy/security concerns are some of the reasons for the slow transition to EMRs.

In most practices, whether paper or electronic medical records are in use, billing is handled with a patient management program. When most of the clinical record keeping is on paper, providers' notes are usually written on the patients' records or transcribed from dictation and placed in the record, where they are signed and dated by the responsible provider. Lab test results are printed; X-rays, ECGs , and other routine test results are included.

In electronic medical records, documents may be created in a variety of ways, but they are ultimately viewed on a computer screen. For example, one general practice uses about 150 medical-history-taking templates for gathering and recording consistent history and physical information from patients. The computer-based templates range in focus from abdominal pain to depression, with from ten to twenty questions each. The on-screen templates are filled out in the exam rooms. Responsible providers then sign the entries, using technology for electronic signatures that verifies the identity of the signer.

Thinking It Through — 2.1

Nicholas J. Kramer, MD
2200 Carriage Lane
Currituck, CT 07886

Consultation Report
on John W. Wu
(Birth date 12/06/1933)

Dear Dr. Kramer:

At your request, I saw Mr. Wu today. This is a sixty-five-year-old male who stopped smoking cigarettes twenty years ago but continues to be a heavy pipe smoker. He has had several episodes of hemoptysis; a small amount of blood was produced along with some white phlegm. He denies any upper respiratory tract infection or symptoms on those occasions. He does not present with chronic cough, chest pain, or shortness of breath. I reviewed the chest X-ray done by you, which exhibits no acute process. His examination was normal.

A bronchoscopy was performed, which produced some evidence of laryngitis, tracheitis, and bronchitis, but no tumor was noted. Bronchial washings were negative.

I find that his bleeding is caused by chronic inflammation of his hypopharynx and bronchial tree, which is related to pipe smoking. There is no present evidence of malignancy.

Thank you for requesting this consultation.

Sincerely,

Mary Lakeland Georges, MD

1. This letter is in the patient medical record of John W. Wu.

What is the purpose of the letter?

How does it demonstrate the use of a patient medical record for continuity of care?

2. The federal government is a leader in promoting the idea of a personal medical record, or PMR. This record, like a physician's record, will contain an individual's lifelong health history, will be accessible on the Internet, and will be capable of being used among hospitals, physician offices, and clinics. In your opinion, will the PMR will help ensure continuity of care for patients? If so, how?

EMRs offer both patients and providers significant advantages over paper records:

- *Immediate access to health information:* The EMR is simultaneously accessible from computers in the office and in other sites such as hospitals. Compared to sorting through papers in a paper folder, an EMR database can save time when vital patient information is needed. Once information is updated in a patient record, it is available to all who need access, whether across the hall or across town.

- *Computerized physician order management:* Physicians can enter orders for prescriptions, tests, and other services at any time. This information is then transmitted to the staff for implementation or directly to pharmacies linked to the practice.
- *Clinical decision support:* An EMR system can provide access to the latest medical research on approved medical websites to help medical decision making.
- *Automated alerts and reminders:* The system can provide medical alerts and reminders for office staff to ensure that patients are scheduled for regular screenings and other preventive practices. Alerts can also be created to identify patient safety issues, such as possible drug interactions.
- *Electronic communication and connectivity:* An EMR system can provide a means of secure and easily accessible communication between physicians and staff and in some offices between physicians and patients.
- *Patient support:* Some EMR programs allow patients to access their medical records and request appointments. These programs also offer patient education on health topics and instructions on preparing for common medical tests, such as an HDL cholesterol test.
- *Administration and reporting:* The EMR may include administrative tools, including reporting systems that enable medical practices to comply with federal and state reporting requirements.
- *Error reduction:* An EMR can decrease medical errors that result from illegible chart notes, since notes are entered electronically on a computer or a handheld device. Nevertheless, the accuracy of the information in the EMR is only as good as the accuracy of the person entering the data; it is still possible to click the wrong button or enter the wrong letter.

Billing Tip

Documentation and Billing: A Vital Connection for Compliance
The connection between documentation and billing is essential. If a service is not documented, it cannot be billed.

Health Care Regulation

To protect consumers' health, both federal and state governments pass laws that affect the medical services that must be offered to patients. To protect the privacy of patients' health information, additional laws cover the way health care plans and providers exchange this information as they conduct business.

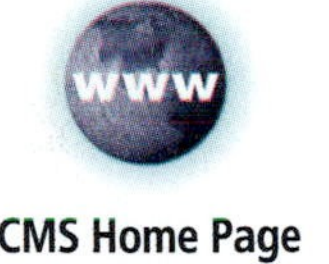

CMS Home Page
http://www.cms.hhs.gov

Federal Regulation

The main federal government agency responsible for health care is the **Centers for Medicare and Medicaid Services**, known as **CMS** (formerly the Health Care Financing Administration, or HCFA). An agency of the Department of Health and Human Services (HHS), CMS administers the Medicare and Medicaid programs to more than 90 million Americans. CMS implements annual federal budget acts and laws such as the Medicare Prescription Drug, Improvement, and Modernization Act that has created help in paying for drugs and for an annual physical examination for Medicare beneficiaries.

CMS also performs activities to ensure the quality of health care, such as:

- Regulating all laboratory testing other than research performed on humans
- Preventing discrimination based on health status for people buying health insurance
- Researching the effectiveness of various methods of health care management, treatment, and financing
- Evaluating the quality of health care facilities and services

CMS policy is often the model for the health care industry. When a change is made in Medicare rules, for example, private payers often adopt a similar rule.

The most important recent legislation is called the **Health Insurance Portability and Accountability Act (HIPAA) of 1996**. This law is designed to:

- Protect peoples' private health information
- Ensure health insurance coverage for workers and their families when they change or lose their jobs
- Uncover fraud and abuse
- Create standards for electronic transmission of health care transactions

> **Billing Tip**
>
> **State-Mandated Benefits**
> States may require benefits that are not mandated in federal regulations. For example, fifteen states mandate coverage of infertility treatments for women.

State Regulation

States are also major regulators of the health care industry. Operating an insurance company without a license is illegal in all states. State commissioners of insurance investigate consumer complaints about the quality and financial aspects of health care. State laws ensure the solvency of insurance companies and managed care organizations, so that they will be able to pay enrollees' claims. States may also restrict price increases on premiums and other charges to patients, require that policies include a guaranteed renewal provision, and control the situations in which an insurer can cancel a patient's coverage.

> **Billing Tip**
>
> **Any Willing Provider**
> Many states have "any willing provider" laws that require a managed care organization to accept all qualified physicians who wish to participate in its plan. This regulation helps reduce the number of patients who have to switch physicians if they change from one plan to another.

HIPAA Rules

Patients' medical records—the actual progress notes, reports, and other clinical materials—are legal documents that belong to the provider who created them. But the provider cannot withhold the information in the records unless providing it would be detrimental to the patient's health. The information belongs to the patient.

Patients control the amount and type of information that is released, except for the use of the data to treat them or to conduct the normal business transactions of the practice. Only patients or their legally appointed representatives have the authority to authorize the release of information to anyone not directly involved in their care.

Medical insurance specialists handle issues such as requests for information from patients' medical records. They need to know what information can be released about patients' conditions and treatments. What information can be legally shared with other providers and health plans? What information must the patient specifically authorize to be released ? The answers to these questions are based on the HIPAA Administrative Simplification provisions.

Congress passed the Administrative Simplification provisions partly because of rising health care costs. A significant portion of every health care dollar is spent on administrative and financial tasks. These costs can be controlled if the business transactions of health care are standardized and handled electronically.

Electronic Data Interchange

The Administrative Simplification provisions encourage the use of **electronic data interchange (EDI)**. EDI is the computer-to-computer exchange of routine business information using publicly available standards. Practice staff members use EDI to exchange health information about their practices' patients with payers and clearinghouses. Each electronic exchange is a **transaction**, which is the electronic equivalent of a business document.

EDI transactions are not visible in the way that an exchange of paperwork, such as a letter, is. An example of a nonmedical transaction is the process of getting cash from an ATM. In an ATM transaction, the computer-to-computer exchange is made up of computer language that is sent and answered between the machines. This exchange happens behind the scenes. It is documented on the customer's end with the transaction receipt that is printed; the bank also has a record at its location.

The Three Administrative Simplification Provisions

There are three parts to HIPAA's Administrative Simplification provisions:

1. *HIPAA Privacy Rule:* The privacy requirements cover patients' health information.
2. *HIPAA Security Rule:* The security requirements state the administrative, technical, and physical safeguards that are required to protect patients' health information.
3. *HIPAA Electronic Transaction and Code Sets Standards:* These standards require every provider who does business electronically to use the same health care transactions, code sets, and identifiers.

> **HIPAA Tip**
>
> **Staying Current with HIPAA**
>
> *HIPAA laws have a lengthy review process before being released as final rules. Future changes are expected. Medical insurance specialists need to stay current with those that affect their areas of responsibility.*

Complying with HIPAA

Health care organizations that are required by law to obey the HIPAA regulations are called **covered entities**. A covered entity is an organization that electronically transmits any information that is protected under HIPAA. Other organizations that work for the covered entities must also agree to follow the HIPAA rules.

CMS HIPAA Home Page

http://www.cms.hhs.gov/hipaa/hipaa2/

Covered Entities

Under HIPAA, three types of covered entities must follow the regulations:

- *Health plans*: The individual or group plan that provides or pays for medical care
- *Health care* ***clearinghouses***: Companies that help providers handle such electronic transactions as submitting claims and that manage electronic medical record systems
- *Health care providers*: People or organizations that furnish, bill, or are paid for health care in the normal course of business

Many physician practices are included under HIPAA. Excepted providers are only those that do not send any claims (or other HIPAA transactions) electronically *and* do not employ any other firm to send electronic claims for them. Since CMS requires practices to send Medicare claims electronically unless they employ fewer than ten full-time or equivalent employees,, many practices have moved to electronic claims. Electronic claims have the advantage of being paid more quickly, too, so practices may use them even when they are not required.

Business Associates

HIPAA also affects many others in the health care field. For instance, outside medical billers are not covered entities; they are not themselves required to comply with the law. However, they must follow HIPAA's rules in order to do business with covered entities. In HIPAA terms, they are **business associates**, a category that includes law firms, accountants, information technology (IT) contractors, transcription companies, compliance consultants, and collection agencies. Through agreements with their business associates, covered entities make sure that they will perform their work as required by HIPAA.

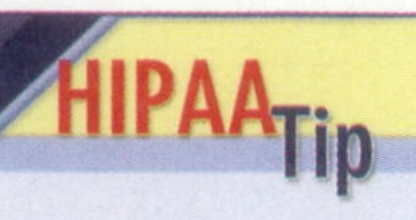

45 CFR Parts 160 and 164

The HIPAA Privacy Rule is also often referred to by its number in the Federal Register, which is 45 CFR Parts 160 and 164.

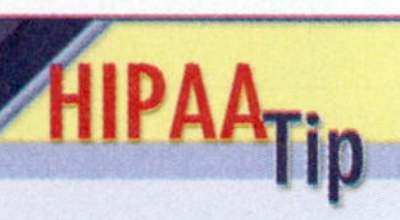

Privacy Officers

The privacy official at a small physician practice may be the office manager who also has other duties. At a large health plan, the position of privacy official may be full time.

HIPAA Privacy Rule

The HIPAA Standards for Privacy of Individually Identifiable Health Information rule is known as the **HIPAA Privacy Rule**. It was the first comprehensive federal protection for the privacy of health information. Its national standards protect individuals' medical records and other personal health information. Before the HIPAA Privacy Rule became law, the personal information stored in hospitals, physicians' practices, and health plans was governed by a patchwork of federal and state laws. Some state laws were strict, but others were not.

The privacy rule says that covered entities must:

- Have a set of privacy practices that are appropriate for its health care services
- Notify patients about their privacy rights and how their information can be used or disclosed
- Train employees so that they understand the privacy practices
- Appoint a privacy official responsible for seeing that the privacy practices are adopted and followed
- Safeguard patients' records

Protected Health Information

The HIPAA privacy rule covers the use and disclosure of patients' **protected health information (PHI)**. PHI is defined as individually identifiable health information that is transmitted or maintained by electronic media, such as over the Internet, by computer modem, or on magnetic tape or compact disks. This information includes a person's:

- Name
- Address (including street address, city, county, ZIP code)
- Names of relatives and employers
- Birth date
- Telephone numbers
- Fax number
- E-mail address
- Social Security number
- Medical record number
- Health plan beneficiary number
- Account number
- Certificate or license number
- Serial number of any vehicle or other device
- Website address
- Fingerprints or voiceprints
- Photographic images

Disclosure for Treatment, Payment, and Health Care Operations

Patients' PHI under HIPAA can be used and disclosed by providers for treatment, payment, and health care operations. *Use of PHI* means sharing or analysis *within* the entity that holds the information. *Disclosure of PHI* means the release, transfer, provision of access to, or divulging of PHI *outside* the entity holding the information.

Both use and disclosure of PHI are necessary and permitted for patients' **treatment, payment, and health care operations (TPO)**. *Treatment* means providing and coordinating the patient's medical care; *payment* refers to the exchange of information with health plans; and *health care operations* are the general business management functions.

Minimum Necessary Standard When using or disclosing protected health information, a covered entity must try to limit the information to the minimum amount of PHI necessary for the intended purpose. The **minimum necessary standard** means taking reasonable safeguards to protect PHI from incidental disclosure.

Examples of complying with HIPAA

A medical insurance specialist does not disclose a patient's history of cancer on a workers' compensation claim for a sprained ankle. Only the information the recipient needs to know is given.

A physician's assistant faxes appropriate patient cardiology test results before scheduled surgery.

A physician sends an e-mail message to another physician requesting a consultation on a patient's case.

A patient's family member picks up medical supplies and a prescription.

Designated Record Set A covered entity must disclose individuals' PHI to them (or to their personal representatives) when they request access to, or an accounting of disclosures of, their PHI. Patients' rights apply to a **designated record set (DRS)**. For a provider, the designated record set means the medical and billing records the provider maintains. It does not include appointment and surgery schedules, requests for lab tests, and birth and death records. It also does not include mental health information, psychotherapy notes, and genetic information. For a health plan, the designated record set includes enrollment, payment, claim decisions, and medical management systems of the plan.

Within the designated record set, patients have the right to:

- Access, copy, and inspect their PHI
- Request amendments to their health information
- Obtain accounting of most disclosures of their health information
- Receive communications from providers via other means, such as in Braille or in foreign languages
- Complain about alleged violations of the regulations and the provider's own information policies

Notice of Privacy Practices Covered entities must give each patient a notice of privacy practice at the first contact or encounter. To meet this requirement, physician practices give patients their **Notice of Privacy Practices (NPP)** (see Figure 2.7 on pages 50 and 51) and ask them to sign an acknowledgment that they have received it (see Chapter 3). The notice explains how patients' PHI may be used and describes their rights.

Practices may choose to use a layered approach to giving patients the notice. On top of the information packet is a short notice, like the one shown in Figure 2.7, that briefly describes the uses and disclosures of PHI and the person's rights. The longer notice is placed beneath it.

HIPAA Tip

HIPAA Exemptions

Certain benefits are always exempt from HIPAA, including coverage only for accident, disability income coverage, liability insurance, workers' compensation, automobile medical payment and liability insurance, credit-only insurance (such as mortgage insurance), and coverage for on-site medical clinics.

HIPAA Tip

PHI and Release of Information Document

A patient release of information document is not needed when PHI is shared for TPO under HIPAA. However, state law may require authorization to release data, so many practices continue to ask patients to sign releases.

HIPAA Tip

Health Care Providers and the Minimum Necessary Standard

The minimum necessary standard does not apply to any type of disclosure—oral, written, phone, fax, e-mail, or other—among health care providers for treatment purposes.

HIPAA Tip

Patient Complaints

Patients who observe privacy problems in their providers' offices can complain either to the practice or to the Office for Civil Rights of the Department of Health and Human Services (HHS). Complaints must be put in writing, either on paper or electronically, and sent to OCR within 180 days.

Valley Associates, P.C.

NOTICE OF PRIVACY PRACTICES

THIS NOTICE DESCRIBES HOW MEDICAL INFORMATION ABOUT YOU MAY BE USED AND DISCLOSED AND HOW YOU CAN GET ACCESS TO THIS INFORMATION. PLEASE REVIEW IT CAREFULLY.

WHY ARE YOU GETTING THIS NOTICE?

Valley Associates, P.C. is required by federal and state law to maintain the privacy of your health information. The use and disclosure of your health information is governed by regulations under the Health Insurance Portability and Accountability Act of 1996 (HIPAA) and the requirements of applicable state law. For health information covered by HIPAA, we are required to provide you with this Notice and will abide by this Notice with respect to such health information. If you have questions about this Notice, please contact our Privacy Officer at 877-555-1313. We will ask you to sign an "acknowledgment" indicating that you have been provided with this notice.

WHAT HEALTH INFORMATION IS PROTECTED?

We are committed to protecting the privacy of information we gather about you while providing health-related services. Some examples of protected health information are:

- Information indicating that you are a patient receiving treatment or other health-related services from our physicians or staff;
- Information about your health condition (such as a disease you may have);
- Information about health care products or services you have received or may receive in the future (such as an operation); or
- Information about your health care benefits under an insurance plan (such as whether a prescription is covered);

when combined with:

- Demographic information (such as your name, address, or insurance status);
- Unique numbers that may identify you (such as your Social Security number, your phone number, or your driver's license number); and
- Other types of information that may identify who you are.

SUMMARY OF THIS NOTICE

This summary includes references to paragraphs throughout this notice that you may read for additional information.

1. Written Authorization Requirement

We may use your health information or share it with others in order to treat your condition, obtain payment for that treatment, and run our business operations. We generally need your written authorization for other uses and disclosures of your health information, unless an exception described in this Notice applies.

2. Authorizing Transfer of Your Records

You may request that we transfer your records to another person or organization by completing a written authorization form. This form will specify what information is being released, to whom, and for what purpose. The authorization will have an expiration date.

3. Canceling Your Written Authorization

If you provide us with written authorization, you may revoke, or cancel, it at any time, except to the extent that we have already relied upon it. To revoke a written authorization, please write to the doctor's office where you initially gave your authorization.

4. Exceptions to Written Authorization Requirement

There are some situations in which we do not need your written authorization before using your health information or sharing it with others. They include:

Treatment, Payment and Operations
As mentioned above, we may use your health information or share it with others in order to treat your condition, obtain payment for that treatment, and run our business operations.

Family and Friends
If you do not object, we will share information about your health with family and friends involved in your care.

FIGURE 2.7 Example of a Notice of Privacy Practices

Research
Although we will generally try to obtain your written authorization before using your health information for research purposes, there may be certain situations in which we are not required to obtain your written authorization.

De-Identified Information
We may use or disclose your health information if we have removed any information that might identify you. When all identifying information is removed, we say that the health information is "completely de-identified." We may also use and disclose "partially de-identified" information if the person who will receive it agrees in writing to protect your privacy when using the information.

Incidental Disclosures
We may inadvertently use or disclose your health information despite having taken all reasonable precautions to protect the privacy and confidentiality of your health information.

Emergencies or Public Need
We may use or disclose your health information in an emergency or for important public health needs. For example, we may share your information with public health officials at the State or city health departments who are authorized to investigate and control the spread of diseases.

5. How to Access Your Health Information

You generally have the right to inspect and get copies of your health information.

6. How to Correct Your Health Information

You have the right to request that we amend your health information if you believe it is inaccurate or incomplete.

7. How to Identify Others Who Have Received Your Health Information

You have the right to receive an "accounting of disclosures." This is a report that identifies certain persons or organizations to which we have disclosed your health information. All disclosures are made according to the protections described in this Notice of Privacy Practices. Many routine disclosures we make (for treatment, payment, or business operations, among others) will not be included in this report. However, it will identify any non-routine disclosures of your information.

8. How to Request Additional Privacy Protections

You have the right to request further restrictions on the way we use your health information or share it with others. However, we are not required to agree to the restriction you request. If we do agree with your request, we will be bound by our agreement.

9. How to Request Alternative Communications

You have the right to request that we contact you in a way that is more confidential for you, such as at home instead of at work. We will try to accommodate all reasonable requests.

10. How Someone May Act On Your Behalf

You have the right to name a personal representative who may act on your behalf to control the privacy of your health information. Parents and guardians will generally have the right to control the privacy of health information about minors unless the minors are permitted by law to act on their own behalf.

11. How to Learn about Special Protections for HIV, Alcohol and Substance Abuse, Mental Health and Genetic Information

Special privacy protections apply to HIV-related information, alcohol and substance abuse treatment information, mental health information, psychotherapy notes and genetic information.

12. How to Obtain A Copy of This Notice

If you have not already received one, you have the right to a paper copy of this notice. You may request a paper copy at any time, even if you have previously agreed to receive this notice electronically. You can request a copy of the privacy notice directly from your doctor's office. You may also obtain a copy of this notice from our website or by requesting a copy at your next visit.

13. How to Obtain A Copy of Revised Notice

We may change our privacy practices from time to time. If we do, we will revise this notice so you will have an accurate summary of our practices. You will be able to obtain your own copy of the revised notice by accessing our website or by calling your doctor's office. You may also ask for one at the time of your next visit. The effective date of the notice is noted in the top right corner of each page. We are required to abide by the terms of the notice that is currently in effect.

14. How To File A Complaint

If you believe your privacy rights have been violated, you may file a complaint with us or with the federal Office of Civil Rights. To file a complaint with us, please contact our Privacy Officer.

No one will retaliate or take action against you for filing a complaint.

HIPAA Tip

PHI and Medical Office Staff

Be careful not to discuss patients' cases with anyone outside the office, including family and friends. Avoid talking about cases, too, in the practice's reception areas where other patients might hear. Close charts on desks when they are not being worked on. Position computer screens so that only the person working with a file can view it.

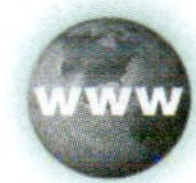

Questions and Answers on HIPAA Privacy Policies

http://answers.hhs.gov

HIPAA Tip

Charging for Copying

Practices may charge patients a fee for supplying copies of their records, but cannot hold records "hostage" while awaiting payment.

PHI and Accounting for Disclosures Patients have the right to an accounting of disclosures of their PHI other than for TPO (see Figure 2.8). When a patient's PHI is accidentally disclosed, the disclosure should be documented in the individual's medical record, since the individual did not authorize it and it was not a permitted disclosure. An example is faxing a discharge summary to the wrong physician's office.

Authorizations

For use or disclosure other than for TPO, the covered entity must have the patient sign an **authorization** to release the information. Information about substance (alcohol and drug) abuse, sexually transmitted diseases (STDs) or human immunodeficiency virus (HIV), and behavioral/mental health services

PATIENT REQUEST FOR ACCOUNTING OF DISCLOSURES

Patient Name

Patient Address

Medical Record # Date of Birth

Name & Address of Requestor if not patient

"Please consider this a request for an accounting of all disclosures for the time frames indicated below (Maximum time frame that can be requested is six years prior to the date of the request, but not before April 14, 2003). I understand that there is a fee for this accounting and wish to proceed. I understand that the accounting will be provided to me within sixty days unless I am notified in writing that an extension of up to thirty days is necessary."

Patient or Requestor to Complete:			Practice to Complete:		
From Date(s):	To Date(s):	Purpose of Disclosure:	Date Request In	Date Information to Patient	Fee
Date:	Signature of Patient or Legal Representative:				
Date:	Signature of Patient or Legal Representative:				

FIGURE 2.8 Example of a Patient Request for Accounting of Disclosures Form

may not be released without a specific authorization from the patient. The authorization document must be in plain language and include the following:

- A description of the information to be used or disclosed
- The name or other specific identification of the person(s) authorized to use or disclose the information
- The name of the person(s) or group of people to whom the covered entity may make the use or disclosure
- A description of each purpose of the requested use or disclosure
- An expiration date
- The signature of the individual (or authorized representative) and the date

In addition, the rule states that a valid authorization must include:

- A statement of the individual's right to revoke the authorization in writing
- A statement about whether the covered entity is able to base treatment, payment, enrollment, or eligibility for benefits on the authorization
- A statement that information used or disclosed after the authorization may be disclosed again by the recipient and may no longer be protected by the rule

A sample authorization form is shown in Figure 2.9 on page 54.

Uses or disclosures for which the covered entity has received specific authorization from the patient do not have to follow the minimum necessary standard. Incidental use and disclosure are also allowed. For example, the practice may use reception-area sign-in sheets.

HIPAA Tip

PHI and Authorization to Release

To legally release PHI for purposes other than treatment, payment, or health care operations, a signed authorization document is required.

Requests for Information Other Than for TPO

There are a number of exceptions to the usual rules for release:

- Court orders
- Workers' compensation cases
- Statutory reports
- Research

All these types of disclosures must be logged, and the release information must be available to the patient who requests it.

Release Under Court Order If the patient's PHI is required as evidence by a court of law, the provider may release it without the patient's approval if a judicial order is received. In the case of a lawsuit, a court sometimes decides that a physician or medical practice staff member must provide testimony. The court issues a **subpoena**, an order of the court directing a party to appear and testify. If the court requires the witness to bring certain evidence, such as a patient medical record, it issues a **subpoena *duces tecum*,** which directs the party to appear, to testify, and to bring specified documents or items.

Workers' Compensation Cases State law may provide for release of records to employers in workers' compensation cases (see Chapter 13). The law may also authorize release to the state workers' compensation administration board and to the insurance company that handles these claims for the state.

Statutory Reports Some specific types of information are required by state law to be released to state health or social services departments. For example, physicians must make statutory reports for patients' births and deaths and for cases of abuse. Because of the danger of harm to patients or others, communicable diseases such as tuberculosis, hepatitis, and rabies must usually be reported.

A special category of communicable disease control is applied to patients with diagnoses of human immunodeficiency virus (HIV) infection and acquired

HIPAA Tip

PHI and Practice Policy

The release of protected health information must follow the practice's policies and procedures. The practice's privacy official trains medical insurance specialists on how to verify the identity and authority of a person requesting PHI.

What specific information can be released

To whom

For what purpose

Patient Name: ____________________

Health Record Number: ____________________

Date of Birth: ____________________

1. I authorize the use or disclosure of the above named individual's health information as described below.

2. The following individual(s) or organization(s) are authorized to make the disclosure: ____________________

3. The type of information to be used or disclosed is as follows (check the appropriate boxes and include other information where indicated)

- ❑ problem list
- ❑ medication list
- ❑ list of allergies
- ❑ immunization records
- ❑ most recent history
- ❑ most recent discharge summary
- ❑ lab results (please describe the dates or types of lab tests you would like disclosed): ____________________
- ❑ x-ray and imaging reports (please describe the dates or types of x-rays or images you would like disclosed): ____________________
- ❑ consultation reports from (please supply doctors' names): ____________________
- ❑ entire record
- ❑ other (please describe): ____________________

4. I understand that the information in my health record may include information relating to sexually transmitted disease, acquired immunodeficiency syndrome (AIDS), or human immunodeficiency virus (HIV). It may also include information about behavioral or mental health services, and treatment for alcohol and drug abuse.

5. The information identified above may be used by or disclosed to the following individuals or organization(s):

Name: ____________________

Address: ____________________

Name: ____________________

Address: ____________________

6. This information for which I'm authorizing disclosure will be used for the following purpose:

- ❑ my personal records
- ❑ sharing with other health care providers as needed/other (please describe): ____________________

7. I understand that I have a right to revoke this authorization at any time. I understand that if I revoke this authorization, I must do so in writing and present my written revocation to the health information management department. I understand that the revocation will not apply to information that has already been released in response to this authorization. I understand that the revocation will not apply to my insurance company when the law provides my insurer with the right to contest a claim under my policy.

8. This authorization will expire (insert date or event): ____________________

If I fail to specify an expiration date or event, this authorization will expire six months from the date on which it was signed.

9. I understand that once the above information is disclosed, it may be redisclosed by the recipient and the information may not be protected by federal privacy laws or regulations.

10. I understand authorizing the use or disclosure of the information identified above is voluntary. I need not sign this form to ensure health care treatment.

Signature of patient or legal representative: ____________________ Date: ____________

If signed by legal representative, relationship to patient

Signature of witness: ____________________ Date: ____________

Distribution of copies: Original to provider; copy to patient; copy to accompany use or disclosure

Note: This sample form was developed by the American Health Information Management Association for discussion purposes. It should not be used without review by the issuing organization's legal counsel to ensure compliance with other federal and state laws and regulations.

FIGURE 2.9 Example of an Authorization to Use or Disclose Health Information

immunodeficiency syndrome (AIDS). Every state requires AIDS cases to be reported. Most states also require reporting of the HIV infection that causes the syndrome. However, state law varies concerning whether just the fact of a case is to be reported or if the patient's name must also be reported. The practice guidelines reflect the state laws and must be strictly observed, as all these regulations should be, to protect patients' privacy and to comply with the regulations.

Research Data PHI may be made available to researchers approved by the practice. For example, if a physician is conducting clinical research on a type of diabetes, the practice may share information from appropriate records for analysis. When the researcher issues reports or studies based on the information, specific patients' names may not be identified.

De-Identified Health Information

There are no restrictions on the use or disclosure of **de-identified health information** that neither identifies nor provides a reasonable basis to identify an individual. For example, these identifiers must be removed: names, medical record numbers, health plan beneficiary numbers, device identifiers (such as pacemakers), and biometric identifiers, such as fingerprints and voiceprints.

Psychotherapy Notes

Psychotherapy notes have special protection under HIPAA. According to the American Health Information Management Association Practice Brief on Legal Process and Electronic Health Records,

Under the HIPAA Privacy Rule, psychotherapy notes are those recorded (in any medium) by a healthcare provider who is a mental health professional documenting or analyzing the content of conversation during a private counseling session or a group, joint, or family counseling session and that are separated from the rest of the individual's medical record. Notes exclude medication prescription and monitoring, counseling session start or stop times, the modalities and frequencies of treatment furnished, results of clinical tests, and any summary of diagnosis, functional status, the treatment plan, symptoms, prognosis, and progress to date. The privacy rule gives such notes extra protection as may state law. (Available online at http://www.ahima.org under Resources)

State Statutes

Some state statues are more stringent than HIPAA specifications. Areas in which state statutes may differ from HIPAA include the following:

- Designated record set
- Psychotherapy notes

Thinking It Through — 2.2

Based on the information in Figure 2.7:

1. What document is required when a patient asks Valley Associates to transfer a record to another person or organization?
2. Is written authorization from a patient needed to use or disclose health information in an emergency?
3. What is the purpose of an "accounting of disclosures"?

HIPAA Tip

PHI and Answering Machines

If possible, ask patients whether staff members may leave messages on answering machines or with friends or family during their initial visits. If this is not done, messages should follow the minimum necessary standard; the staff member should leave a phone number and a request for the patient to call back. For example: "This is the doctor's office with a message for Mr. Warner. Please call us at 203-123-4567."

HIPAA Tip

PHI and Reports

The Association for Integrity of Healthcare Documentation (formerly the American Association for Medical Transcription) advises against using a patient's name in the body of a medical report. Instead, place identification information only in the demographic section, where it can be easily deleted when the report data are needed for research.

Billing Tip

Internet Security Symbol On the Internet, when an item is secure, a small padlock appears in the status bar at the bottom of the browser window.

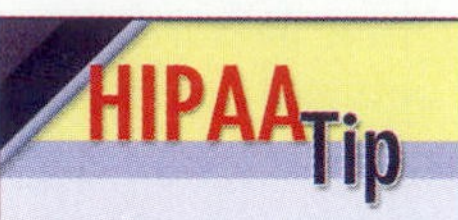

Selecting Good Passwords

- *Always use a combination of at least six letters and numbers that are not real words and also are not obvious (such as a number string like 123456 or a birth date).*
- *Do not use a user ID (logon, sign-on) as a password. Even if an ID has both numbers and letters, it is not secret.*
- *Select a mixture of uppercase and lowercase letters if the system permits, and include special characters, such as @, $, or &, if possible.*
- *Change passwords periodically, but not too often. Forcing frequent changes can actually make security worse because users are more likely to write down passwords.*

- Rights of inmates
- Information complied for civil, criminal, or administrative court cases

Each practice's privacy official reviews state laws and develops policies and procedures for compliance with the HIPAA Privacy Rule. The tougher rules are implemented.

HIPAA Security Rule

The **HIPAA Security Rule** requires covered entities to establish safeguards to protect PHI. The security rule specifies how to secure such protected health information on computer networks, the Internet, and storage disks such as floppy disks or CDs.

Encryption Is Required

Information security is needed when computers exchange data over the Internet. Security measures rely on **encryption**, the process of encoding information in such a way that only the person (or computer) with the key can decode it. Practice management programs (PMPs) encrypt data traveling between the office and the Internet, such as patients' Social Security numbers, so that the information is secure.

Security Measures

A number of other security measures help enforce the HIPAA Security Rule. These include:

- Access control, passwords, and log files to keep intruders out
- Backups to replace items after damage
- Security policies to handle violations that do occur

Access Control, Passwords, and Log Files

Most practices use role-based access, meaning that only people who need information can see it. Once access rights have been assigned, each user is given a key to the designated databases. Users must enter a user ID and a **password** (the key) to see files to which they have been granted access rights.

For example, receptionists may view the names of patients coming to the office on one day, but they should not see those patients' medical records. However, the nurse or physician needs to view the patient records. Receptionists are given individual computer passwords that let them view the day's schedule but that denies entry to patient records. The physicians and nurses possess computer passwords that allow them to see all patient records.

The PMP also creates activity logs of who has accessed—or tried to access—information, and passwords prevent unauthorized users from gaining access to information on a computer or network.

Figure 2.10 shows how a practice management program is used to set up security. Each person who will be using the program is given a login name and has a password. The person has also been assigned an access level based on the information he or she needs to use, as shown in the Security Setup screen. The Security Warning screen illustrates the PMP's access denial message.

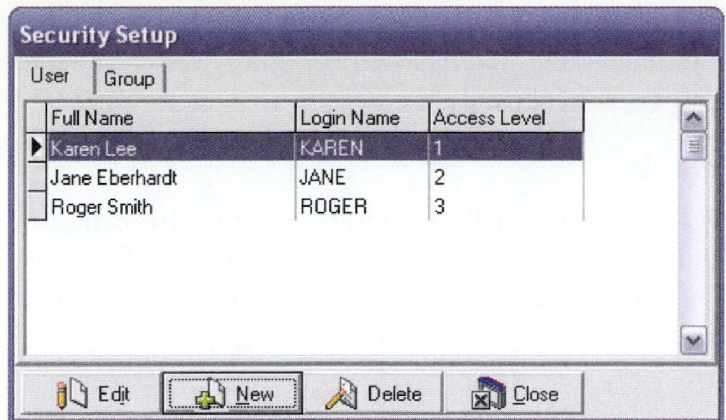

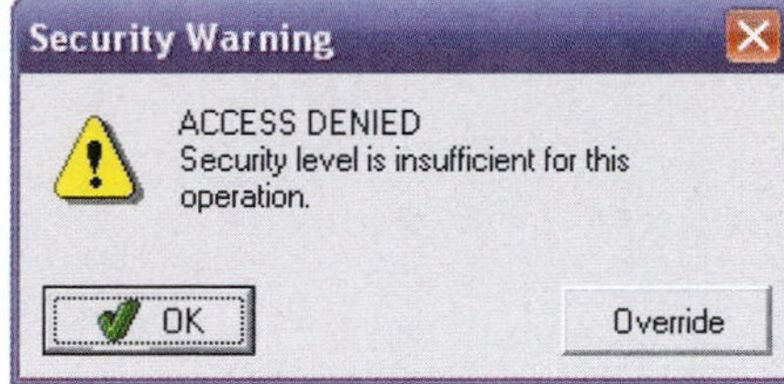

FIGURE 2.10 Medisoft Security Setup and Security Warnings Screens

Thinking It Through — 2.3

1. Imagine that you are employed as a medical insurance specialist for Family Medical Center. Make up a password that you will use to keep your files secure.
2. As an employee, how would you respond to another staff member who asked to see your latest claim files in order to see how you handled a particular situation?

Backups

Backing up is the activity of copying files to another medium so that they will be preserved in case the originals are no longer available. A successful backup plan is critical in recovering from either a minor or major security incident that jeopardizes critical data.

Security Policy

Practices have security policies which inform employees about their responsibilities for protecting electronically stored information. Many practices include this information in handbooks distributed to all employees. These handbooks contain general information about the organizations, their structures, and their policies as well as specific information about employee responsibilities.

HIPAA Electronic Health Care Transactions and Code Sets

The **HIPAA Electronic Health Care Transactions and Code Sets** (TCS) standards make it possible for physicians and health plans to exchange electronic data using a standard format and standard code sets.

Standard Transactions

The HIPAA transactions standards apply to the electronic data that are regularly sent back and forth between providers, health plans, and employers. Each standard is labeled with both a number and a name. Either the number (such as "the 837") or the name (such as the "HIPAA Claim") may be used to refer to the particular electronic document format.

Number	*Official Name*
X12 837	Health Care Claims or Equivalent Encounter Information/Coordination of Benefits—coordination of benefits refers to an exchange of information between payers when a patient has more than one health plan
X12 276/277	Health Care Claim Status Inquiry/Response
X12 270/271	Eligibility for a Health Plan Inquiry/Response
X12 278	Referral Authorization Inquiry/Response
X12 835	Health Care Payment and Remittance Advice
X12 820	Health Plan Premium Payments
X12 834	Health Plan Enrollment and Disenrollment

Medical insurance specialists use the first five transactions in performing their jobs. Each of these is covered in later text chapters.

Standard Code Sets

Under HIPAA, a **code set** is any group of codes used for encoding data elements, such as tables of terms, medical concepts, medical diagnosis codes, or medical procedure codes. Medical code sets used in the health care industry include coding systems for diseases; treatments and procedures; and supplies or other items used to perform these actions. These standards, listed in Table 2.2, are covered in Chapters 4, 5, 6, and 16.

HIPAA National Identifiers

HIPAA National Identifiers are for:

- Employers
- Health care providers
- Health plans
- Patients

Identifiers are numbers of predetermined length and structure, such as a person's Social Security number. They are important because the unique numbers can be used in electronic transactions. These unique numbers can replace the

TABLE 2.2 HIPAA Standard Code Sets

Purpose	Standard
Codes for diseases, injuries, impairments, and other health-related problems	*International Classification of Diseases*, Ninth Revision, *Clinical Modification* (ICD-9-CM), Volumes 1 and 2
Codes for procedures or other actions taken to prevent, diagnose, treat, or manage diseases, injuries, and impairments	Physicians' Services: *Current Procedural Terminology* (CPT) Inpatient Hospital Services: *International Classification of Diseases*, Ninth Revision, *Clinical Modification*, Volume 3: *Procedures*
Codes for dental services	*Current Dental Terminology* (CDT-4)
Codes for other medical services	Healthcare Common Procedures Coding System (HCPCS)

many numbers that are currently used. Two identifiers have been set up, and two are to be established in the future.

Employer Identification Number (EIN)

The employer identifier is used when employers enroll or disenroll employees in a health plan (X12 834) or make premium payments to plans on behalf of their employees (X12 820). The Employer Identification Number (EIN) issued by the Internal Revenue Service is the HIPAA standard.

National Provider Identifier (NPI)

The **National Provider Identifier (NPI)** is the standard for the identification of providers when filing claims and other transactions. The NPI will replace other identifying numbers that have been in use, such as the UPIN for Medicare and the numbers that have been assigned by each payer to the provider.

The NPI has nine numbers and a check digit, for a total of ten numbers. The numbers are assigned by the federal government to individual providers, such as physicians and nurses, and also to provider organizations such as hospitals, pharmacies, and clinics. Once assigned, the NPI will not change; it remains with the provider regardless of job or location changes.

All health care providers who transmit health information electronically must obtain NPIs, even if they use business associates to prepare the transactions. Most health plans, including Medicare, Medicaid, and private payers, and all clearinghouses must accept and use NPIs in HIPAA transactions by May 23, 2007. Small health plans have until May 23, 2008.

Billing Tip

Physician and Group NPIs
If a physician is in a group practice, both the individual doctor and the group have NPIs.

Fraud and Abuse Regulations

Almost everyone involved in the delivery of health care is trustworthy and is devoted to patients' welfare. However, some people are not. Health care fraud and abuse laws help control cheating in the health care system. Is this really necessary? The evidence says that it is. From 1998 to 2003, the federal government recovered an estimated $5.3 billion in fraud-related judgments and settlements. The National Health Care Anti-Fraud Association has estimated that of the $1.7 trillion spent on health care in 2003, from 3 to 5 percent was lost to fraud.

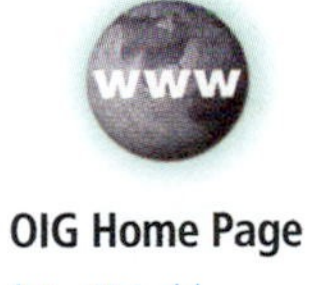

OIG Home Page
http://oig.hhs.gov

Thinking It Through — 2.4

Gloria Traylor, an employee of National Bank, called Marilyn Rennagel, a medical insurance specialist who works for Dr. Judy Fisk. The bank is considering hiring one of Dr. Fisk's patients, Juan Ramirez, and Ms. Traylor would like to know if he has any known medical problems. Marilyn, in a hurry to complete the call and get back to work on this week's claims, quickly explains that she remembers that Mr. Ramirez was treated for depression some years ago, but that he has been fine since that time. She adds that she thinks he would make an excellent employee.

In your opinion, did Marilyn handle this call correctly?

What problems might result from her answers?

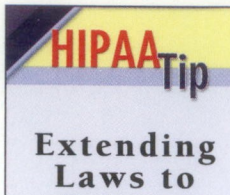

Extending Laws to Private Payers

HIPAA extended existing laws governing fraud in the Medicare and Medicaid programs to all health plans.

The Health Care Fraud and Abuse Control Program

HIPAA created the **Health Care Fraud and Abuse Control Program** to uncover and prosecute fraud and abuse. The HHS **Office of the Inspector General (OIG)** has the task of detecting health care fraud and abuse and enforcing all laws relating to them. The OIG works with the U.S. Department of Justice (DOJ), which includes the Federal Bureau of Investigation (FBI), under the direction of the U.S. Attorney General to prosecute those suspected of medical fraud and abuse. In 2005, the OIG reported nearly 4,000 fraud and abuse exclusions, 537 criminal actions against individuals or facilities, and 262 civil actions. Two large settlements were a $325 million-plus fraud settlement with HealthSouth Corporation related to Medicare fraud and a $532 million refund from the State of New York related to Medicaid audits.

Federal False Claims Act (31 USC § 3729)

The federal False Claims Act (FCA), a related law, prohibits submitting a fraudulent claim or making a false statement or representation in connection with a claim. It also encourages reporting suspected fraud and abuse against the government by protecting and rewarding people involved in ***qui tam***, or whistleblower, cases. The person who makes the accusation of suspected fraud is called the **relator**. Under the law, the relator is protected against employer retaliation. If the lawsuit results in a fine paid to the federal government, the whistle-blower may be entitled to 15 to 25 percent of the amount paid. People who blow the whistle are current or former employees of insurance companies or medical practices, program beneficiaries, and independent contractors.

Additional Laws

Additional laws relating to health care fraud and abuse control include:

- An antikickback statute that makes it illegal to knowingly offer incentives to induce referrals for services that are paid by government health care programs. Many financial actions are considered to be incentives, including illegal direct payments to other physicians and routine waivers of coinsurance and deductibles.
- Self-referral prohibitions (called Stark rules) that make it illegal for physicians (or members of their immediate families) to have financial relationships with clinics to which they refer their patients, such as radiology service clinics and clinical laboratory services. (Note, however, that there are many legal exceptions to this prohibition under various business structures.)
- The Sarbanes-Oxley Act of 2002 that requires publicly traded corporations to attest that their financial management is sound. These provisions apply to for-profit health care companies. The act includes whistle-blower protection so that employees can report wrongdoing without fear of retaliation.

■ Case

OIG Enforcement Actions for Fraud, Kickbacks and Theft

Those were crimes at the center of three enforcement actions recently announced by the OIG. The enforcement actions are as follows:

- In South Carolina, a physical therapist was sentenced to nineteen months and was fined $400,000 for health care fraud. The therapist billed Medicare as a private insurer for three to five hours of therapy, but performed only one hour.

- In Florida, a durable medical equipment company owner was sentenced to prison for antikickback violations after he received kickbacks from the owner of a pharmacy in exchange for referring patients in need of aerosol medications. The company owner was sentenced to five months in prison and five months of home detention. He was also fined $15,000.
- In Maryland, a former National Institutes of Health purchasing agent was fined $2,400 after she pled guilty to theft of government property. The woman used her government credit card to secure rental cars for personal use. ■

Definition of Fraud and Abuse

Fraud is an act of deception used to take advantage of another person. For example, misrepresenting professional credentials and forging another person's signature on a check are fraudulent. Pretending to be a physician and treating patients without a valid medical license is also fraudulent. Fraudulent acts are intentional; the individual expects an illegal or unauthorized benefit to result.

Claims fraud occurs when health care providers or others falsely report charges to payers. A provider may bill for services that were not performed, overcharge for services, or fail to provide complete services under a contract. A patient may exaggerate an injury to get a settlement from an insurance company or may ask a medical insurance specialist to change a date on a chart so that a service is covered by a health plan.

In federal law, **abuse** means an action that misuses money that the government has allocated, such as Medicare funds. Abuse is illegal because taxpayers' dollars are misspent. An example of abuse is an ambulance service that billed Medicare for transporting a patient to the hospital when the patient did not need ambulance service. This abuse—billing for services that were not medically necessary—resulted in improper payment for the ambulance company. Abuse is not necessarily intentional. It may be the result of ignorance of a billing rule or of inaccurate coding.

Billing Tip

Fraud versus Abuse
To bill when the task was not done is fraud; to bill when it was not necessary is abuse. Remember the rule: If a service was not documented, in the view of the payer it was not done and cannot be billed. To bill for undocumented services is fraudulent.

■ Case

A billing manager for a plastic surgeons' group pleaded guilty to falsifying medical records to obtain insurance coverage for patients. She admitted that she falsified CT scan reports used to preauthorize insurance coverage for certain sinus-related surgeries. In some cases, when patients' underlying conditions were not serious enough to justify insurance payment for surgery, she falsified the report forms by cutting and pasting from her own personal CT scan report, which reflected a more serious underlying sinus condition. The billing manager faced a jail sentence and a criminal fine. ■

Examples of Fraudulent or Abusive Acts

A number of billing practices are fraudulent or abusive. Investigators reviewing physicians' billing work look for patterns like these:

- Intentionally billing for services that were not performed or documented

  Example A lab bills Medicare for two tests when only one was done.

  Example A physician asks a coder to report a physical examination that was just a telephone conversation.

- Reporting services at a higher level than was carried out

  Example After a visit for a flu shot, the provider bills the encounter as a comprehensive physical examination plus a vaccination.

- Performing and billing for procedures that are not related to the patient's condition and therefore not medically necessary

  Example After reading an article about Lyme disease, a patient is worried about having worked in her garden over the summer, and she requests a Lyme disease diagnostic test. Although no symptoms or signs have been reported, the physician orders and bills for the *Borrelia burgdorferi* (Lyme disease) confirmatory immunoblot test.

■ Case

Steven Bander, MD, a former chief medical officer for Gambro Healthcare U.S.A., was awarded $56 million of a $350.5 million settlement for blowing the whistle on the dialysis center operator's Medicare and Medicaid fraud in 2001, the *Jefferson City* (Missouri) *News Tribune* reported on March 27.

Bander, a St. Louis kidney specialist, filed his own lawsuit in 2001, which prompted the Justice Department to get involved. The result of the federal case against Gambro is the fifth largest health care fraud settlement in history.

According to the lawsuits, Gambro created a false company to inflate its billings by $500 per patient per month, the *News Tribune* reported. At the time, the company treated more than 40,000 patients per year.

According to U.S. Attorney Jim Martin, Bander filed suit after trying to stop the fraud himself. Martin also told the *News Tribune* that although the sum designated for Bander is large, the government wouldn't have known about the fraud without his contributions. "We collected $350 million from Gambro Healthcare specifically because this man initiated the whistle-blower lawsuit that he did," Martin said. ■

Enforcement And Penalties

HIPAA regulations are enforced by the **Office for Civil Rights (OCR)**. When OCR investigates a complaint, the covered entity must cooperate and provide access to its facilities, books, records, and systems, including relevant protected health information. People who do not comply with HIPAA may be fined. Civil penalties for HIPAA violations—are for covered entities, not business associates—can be up to $100 for each offense, with an annual cap of

$25,000 for repeated violations of the same requirement. Criminal penalties, which also apply to the covered entity but not necessarily to staff or business associates, include larger fees and/or prison sentences. Physicians can also lose their contracts with payers and can be excluded from participation as providers in all government health care programs.

WWW

OCR Privacy Fact Sheets
http://www.hhs.gov/ocr/hipaa/

The Office of the Inspector General (OIG) enforces rules relating to fraud and abuse. Most billing-related accusations under the False Claims Act are based on the guideline that providers who *knew or should have known* that a claim for service was false can be held liable. The intent to commit fraud does not have to be proved by the accuser in order for the provider to be found guilty. Actions that might be viewed as errors or occasional slips might also be seen as establishing a pattern of violations, which constitute the knowledge meant by "providers knew or should have known."

Compliance Guideline

Ongoing Compliance Education
As explained in the next section, medical office staff members receive ongoing training and education in current rules, so that they can avoid even the appearance of fraud.

OIG has the authority to investigate suspected fraud cases and to **audit** the records of physicians and payers. In an audit, which is a methodical examination, investigators review selected medical records to see if the documentation matches the billing. The accounting records are often reviewed as well. When problems are found, the investigation proceeds and may result in charges of fraud or abuse against the practice.

Although the OIG says that "under the law, physicians are not subject to civil, administrative, or criminal penalties for innocent errors, or even negligence," decisions about whether there are clear patterns and inadequate internal procedures can be subjective at times, making the line between honest mistakes and fraud very thin. Medical practice staff members must avoid any actions that could be perceived as noncompliant.

Compliance Plans

Because of the risk of fraud and abuse liability, medical practices must be sure that billing rules are followed by all staff members. In addition to responsibility for their own actions, physicians are liable for the professional actions of employees they supervise. This responsibility is a result of the law of ***respondeat superior***, which states that an employer is responsible for an employee's actions. Physicians are held to this doctrine, so they can be charged for the fraudulent behavior of any staff member.

A wise slogan is that "the best defense is a good offense." For this reason, medical practices write and implement **compliance plans** to uncover compliance problems and correct them to avoid risking liability. A compliance plan is a process for finding, correcting, and preventing illegal medical office practices. It is a written document prepared by a compliance officer and committee that sets up the steps needed to (1) audit and monitor compliance with government regulations, especially in the area of coding and billing, (2) have policies and procedures that are consistent, (3) provide for ongoing staff training and communication, and (4) respond to and correct errors.

The goals of the compliance plan are to:

- Prevent fraud and abuse through a formal process to identify, investigate, fix, and prevent repeat violations relating to reimbursement for health care services
- Ensure compliance with applicable federal, state, and local laws, including employment and environmental laws as well as antifraud laws
- Help defend the practice if it is investigated or prosecuted for fraud by substantiating the desire to behave compliantly and thus reduce any fines or criminal prosecution

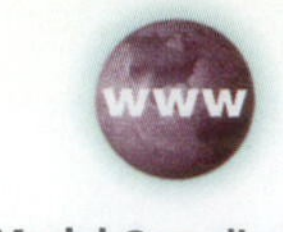

Model Compliance Programs

http://oig.hhs.gov/fraud/compliancequidance.html

Having a compliance plan demonstrates to outside investigators that the practice has made honest, ongoing attempts to find and fix weak areas.

Compliance plans cover more that just coding and billing. They also cover all areas of government regulation of medical practices, such as Equal Employment Opportunity (EEO) regulations (for example, hiring and promotion policies) and Occupational Safety and Health Administration (OSHA) regulations (for example, fire safety and handling of hazardous materials such as blood-borne pathogens).

Parts of a Compliance Plan

Generally, according to the OIG, voluntary plans should contain seven elements:

1. Consistent written policies and procedures
2. Appointment of a compliance officer and committee
3. Training
4. Communication
5. Disciplinary systems
6. Auditing and monitoring
7. Responding to and correcting errors

Following the OIG's guidance can help in the defense against a false claims accusation. Having a plan in place shows that efforts are made to understand the rules and correct errors. This indicates to the OIG that the problems may not add up to a pattern or practice of abuse, but may simply be errors.

Compliance Guideline

Medical Liability Insurance
Medical liability cases for fraud often result in lawsuits. Physicians purchase professional liability insurance to cover such legal expenses. Although they are covered under the physician's policy, other medical professionals often purchase their own liability insurance. Medical coders and medical insurance specialists who perform coding tasks are advised to have professional liability insurance called error and omission (E&O) insurance, which protects against financial loss due to intentional or unintentional failure to perform work correctly.

Compliance Officer and Committee

To establish the plan and follow up on its provisions, most medical practices appoint a compliance officer who is in charge of the ongoing work. The compliance officer may be one of the practice's physicians, the practice manager, or the billing manager. A compliance committee is also usually established to oversee the program.

Code of Conduct

The practice's compliance plan emphasizes the procedures that are to be followed to meet existing documentation, coding, and medical necessity requirements. It also has a code of conduct for the members of the practice, which covers:

- Procedures for ensuring compliance with laws relating to referral arrangements
- Provisions for discussing compliance during employees' performance reviews and for disciplinary action against employees, if needed
- Mechanisms to encourage employees to report compliance concerns directly to the compliance officer so as to reduce the risk of whistle-blower actions

Promoting ethical behavior in the practice's daily operations can also reduce employee dissatisfaction and turnover by showing employees that the practice has a strong commitment to honest, ethical conduct.

Compliance Guideline

Have It in Writing!
Do not code or bill services that are not supported by documentation, even if instructed to so do by a physician. Instead, report this kind of situation to the practice's compliance officer.

Thinking It Through — 2.5

Mary Kelley, a patient of the Good Health Clinic, asked Kathleen Culpepper, the medical insurance specialist, to help her out of a tough financial spot. Her medical insurance authorized her to receive four radiation treatments for her condition, one every thirty-five days. Because she was out of town, she did not schedule her appointment for the last treatment until today, which is one week beyond the approved period. The insurance company will not reimburse Mary for this procedure. She asks Kathleen to change the date on the record to last Wednesday so that it will be covered, explaining that no one will be hurt by this change and, anyway, she pays the insurance company plenty.

What type of action is Mary asking Kathleen to do?

How should Kathleen handle Mary's request ?

Ongoing Training

Physician Training

Part of the compliance plan is a commitment to keep physicians trained in pertinent coding and regulatory matters. Often the medical insurance specialist or medical coder is assigned the task of briefing physicians on changed codes or medical necessity regulations. The following guidelines are helpful in conducting physician training classes:

- Keep the presentation as brief and straightforward as possible.
- In a multispecialty practice, issues should be discussed by specialty; all physicians do not need to know changed rules on dermatology, for example.
- Use actual examples, and stick to the facts when presenting material.
- Explain the benefits of coding compliance to the physicians, and listen to their feedback to improve job performance.
- Set up a way to address additional changes during the year, such as an office newsletter or compliance meetings.

Staff Training

An important part of the compliance plan is a commitment to train medical office staff members who are involved with coding and billing. Ongoing training also requires having the current annual updates, reading health plans' bulletins and periodicals, and researching changed regulations. Compliance officers often conduct refresher classes in proper coding and billing techniques.

Review

Steps to Success

- ❐ Read this chapter and review the Key Terms and the Chapter Summary.
- ❐ Answer the Review Questions and Applying Your Knowledge in the Chapter Review.
- ❐ Access the chapter's websites and complete the Internet Activities to learn more about available professional resources.
- ❐ Complete the related chapter in the *Medical Insurance Workbook* to reinforce your understanding of HIPAA and medical records.

Chapter Summary

1. Patients' medical records, which contain the complete, chronological, and comprehensive documentation of their health history and status, are used by providers to communicate and coordinate health care. The records are used by medical insurance specialists to prepare and support health care claims. Documentation of an examination includes the chief complaint (CC), the history, the examination, the diagnosis, and the treatment plan. The process leading to the patient's informed consent for procedures is also documented. A progress report documents a patient's response to a treatment plan and provides justification for continued treatment. At the end of a treatment plan, a discharge summary documents the patient's final status and prognosis. If the provider-patient relationship is terminated, the reasons for termination and the status of the patient's treatment plan are documented, and the patient is informed in writing.
2. Electronic medical records and paper records are each forms of medical documentation. EMRs have the advantage of immediate access to health information, computerized physician order management, clinical decision support, automated alerts and reminders, electronic communication and connectivity, patient support, administration and reporting, and error reduction.
3. The HIPAA Privacy Rule, a part of the Administrative Simplification provisions, regulates the use and disclosure of patients' protected health information (PHI).
4. Under HIPAA, a covered entity is a health plan, health care clearinghouse, or health care provider that transmits any health information in electronic form in connection with a HIPAA transaction. A business associate, such as a law firm or billing service that performs work for a covered entity, must agree to follow applicable HIPAA regulations to safeguard protected health information.
5. Protected health information (PHI) is individually identifiable health information that is transmitted or maintained by electronic media, including data such as a patient's name, Social Security number, address, and phone number.
6. For use or disclosure for treatment, payment, or health care operations (TPO), no release is required from the patient. To release PHI for other than TPO, a covered entity must have an authorization signed by the patient. The authorization document must be in plain language and have a description of the information to be used, who can disclose it and for what purpose, who will receive it, an expiration date, and the patient's signature.
7. The HIPAA Security Rule, a part of the Administrative Simplification provisions, requires covered entities to establish administrative, physical, and technical safeguards to protect the confidentiality, integrity, and availability of health information.
8. The HIPAA Electronic Health Care Transactions and Code Sets establish standards for the exchange of financial and administrative data among covered entities. The standards

require the covered entities to use common electronic transaction methods and code sets. The four National Identifiers are for employers, health care providers, health plans, and patients.

9. The Health Care Fraud and Abuse Control Program, part of HIPAA, was enacted to prevent fraud and abuse in health care billing. This law, as well as the Federal False Claims Act and other related laws are enforced by the Office of Inspector General (OIG).

10. A medical practice compliance plan includes consistent written policies and procedures, appointment of a compliance officer and committee, training plans, communication guidelines, disciplinary systems, ongoing monitoring and auditing of claim preparation, and responding to and correcting errors. Each part of the plan addresses compliance concerns of government and private payers. Having a formal process in place is a sign that the practice has made a good-faith effort to achieve compliance.

Review Questions

Match the key terms with their definitions.

A. HIPAA Privacy Rule
B. authorization
C. minimum necessary standard
D. business associate
E. clearinghouse
F. Notice of Privacy Practices
G. code set
H. HIPAA Security Rule
I. covered entity
J. documentation

____ 1. Law under the Administrative Simplification provisions of HIPAA requiring covered entities to establish administrative, physical, and technical safeguards to protect the confidentiality, integrity, and availability of health information

____ 2. The systematic, logical, and consistent recording of a patient's health status—history, examinations, tests, results of treatments, and observations—in chronological order in a patient's medical record

____ 3. A person or organization that performs a function or activity for a covered entity but is not part of its workforce

____ 4. The principle that individually identifiable health information should be disclosed only to the extent needed to support the purpose of the disclosure

____ 5. Under HIPAA, a health plan, health care clearinghouse, or health care provider that transmits any health information in electronic form in connection with a HIPAA transaction

____ 6. Law under the Administrative Simplification provisions of HIPAA regulating the use and disclosure of patients' protected health information—individually identifiable health information that is transmitted or maintained by electronic media

____ 7. A HIPAA-mandated document that presents a covered entity's principles and procedures related to the protection of patients' protected health information

____ 8. A coding system used to encode elements of data

____ 9. A company that offers providers, for a fee, the service of receiving electronic or paper claims, checking and preparing them for processing, and transmitting them in proper data format to the correct carriers

____ 10. Document signed by a patient that permits release of medical information under the specific stated conditions

Decide whether each statement is true or false.

_____ 1. Electronic medical records offer advantages over paper records.

_____ 2. Fraud is not intentional.

_____ 3. The chief complaint is usually documented using clinical terminology.

_____ 4. The three major parts of the Administrative Simplification provisions are the privacy requirements, the security requirements, and the electronic transactions and code sets.

_____ 5. When federal and state privacy laws disagree, the federal rule is always followed.

_____ 6. Under HIPAA regulations, each medical practice must appoint a privacy official.

_____ 7. Protected health information includes the various numbers assigned to patients, such as their medical record numbers and their health plan beneficiary numbers.

_____ 8. The minimum necessary standard does not refer to the patient's health history.

_____ 9. Patients have the right to access, copy, inspect, and request amendment of their medical and billing records.

_____10. A patient's authorization is needed to disclose protected information for payment purposes.

Select the letter that best completes the statement or answers the question.

1. Under the HIPAA Privacy Rule, physician practices must
   A. train employees about the practice's privacy policy
   B. appoint a staff member as the privacy officer
   C. both A and B
   D. neither A nor B

2. A Notice of Privacy Practices is given to
   A. a practice's patients
   B. a practice's business associates
   C. the health plans with which a practice contracts
   D. none of the above

3. Patients' PHI may be released without authorization to
   A. local newspapers
   B. employers in workers' compensation cases
   C. social workers
   D. family and friends

4. Which government group has the authority to enforce the HIPAA Privacy Rule?
   A. CIA
   B. OIG
   C. OCR
   D. Medicaid

5. Patients always have the right to
   A. withdraw their authorization to release information
   B. alter the information in their medical records
   C. block release of information about their communicable diseases to the state health department
   D. none of the above

6. The authorization to release information must specify
   A. the number of pages to be released
   B. the Social Security number of the patient
   C. the entity to whom the information is to be released
   D. the name of the treating physician

7. Health information that does not identify an individual is referred to as
   A. protected health information
   B. authorized health release
   C. statutory data
   D. de-identified health information

8. Violating the HIPAA Privacy Rule can result in
   A. civil penalties
   B. criminal penalties
   C. both civil and criminal penalties
   D. neither civil nor criminal penalties

9. The main purpose of the HIPAA Security Rule is to
   A. regulate electronic transactions
   B. protect research data
   C. control the confidentiality and integrity of and access to protected health information
   D. protect medcal facilities from criminal acts such as robbery

10. A compliance plan contains
   A. consistent written policies and procedures
   B. medical office staff names
   C. the practice's main health plans
   D. all of the above

Answer the following question.

1. Define the following abbreviations:
   A. OCR
   B. PHI
   C. TCS
   D. DRS
   E. EMR
   F. CC
   G. NPI
   H. NPP
   I. OIG

Applying Your Knowledge

Case 2.1 Working With HIPAA

In each of these cases of release of PHI, was the HIPAA Privacy Rule followed? Why or why not?

A. A laboratory communicates a patient's medical test results to a physician by phone.

____

____

B. A physician mails a copy of a patient's medical record to a specialist who intends to treat the patient.

____

____

C. A hospital faxes a patient's health care instructions to a nursing home to which the patient is to be transferred. ______________________________

____

____

D. A doctor discusses a patient's condition over the phone with an emergency room physician who is providing the patient with emergency care. ____

____

____

E. A doctor orally discuss a patient's treatment regimen with a nurse who will be involved in the patient's care. ____

____

____

F. A physician consults with another physician by e-mail about a patient's condition.

____

____

____

G. A hospital shares an organ donor's medical information with another hospital treating the organ recipient.

____

____

H. A medical insurance specialist answers questions over the phone from a health plan about a patient's dates of service on a submitted claim. ____

____

____

Case 2.2 Applying HIPAA

Rosalyn Ramirez is a medical insurance specialist employed by Valley Associates, P.C., a midsized multispecialty practice with an excellent record of complying with HIPAA rules. Rosalyn answers the telephone and hears this question:

"This is Jane Mazloum, I'm a patient of Dr. Olgivy. I just listened to a phone message from your office about coming in for a checkup. My husband and I were talking about this. Since this is my first pregnancy and I am working, we really don't want anyone else to know about it yet. Has this information been given to anybody outside the clinic?" How do you recommend that she respond?

Case 2.3 Handling Authorizations

Angelo Diaz signed the authorization form below. When his insurance company called for an explanation of a reported procedure that Dr. Handlesman performed to treat a stomach ulcer, George Welofar, the clinic's registered nurse, released copies of his complete file. On reviewing Mr. Diaz's history of treatment for alcohol abuse, the insurance company refused to pay the claim, stating that Mr. Diaz's alcoholism had caused the condition. Mr. Diaz complained to the practice manager about the situation.

Should the information have been released?

Patient Name: Angelo Diaz

Health Record Number: ADI00

Date of Birth: 10-12-1945

1. I authorize the use or disclosure of the above named individual's health information as described below.

2. The following individual(s) or organization(s) are authorized to make the disclosure: Dr. L. Handlesman

3. The type of information to be used or disclosed is as follows (check the appropriate boxes and include other information where indicated)

- ☐ problem list
- ☐ medication list
- ☐ list of allergies
- ☐ immunization records
- ☑ most recent history
- ☐ most recent discharge summary
- ☐ lab results (please describe the dates or types of lab tests you would like disclosed): ____________
- ☑ x-ray and imaging reports (please describe the dates or types of x-rays or images you would like disclosed): ____________
- ☐ consultation reports from (please supply doctors' names): ____________
- ☐ entire record
- ☑ other (please describe): Progress notes

4. I understand that the information in my health record may include information relating to sexually transmitted disease, acquired immunodeficiency syndrome (AIDS), or human immunodeficiency virus (HIV). It may also include information about behavioral or mental health services, and treatment for alcohol and drug abuse.

5. The information identified above may be used by or disclosed to the following individuals or organization(s):

Name: Blue Cross & Blue Shield

Address: ____________

Name: ____________

Address: ____________

6. This information for which I'm authorizing disclosure will be used for the following purpose:

- ☐ my personal records
- ☐ sharing with other health care providers as needed/other (please describe): ____________

7. I understand that I have a right to revoke this authorization at any time. I understand that if I revoke this authorization, I must do so in writing and present my written revocation to the health information management department. I understand that the revocation will not apply to information that has already been released in response to this authorization. I understand that the revocation will not apply to my insurance company when the law provides my insurer with the right to contest a claim under my policy.

8. This authorization will expire (insert date or event): ____________

If I fail to specify an expiration date or event, this authorization will expire six months from the date on which it was signed.

9. I understand that once the above information is disclosed, it may be redisclosed by the recipient and the information may not be protected by federal privacy laws or regulations.

10. I understand authorizing the use or disclosure of the information identified above is voluntary. I need not sign this form to ensure healthcare treatment.

Signature of patient or legal representative: *Angelo Diaz* Date: 3-1-2008

If signed by legal representative, relationship to patient

Signature of witness: ____________ Date: ____________

Distribution of copies: Original to provider; copy to patient; copy to accompany use or disclosure

Note: This sample form was developed by the American Health Information Management Association for discussion purposes. It should not be used without review by the issuing organization's legal counsel to ensure compliance with other federal and state laws and regulations.

Case 2.4 Working With Medical Records

The following chart note contains typical documentation abbreviations and shortened forms for words.

> 65-yo female; hx of right breast ca seen in SurgiCenter for bx of breast mass. Frozen section reported as benign tumor. Bleeding followed the biopsy. Reopened the breast along site of previous incision with coagulation of bleeders. Wound sutured. Pt adm. for observation of post-op bleeding. Discharged with no bleeding recurrence.
>
> Final Dx: Benign neoplasm, left breast.

Research the meaning of each abbreviation (see the Abbreviations list at the end of the text), and write their meanings:

A. yo

B. hx

C. ca

D. bx

E. Pt

F. adm.

G. op

H. Dx

Internet Activities

1. State insurance commissions protect consumers in the area of health insurance. For example, many states set up ombudsman offices to provide information on managed care. Locate the organization in your state that provides health insurance help, or visit http://www.omc.state.ct.us to explore the state's information.
2. Both the Computer-based Patient Record Institute (CPRI) and the Medical Record Institute promote the development of the electronic (computer-based) medical record. Go to http://www.cpri.org/ and http://www.medrecinst.com/, and research the present status of electronic medical records in the United States. From your reading, explain how electronic records can improve patient care.
3. Visit the website of the American Medical Association at http://www.ama-assn.org. Do a site search for medical records, and report on the summary findings of a recent study on this subject.
4. Visit the website of the Centers for Medicare and Medicaid Services (CMS) to research the current status of HIPAA National Identifiers. Determine whether standards have been adopted for health plan or patient identifiers.

Chapter 3

Patient Encounters and Billing Information

CHAPTER OUTLINE

Gathering Patient Information

Establishing Financial Responsibility

Updating Patient Diagnosis, Procedures, and Charges

Collecting Time-of-Service Payments and Checking Out Patients

Learning Outcomes

After studying this chapter, you should be able to:

1. Explain the method used to classify patients as new or established.
2. Describe the information that new and returning patients provide before their encounters.
3. Discuss the purpose of the Assignment of Benefits.
4. Explain the purpose of the HIPAA Acknowledgment of Receipt of Notice of Privacy Practices.
5. Describe the procedures for verifying patients' eligibility for insurance benefits and for requesting referral or preauthorization approval.
6. Explain how to determine the primary insurance for patients who have more than one health plan.
7. Discuss the use and typical formats of encounter forms.
8. List the four types of charges that are collected from patients at the time of service.
9. Describe the billing procedures and transactions that follow patients' encounters.
10. Explain the importance of communication skills in working with patients, payers, and providers.

Key Terms

accept assignment
Acknowledgment of Receipt of Notice of Privacy Practices
adjustment
assignment of benefits
birthday rule
certification number
charge capture
chart number
coordination of benefits (COB)
direct provider
encounter form
established patient (EP)
financial policy
gender rule
guarantor
HIPAA Coordination of Benefits
HIPAA Eligibility for a Health Plan
HIPAA Referral Certification and Authorization
indirect provider
insured
new patient (NP)
nonparticipating provider (nonPAR)
participating provider (PAR)
patient information form
primary insurance
prior authorization number
referral number
referral waiver
referring physician
secondary insurance
self-pay patient
subscriber
superbill
supplemental insurance
tertiary insurance
trace number
walkout receipt

Successful billing and reimbursement begins with establishing financial responsibility for medical services. Determining the patient's and the health plan's obligations for payment, as explained in this chapter, is a cornerstone of reimbursement. Cutting corners or making mistakes here will lead to collection problems later.

Processing encounters for billing purposes has three parts. First, information about patients and their insurance coverage is gathered and verified. Then data about the diagnoses and procedures are documented by the provider and used by the medical insurance specialist to update the patient's account. Finally, time-of-service charges are collected from patients. Patients leave the encounter with a clear understanding of the next steps in the payment process: claims, insurance payments, and paying the bills they will receive for balances due.

Gathering Patient Information

To gather accurate information for billing and medical care, practices ask patients to supply information and then double-check key data. Patients who are new to the medical practice complete many forms before their first appointment. A **new patient (NP)** is someone who has not received any services from the provider (or another provider of the same specialty who is a member of the same practice) within the past three years. A returning patient is called an **established patient (EP)**. This patient has seen the provider (or another provider in the practice who has the same specialty) within the past three years. Established patients review and update the information that is on file about them. Figure 3.1 illustrates how to decide which category fits the patient.

Information for New Patients

When the patient is new to the practice, five types of information are important:

1. Preregistration and scheduling information
2. Medical history
3. Patient/guarantor information and insurance information
4. Assignment of benefits
5. Acknowledgment of Receipt of Notice of Privacy Practices

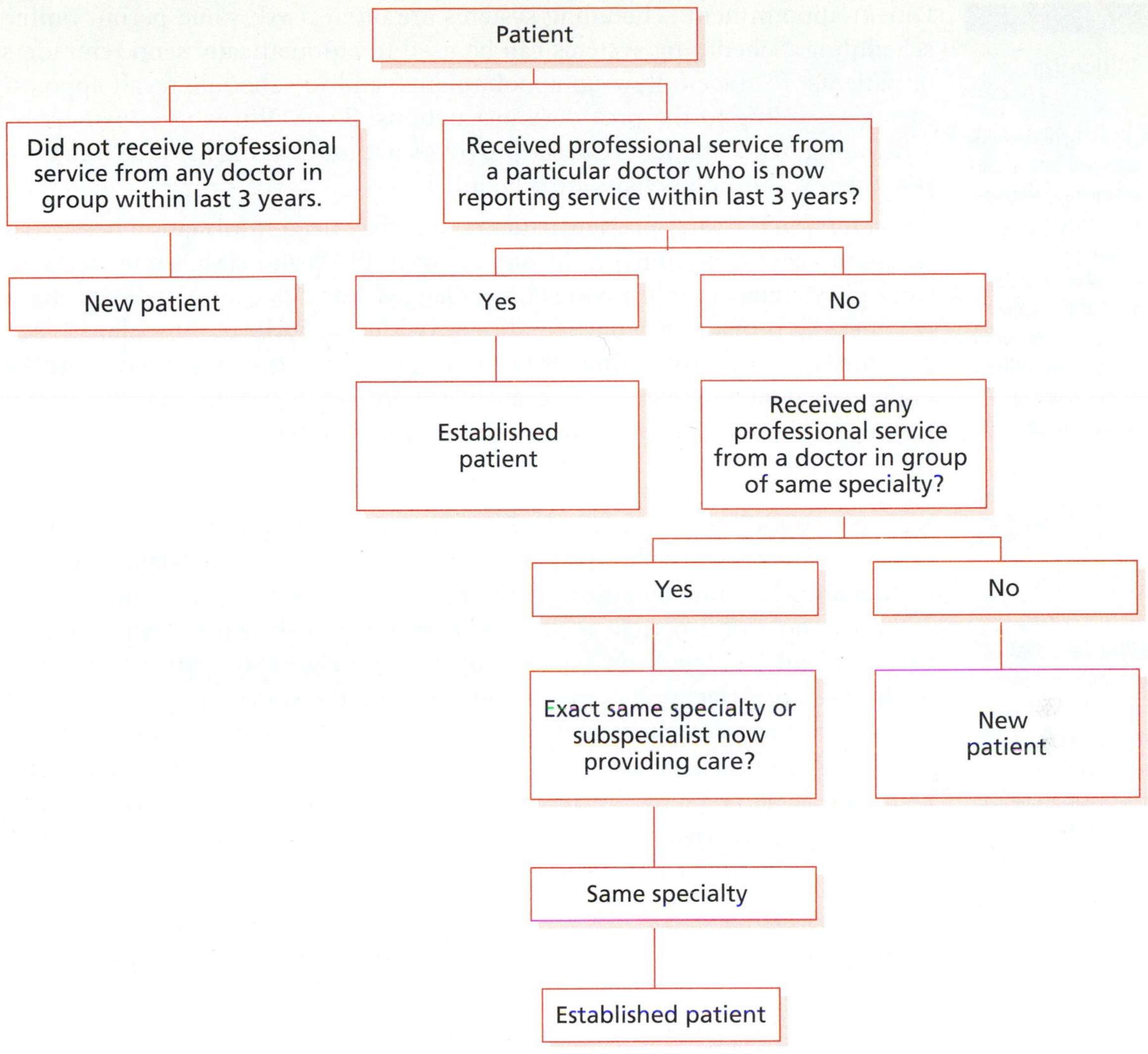

Figure 3.1 Decision Tree for New versus Established Patients

Preregistration and Scheduling Information

The collection of information begins before the patient presents at the front desk for an appointment. Most medical practices have a preregistration process to check that patients' health care requirements are appropriate for the medical practice and to schedule appointments of the correct length.

Preregistration Basics When new patients call for appointments, basic information is usually gathered:

- Full name
- Telephone number
- Address
- Date of birth
- Gender
- Reason for call or nature of complaint, including information about previous treatment
- If insured, the name of the health plan and whether a copay is required
- If referred, the name of the referring physician

Billing Tip

Referring Physician
A referring physician sends a patient to another physician for treatment.

Scheduling Appointments Front office employees handle appointments and scheduling in most practices and may also handle prescription refill requests.

Patient-appointment scheduling systems are often used; some permit online scheduling. Scheduling systems can be used to automatically send reminders to patients, to trace follow-up appointments, and to schedule recall appointments according to the provider's instructions. Some offices use open-access scheduling, where patients can see providers without having made advance appointments; follow-up visits are scheduled.

Provider Participation New patients, too, may need information before deciding to make appointments. Most patients in PPOs and HMOs must use network physicians to avoid paying higher charges. For this reason, patients check whether the provider is a **participating provider**, or **PAR**, in their plan. When patients see **nonparticipating**, or **nonPAR**, **providers**, they must pay more—a higher copayment, greater coinsurance, or both—so a patient may choose not to make an appointment because of the additional expense.

> **Billing Tip**
>
> **MCOs and Appointments**
> Many managed care organizations require participating physicians to see enrolled patients within a short time of their calling for appointments. Some also require PCPs to handle emergencies in the office, rather than sending patients to the emergency department.

Medical History

New patients complete medical history forms. Some practices give printed forms to patients when they come in. Others make the form available for completion ahead of time by posting it online or mailing it to the patient.

An example of a patient medical history form is shown in Figure 3.2 on pages 77 and 78. The form asks for information about the patient's personal medical history, the family's medical history, and the social history. Social history covers lifestyle factors such as smoking, exercise, and alcohol use. Many specialists use less-detailed forms that cover the histories needed for treatment.

The physician reviews the information on the medical history form with the patient during the visit. The patient's answers and the physician's notes are documented in the medical record.

> **Billing Tip**
>
> **Know Plan Participation**
> Administrative staff members must know what plans the providers participate in. A summary of these plans should be available during patient registration.

Patient Information

A new patient arriving at the front desk for an appointment completes a **patient information form** (see Figure 3.3 on page 79). This form is also called a patient registration form. It is used to collect the following demographic information about the patient:

- First name, middle initial, and last name.
- Gender (*F* for female or *M* for male).
- Marital status (*S* for single, *M* for married, *D* for divorced, *W* for widowed).
- Birth date, using four digits for the year.
- Home address and telephone number (area code with seven-digit number).
- Social Security number.
- Employer's name, address, and telephone number.
- For a married patient, the name and employer of the spouse.
- A contact person for the patient in case of a medical emergency.
- If the patient is a minor (under the age of majority according to state law) or has a medical power of attorney in place (such as a person who is handling the medical decisions of another person), the responsible person's name, gender, marital status, birth date, address, Social Security number, telephone number, and employer information. If a minor, the child's status if a full-time or part-time student is recorded. In most cases, the responsible person is a parent, guardian, adult child, or other person acting with legal authority to make health care decisions on behalf of the patient.
- The name of the patient's health plan.
- The health plan's policyholder's name (the policyholder may be a spouse, divorced spouse, guardian, or other relation), birth date, plan type, Social Security number, policy number or group number, telephone number, and employer.

> **Billing Tip**
>
> **Subscriber, Insured, or Guarantor: All Mean Policyholder**
> Other terms for policyholder are insured, subscriber, and guarantor. This person is the holder of the insurance policy that covers the patient and is not necessarily also a patient of the practice.

PATIENT HEALTH SURVEY

NAME PLATE

NAME ______ AGE ______ M ______ F ______ DATE ______

ADDRESS ______ PHONE ______

HISTORY OF PAST ILLNESS: Have you had

Childhood:
- ☐ Measles ☐ Mumps ☐ Chicken Pox
- ☐ Congenital Abnormalities ☐ Rheumatic fever or heart disease

Adult:
- ☐ Asthma ☐ High Blood Pressure ☐ Cancer (Site______)
- ☐ Diabetes ☐ Ulcer or Gastritis ☐ Thyroid Problems
- ☐ Tuberculosis ☐ Kidney Problem ☐ Liver Problems
- ☐ Blood Problem ☐ Venereal Disease ☐ Heart Failure
- ☐ Heart Attack ☐ Abnormal Heart Rhythm

Have you had any serious illness? No Yes
Have you ever had a transfusion? No Yes
Have you ever been hospitalized or been under medical care for very long? No Yes

If Yes, for what reason? ______

Most recent immunizations:
Hepatitis B______(date) Flu Vaccine______(date)
Pneumovax______(date) Tetanus______(date)

OPERATIONS:
Have you ever had any surgery? No Yes

List:
- ☐ Appendectomy ☐ Hysterectomy (If so, reason______)
- ☐ Ovaries Removed ☐ Joint Replacement
- ☐ Gallbladder ☐ Bypass (If so, what______)
- ☐ Other ______

ALLERGIES:

MEDICATIONS:

INJURIES:
Have you ever been seriously injured in a motor vehicle accident? No Yes
Have you had any head concussions or injuries? No Yes
Have you ever been knocked unconscious? No Yes

SOCIAL HISTORY:
Circle One: Single Married Separated Divorced Widowed Significant Other

With whom do you live? ______

Recreational Drug Usage? No Yes
Do you have any problems with sexual function? No Yes

Foreign travel within last year______

Coffee______ Tea______ Cola's______ (per day)

Alcoholic Beverages: Never______ 1-5 per week______ < 1 per week______ Other______

Tobacco: ☐ Never Smoked ☐ Years smoked______ ☐ Quit______years ago ☐ Packs per day______

84168 (12/01)

SOCIAL HISTORY: (continued)

Are you employed? Full Time______ Part Time______

What is your job? ______

Are you exposed to fumes, dusts or solvents? ______

How much time have you lost from work because of your health during the past?
Six Months______ One Year______ Five Years______

Education: (Years)
Grade School______ College______ Postgraduate______

Do you wear seatbelts? ☐ Always ☐ Sometimes ☐ Never

FAMILY HISTORY:	Age	Health	If Deceased, Age at Death	Cause of Death
Father				
Mother				
Brother/Sister				
Husband/Wife				
Son/Daughter				

Has either parent, sister, brother, child or grandparent ever had?

Stroke	No	Yes	Heart Trouble	No	Yes
Tuberculosis	No	Yes	High Blood Pressure	No	Yes
Diabetes	No	Yes			

Has any blood relative ever had?

Cancer	No	Yes	Bleeding Tendancy	No	Yes
Type:			Gout or other crippling arthritis		
Suicide	No	Yes		No	Yes
Mental Illness	No	Yes	Hereditary Defects	No	Yes

Figure 3.2 Medical History Form

- If the patient is covered by another health plan, the name and policyholder information for that plan.

The patient information form is filed in both the patient medical and billing records.

PATIENT HEALTH SURVEY

NAME PLATE

CIRCLE NO OR YES FOR THOSE THAT APPLY

SYSTEMIC REVIEW: Do you have any of the following?
General: Maximum weight________ Minimum weight________
Recent weight change? .... No Yes
Have you been in good general health most of your life? .... No Yes
Have you recently had?
☐ Weakness ☐ Fever ☐ Chills ☐ Night Sweats
☐ Fainting ☐ Problems Sleeping

Skin:
Skin Disease .... No Yes
Jaundice .... No Yes
Hives, eczema or rash .... No Yes

Head-Eyes-Ears-Nose-Throat (cont'd):
Dry eyes or mouth .... No Yes
Bleeding Gums - Frequent or Constant .... No Yes
Blurred Vision .... No Yes
Date of Last Eye Exam ________
Sneezing or runny nose .... No Yes
Nosebleeds - Frequent .... No Yes
Chronic sinus trouble .... No Yes
Ear disease .... No Yes
Impaired hearing .... No Yes
Dizziness or sensation of room spinning .... No Yes
Frequent or severe headaches .... No Yes

Respiratory:
Asthma or Wheezing .... No Yes
Difficulty breathing .... No Yes
Any trouble with lungs .... No Yes
Pleurisy or Pneumonia .... No Yes
Cough up Blood (ever) .... No Yes

Cardiovascular:
Chest pain, pressure, or tightness .... No Yes
Shortness of breath with walking or lying down .... No Yes
Difficulty walking two blocks .... No Yes
Palpitations .... No Yes
Swelling of hands, feet or ankles .... No Yes
Awakening in the nights smothering .... No Yes
Heart murmur .... No Yes

Gastrointestinal:
Vomiting blood or food .... No Yes
Gallbladder disease .... No Yes
Change in appetite .... No Yes
Hepatitis/Jaundice .... No Yes
Painful bowel movements .... No Yes
Bleeding with bowel movements .... No Yes
Black stools .... No Yes
Hemorrhoids or piles .... No Yes
Recent change in bowel habits .... No Yes
Frequent diarrhea .... No Yes
Heartburn or indigestion .... No Yes
Cramping or pain in the abdomen .... No Yes
Does food stick in throat .... No Yes

Endocrine:
Hormone therapy .... No Yes
Any change in hat or glove size .... No Yes
Any change in hair growth .... No Yes
Have you become colder than before - or skin become dryer .... No Yes

Neck:
Stiffness .... No Yes
Enlarged glands .... No Yes

Genitourinary:
Loss of urine .... No Yes
Blood in urine .... No Yes
Frequent urination .... No Yes
Burning or painfu .... No Yes
Night time urinating .... No Yes
Kidney trouble .... No Yes
Problem stopping/starting flow of urine .... No Yes
Testicular mass .... No Yes
Testicular pain .... No Yes
Prostate problem .... No Yes
Sexual Dysfunction .... No Yes
STD / AIDS Risk .... No Yes

Gynecological:
First day of last period ________
Age periods started ________
How long do periods last? ________ Days
Frequency of periods every ________ Days
Pain with periods .... No Yes
Number of pregnancies ________
Number of miscarriages ________
Date of last cancer smear and results ________
Breast Lump .... No Yes
Abnormal Vaginal Discharge .... No Yes
Breast Discharge .... No Yes
Pain with Intercourse .... No Yes
Skin change of Breast .... No Yes
Nipple retraction .... No Yes

Locomotor-Musculoskeletal:
Stiffness or pain in joints (check all that apply)
☐Finger ☐Hands ☐Wrist ☐Elbows ☐Shoulders ☐Neck ☐Back
☐Hip ☐Knee ☐Toes ☐Foot ☐Temporomandibular Joint
Weakness of muscles or joints .... No Yes
Any difficulty in walking .... No Yes
Any pain in calves or buttocks on walking relieved by rest .... No Yes

Neuro-Psychiatric:
☐Transient blindness ☐Tremor ☐Numbness in fingers ☐ Weakness
Have you ever had counselling for your mental health? ... No Yes
Have you ever been advised to see a psychiatrist? ...... No Yes
Do you ever have, or have had, fainting spells? .... No Yes
Convulsions .... No Yes
Paralysis .... No Yes
Problem with coordination .... No Yes
Domestic violence .... No Yes
Depression Symptoms (difficulty sleeping, loss of appetite loss of interest in activities, feelings of hopelessness) .... No Yes

Hematologic:
Are you slow to heal after cuts? .... No Yes
Anemia .... No Yes
Phlebitis or Blood Clots in veins .... No Yes
Have you had difficulty with bleeding excessively after tooth extraction or surgery? .... No Yes
Have you had abnormal bruising or bleeding? .... No Yes

Source of information, if other than patient: ________

Signature of person acquiring this information: ________

________ Provider ________ Date ________ Signature of Patient

Figure 3.2 Continued

Insurance Cards

For an insured new patient, the front and the back of the insurance card are scanned or photocopied. All data from the card that the patient has written on the patient information form is double-checked for accuracy.

VALLEY ASSOCIATES, PC
1400 West Center Street
Toledo, OH 43601-0123
614-321-0987

PATIENT INFORMATION FORM

THIS SECTION REFERS TO PATIENT ONLY			
Name:	Sex:	Marital Status: ☐S ☐M ☐D ☐W	Birth Date:
Address:	SS#:		
City: State: Zip:	Employer:		Phone:
Home Phone:	Employer's Address:		
Work Phone:	City:	State:	Zip:
Spouse's Name:	Spouse's Employer:		
Emergency Contact:	Relationship:		Phone #:

FILL IN IF PATIENT IS A MINOR			
Parent/Guardian's Name:	Sex:	Marital Status: ☐S ☐M ☐D ☐W	Birth Date:
Phone:	SS#:		
Address:	Employer:		Phone:
City: State: Zip:	Employer's Address:		
Student Status:	City:	State:	Zip:

INSURANCE INFORMATION			
Primary Insurance Company:		Secondary Insurance Company:	
Subscriber's Name:	Birth Date:	Subscriber's Name:	Birth Date:
Plan:	SS#:	Plan:	
Policy #:	Group #:	Policy #:	Group #:
Copayment/Deductible:	Price Code:		

OTHER INFORMATION	
Reason for visit:	Allergy to Medication (list):
Name of referring physician:	If auto accident, list date and state in which it occurred:

I authorize treatment and agree to pay all fees and charges for the person named above. I agree to pay all charges shown by statements, promptly upon their presentation, unless credit arrangements are agreed upon in writing.

I authorize payment directly to VALLEY ASSOCIATES, PC of insurance benefits otherwise payable to me. I hereby authorize the release of any medical information necessary in order to process a claim for payment in my behalf.

________________________________ ________________________________
(Patient's Signature/Parent or Guardian's Signature) (Date)

I plan to make payment of my medical expenses as follows (check one or more):

_____Insurance (as above) _____Cash/Check/Credit/Debit Card _____Medicare _____Medicaid _____ Workers' Comp.

Figure 3.3 Patient Information (Registration) Form

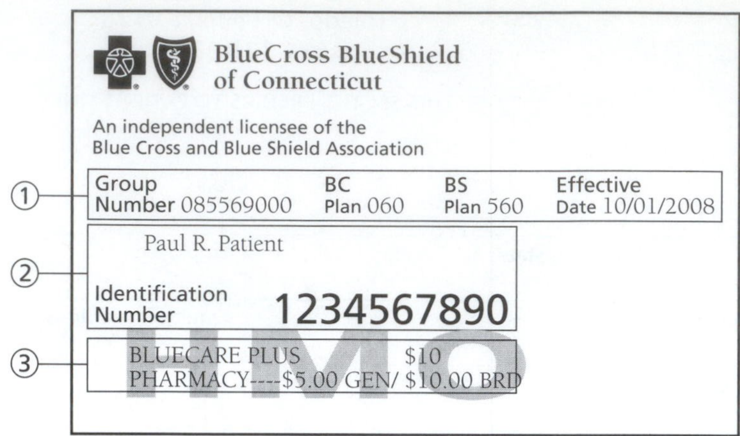
BlueCross BlueShield
of Connecticut
An independent licensee of the
Blue Cross and Blue Shield Association
Group Number 085569000
BC Plan 060
BS Plan 560
Effective Date 10/01/2008
Paul R. Patient
Identification Number 1234567890
BLUECARE PLUS $10
PHARMACY----$5.00 GEN/ $10.00 BRD
HMO
①
②
③

1. ***Group identification number***
   The 9-digit number used to identify the member's employer.

   Blue Cross Blue Shield plan codes
   The numbers used to identify the codes assigned to each plan by the Blue Cross Blue Shield Association: used for claims submissions when medical services are rendered out-of-state.

   Effective date
   The date on which the member's coverage became effective.
2. ***Member name***
   The full name of the cardholder.

   Identification number
   The 10-digit number used to identify each Anthem Blue Cross and Blue Shield of Connecticut or BlueCare Health Plan member.
3. ***Health plan***
   The name of the health plan and the type of coverage; usually lists any copayment amounts, frequency limits or annual maximums for home and office visits; may also list the member's annual deductible amount.

   Riders
   The type(s) of riders that are included in the member's benefits (DME, Visions).

   Pharmacy
   The type of prescription drug coverage; lists copayment amounts

Figure 3.4 An Example of an Insurance Card

> **Billing Tip**
>
> **Matching the Patient's Name**
> Payers want the name of the patient on a claim to be exactly as it is shown on the insurance card. Do not use nicknames, skip middle initials, or make any other changes. Compare the patient information form carefully with the insurance card, and resolve any discrepancies before the encounter.

Most insurance cards have the following information (see Figure 3.4):

- Group identification number
- Date on which the member's coverage became effective
- Member name
- Member identification number
- The health plan's name, type of coverage, copayment requirements, and frequency limits or annual maximums for services; sometimes the annual deductible
- Optional items, such as prescription drugs that are covered, with the copayment requirements

Photo Identification

Many practices also require the patient to present a photo ID card, such as a driver's license, which the practice copies for the chart.

Assignment of Benefits

I hereby assign to Valley Associates, PC, any insurance or other third-party benefits available for health care services provided to me. I understand that Valley Associates has the right to refuse or accept assignment of such benefits. If these benefits are not assigned to Valley Associates, I agree to forward to Valley Associates all health insurance and other third-party payments that I receive for services rendered to me immediately upon receipt.

Signature of Patient/Legal Guardian: ______________________________

Date: __________________

Figure 3.5 Assignment of Benefits Form

Assignment of Benefits

Physicians usually submit claims for patients and receive payments directly from the payers. This saves patients paperwork; it also benefits providers, since payments are faster. The policyholder must authorize this procedure by signing and dating an **assignment of benefits** statement. This may be a separate form, as in Figure 3.5, or an entry on the patient information form, as in Figure 3.3 on page 79. The assignment of benefits statement is filed in both the patient medical and billing records.

Acknowledgment of Receipt of Notice of Privacy Practices

Under the HIPAA Privacy Rule (see Chapter 2), providers do not need specific authorization in order to release patients' PHI for treatment, payment, and operations (TPO) purposes. These uses are defined as:

1. *Treatment:* This purpose primarily consists of discussion of the patient's case with other providers. For example, the physician may document the role of each member of the health care team in providing care. Each team member then records actions and observations so that the ordering physician knows how the patient is responding to treatment.
2. *Payment:* Practices usually submit claims on behalf of patients; this involves sending demographic and diagnostic information.
3. *Operations:* This purpose includes activities such as staff training and quality improvement.

Providers must have patients' authorization to use or disclose information that is not for TPO purposes. For example, a patient who wishes a provider to disclose PHI to a life insurance company must complete an authorization form (see Chapter 2, Figure 2.9) to do so.

Under HIPAA, providers must inform each patient about their privacy practices one time. The most common method is to give the patient a copy of the medical office's privacy practices to read, and then to have the patient sign a separate form called an **Acknowledgment of Receipt of Notice of Privacy Practices** (see Figure 3.6 on page 82). This form states that the patient has read the privacy practices and understands how the provider intends to protect the patient's rights to privacy under HIPAA.

The provider must make a good-faith effort to have patients sign this document. The provider must also document—in the medical record—whether the

Compliance Guideline

State Law on Assignment of Benefits
The following states have laws mandating that the payer must pay the provider of services (rather than the patient) if a valid assignment of benefits is on file and the payer has been notified of the assignment of benefits: Alabama, Alaska, Colorado, Connecticut, Georgia, Idaho, Louisiana, Maine, Missouri, Nevada, New Jersey, North Dakota, Ohio, Oklahoma, South Dakota, Tennessee, Texas, and Virginia.

Billing tip

Release Document
As noted in Chapter 2, state law may be more stringent than HIPAA and demand an authorization to release TPO information. Many practices routinely have patients sign release of information statements.

HIPAA Tip

Who is Requesting PHI?

Although the HIPAA Privacy Rule permits sharing PHI for TPO purposes without authorization, it also requires verification of the identity of the person who is asking for the information. The person's authority to access PHI must also be verified. If the requestor's right to the information is not certain, the best practice is to have the patient authorize the release of PHI.

HIPAA Tip

Keeping Acknow-ledgments on File

Providers must retain signed acknowledgments as well as documentation about unsuccessful attempts to obtain them for six years.

Acknowledgment of Receipt of Notice of Privacy Practices

I understand that the providers of Valley Associates, PC, may share my health information for treatment, billing and healthcare operations. I have been given a copy of the organization's notice of privacy practices that describes how my health information is used and shared. I understand that Valley Associates has the right to change this notice at any time. I may obtain a current copy by contacting the practice's office or by visiting the website at www.xxx.com.

My signature below constitutes my acknowledgment that I have been provided with a copy of the notice of privacy practices.

____

Signature of Patient or Legal Representative Date

If signed by legal representative,
relationship to patient:______________________

Figure 3.6 Acknowledgment of Receipt of Notice of Privacy Practices

patient signed the form. The format for the acknowledgment is up to the practice. Only a **direct provider**, one who directly treats the patient, is required to have patients sign an acknowledgment. An **indirect provider**, such as a pathologist, must have a privacy notice but does not have to secure additional acknowledgments.

If a patient who has not received a privacy notice or signed an Acknowledgment calls for a prescription refill, the recommended procedure is to mail the patient a copy of the privacy notice, along with an acknowledgment of receipt form, and to document the mailing to show a good-faith effort that meets the office's HIPAA obligation in the event that the patient does not return the signed form.

HIPAA does not require the parent or guardian of a minor to sign. If a child is accompanied by a parent or guardian who is completing other paperwork on behalf of the minor, it is reasonable to ask that adult to sign the Acknowledgment of receipt. On the other hand, if the child or teen is unaccompanied, the minor patient may be asked to sign.

Information for Established Patients

When established patients present for appointments, the front desk asks whether any pertinent personal or insurance information has changed. This update process is important because different employment, marital status, dependent status, or plans may affect patients' coverage. Patients may also phone in changes, such as new addresses or employers.

To double-check that information is current, most practices periodically ask established patients to review and sign off on their patient information forms when they come in. This review should be done at least once a year. A good time is an established patient's first appointment in a new year. The file is also checked to be sure that the patient has been given a current Notice of Privacy Practices.

If the insurance of an established patient has changed, both sides of the new card are copied, and all data are checked. Many practices routinely scan or copy the card at each visit as a safeguard.

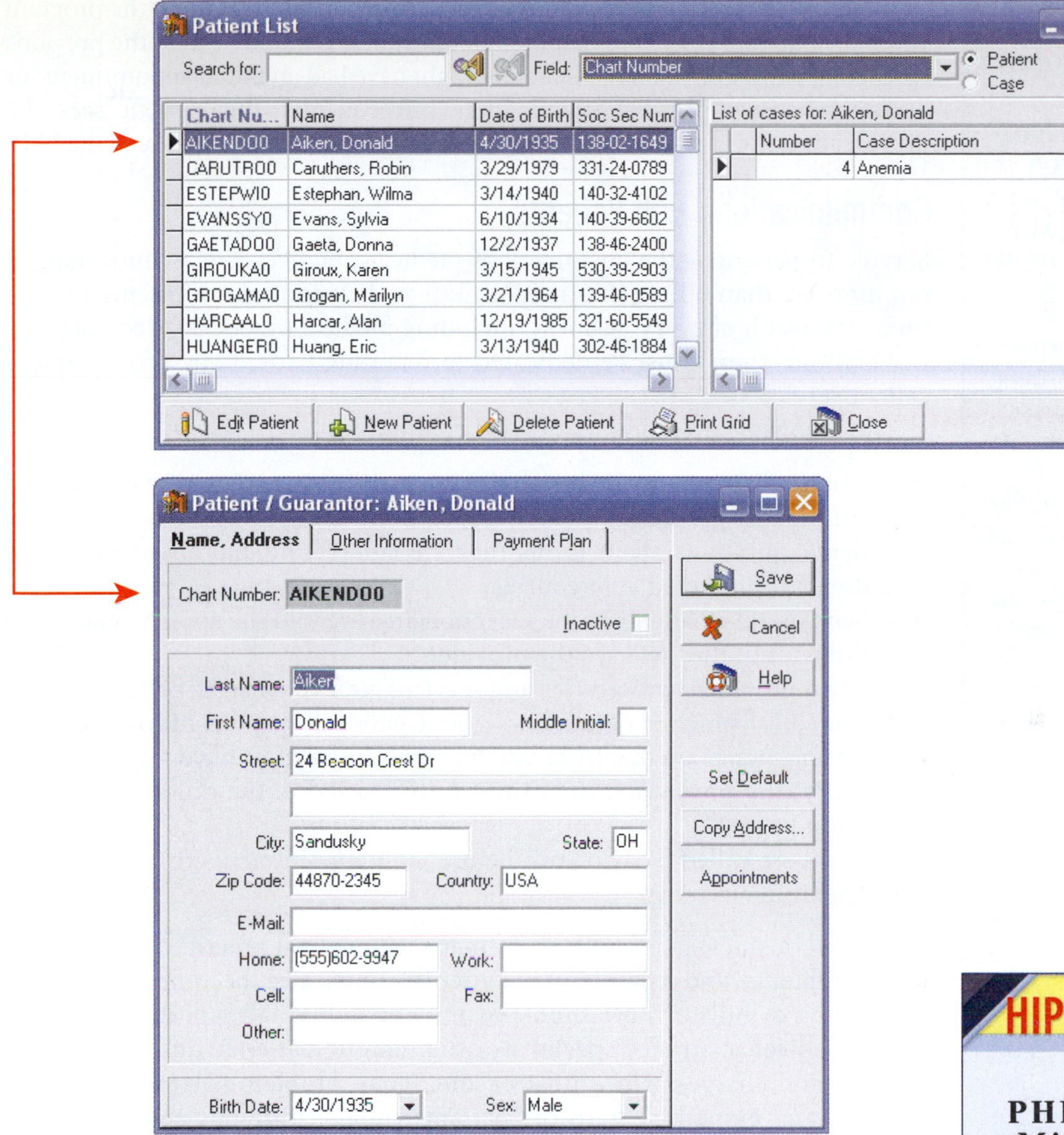

Figure 3.7 (a) Patient List, (b) Patient/Guarantor Dialog

Entering Patient Information in the Practice Management Program

A practice management program (PMP) is set up with databases about the practice's income and expense accounting. The provider database has information about physicians and other health professionals who work in the practice, such as their medical license numbers, tax identification numbers, and office hours. A database of common diagnosis and procedure codes is also built in the PMP. After these databases are set up, the medical insurance specialist can enter patients' demographic and visit information to begin the process of billing.

The database of patients in the practice management program must be continually kept up to date. For each new patient, a new file and a new **chart number** are set up. The chart number is a unique number that identifies the patient. It links all the information that is stored in the other databases—providers, insurance plans, diagnoses, procedures, and claims—to the case of the particular patient. Figure 3.7 shows a sample of a PMP screen used to enter a new patient into the patient database.

> **HIPAA Tip**
>
> **PHI and Minors**
>
> *A covered entity may choose to provide or deny a parent access to a minor's personal health information (PHI) if doing so is consistent with state or other applicable law and provided that the decision is made by a licensed health care professional. These options apply whether or not the parent is the minor's personal representative.*

HIPAA Tip

Observing HIPAA Privacy and Security Requirements

Front office staff members follow HIPAA requirements in dealing with patients. They use reasonable safeguards, such as speaking softly and never leaving handheld dictation devices unattended, to prevent others from hearing PHI. Computer monitors, medical records, and other documents are not visible to patients who are checking in or to others in the waiting room.

Usually, a new *case* or record for an established patient is set up in the program when the patient's chief complaint for an encounter is different than the previous chief complaint. For example, a patient might have had an initial appointment for a comprehensive physical examination. Subsequently, this patient sees the provider because of stomach pain. Each visit is set up as a separate case in the PMP.

Communications with Patients

Service to patients—the customers of medical practices—is as important, if not more so, than billing information. Satisfied customers are essential to the financial health of every business, including medical practices. Medical practice staff members must be dedicated to retaining patients by providing excellent service.

The following are examples of good communication:

- Established and new patients who call or arrive for appointments are always given friendly greetings and are referred to by name.
- Patients' questions about forms they are completing and about insurance matters are answered with courtesy.
- When possible, patients in the reception area are told the approximate waiting time until they will see the provider.
- Fees for providers' procedures and services are explained to patients.
- The medical practice's guidelines about patients' responsibilities, such as when payments are due from patients and the need to have referrals from primary care physicians, are prominently posted in the office (see Figure 3.12 on page 97).
- Patients are called a day or two before their appointments to remind them of appointment times.

Like all businesses, even the best-managed medical practices have to deal with problems and complaints. Patients sometimes become upset over scheduling or bills or have problems understanding lab reports or instructions. Medical insurance specialists often handle patients' questions about benefits and charges. They must become good problem solvers, willing to listen to and empathize with the patient while sorting out emotions from facts to get accurate information. Phrases such as these reduce patients' anger and frustration:

"I'm glad you brought this to our attention. I will look into it further."

"I can appreciate how you would feel this way."

"It sounds like we have caused some inconvenience, and I apologize."

"I understand that you are angry. Let me try to understand your concerns so we can address the situation."

"Thank you for taking the time to tell us about this. Because you have, we can resolve issues like the one you raised."

Medical insurance specialists need to use the available resources and to investigate solutions to problems. Following through on promised information is also critical. A medical insurance specialist who says to a patient "I will call you by the end of next week with that information" must do exactly that. Even if the problem is not solved, the patient needs an update on the situation within the stated time frame.

Thinking It Through — 3.1

1. Review these multiple versions of the same name:

   Ralph Smith
   Ralph P. Smith
   Ralph Plane Smith
   R. Plane Smith
   R. P. Smith

   If "Ralph Plane Smith" appears on the insurance card and his mother writes "Ralph Smith" on the patient information form, which version should be used for the medical practice's records? Why?

2. Refer to the patient information form below. According to the information supplied by the patient, who is the policyholder? What is the patient's relationship to the policyholder?

PATIENT INFORMATION FORM

THIS SECTION REFERS TO PATIENT ONLY			
Name: Mary Anne C. Kopelman	Sex: F	Marital status: ☐S ☒M ☐D ☐W	Birth date: 9/7/73
Address: 45 Mason Street	SS#: 465-99-0022		
City: Hopewell State: OH Zip: 43800	Employer:		
Home phone: 999-555-6877	Employer's address:		
Work phone:	City: State: Zip:		
Spouse's name: Arnold B. Kopelman	Spouse's employer: U.S. Army, Fort Tyrone		
Emergency contact: Arnold B. Kopelman	Relationship: husband	Phone #: 999-555-0018	

INSURANCE INFORMATION	
Primary insurance company: TriCare	Secondary insurance company:
Policyholder's name: Arnold B. Kopelman Birth date: 4/10/73	Policyholder's name: Birth date:
Plan: TriCare SS#: 230-56-9874	Plan:
Policy #: 230-56-9874 Group #: USA9947	Policy #: Group #:

Establishing Financial Responsibility

To be paid for services, medical practices need to establish financial responsibility. Medical insurance specialists are vital employees in this process. For insured patients, they follow three steps to establish financial responsibility:

1. Verify the patient's eligibility for insurance benefits
2. Determine preauthorization and referral requirements
3. Determine the primary payer if more than one insurance plan is in effect

Verify Patient Eligibility for Insurance Benefits

The first step is to verify patients' eligibility for benefits. Medical insurance specialists abstract information about the patient's payer/plan from the patient's information form (PIF) and the insurance card. They then contact the payer to verify three points:

1. Patients' general eligibility for benefits
2. The amount of the copayment, if one is required
3. Whether the planned encounter is for a covered service that is medically necessary under the payer's rules

These items are checked before an encounter except in a medical emergency, where care is provided immediately and insurance is checked after the encounter.

Factors Affecting General Eligibility

General eligibility for benefits depends on a number of factors. If premiums are required, patients must have paid them on time. For government-sponsored plans where income is the criterion, like Medicaid, eligibility can change monthly. For patients with employer-sponsored health plans, employment status can be the deciding factor:

- Coverage may end on the last day of the month in which the employee's active full-time service ends, such as for disability, layoff, or termination.
- The employee may no longer qualify as a member of the group. For example, some companies do not provide benefits for part-time employees. If a full-time employee changes to part-time employment, the coverage ends.
- An eligible dependent's coverage may end on the last day of the month in which the dependent status ends, such as reaching the age limit stated in the policy.

If the plan is an HMO that requires a primary care provider (PCP), a general or family practice must verify that (1) the provider is a plan participant, (2) the patient is listed on the plan's enrollment master list, and (3) the patient is assigned to the PCP as of the date of service.

The medical insurance specialist checks with the payer to confirm whether the patient is currently covered. If online access is used, Web information and e-mail messages are exchanged with provider representatives. If the payer requires the use of the telephone, the provider representative is called. Based on the patient's plan, eligibility for these specific benefits may also need checking:

- Office visits
- Lab coverage
- Diagnostic X-rays
- Maternity coverage
- Pap smear coverage
- Coverage of psychiatric visits
- Physical or occupational therapy

Billing Tip

Plan Information
Be aware of the copayments, precertification and referral requirements, and noncovered services for plans in which the practice participates.

Billing Tip

Payers' Rules for Medical Necessity
Medicare requires patients to be notified if their insurance is not going to cover a visit, as detailed in Chapter 10. Other payers have similar rules.

Billing Tip

Getting Online Information About Patients
A portal is a website that is an entry point to other websites. Many insurers have portals to be used to check patient eligibility for coverage, get information on copayments and deductibles, process claims, and submit preauthorization requests.

Billing Tip

Check the Lab Requirements
Because many MCOs specify which laboratory must be used, patients should be notified that they are responsible for telling the practice about their plans' lab requirements, so that if specimens are sent to the wrong lab, the practice is not responsible for the costs.

- Durable medical equipment (DME)
- Foot care

Checking Out-Of-Network Benefits

If patients have insurance coverage but the practice does not participate in their plans, the medical insurance specialist checks the out-of-network benefit. When the patient has out-of-network benefits, the payer's rules concerning copayments and coverage are followed. If a patient does not have out-of-network benefits, as is common when the health plan is an HMO, the patient is responsible for the entire bill, rather than simply a copayment.

Verifying the Amount of the Copayment

The amount of the copayment, if required, must be checked. It is sometimes the case that the copay on the insurance card is out of date, and the correct copay needs to be collected.

Determining Whether the Planned Encounter Is for a Covered Service

The medical insurance specialist also must attempt to determine whether the planned encounter is for a covered service. If the service will not be covered, that patient can be informed and made aware of financial responsibility in advance.

The resources for covered services include knowledge of the major plans held by the practice's patients, information from the provider representative and payer websites, and the electronic benefit inquires described below. Medical insurance specialists are familiar with what the plans cover in general. For example, most plans cover regular office visits, but they may not cover preventive services or some therapeutic services. Unusual or unfamiliar services must be researched, and the payer must be queried.

Electronic Benefit Inquiries and Responses

An electronic transaction, a telephone call, or a fax or e-mail message may be used to communicate with the payer. Electronic transactions are the most efficient. When an eligibility benefits transaction is sent, the computer program assigns a unique **trace number** to the inquiry. Often, eligibility transactions are sent the day before patients arrive for appointments. If the PMP has this feature, the eligibility transaction can be sent automatically.

The health plan responds to an eligibility inquiry with this information:

- Trace number, as a double-check on the inquiry
- Benefit information, such as whether the insurance coverage is active
- Covered period—the period of dates that the coverage is active
- Benefit units, such as how many physical therapy visits
- Coverage level—that is, who is covered, such as spouse and family or individual

The following information may also be transmitted:

- The copay amount
- The yearly deductible amount
- The coinsurance amount
- The out-of-pocket expenses
- The health plan's information on the insured's/patient's first and last names, dates of birth, and identification numbers
- Primary care provider

Procedures When the Patient Is Not Covered

If an insured patient's policy does not cover a planned service, this situation is discussed with the patient. Patients should be informed that the payer does not

HIPAA Tip

X12 270/271 Eligibility for a Health Plan Inquiry/Response

The HIPAA Eligibility for a Health Plan transaction is also called the X12 270/271. The number 270 refers to the inquiry that is sent, and 271 to the answer returned by the payer.

Billing Tip

Double-Checking Patients' Information
Review the payer's spelling of the insured's and the patient's first and last names as well as the dates of birth and identification numbers. Correct any mistakes in the record, so that when a health care claim is later transmitted for the encounter, it will be accepted for processing.

Service to be performed: ______________________
Estimated charge: ______________________
Date of planned service: ______________________
Reason for exclusion: ______________________
____

I, ____________, a patient of _____________, understand the service described above is excluded from my health insurance. I am responsible for payment in full of the charges for this service.

Figure 3.8 Sample Financial Agreement for Patient Payment of Noncovered Services

> **Billing Tip**
>
> **Processing the Patient Financial Agreement**
> Patients should be given copies of their financial agreements. A signed original is filed in the patient's record.

pay for the service and that they are responsible for the charges. For example, some plans do not pay for preventive services such as annual physical examinations. Many patients, however, consider preventive services a good idea and are willing to pay for them.

Some payers require the physician to use specific forms to tell the patient about uncovered services. These financial agreement forms, which patients must sign, prove that patients have been told about their obligation to pay the bill *before* the services are given. Figure 3.8 is an example of a form used to tell patients in advance of the probable cost of procedures that are not going to be covered by their plan and to secure their agreement to pay.

Determine Preauthorization and Referral Requirements

Preauthorization

A managed care payer often requires preauthorization before the patient sees a specialist, is admitted to the hospital, or has a particular procedure. The medical insurance specialist may request preauthorization over the phone, by e-mail or fax, or by an electronic transaction. If the payer approves the service, it issues a **prior authorization number** that must be entered in the practice management program so it will stored and appear later on the health care claim for the encounter. (This number may also be called a **certification number**.)

> **HIPAA Tip**
>
> **HIPAA Referral Certification and Authorization**
>
> *If an electronic transaction is used for referrals and preauthorizations, it must be the HIPAA Referral Certification and Authorization transaction, also called the X12 278.*

Referrals

Often, a physician needs to send a patient to another physician for evaluation and/or treatment. For example, an internist might send a patient to a cardiologist to evaluate heart function. If a patient's plan requires it, the patient is given a **referral number** and a referral document, which is a written request for the medical service. The patient is usually responsible for bringing these items to the encounter with the specialist.

A paper referral document (see Figure 3.9) describes the services the patient is certified to receive. (This approval may instead be communicated electronically using the HIPAA referral transaction.) The specialist's office handling a referred patient must:

- Check that the patient has a referral number
- Verify patient enrollment in the plan
- Understand restrictions to services, such as regulations that require the patient to visit a specialist in a specific period of time after receiving the

Referral Form

Label with Patient's Demographic & Insurance Information

Physician referred to ______________________________

Referred for:

❑ Consult only
❑ Follow-up
❑ Lab
❑ X-Ray
❑ Procedure
❑ Other

Reason for visit ______________________________

Number of visits __________

Appointment Requested: Please contact patient; phone: ____________

Primary care physician

Name ______________________________

Signature ______________________________

Phone ______________________________

Figure 3.9 Referral

referral or that limit the number of times the patient can receive services from the specialist

Two other situations arise with referrals:

1. A managed care patient may "self-refer"—come for specialty care without a referral number when one is required. The medical insurance specialist then asks the patient to sign a form acknowledging responsibility for the services. A sample form is shown in Figure 3.10a on page 90.
2. A patient who is required to have a referral document does not bring one. The medical insurance specialist then asks the patient to sign a document such as that shown in Figure 3.10 b on page 90. This **referral waiver** ensures that the patient will pay for services received if in fact a referral is not documented in the time specified.

Determine the Primary Insurance

The medical insurance specialist also examines the patient information form and insurance card to see if other coverage is in effect. A patient may have more than one health plan. The specialist then decides which is the **primary insurance**—the plan that pays first when more than one plan is in effect—and which is the **secondary insurance**—an additional policy that provides benefits. **Tertiary insurance**, a third payer, is possible. Some patients have **supplemental insurance**, a "fill-the-gap" insurance plan that covers parts of expenses, such as coinsurance, that they must otherwise pay under the primary plan.

Billing Tip

Billing Supplemental Plans

Supplemental insurance held with the same payer can be billed on a single claim. Claims for supplemental insurance held with other than the primary payer are sent after the primary payer's payment is posted, just as secondary claims are.

Member Self-Referral Acknowledgment

I, _______________________, understand that I am seeking the care of this specialty physician or health care provider, _______________, without a referral from my primary care physician. I understand that the terms of my Plan coverage require that I obtain that referral, and that if I fail to do so, my Plan will not cover any part of the charges, costs or expenses related to this specialist's services to me.

Signed,

_______________________ _______________

(member's name) (date)

****

Specialty physician or other health care provider:

Please keep a copy of this form in your patient's file

(a)

Referral Waiver

I did not bring a referral for the medical services I will receive today. If my primary care physician does not provide a referral within two days, I understand that I am responsible for paying for the services I am requesting.

Signature: _______________________________

Date: _______________

(b)

Figure 3.10 (a) Self-Referral Document, (b) Referral Waiver

> **HIPAA Tip**
>
> **HIPAA Coordination of Benefits**
>
> *The HIPAA Coordination of Benefits transaction is used to send the necessary data to payers. This transaction is also called the X12 837—the same transaction used to send health care claims electronically—because it goes along with the claim.*

As a practical matter for billing, determining the primary insurance is important because this payer is sent the first claim for the encounter. A second claim is sent to the secondary payer after the payment is received for the primary claim.

Deciding which payer is primary is also important because insurance policies contain a provision called **coordination of benefits (COB)**. The coordination of benefits guidelines ensure that when a patient has more than one policy, maximum appropriate benefits are paid, but without duplication. Under the law, to protect the insurance companies, if the patient has signed an assignment of benefits statement, the provider is responsible for reporting any additional insurance coverage to the primary payer.

Coordination of benefits in government-sponsored programs follows specific guidelines. Primary and secondary coverage under Medicare, Medicaid, and other programs is discussed in Chapters 10, 11, and 12. Note that COB information can also be exchanged between provider and health plan or between a health plan and another payer, such as auto insurance.

Guidelines for Determining the Primary Insurance

How do patients come to have more than one plan in effect? Possible answers are that a patient may have coverage under more than one group plan, such as

TABLE 3.1 Determining Primary Coverage
• If the patient has only one policy, it is primary. • If the patient has coverage under two plans, the plan that has been in effect for the patient for the longest period of time is primary. However, if an active employee has a plan with the present employer and is still covered by a former employer's plan as a retiree or a laid-off employee, the current employer's plan is primary.
• If the patient is also covered as a dependent under another insurance policy, the patient's plan is primary.
• If an employed patient has coverage under the employer's plan and additional coverage under a government-sponsored plan, the employer's plan is primary. For example, if a patient is enrolled in a PPO through employment and is also on Medicare, the PPO is primary.
• If a retired patient is covered by a spouse's employer's plan and the spouse is still employed, the spouse's plan is primary, even if the retired person has Medicare.
• If the patient is a dependent child covered by both parents' plans and the parents are not separated or divorced (or if the parents have joint custody of the child), the primary plan is determined by the birthday rule.
• If two or more plans cover dependent children of separated or divorced parents who do not have joint custody of their children, the children's primary plan is determined in this order: — The plan of the custodial parent — The plan of the spouse of the custodial parent if remarried — The plan of the parent without custody

a person who has both employer-sponsored insurance and a policy from union membership. A person may have primary insurance coverage from an employer but also be covered as a dependent under a spouse's insurance, making the spouse's plan the person's additional insurance.

General guidelines for determining the primary insurance are shown in Table 3.1.

Guidelines for Children with More than One Insurance Plan

A child's parents may each have primary insurance. If both parents cover dependents on their plans, the child's primary insurance is usually determined by the **birthday rule**. This rule states that the parent whose day of birth is earlier in the calendar year is primary. For example, Rachel Foster's mother and father both work and have employer-sponsored insurance policies. Her father, George Foster, was born on October 7, 1971, and her mother, Myrna, was born on May 15, 1972. Since the mother's date of birth is earlier in the calendar year (although the father is older), her plan is Rachel's primary insurance. The father's plan is secondary for Rachel. Note that if a dependent child's primary insurance does not provide for the complete reimbursement of a bill, the balance may usually be submitted to the other parent's plan for consideration.

Another, much less common, way to determine a child's primary coverage is called the **gender rule**. When this rule applies, if the child is covered by two health plans, the father's plan is primary. In some states, insurance regulations require a plan that uses the gender rule to be primary to a plan that follows the birthday rule.

The insurance policy also covers which parent's plan is primary for dependent children of separated or divorced parents. If the parents have joint custody, the birthday rule usually applies. If the parents do not have joint custody of the child, unless otherwise directed by a court order, usually the primary benefits are determined in this order:

- The plan of the custodial parent
- The plan of the spouse of the custodial parent, if the parent has remarried
- The plan of the parent without custody

Entering Insurance Information in the Practice Management Program

The practice management program contains a database of the payers from whom the medical practice usually receives payments. The database contains each payer's name and the contact's name; the plan type, such as HMO, PPO, Medicare, Medicaid, or other; and telephone and fax numbers. Like the patient database, the payer database must be updated to reflect changes, such as new participation agreements or a new payer representative contact information.

The medical insurance specialist selects the payer that is the patient's primary insurance coverage from the insurance database. If the particular payer has not already been entered, the PMP is updated with the payer's information. Secondary coverage is also selected for the patient as applicable. Other related facts, such as policy numbers, effective dates, and referral numbers, are entered for each patient.

Communications with Payers

Communications with payers' representatives—whether to check on eligibility, receive referral certification, or resolve billing disputes—are frequent and are vitally important to the medical practice. Getting answers quickly means quicker payment for services. Medical insurance specialists follow these guidelines for effective communication:

- Learn the name, telephone number/extension, and e-mail address of the appropriate representative at each payer. If possible, invite the representative to visit the office and meet the staff.
- Use a professional, courteous telephone manner or writing style to help build good relationships.
- Keep current with changing reimbursement policies and utilization guidelines by regularly reviewing information from payers. Usually, the medical practice receives Internet or printed bulletins or newsletters that contain up-to-date information from health plans and government-sponsored programs.

All communications with payer representatives should be documented in the patient's financial record. The representative's name, the date of the communication, and the outcome should be described. This information is sometimes needed later to explain or defend a charge on a patient's insurance claim.

Compliance Guideline

Payer Communications
Payer communications are documented in the financial record rather than the medical (clinical) record.

Updating Patient Diagnoses, Procedures, and Charges

After the registration process is complete, patients are shown to rooms for their appointments with providers. In offices using traditional medical records, the provider documents the encounter in the patient's chart. If the office uses electronic medical records, a suitable template is completed by the provider. After the visit, the medical insurance specialist uses the documented diagnoses and procedures to update the practice management program and to total charges for the visit.

Encounter Forms

During or just after a visit, an **encounter form** – either electronic or paper — is completed by a provider to summarize billing information for a patient's visit. This may be done using a device such as a laptop computer, tablet PC, or PDA (personal digital assistant), or by checking off items on a paper form. Physicians should sign and date the completed encounter forms for their patients.

VALLEY ASSOCIATES, PC
Christopher M. Connolly, MD - Internal Medicine
555-967-0303
FED I.D. #16-1234567

PATIENT NAME				APPT. DATE/TIME			
Deysenrothe, Mae J.				10/6/2008 9:30 am			
PATIENT NO.				**DX**			
DEYSEMA0				1. V70.0 Exam, Adult 2. 3. 4.			
DESCRIPTION	**✓**	**CPT**	**FEE**	**DESCRIPTION**	**✓**	**CPT**	**FEE**
OFFICE VISITS				**PROCEDURES**			
New Patient				Diagnostic Anoscopy		46600	
LI Problem Focused		99201		ECG Complete	✓	93000	70
LII Expanded		99202		I&D, Abscess		10060	
LIII Detailed		99203		Pap Smear		88150	
LIV Comp./Mod.		99204		Removal of Cerumen		69210	
LV Comp./High		99205		Removal 1 Lesion		17000	
Established Patient				Removal 2-14 Lesions		17003	
LI Minimum		99211		Removal 15+ Lesions		17004	
LII Problem Focused		99212		Rhythm ECG w/Report		93040	
LIII Expanded		99213		Rhythm ECG w/Tracing		93041	
LIV Detailed		99214		Sigmoidoscopy, diag.		45330	
LV Comp./High		99215					
				LABORATORY			
PREVENTIVE VISIT				Bacteria Culture		87081	
New Patient				Fungal Culture		87101	
Age 12-17		99384		Glucose Finger Stick		82948	
Age 18-39		99385		Lipid Panel		80061	
Age 40-64	✓	99386	180	Specimen Handling		99000	
Age 65+		99387		Stool/Occult Blood		82270	
Established Patient				Tine Test		85008	
Age 12-17		99394		Tuberculin PPD		85590	
Age 18-39		99395		Urinalysis	✓	81000	17
Age 40-64		99396		Venipuncture		36415	
Age 65+		99397					
				INJECTION/IMMUN.			
CONSULTATION: OFFICE/OP				Immun. Admin.	✓	90471	20
Requested By:				Ea. Addl.		90472	
LI Problem Focused		99241		Hepatitis A Immun		90632	
LII Expanded		99242		Hepatitis B Immun		90746	
LIII Detailed		99243		Influenza Immun	✓	90659	68
LIV Comp./Mod.		99244		Pneumovax		90732	
LV Comp./High		99245					
				TOTAL FEES			355

Figure 3.11 Completed Encounter Form

Encounter forms record the services provided to a patient, as shown in the completed office encounter form in Figure 3.11. These forms (also called **superbills**, charge slips, or routing slips) list the medical practice's most frequently performed procedures with their procedure codes. It also often has blanks where the diagnosis and its code(s) are filled in. (Some forms include a list of the diagnoses that are most frequently made by the practice's physicians.)

Thinking it Through — 3.2

When a patient has secondary insurance, the claim for that payer is sent after the claim to the primary payer is paid. Why is that the case? What information do you think the medical insurance specialist provides to the secondary payer?

Billing Tip

Encounter Forms for Hospital Visits
Specially designed encounter forms (sometimes called hospital charge tickets) are used when the provider sees patients in the hospital. These forms list the patient's identification and date of service, but they may show different diagnoses and procedure codes for the care typically provided in the hospital setting.

Billing Tip

Numbering Encounter Forms
Encounter forms should be prenumbered to make sure that all the days' appointments jibe with the day's encounter forms. This provides a check that all visits have been entered in the practice management program for accurate charge capture.

Other information is often included on the form:

- A checklist of managed care plans under contract and their utilization guidelines
- The patient's prior balance due, if any
- Check boxes to indicate the timing and need for a follow-up appointment to be scheduled for the patient during checkout

Preprinted or Computer-Generated Encounter Forms

The paper form may be designed by the practice manager and/or physicians based on analysis of the practice's medical services. It is then printed, usually with carbonless copies available for distribution according to the practice's policy. For example, the top copy may be filed in the medical record; the second copy may be filed in the financial record; and the third copy may be given to the patient.

Alternatively, the form may be printed for each patient's appointment using the practice management program. A customized encounter form lists the date of the appointment, the patient's name, and the identification number assigned by the medical practice. It can also be designed to show the patient's previous balance, the day's fees, payments made, and the amount due.

Communications with Providers

At times, medical insurance specialists find incorrect or conflicting data on encounter forms. It may be necessary to check the documentation and, if still problematic, with the physician to clear up the discrepancies. In such cases, it is important to remember that medical practices are extremely busy places. Providers often have crowded schedules, especially if they see many patients, and have little time to go over billing and coding issues. Questions must be kept to those that are essential for correct billing.

Also, encounter forms (and practice management programs) list procedure codes and, often, diagnosis codes that change periodically. Medical insurance specialists must be sure that these databases are updated when new codes are issued and old codes are modified or dropped (see Chapters 4, 5, and 6). They also bring key changes in codes or payers' coverage to the providers' attention. Usually the practice manager arranges a time to discuss such matters with the physicians.

Thinking it Through — 3.3

Review the completed encounter form shown in Figure 3.11 on page 93.

1. What is the age range of the patient?
2. Is this a new or an established patient?
3. What procedures were performed during the encounter?
4. What laboratory tests were ordered?

Collecting Time-of-Service Payments and Checking Out Patients

The practice management program is used to record the financial transactions that result from patients' visits:

- Charges—the amounts that providers bill for services performed
- Payments—monies the practice receive from health plans and patients
- **Adjustments**—changes to patients' accounts, such as returned check fees

Information from the encounter form is entered in the program to calculate charges. The program is also used to record patients' payments, print receipts, and compute patients' outstanding account balances. Later, when insurance payments are received for insured patients, the amounts are posted to the patient's account in the program, reducing the balance that the patient owes.

Collections at the Time of Service

Up-front collection—money collected before the patient leaves the office—is an important part of cash flow. Practices routinely collect the following charges at the time of service:

- Copayments
- Noncovered or overlimit fees
- Charges of nonparticipating providers
- Charges for self-pay patients

Some practices also collect deductibles at the time of service.

Copayments

Copayments are always collected at the time of service. In some practices, they are collected before the encounter; in others, right after the encounter.

The copayment amount depends on the type of service and on whether the provider is in the patient's network. Copays for out-of-network providers are usually higher than for in-network providers. Specific copay amounts may be required for office visits to PCPs versus specialists and for lab work, radiology services such as X-rays, and surgery.

When a patient receives more than one covered service in a single day, the health plan may permit multiple copayments. For example, copays for both an annual physical exam and for lab tests may be due from the patient. Review the terms of the policy to determine whether multiple copays should be collected on the same day of service.

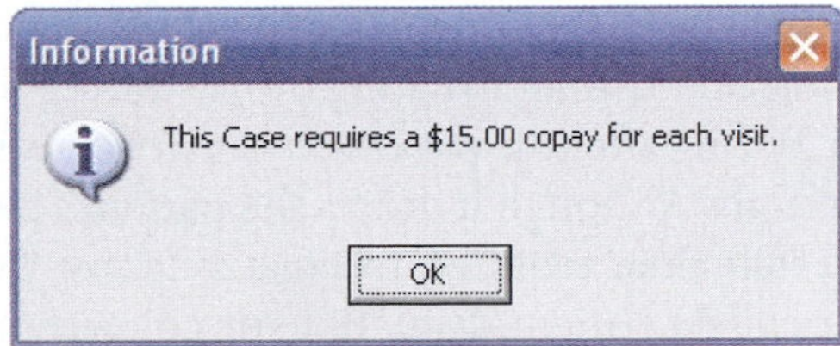

Charges for Noncovered/Overlimit Services

Insurance policies require patients to pay for noncovered (excluded) services, and payers do not control what the providers charge for noncovered services. Likewise, if the plan has a limit on the usage of certain covered services, patients are responsible for paying for visits beyond the allowed number. For example,

Billing Tip

Collecting Copays

- Many offices tell patients who are scheduling visits what copays they will owe at the time of service.
- Keep change to make it easier for cash patients to make time-of-service payments.
- Ask for payment. "We verified your insurance coverage, and there is a copay that is your responsibility. Would you like to pay by cash, check, or credit or debit card?"

HIPAA Tip

Billing for Medical Record Copies

Under HIPAA, it is permissible to bill patients a reasonable charge for supplying copies of their medical records. Costs include labor, supplies, postage, and time to prepare record summaries. Practices must check state laws, however, to see if there is a per-page charge limit.

Billing Tip

Copayment Reminder

Many practice management programs have a copayment reminder feature that shows the copayment that is due.

if five physical therapy encounters are permitted annually, the patient must pay for any additional visits. Practices usually collect these charges from patients at the time of service.

Charges of Nonparticipating Providers

As noted earlier in this chapter, when patients have encounters with a provider who participates in the plan under which they have coverage—such as a Medicare-participating provider—they sign assignment of benefits statements. This authorizes the provider to **accept assignment** for the patients—that is, to file claims for the patient and receive payments directly from the payer. If the provider is nonparticipating but the practice is billing the plan for the patient to receive out-of-network benefits, the patient is usually asked to assign benefits so that payment can be collected directly. However, note that some nonparticipating physicians require full payment from patients and do not file claims on their behalf.

Charges for Services to Self-Pay Patients

Patients who do not have insurance coverage are called **self-pay patients**. Since more than 45 million Americans do not have insurance, self-pay patients present for office visits daily. Medical insurance specialists follow the practice's procedures for informing patients of their responsibility for paying their bills. Practices may require self-pay patients to pay their bills in full at the time of service.

Deductibles

Some practices have the policy of collecting patients' annual deductibles at the time of service. If this is the case, the medical insurance specialist researches the amount of the deductible and the amount the patient has already paid.

Deciding When to Bill Patients: Before or After Insurance Payments?

The practice must decide whether to collect patient charges other than the four types discussed above. There are two options:

1. *Collect all charges at the time of service*: Calculate charges based on the physician's usual fees or estimate the payer's likely reimbursement, and collect payment from patients before claims are sent and payment is received.
2. *Bill charges after claims are paid:* Submit claims and bill patients after payment is made by the payer.

The first option has the advantage of producing payments from patients faster. It is problematic, though, because the payer's reimbursement is almost always different from the physician's usual fees due to contracted fee schedules. If patients pay before claims are paid, they often must be billed again or sent a refund, requiring more staff time and risking irritating or frustrating the patient.

The second option, billing after the payer's payment is received, ensures that patients are billed correctly. Although it delays the patient's payment, it also reduces the amount of staff time required to create claims. For these reasons, most practices do not collect patient deductible or coinsurance charges at the time of service. Usually, patients are billed after payers' reimbursements are received (see Chapters 14 and 15).

Compliance Guideline

Collecting Charges
Some payers (especially government programs) do not permit providers to collect any charges except copayments from patients until insurance claims are adjudicated. Be sure to comply with the payer's rules.

Financial Policy

Patients should always be reminded of their financial obligations according to practice procedures. The practice's **financial policy** on payment for services is usually either displayed on the wall of the reception area or included in a new patient information packet. A sample of a financial policy is shown in Figure 3.12.

The policy should explain what is required of the patient and when payment is due. For example, the policy may state the following:

For unassigned claims: Payment for the physician's services is expected at the end of your appointment unless you have made other arrangements with our practice manager.

For assigned claims: After your insurance claim is processed by your insurance company, you will be billed for any amount you owe. You are responsible for any part of the charges that are denied or not paid by the carrier. All patient accounts are due within thirty days of the date of the invoice.

Copayments: Copayments must be paid before patients leave the office.

We sincerely wish to provide the best possible medical care. This involves mutual understanding between the patients, doctors, and staff. We encourage, you, our patient, to discuss any questions you may have regarding this payment policy.

Payment is expected at the time of your visit for services not covered by your insurance plan. We accept cash, check, MasterCard, and Visa.

Credit will be extended as necessary.

Credit Policy
Requirements for maintaining your account in good standing are as follows:

1. All charges are due and payable within 30 days of the first billing.
2. For services not covered by your health plan, payment at the time of service is necessary.
3. If other circumstances warrant an extended payment plan, our credit counselor will assist you in these special circumstances at your request.

We welcome early discussion of financial problems. A credit counselor will assist you.

An itemized statement of all medical services will be mailed to you every 30 days. We will prepare and file your claim forms to the health plan. If further information is needed, we will provide an additional report.

Insurance
Unless we have a contract directly with your health plan, we cannot accept the responsibility of negotiating claims. You, the patient, are responsible for payment of medical care regardless of the status of the medical claim. In situations where a claim is pending or when treatment will be over an extended period of time, we will recommend that a payment plan be initiated. Your health plan is a contract between you and your insurance company. We cannot guarantee the payment of your claim. If your insurance company pays only a portion of the bill or denies the claim, any contact or explanation should be made to you, the policyholder. Reduction or rejection of your claim by your insurance company does not relieve the financial obligation you have incurred.

Figure 3.12 Example of a Financial Policy

Estimating What the Patient Will Owe

Many times, patients want to know what their bills will be. For practices that collect patient accounts at the time of service and for high-deductible insurance plans, the physician practice also wants to know what a patient owes so that a payment plan can be agreed to.

To estimate these charges, the medical insurance specialist verifies:

- The patient's deductible amount and whether it has been paid in full, the covered benefits, and coinsurance or other patient financial obligations
- The payer's allowed charges for the planned or provided services

Based on these facts, the specialist calculates the probable bill for the patient.

There are other tools that can be used to estimate charges. Some payers have a swipe-card reader (like a credit card processing device) that can be installed in the reception area and used by patients to learn what the insurer will pay and what the patient owes. Most practice management programs have a feature that permits estimating the patient's bill, as shown below:

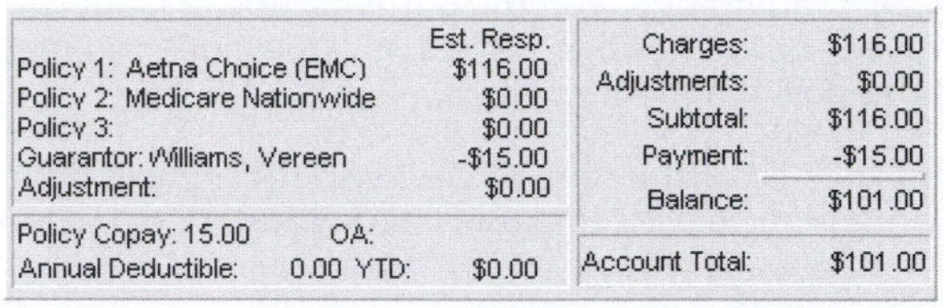

	Est. Resp.
Policy 1: Aetna Choice (EMC)	$116.00
Policy 2: Medicare Nationwide	$0.00
Policy 3:	$0.00
Guarantor: Williams, Vereen	-$15.00
Adjustment:	$0.00
Policy Copay: 15.00 OA:	
Annual Deductible: 0.00 YTD:	$0.00

Charges:	$116.00
Adjustments:	$0.00
Subtotal:	$116.00
Payment:	-$15.00
Balance:	$101.00
Account Total:	$101.00

Financial Arrangements for Large Bills

If patients have large bills that they must pay over time, a financial arrangement for a series of payments may be made (see Figure 3.13). The payments may begin with a prepayment followed by monthly amounts. Such arrangements usually require the approval of the practice manager. They may also be governed by state laws. Payment plans are covered in greater depth in Chapter 15.

Checkout Procedures

After the patient's encounter, the medical insurance specialist posts (that is, enters in the PMP) the patient's case information and diagnosis. Then the day's procedures are posted, and the program calculates the charges. Payments from the patient are entered, and the account is brought up to date.

Billing Tip

Use of Credit and Debit Cards
Accepting credit or debit cards requires paying a fee to the credit card carrier. It is generally considered worth the cost because payments are made immediately and are more convenient for the patient.

Payment Methods: Cash, Check, and Credit or Debit Card

The medical insurance specialist handles patients' payments as follows:

- *Cash:* If payment is made by cash, a receipt is issued.
- *Check:* If payment is made with a check, the amount of the payment and the check number are entered on the encounter form, and a receipt is offered.
- *Credit or debit card:* If the bill is paid with a credit or debit card, the card slip is filled out, and the card is passed through the card reader. A transaction authorization number is received from the card issuer, and the approved card slip is signed by the person paying the bill. The patient is usually offered a receipt in addition to the copy of the credit card sales

Patient Name and Account Number

Total of All Payments Due

FEE	$__________	
PARTIAL PAYMENT	$__________	
UNPAID BALANCE	$__________	
AMOUNT FINANCED	$__________	(amount of credit we have provided to you)
FINANCE CHARGE	$__________	(dollar amount the interest on credit will cost)
ANNUAL PERCENTAGE RATE	$__________	(cost of your credit as a yearly rate)
TOTAL OF PAYMENTS DUE	$__________	(amount paid after all payments are made)

Rights and Duties

I (we) have reviewed the above fees. I agree to make ________ payments in monthly installments of $ ________, due on the _____ day of each month payable to ________, until the total amount is paid in full. The first payment is due on ________. I may request an itemization of the amount financed.

Delinquent Accounts

I (we) understand that I am financially responsible for all fees as stated. My account will be overdue if my scheduled payment is more than 7 days late. There will be a late payment charge of $________ or _____% of the payment, whichever is less. I understand that I will be legally responsible for all costs involved with the collection of this account including all court costs, reasonable attorney fees, and all other expenses incurred with collection if I default on this agreement.

Prepayment Penalty

There is no penalty if the total amount due is paid before the last scheduled payment.

I (we) agree to the terms of the above financial contract.

______________________________ ______________
Signature of Patient, Parent or Legal Representative Date

______________________________ ______________
Witness Date

______________________________ ______________
Authorizing Signature Date

Figure 3.13 Financial Arrangement for Services Form

slip. Telephone approval may be needed if the amount is over a specified limit.

Some practices ask a patient who wants to use a credit or debit card to complete a preauthorization form (see Figure 3.14 on page 100). The patient can authorize charging copays, deductibles, and balances for all visits during a year. The authorization should be renewed according to practice policy.

Walkout Receipts

If the provider has not accepted assignment and is not going to file a claim for a patient, the PMP is used to create a walkout receipt for the patient. The **walkout receipt** summarizes the services and charges for that day as well as any

HIPAA Tip

Identity Theft

To avoid the risk of identity theft, the HIPAA Security Rule requires medical practices to protect patients' credit/debit card information.

Provider's name:____

Provider's tax ID no.: ____

I assign my insurance benefits to the provider listed above. This credit card authorization form is valid for one year unless I cancel the authorization through written notice to the provider.

Patient name	Cardholder name
Billing address	
City	State / Zip
Credit card account number	Expiration date
Cardholder signature	Date

I authorize ______________________________ (provider) to keep my signature/account number on file and to charge my American Express/Discover/Visa/Mastercard/Other credit card account number listed above for the balance of charges not paid by insurance within 90 days and not to exceed $_______.

Figure 3.14 Preauthorized Credit Card Payment Form

payment the patient made (see Figure 3.15). Practices generally handle unassigned claims in one of two ways:

1. The payment is collected from the patient at the time of service (at the end of the encounter). The patient then uses the walkout receipt to report the charges and payments to the insurance company. The insurance company repays the patient (or insured) according to the terms of the plan.
2. The practice collects payment from the patient at the time of service and then sends a claim to the plan on behalf of the patient. The insurance company sends a refund check to the patient with an explanation of benefits.

Thinking it Through — 3.4

1. Why are up-front collections important to the practice?
2. Read the financial policy shown in Figure 3.12. If a patient presents for noncovered services, when is payment expected? Does the provider accept assignment for plans in which it is nonPAR?

Valley Associates, P.C.
1400 West Center Street
Toledo, OH 43601-0123
(555)321-0987

Page: 1 10/1/2008

Patient: Walter Williams
17 Mill Rd
Brooklyn, OH 44144-4567

Chart #: WILLIWA0
Case #: 8

Instructions:
Complete the patient information portion of your insurance claim form. Attach this bill, signed and dated, and all other bills pertaining to the claim. If you have a deductible policy, hold your claim forms until you have met your deductible. Mail directly to your insurance carrier.

Date	Description	Procedure	Modify	Dx 1	Dx 2	Dx 3	Dx 4	Units	Charge
10/1/2008	EP Problem Focused	99212		401.1	780.7			1	46.00
10/1/2008	ECG Complete	93000		401.1	780.7			1	70.00
10/1/2008	Aetna Copayment	AETCPAY						1	-15.00

Provider Information

Provider Name:	Christopher Connolly M.D.
License:	37C4629
Commercial PIN:	
SSN or EIN:	16-1234567

Total Charges:	$ 116.00
Total Payments:	-$ 15.00
Total Adjustments:	$ 0.00
Total Due This Visit:	**$ 101.00**
Total Account Balance:	$ 101.00

Assign and Release: I hereby authorize payment of medical benefits to this physician for the services described above. I also authorize the release of any information necessary to process this claim.

Patient Signature: ________________________ Date: __________

Figure 3.15 Walkout Receipt

Review

Steps to Success

- ❒ Read this chapter and review the Key Terms and the Chapter Summary.
- ❒ Answer the Review Questions and Applying Your Knowledge in the Chapter Review.
- ❒ Access the chapter's websites and complete the Internet Activities to learn more about available professional resources.
- ❒ Complete the related chapter in the *Medical Insurance Workbook* to reinforce your understanding of patient encounters and billing information.

Chapter Summary

1. A new patient (NP) has not received any services from the provider (or another provider of the same specialty who is a member of the same practice) within the past three years. An established patient (EP) has seen the provider (or another provider in the practice who has the same specialty) within the past three years.
2. During preregistration, basic information about the patient is gathered to check that the patient's health care requirements are appropriate for the medical practice, to schedule an appointment of the correct length, and to determine whether the physician participates in the caller's health plan in order to establish responsibility for payment. When a patient arrives for an appointment, a medical history form is completed for the physician's use. The patient information form is completed to gather demographic information such as personal, biographical, and employment information; insurance coverage; and emergency contact and related information. Patient information forms are reviewed annually by established patients to confirm the information. The insurance card is scanned or photocopied; all information is double-checked against the patient information form.
3. An assignment of benefits statement may also be signed by a patient or policyholder. This form authorizes the provider to receive payments for medical services directly from payers.
4. Every patient must be given the office's Notice of Privacy Practices once and must be asked to sign an Acknowledgment of Receipt of Notice of Privacy Practices. This process is followed and documented to show that the office has made a good-faith effort to inform patients of the privacy practices.
5. Medical insurance specialists contact payers to verify patients' plan enrollment and eligibility for benefits. If done electronically, the HIPAA Eligibility for a Health Plan transaction is used. Patients' insurance cards are scanned or photocopied, and their patient information or update forms are checked against the cards. Covered services, restrictions to benefits, various copayment requirements, and/or deductible status may also be checked. Referrals and authorizations for services are handled electronically with the HIPAA Referral Certification and Authorization transaction.
6. Primary insurance coverage is determined when more than one policy is in effect. This determination is based on coordination of benefits rules. The HIPAA Coordination of Benefits transaction may be used to transmit data to payers.
7. Encounter forms are lists of the medical practice's most commonly performed services and procedures and often of frequent diagnoses. The provider checks off the services and proce-

dures a patient received. The encounter form is then used for billing.

8. Patients may be responsible for copayments, excluded services, overlimit usage, and coinsurance. Patients often must meet deductibles before receiving benefits, and some offices collect this, too.
9. After a patient encounter, the medical insurance specialist uses the completed encounter form and the patient medical record to code or verify assigned codes and to analyze the billable services. The charges for these services are calculated; copayments and other fees are collected from patients according to practice policy; and patients' accounts are updated. Walkout receipts are given for any payments patients make.
10. Throughout the billing and reimbursement cycle, communication skills are critical to keeping patients satisfied. Equally important are good relationships with third-party payer representatives who can help smooth the payment process. Medical insurance specialists also communicate important changes in payers' policies to providers and work with the health care team to answer patients' billing questions.

Review Questions

Match the key terms with their definitions.

A. direct provider
B. assignment of benefits
C. new patient
D. secondary insurance
E. encounter form
F. established patient
G. insured
H. coordination of benefits
I. walkout receipt
J. patient information form

____ 1. Form used to summarize the treatments and services patients receive during visits

____ 2. Policyholder, guarantor, or subscriber

____ 3. Authorization by a policyholder that allows a payer to pay benefits directly to a provider

____ 4. The insurance plan that pays benefits after payment by the primary payer when a patient is covered by more than one medical insurance plan

____ 5. The provider who treats the patient

____ 6. A clause in an insurance policy that explains how the policy will pay if more than one insurance policy applies to the claim

____ 7. A patient who has received professional services from a provider, or another provider in the same practice with the same specialty, in the past three years

____ 8. Form completed by patients that summarizes their demographic and insurance information

____ 9. A patient who has not received professional services from a provider, or another provider in the same practice with the same specialty, in the past three years

____10. Document given to a patient who makes a payment

Decide whether each statement is true or false.

____ 1. The HIPAA Health Care Claims or Equivalent Encounter Information/Coordination of Benefits transaction is used for both health care claims and coordination of benefits because secondary payer information goes along with the claim to the primary payer.

____ 2. If both of Gary's parents have primary medical insurance, his father's date of birth is February 13, 1969, and his mother's date of birth is March 4, 1968, his mother's plan is Gary's primary insurance under the birthday rule.

____ 3. Accepting assignment of benefits means that the physician bills the payer on behalf of the patient and receives payment directly.

____ 4. A provider may not treat a patient unless the patient has first signed an Acknowledgment of Receipt of Notice of Privacy Practices.

____ 5. The provider does not need authorization to release a patient's PHI for treatment, payment, or operations purposes.

____ 6. The HIPAA Eligibility for a Health Plan transaction may be used to determine a patient's insurance coverage.

____ 7. Patients' dates of birth should be recorded using all four digits of the year of birth.

____ 8. Patients' insurance benefits are usually verified after provider encounters.

____ 9. The policyholder and the patient are always the same individual.

____ 10. Copayments are collected at the time of service.

Select the letter that best completes the statement or answers the question.

____ 1. A patient's group insurance number written on the patient information or update form must match:
   A. the patient's Social Security number
   B. the number on the patient's insurance card
   C. the practice's identification number for the patient
   D. the diagnosis codes

____ 2. If a health plan member receives medical services from a provider who does not participate in the plan, the cost to the member is:
   A. lower
   B. higher
   C. the same
   D. negotiable

____ 3. What information does a patient information form gather?
   A. the patient's personal information, employment data, and insurance information
   B. the patient's history of present illness, past medical history, and examination results
   C. the patient's chief complaint
   D. the patient's insurance plan deductible and/or copayment requirements

____ 4. If a husband has an insurance policy but is also eligible for benefits as a dependent under his wife's insurance policy, the wife's policy is considered _____ for him.
   A. primary
   B. participating
   C. secondary
   D. coordinated

____ 5. A certification number for a procedure is the result of which transaction and process?
   A. claim status
   B. health care payment and remittance advice
   C. coordination of benefits
   D. referral and authorization

____ 6. A completed encounter form contains:

A. information about the patient's diagnosis

B. information on the procedures performed during the encounter

C. both A and B

D. neither A nor B

____ 7. The encounter form is a source of _____ information for the medical insurance specialist.

A. billing

B. treatment plan

C. third-party payment

D. credit card

____ 8. Under HIPAA, what must be verified about a person who requests PHI?

A. identity

B. authorization to access the information

C. either A or B

D. both A and B

____ 9. Which charges are usually collected at the time of service?

A. copayments, lab fees, and therapy charges

B. copayments, noncovered or overlimit fees, charges of nonparticipating providers, and charges for self-pay patients

C. deductibles and lab fees

D. coinsurance

____ 10. The tertiary insurance pays:

A. after the first and second payers

B. after the first payer

C. after receipt of the claim

D. none of the above

Answer the following questions.

1. Define the following abbreviations:

A. nonPAR ____

____

B. COB ____

____

C. PAR ____

____

D. NP ____

____

E. EP ____

____

Applying Your Knowledge

Case 3.1 Abstracting Insurance Information

Carol Viragras saw Dr. Alex Roderer, a gynecologist with the Alper Group, a multispecialty practice of 235 physicians, on October 24, 2007. On December 3, 2009, she made an appointment to see Dr. Judy Fisk, a gastroenterologist also with the Alper Group. Did the medical insurance specialist handling Dr. Fisk's patients classify Carol as a new or an established patient?

Case 3.2 Documenting Communications

Harry Cornprost, a patient of Dr. Connelley, calls on October 25, 2007, to cancel his appointment for October 31 because he will be out of town. The appointment is rescheduled for December 4. How would you document this call?

Case 3.3 Coordinating Benefits

Based on the information provided, determine the primary insurance in each case.

A. George Rangley enrolled in the ACR plan in 2008 and in the New York Health plan in 2006.

   George's primary plan: ____________________

B. Mary is the child of Gloria and Craig Bivilaque, who are divorced. Mary is a dependent under both Craig's and Gloria's plans. Gloria has custody of Mary.

   Mary's primary plan: ____________________

C. Karen Kaplan's date of birth is 10/11/1970; her husband Carl was born on 12/8/1971. Their child Ralph was born on 4/15/2000. Ralph is a dependent under both Karen's and Carl's plans.

   Ralph's primary plan: ____________________

D. Belle Estaphan has medical insurance from Internet Services, from which she retired last year. She is on Medicare but is also covered under her husband Bernard's plan from Orion International, where he works.

   Belle's primary plan: ____________________

E. Jim Larenges is covered under his spouse's plan and also has medical insurance through his employer.

   Jim's primary plan: ____________________

Case 3.4 Calculating Insurance Math

A. A patient's insurance policy states:

   Annual deductible: $300.00
   Coinsurance: 70/30

   This year the patient has made payments totaling $533.00 to all providers. Today the patient has an office visit (fee: $80.00). The patient presents a credit card for payment of today's bill. What is the amount that the patient should pay?

B. A patient is a member of a health plan with a 15 percent discount from the provider's usual fees and a $10.00 copay. The days' charges are $480.00. What are the amounts that the HMO and the patient each pay?

C. A patient is a member of a health plan that has a 20 percent discount from the provider and a 15 percent copay. If the day's charges are $210.00, what are the amounts that the HMO and the patient each pay?

Internet Activities

1. Research new updates on HIPAA rules at the Office of Civil Rights (OCR): http://www.hhs.gov/ocr/hipaa.
2. Investigate the website for your state's Blue Cross and Blue Shield Association member plan. Research the information that is on the patient's ID card in a selected BCBS plan.

Part 2 Claim Coding

Chapter 4
Diagnostic Coding: Introduction to ICD-9-CM

Chapter 5
Procedural Coding: Introduction to CPT

Chapter 6
Procedural Coding: Introduction to HCPCS

Chapter 4

Diagnostic Coding: Introduction to ICD-9-CM

CHAPTER OUTLINE

The ICD-9-CM

New Version: ICD-10-CM

Organization of the ICD-9-CM

The Alphabetic Index

The Tabular List

V Codes and E Codes

Coding Steps

Official Coding Guidelines

Overview of ICD-9-CM Chapters

Learning Outcomes

After studying this chapter, you should be able to:

1. Discuss the purpose of the ICD-9-CM.
2. Explain how to locate the periodic updates to ICD-9-CM codes using the Internet.
3. Describe the structure and content of the Alphabetic Index and the Tabular List.
4. Understand the conventions that are followed in the Alphabetic Index and the Tabular List.
5. Identify the purpose and correct use of V codes.
6. Identify the purpose and correct use of E codes.
7. List the three steps in the diagnostic coding process.
8. Explain how to locate the ICD-9-CM Official Guidelines for Coding and Reporting using the Internet.
9. Describe and provide examples of three key coding guidelines.
10. Analyze diagnostic statements, apply appropriate coding guidelines, and assign correct ICD-9-CM codes.

Key Terms

acute
addenda
adverse effect
Alphabetic Index
category
chief complaint (CC)
chronic
coexisting condition
combination code
convention
crosswalk
diagnostic statement
E code
eponym
etiology
ICD-9-CM
ICD-9-CM Official Guidelines for Coding and Reporting
late effect
main term
manifestation
NEC (not elsewhere classified)
NOS (not otherwise specified)
primary diagnosis
subcategory
subclassification
subterm
supplementary term
Table of Drugs and Chemicals
Tabular List
unspecified
V code

Scientists and medical researchers have long gathered information from medical records about patients' illnesses and causes of death. In place of written descriptions of many different symptoms and conditions, standardized diagnosis codes have been developed. A coding system provides an accurate way to collect statistics to keep people healthy and to plan for needed health care resources as well as to record morbidity (disease) and mortality (death) data.

In physicians' practices, diagnosis codes are used to report patients' conditions on claims. The physician determines the diagnosis. The physician, medical coder, insurance or billing specialist, or medical assistant may be responsible for assigning the code for the diagnosis. Expertise in diagnostic coding requires knowledge of medical terminology, pathophysiology, and anatomy as well as experience in correctly applying the guidelines for assigning codes.

This chapter provides a fundamental understanding of current diagnostic coding principles and guidelines—and how to keep up with changing codes—so that medical insurance specialists can work effectively with health care claims.

The ICD-9-CM

The diagnosis codes used in the United States are based on the *International Classification of Diseases* (ICD). The ICD lists diseases and three-digit codes according to a system created by the World Health Organization of the United Nations. Since the coding system was first developed more than a hundred years ago, it has been revised a number of times. The ICD is the classification used by the federal government to categorize mortality data from death certificates.

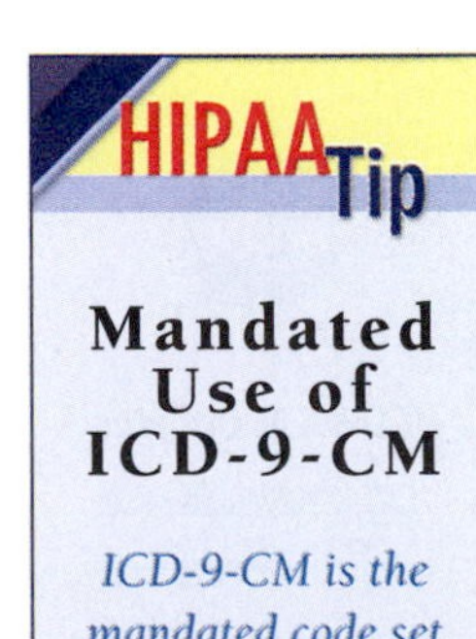

Mandated Use of ICD-9-CM

ICD-9-CM is the mandated code set for diagnoses under the HIPAA Electronic Health Care Transactions and Code Sets standards. Codes must be current as of the date of service.

History

A U.S. version of the ninth edition of the ICD (ICD-9) was published in 1979. A committee of physicians from various organizations and specialties prepared this version, which is called the ICD-9's *Clinical Modification*, or **ICD-9-CM**. It is used to code and classify morbidity data from patient medical records, physician offices, and surveys conducted by the National Center for Health Statistics. Codes in the ICD-9-CM describe conditions and illnesses more precisely than does the World Health Organization's ICD-9 because the codes are intended to provide a more complete picture of patients' conditions.

Billing Tip

Compliant Billing Using New Codes
Update encounter forms and ICD-9-CM databases when the addenda are released and inform providers about changed codes. But before updating the codes, the recommended procedure is to process and submit all claims from before the date that the codes changes go into effect. This ensures using the correct codes for visits previous to the effective date for code updates. Some practice management programs can be set up to warn the user when a diagnosis code entered for a claim is out of date for that date of service.

Thinking It Through — 4.1

Each year, the ICD-9-CM has many new categories, in part for diseases that have been discovered since the previous revision. What are examples of diseases that have been diagnosed in the last two decades?

The Medicare Catastrophic Coverage Act of 1988 mandated the change from written diagnoses to ICD-9-CM diagnosis codes for Medicare claims. After the Medicare ruling, private payers also began to require physicians to report diagnoses with ICD-9-CM codes. Using these diagnosis codes is now law under the Health Insurance Portability and Accountability Act of 1996 (HIPAA).

An ICD-9-CM diagnosis code has either three, four, or five digits plus a description. The system is built on categories for diseases, injuries, and symptoms. A category has three digits. Most categories have subcategories of four-digit codes. Some codes are further subclassified into five-digit codes. For example:

Category 415: Acute pulmonary heart disease (three digits)
Subcategory 415.1: Pulmonary embolism and infarction (four digits)
Subclassification: 415.11: Iatrogenic pulmonary embolism and infarction (five digits)

This structure enables coders to assign the most specific diagnosis that is documented in the patient medical record. A fifth digit is more specific than a fourth digit, and a fourth digit is more specific than a three-digit code. When fourth and fifth digits are in the ICD-9-CM, they are not optional; they must be used. For example, Centers for Medicare and Medicaid Services (CMS) rules state that a Medicare claim will be rejected when the most specific code available is not used.

Updates

The National Center for Health Statistics and the CMS release ICD-9-CM updates called the **addenda** that take effect on October 1 and April 1 of every year. The October 1 changes are the major updates; April 1 is used to catch up on codes that were not included in the major changes. The major new, invalid, and revised codes are posted on the website of NCHS by the beginning of July for mandated use as of October 1 of the year.

New codes must be used as of the date they go into effect, and invalid (deleted) codes must not be used. The U.S. Government Printing Office (GPO) publishes the official ICD-9-CM on the Internet and in CD-ROM format every year. Various commercial publishers include the updated codes in annual coding books that are printed soon after the July updates are released. Practices must ensure that the current reference is available and that the current codes are in use.

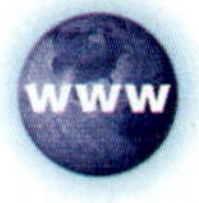

ICD-9-CM Updates
http://www.cdc.gov/nchs/icd9.htm

Organization of the ICD-9-CM

The ICD-9-CM has three parts:

1. *Diseases and Injuries: Tabular List—Volume 1:* The **Tabular List** is made up of seventeen chapters of disease descriptions and codes with two supplementary classifications and five appendixes.
2. *Diseases and Injuries: Alphabetic Index—Volume 2:* The **Alphabetic Index** provides (a) an index of the disease descriptions in the Tabular List, (b) an index in table format of drugs and chemicals that cause poisoning, and (c) an index of external causes of injury, such as accidents.

New Version: ICD-10-CM

The tenth edition of the ICD was published by the World Health Organization in 1990. In the United States, the new *Clinical Modification* (ICD-10-CM) data set is being reviewed by health care professionals. ICD-10-CM is expected to be adopted as the mandatory U.S. diagnosis code set within a few years. (Other countries, such as Australia and Canada, already use their own modifications of ICD-10.) The major changes are:

- The ICD-10 contains more than two thousand categories of diseases, many more than the ICD-9. This creates more codes to permit more-specific reporting of diseases and newly recognized conditions.
- Codes are alphanumeric, containing a letter followed by up to five numbers.
- A sixth digit is added to capture clinical details. For example, all codes that relate to pregnancy, labor, and childbirth include a digit that indicates the patient's trimester.
- Codes are added to show which side of the body is affected for a disease or condition that can be involved with the right side, the left side, or bilaterally. For example, separate codes are listed for a malignant neoplasm of right upper-inner quadrant of the female breast and for a malignant neoplasm of left upper-inner quadrant of the female breast.

When ICD-10-CM is mandated for use, a **crosswalk** will also be available. A crosswalk is a printed or computerized resource that connects two sets of data. The crosswalk connecting ICD-10-CM to ICD-9-CM will be used by medical insurance specialists to relate the two coding systems. For example, here are comparisons of ICD-9-CM and ICD-10-CM codes:

	ICD-9-CM Code	ICD-10-CM Code
Benign Prostatic Hypertrophy (BPH), not otherwise specified	600.00	N40.00
BPH with urinary retention	600.01	N40.01
Prostate polyp with urethral stricture	600.21	N40.21

Although the code numbers look different, the basic systems are very much alike. People who are familiar with the current codes will find that their training quickly applies to the new system.

3. *Procedures: Tabular List and Alphabetic Index—Volume 3:* This volume covers procedures performed chiefly in hospitals by physicians and other practitioners.

Volumes 1 and 2 are used for physician practice (outpatient) diagnostic coding. The use of Volume 3 for hospital coding is covered in Chapter 16.

Although the Tabular List and the Alphabetic Index are labeled Volume 1 and Volume 2, they are related like the parts of a book. First, the Alphabetic Index is used to find a code for a patient's condition or symptom. The index entry provides a pointer to the correct code number in the Tabular List. That code is then located in the Tabular List so that its correct use can be checked. This two-step process must be followed in order to code correctly. This chapter follows this order of use, with the Alphabetic Index discussed first, followed by the Tabular List. (Some publishers' versions of the ICD-9-CM place the Alphabetic Index before the Tabular List for the same reason.)

The Alphabetic Index

The Alphabetic Index contains all the medical terms in the Tabular List classifications. For some conditions, it also lists common terms that are not found in the Tabular List. The index is organized by the condition, not by the body part (anatomical site) in which the condition occurs.

The term *wrist fracture* is located by looking under *fracture* (the condition) and then, below it, *wrist* (the location), rather than under *wrist* to find *fracture*.

The medical term describing the condition for which a patient is receiving care is located in the physician's **diagnostic statement**. For each encounter, the diagnostic statement includes the main reason for the patient encounter. It may also provide descriptions of additional conditions or symptoms that have been treated or that are related to the patient's current illness.

Main Terms, Subterms, and Supplementary Terms

The assignment of the correct code begins with looking up the medical term that describes the patient's condition. Figure 4.1 illustrates the format of the Alphabetic Index. Each **main term** is printed in boldface type and is followed by its code number. For example, if the diagnostic statement is "the patient presents with blindness," the main term *blindness* is located in the Alphabetic Index (see Figure 4.1).

Below the main term, any **subterms** with their codes appear. Subterms are essential in the selection of correct codes. They may show the **etiology** of the disease—its cause or origin—or describe a particular type or body site for the main term. For example, the main term *blindness* in Figure 4.1 includes five subterms, each indicating a different etiology or type—such as color blindness—for that condition.

Blepharitis (eyelid) 373.00
  angularis 373.01
  ciliaris 373.00
    with ulcer 373.01
  marginal 373.00
    with ulcer 373.01
  scrofulous (*see also* Tuberculosis) 017.3
    [373.00]
  squamous 373.02
  ulcerative 373.01
Blepharochalasis 374.34
  congenital 743.62
Blepharoclonus 333.81
Blepharoconjunctivitis (*see also* Conjunctivitis)
    372.20
  angular 372.21
  contact 372.22
Blepharophimosis (eyelid) 374.46
  congenital 743.62
Blepharoplegia 374.89
Blepharoptosis 374.30
  congenital 743.61
Blepharopyorrhea 098.49
Blepharospasm 333.81
Blessig's cyst 362.62
Blighted ovum 631
Blind
  bronchus (congenital) 748.3
  eye—*see also* Blindness
    hypertensive 360.42
    hypotensive 360.41
  loop syndrome (postoperative) 579.2
  sac, fallopian tube (congenital) 752.19
  spot, enlarged 368.42
  tract or tube (congenital) NEC—*see* Atresia
Blindness (acquired) (congenital) (Both eyes)
    369.00
  blast 921.3
    with nerve injury—*see* Injury, nerve, optic
  Brightis — *see* Uremia
  color (congenital) 368.59
    acquired 368.55
    blue 368.53
    green 368.52
    red 368.51
    total 368.54
  concussion 950.9
  cortical 377.75

Figure 4.1 Example of Alphabetic Index Entries

Any **supplementary terms** for main terms or subterms are shown in parentheses on the same line. Supplementary terms are not essential to the selection of the correct code and are often referred to as nonessential modifiers. They help point to the correct term, but they do not have to appear in the physician's diagnostic statement for the coder to correctly select the code. In Figure 4.1, for example, any of the supplementary terms *acquired*, *congenital*, and *both eyes* may modify the main term in the diagnostic statement, such as "the patient presents with blindness acquired in childhood," or none of these terms may appear.

Turnover Lines

If the main term or subterm is too long to fit on one line, as is often the case when many supplementary terms appear, turnover (or carryover) lines are used. Turnover lines are always indented farther to the right than are subterms. It is important to read carefully to distinguish a turnover line from a subterm line. For example, under the main term *blindness* (Figure 4.1) in the Alphabetic Index, a long list of supplementary terms appears before the first subterm. Without close attention, it is possible to confuse a turnover entry with a subterm.

Cross-References

Some entries use cross-references. If the cross-reference *see* appears after a main term, the coder must look up the term that follows the word *see* in the index. The *see* reference means that the main term where the coder first looked is not correct; another category must be used. In Figure 4.1, for example, to code the last subterm under *blind*, the term *atresia* must be found.

See also, another type of cross-reference, points the coder to related index entries. *See also category* indicates that the coder should review the additional categories that are mentioned. For example, in the following entry, the entries between 633.0 and 633.9 should be checked, as well as 639.0:

Sepsis with
    ectopic pregnancy (*see also* categories 633.0–633.9) 639.0

Notes

At times, notes are shown below terms. These boxed, italicized instructions are important because they provide information on selecting the correct code. For example, this note appears in the listings for inguinal hernias (category 550):

Note—Use the following fifth-digit subclassification with category 550:

0 unilateral or unspecified (not specified as recurrent)
1 unilateral or unspecified, recurrent
2 bilateral (not specified as recurrent)
3 bilateral, recurrent

This note also illustrates another **convention** that is followed in the index: Numbered items are listed in numerical order from lowest to highest. Conventions are typographic techniques or standard practices that provide visual guidelines for understanding printed material. For example, numbered items are listed in numerical order whether the items are pure numbers (1, 2, 3) or words (first, second, third).

The Abbreviation NEC

Not elsewhere classified, or **NEC**, appears with a term when there is no code that is specific for the condition. This abbreviation means that no code matches the exact situation. For example:

Hemorrhage, brain, traumatic NEC 853.0

Multiple Codes and Connecting Words

Some conditions may require two codes, one for the etiology and a second for the **manifestation**, the disease's typical signs or symptoms. This is the case when two codes, the second in brackets and italics, appear after a term:

Phlebitis
    gouty 274.89 *[451.9]*

This entry indicates that the diagnostic statement "gouty phlebitis" requires two codes, one for the etiology (gout) and one for the manifestation (phlebitis). The use of italics for codes means that they cannot be used as primary codes; they are listed after the codes for the etiology.

Thinking It Through — 4.2

1. The following entry appears in the Alphabetic Index.
   Kimmelstiel (-Wilson) disease or syndrome
   (Intercapillary glomerulosclerosis) 250.4 [581.81]

   What type of term is Kimmelstiel(-Wilson)?

   ____

   What type of term is shown indented and in parentheses?

   ____

   Does this disease require one or two codes?

   ____

2. Locate the following main terms in the Alphabetic Index. List and interpret any cross-references you find next to the entries.

   La grippe ______________

   Anginoid pain __________

   Branchial ______________

3. Are see cross-references in the Alphabetic Index followed by codes? Why?

   ____

4. Locate the main term Choledocholithiasis in the Alphabetic Index, and explain the purpose of the note beneath it.

   ____

   ____

The use of connecting words, such as *due to*, *during*, *following*, and *with*, may also indicate the need for two codes, or for a single code that covers both conditions. For example, the main term below is followed by a *due to* subterm:

Cowpox (abortive) 051.0
due to vaccination 999.0

When the Alphabetic Index indicates the possible need for two codes, the Tabular List entry is used to determine whether they are needed. In some cases, a **combination code** describing both the etiology and the manifestation is available instead of two codes. For example:

Closed skull fracture with subdural hemorrhage and concussion 803.29

Common Terms

Many terms appear more than once in the Alphabetic Index. Often, the term in common use is listed as well as the accepted medical terminology. For example, there is an entry for *flu*, with a cross-reference to *influenza*.

Eponyms

An **eponym** (pronounced ĕp'- o – nim) is a condition (or a procedure) named for a person. Some eponyms are named for the physicians who discovered or invented them; others are named for patients. An eponym is usually listed both under that name and under the main term *disease* or *syndrome*. For example, Hodgkin's disease appears as a subterm under *disease* and as a key term.

The Tabular List

The Tabular List received its name from the language of statistics; the word *tabulate* means to count, record, or list systematically. The diseases and injuries in the Tabular List are organized into chapters according to etiology or body system. Supplementary codes and appendixes cover other special situations. The organization of the Tabular List and the ranges of codes covered in each part are shown in Table 4.1 on page 118.

Categories, Subcategories, and Subclassifications

Each Tabular List chapter is divided into sections with titles that indicate the types of related diseases or conditions they cover. For example, Chapter 9 has seven sections, one of which is

Hernia of Abdominal Cavity (550–553)

Within each section, there are three levels of codes:

1. A **category** is a three-digit code that covers a single disease or related condition. (See Appendix E of the Tabular List for the complete listing of categories.) For example, the category 551 in Figure 4.2 on page 119 covers "other hernia of abdominal cavity, with gangrene."
2. A **subcategory** is a four-digit subdivision of a category. It provides a further breakdown of the disease to show its etiology, site, or manifestation. For example, the 551 category has six subcategories:

551.0 Femoral hernia with gangrene
551.1 Umbilical hernia with gangrene
551.2 Ventral hernia with gangrene

551.3 Diaphragmatic hernia with gangrene
551.8 Hernia of other specified sites, with gangrene
551.9 Hernia of unspecified site, with gangrene

3. A **subclassification** is a five-digit subdivision of a subcategory. For example, the following fifth digits are to be used with code 551.0:

551.00 Unilateral or unspecified (not specified as recurrent)
551.01 Unilateral or unspecified, recurrent
551.02 Bilateral (not specified as recurrent)
551.03 Bilateral, recurrent

Symbols, Notes, Punctuation Marks, and Abbreviations

Coding correctly requires understanding the conventions—the symbols, instructional notes, and punctuation marks—that appear in the Tabular List.

TABLE 4.1 Tabular List Organization

CLASSIFICATION OF DISEASES AND INJURIES		
Chapter		**Categories**
1	Infectious and Parasitic Diseases	001–139
2	Neoplasms	140–239
3	Endocrine, Nutritional, and Metabolic Diseases, and Immunity Disorders	240–279
4	Diseases of the Blood and Blood-Forming Organs	280–289
5	Mental Disorders	290–319
6	Diseases of the Central Nervous System and Sense Organs	320–389
7	Diseases of the Circulatory System	390–459
8	Diseases of the Respiratory System	460–519
9	Diseases of the Digestive System	520–579
10	Diseases of the Genitourinary System	580–629
11	Complications of Pregnancy, Childbirth, and the Puerperium	630–677
12	Diseases of the Skin and Subcutaneous Tissue	680–709
13	Diseases of the Musculoskeletal System and Connective Tissue	710–739
14	Congenital Anomalies	740–759
15	Certain Conditions Originating in the Perinatal Period	760–779
16	Symptoms, Signs, and Ill-Defined Conditions	780–799
17	Injury and Poisoning	800–999
Supplementary Classifications		
V Codes	Supplementary Classification of Factors Influencing Health Status and Contact with Health Services	V01–V83
E Codes	Supplementary Classification of External Causes of Injury and Poisoning	E800–E999
Appendixes		
Appendix A	Morphology of Neoplasms	
Appendix B	Glossary of Mental Disorders	
Appendix C	Classification of Drugs by American Hospital Formulary Services List Number and Their ICD-9-CM Equivalents	
Appendix D	Classification of Industrial Accidents According to Agency	
Appendix E	List of Three-Digit Categories	

551 Other hernia of abdominal cavity, with gangrene
Includes: that with gangrene (and obstruction)
⑤ **551.0 Femoral hernia with gangrene**
551.00 Unilateral or unspecified (not specified as recurrent)
Femoral hernia NOS with gangrene
551.01 Unilateral or unspecified, recurrent
551.02 Bilateral (not specified as recurrent)
551.03 Bilateral, recurrent
551.1 Umbilical hernia with gangrene
Parumbilical hernia specified as gangrenous
⑤ **551.2 Ventral hernia with gangrene**
551.20 Ventral, unspecified, with gangrene
551.21 Incisional, with gangrene
Hernia:
postoperative } specified as gangrenous
Recurrent, ventral }
551.29 Other
Epigastric hernia specified as gangrenous
551.3 Diaphragmatic hernia with gangrene
Hernia:
hiatal (esophageal) (sliding) }
Paraesophageal } specified as gangrenous
Thoracic stomach }
Excludes: congenital diaphragmatic hernia (756.6)
551.8 Hernia of other specified sites, with gangrene
Any condition classifiable to 553.8 if specified as gangrenous
551.9 Hernia of unspecified site, with gangrene
Any condition classifiable to 553.9 if specified as gangrenous

Figure 4.2 Example of Tabular List Entries

Symbol for Fifth-Digit Requirement

Depending on the publisher of the ICD-9-CM, a section mark (§) or other symbol (such as ⑤ or ✓) appears next to a chapter, a category, or a subcategory that requires a fifth digit to be assigned. (See, for example, the ⑤ that appears next to subcategories 551.0 and 551.2 in Figure 4.2.) These are important reminders to assign the appropriate five-digit subclassification. If the fifth-digit requirement extends beyond the page where this symbol first appears, the symbol is repeated on all other pages where it applies, so that it is easy to notice.

Includes and Excludes Notes

Notes headed by the word *includes* refine the content of the category or section appearing above them. For example, after the three-digit category 461, acute sinusitis, the *include* note states that the category includes abscess, empyema, infection, inflammation, and suppuration.

Notes headed by the word *excludes* (which is boxed and italicized) indicate conditions that are not classifiable to the code above. In the category 461, for example, the *exclude* note states that the category does not include chronic or unspecified sinusitis. The note may also give the code(s) of the excluded condition(s).

Billing Tip

Fifth-Digit Requirement
If the ICD-9-CM indicates that a fifth digit is required, it must be included. But if it is not required, a zero or zeroes should not be added to the four-digit or three-digit code. The use of a fifth digit when it is not required makes the code invalid.

Colons in Includes and Excludes Notes

A colon (:) in an *includes* or *excludes* note indicates an incomplete term. One or more of the entries following the colon is required to make a complete term. Unlike terms in parentheses or brackets, when the colon is used, the diagnostic statement must include one of the terms after the colon to be assigned a code from the particular category. For example, the *excludes* note after the information for *coma* is as follows:

780.0 Alteration of consciousness
Excludes: coma:
diabetic (250.2–250.3)
hepatic (572.2)
originating in the perinatal period (779.2)

For the *excludes* note to apply to *coma*, "diabetic," " hepatic," or "originating in the perinatal period" must appear in the diagnostic statement.

Parentheses

Parentheses ( ) are used around descriptions that do not affect the code—that is, supplementary terms. For example, the subcategory 453.9, other venous embolism and thrombosis, of unspecified site, is followed by the entry "thrombosis (vein)."

Brackets

Brackets [ ] are used around synonyms, alternative wordings, or explanations. They have the same meaning as parentheses. For example, category 460, acute nasopharyngitis, is followed by the entry "[common cold]."

Braces

A brace } encloses a series of terms that is attached to the statement that appears to the right of the brace. It is an alternate format for a long list after a colon and also indicates incomplete terms. For example, the information after code 786.59, Chest pain, other, is as follows:

Discomfort	
Pressure	} in chest
Tightness	

For this code to be applied to a diagnosis of "chest pain, other," "discomfort," "pressure," or "tightness" must appear in the statement.

Lozenge

The lozenge (□) next to a code shows that it is not part of the World Health Organization's ICD. It appears only in the ICD-9-CM. This symbol can be ignored in coding diagnostic statements.

Abbreviations: NEC versus NOS

NEC, not elsewhere classified, is used in the Tabular List as well as in the Alphabetic Index. Another abbreviation, **NOS**, or **not otherwise specified**, means **unspecified**. This term or abbreviation indicates that the code above it should be used when a condition is not completely described in the medical record. For example, the code 827, other, multiple, and ill-defined fractures of lower limb, includes "leg NOS." If the documentation reads "patient suffered a fractured leg," this code is appropriate, since there is not enough information to determine which bone in the leg is involved. Note, however, that third-party payers may deny claims that use unspecified diagnosis codes. When possible, more-specific clinical documentation should be requested of the provider.

New and Revised Text Symbols

Many publishers use a bullet (•) at a code or a line of text to show that the entry is new. A single triangle (▶) or facing triangles (▶◀) are also often used to mean a new or revised description.

Multiple Codes

Some phrases contain instructions about the need for additional codes. The phrases point to situations in which more than one code is required to properly reflect the diagnostic statement. For example, a statement that a condition is "due to" or "associated with" may require an additional code.

Code First Underlying Disease

The instruction *code first underlying disease* appears below a code that must not be used as a primary code. These codes are for symptoms only, never for causes. The codes and their descriptions are in italic type, meaning that the code cannot be listed first even if the diagnostic statement is written that way. The phrase *code first associated disorder* or *code first underlying disorder* may appear below the italicized code and term. At times, a specific instruction is given, such as in this example:

366.31 Glaucomatous flecks (subcapsular)
Code first underlying glaucoma (365.0–365.9)

Billing Tip

NEC or NOS?
Not elsewhere classified (NEC) means that no code matches the diagnostic statement. Not otherwise specified (NOS) means that the diagnostic statement does not have enough information to assign a specific code.

Thinking It Through — 4.3

Provide the following information about codes found in the Tabular List.

1. What agent is excluded from subcategory 972.0, cardiac rhythm regulators?

 ____

2. A brace is located under 562.00. What does the brace mean?

 ____

3. What is the meaning of the symbol in front of category 017?

 ____

4. What types of gastric ulcers are included in category 531?

 ____

5. What is the meaning of the phrase that follows subclassification 466.19?

 ____

6. What is the meaning of the phrase that follows subcategory 730.7?

 ____

Use Additional Code, Code Also, or Use Additional Code, if Desired

If a code is followed by the instruction *use an additional code* or *code also* or by a note saying the same thing, two codes are required. The order of the codes must be the same as shown in the Alphabetic Index: the etiology comes first, followed by the manifestation code.

The phrase *use additional code, if desired,* also means to use an additional code if it can be determined. This instruction may apply to an entire chapter, or it may appear in a subcategory following a code. When the diagnostic statement has sufficient information, an additional code is determined in the same way as *code first underlying disease*. For example, code 711.00, pyogenic arthritis (site unspecified), is followed by the phrase:

Use additional code, if desired, to identify infectious organisms (041.0–041.8)

In this case, if the documentation indicates it, the infectious organism causing the condition is coded.

> **Billing Tip**
>
> **Use V Codes to Show Medical Necessity**
> V codes such as family history or a patient's previous condition help demonstrate why a service was medically necessary.

V Codes And E Codes

Two supplementary classifications follow the chapters of the Tabular List:

- **V codes** identify encounters for reasons other than illness or injury.
- **E codes** identify the external causes of injuries and poisoning.

Both V and E codes are alphanumeric; they contain letters followed by numbers. For example, the code for a complete physical examination of an adult is V70.0. The code for a fall from a ladder is E881.0.

V Codes

V codes are used

- For visits with healthy patients who receive services other than treatments, such as annual checkups, immunizations, and normal childbirth. This use is coded by a V code that identifies the service, such as

  V06.4 Prophylactic vaccination/inoculation against measles-mumps-rubella (MMR)

- For encounters with patients having known conditions for which they are receiving one of three types of treatment: chemotherapy, radiation therapy, and rehabilitation. In these cases, the encounter is coded first with a V code, and the condition is listed second. For example:

  V58.1 Encounter for chemotherapy
  233.0 Breast carcinoma

- Listing the V code first for these three treatments is an exception to general coding rules. Usually, when patients receive therapeutic treatments for already diagnosed conditions, the previously diagnosed condition is used for the primary code.
- For encounters in which a problem not currently affecting the patient's health status needs to be noted. For example, codes V10–V19 cover history. If a person with a family history of colon cancer presents with rectal bleeding, the problem is listed first, and the V code is assigned as an additional code, as is shown here:

  569.3 Hemorrhage of rectum and anus
  V16.0 Family history of malignant neoplasm

- For encounters in which patients are being evaluated preoperatively, a code from category V72.8 is listed first, followed by a code for the condition that is the reason for the surgery. For example:

V72.81 Preoperative cardiovascular examination
414.01 Arteriosclerotic heart disease of native coronary artery

A V code can be used as either a primary code for an encounter or as an additional code. It is researched the same way as other codes, using the Alphabetic Index to point to the term's code and the Supplementary Classification in the Tabular List to verify it. The terms that indicate the need for V codes, however, are not the same as other medical terms. They usually have to do with a reason for an encounter other than a disease or its complications. When found in diagnostic statements, the words listed in Table 4.2 often point to V codes.

E Codes

E (for external) codes are used to classify the injuries resulting from various environmental events, such as transportation accidents, accidental poisoning by drugs or other substances, falls, and fires. An E code is not used alone. It always supplements a code that identifies the injury or condition itself.

E codes are located by first using Section 3 of the Alphabetic Index, Alphabetic Index to External Causes of Injury and Poisoning. This index is organized by main terms describing the accident, circumstance, event, or specific agent (drug or chemical) that caused the injury. Codes are verified in the Supplementary Classifications section of the Tabular List.

E codes are often used in collecting public health information. These categories are important in medical practices:

- *Accidents:* When a patient has an accident, the payer checks the E code that is assigned to verify that the services are covered by the medical insurance policy rather than by an automobile policy or workers' compensation laws.
- *Drug reactions:* The categories E930 to E949 apply to an **adverse effect**, a patient's unintentional, harmful reaction to a proper dosage of a drug. The specific drug is located in the **Table of Drugs and Chemicals** in the Alphabetic Index. Adverse effects are different from poisoning, which refers to the medical result of the incorrect use of a substance. Poisoning codes are found under categories 960–979.

Billing Tip

Use E Codes to Show Who Is Responsible for Payment

E codes for trauma and accidents help payers determine what insurance applies. These codes are especially useful on workers' compensation claims.

TABLE 4.2 Terminology Associated with V Codes

	Example	
Contact	V01.1	Contact with tuberculosis
Contraception	V25.1	Insertion of intrauterine contraceptive device
Counseling	V61.11	Counseling for victim of spousal and partner abuse
Examination	V70	General medical examination
Fitting of	V52	Fitting and adjustment of prosthetic device and implant
Follow-up	V67.0	Follow-up examination following surgery
Health or healthy	V20	Health supervision of infant or child
History (of)	V10.05	Personal history of malignant neoplasm, large intestine
Replacement	V42.0	Kidney replaced by transplant
Screening/test	V73.2	Special screening examination for measles
Status	V44	Artificial opening status
Supervision (of)	V23	Supervision of high-risk pregnancy
Therapy	V57.3	Speech therapy
Vaccination/inoculation	V06	Need for prophylactic vaccination and inoculation against combinations of disease

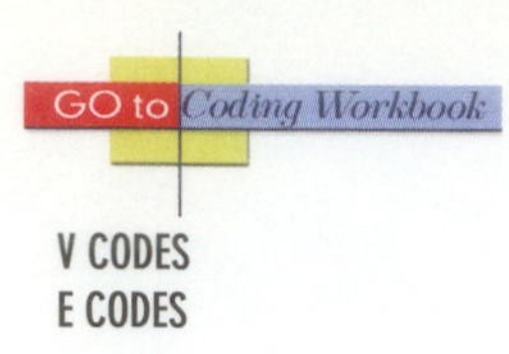

V CODES
E CODES

Note: If the *Medical Insurance Coding Workbook for Physician Practices* is assigned for coding practice, the icon in the margin tells you to test your understanding at certain points by completing exercises. For example, the icon at the left means to turn to the *Coding Workbook* and complete exercises on V codes and E codes.

Coding Steps

The correct procedure for assigning accurate diagnosis codes has three steps.

Step 1 Determine the Reason for the Encounter

In medical practices, diagnosis coding begins with the patient's **chief complaint** (CC). The chief complaint is the medical reason that the patient presents for the particular visit. The code will be assigned based on the physician's diagnosis of the patient's chief complaint. This **primary diagnosis** is documented in the patient's medical record. It is the diagnosis, condition, problem, or other reason that the documentation shows as being chiefly responsible for the services that are provided. This primary diagnosis provides the main term to be coded first.

> If a patient has cancer, the disease is probably the patient's major health problem. However, if that patient sees the physician for an ear infection that is not related to the cancer, the primary diagnosis for that particular claim is the ear infection.

At times, there is more than one diagnosis because many patients have complex conditions. Someone with hypertension (high blood pressure), for example, may also have heart disease. In these cases, the primary diagnosis is listed first on the insurance claim. After that, additional **coexisting condition(s)** may be listed. These are conditions that occur at the same time as the primary diagnosis and affect the treatment or recovery from the primary diagnosis. For example, a patient with diabetes mellitus complains of poor circulation. The diagnosis for this person's office visit to complain of numbness in the fingers and toes would likely include the diabetes as a coexisting condition. Sometimes, a diagnosis code contains both the primary and a coexisting condition. For example, code 365.63 means glaucoma associated with vascular disorders.

Billing Tip

Physician versus Facility Coding
There are different coding rules for physician coding and facility (hospital) coding. One rule affects what diagnosis to code. In hospitals, the patient's condition is called the principal (rather than primary) diagnosis and often it is not known until the end of the hospital stay. This final diagnosis, rather than the admitting diagnosis, is coded for claims. (Hospital coding is covered in Chapter 16.)

Step 2 Locate the Term in the Alphabetic Index

The main term for the patient's primary diagnosis is located in the Alphabetic Index. These guidelines should be observed in choosing the correct term:

- Use any supplementary terms in the diagnostic statement to help locate the main term.
- Read and follow any notes below the main term.
- Review the subterms to find the most specific match to the diagnosis.
- Read and follow any cross-references.
- Make note of a two-code (etiology and/or manifestation) indication.

Billing Tip

Correct Coding Procedure
Never use only the Alphabetic Index or only the Tabular List to code. Either approach causes coding errors.

Step 3 Verify the Code in the Tabular List

The code for the main term is then located in the Tabular List. These guidelines are observed to verify the selection of the correct code:

- Read *include* or *excludes* notes, checking back to see whether any apply to the code's category, section, or chapter.
- Be alert for and follow instructions for fifth-digit requirements.
- Follow any instructions requiring the selection of additional codes (such as "code also" or "code first underlying disease").
- List multiple codes in the correct order.

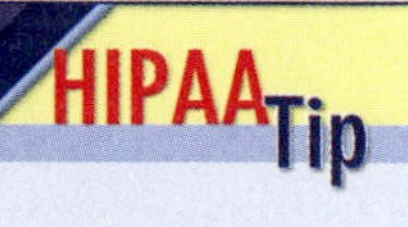

Official Guidelines

HIPAA requires adherence to the Official Guidelines when assigning diagnosis codes.

Thinking It Through — 4.4

1. **Why is it important to use the Alphabetic Index and then the Tabular List to find the correct code? Work through this coding process, and then comment on your result.**
   - A. Double-underline the main term and underline the subterm.
     patient complains of abdominal cramps
   - B. Find the term in the Alphabetic Index, and list its code.
     ______________ ______________________
   - C. Verify the code in the Tabular List, reading all instructions. List the code you have determined to be correct.
     ______________ ______________________
   - D. Did the result of your research in the Tabular List match the main term's code in the Alphabetic Index? Why?
     ____

2. **Place a double underline below the main terms and a single underline below any subterms in each of the following statements, and then determine the correct codes.**
   - A. cerebral atherosclerosis
   - B. spasmodic asthma with status asthmaticus
   - C. congenital night blindness
   - D. recurrent inguinal hernia with obstruction
   - E. incomplete bundle branch heart block
   - F. acute bacterial food poisoning
   - G. malnutrition following gastrointestinal surgery
   - H. skin test for hypersensitivity
   - I. frequency of urination disturbing sleep

Official Coding Guidelines

Diagnosis coding in health care follows specific guidelines. These **ICD-9-CM Official Guidelines for Coding and Reporting** (the Official Guidelines) are developed by a group known as the four cooperating parties. The group is made up of CMS advisers and participants from the American Hospital Association (AHA), the American Health Information Management Association (AHIMA), and the National Center for Health Statistics (NCHS) [IA] http://www.cdc.gov/nchs/ICD-9-htm.

The Official Guidelines have sections for general rules as well as for inpatient (hospital) and outpatient (physician office/clinic) coding. Figure 4.3 on page 126 presents Section IV, "Diagnostic Coding and Reporting for Outpatient Services," of the Official Guidelines. This section covers physician office/clinic

Section IV. Diagnostic Coding and Reporting Guidelines for Outpatient Services

These coding guidelines for outpatient diagnoses have been approved for use by hospitals/providers in coding and reporting hospital-based outpatient services and provider-based office visits.

Information about the use of certain abbreviations, punctuation, symbols, and other conventions used in the ICD-9-CM Tabular List (code numbers and titles), can be found in Section IA of these guidelines, under "Conventions Used in the Tabular List." Information about the correct sequence to use in finding a code is also described in Section I.

The terms encounter and visit are often used interchangeably in describing outpatient service contacts and, therefore, appear together in these guidelines without distinguishing one from the other.

Though the conventions and general guidelines apply to all settings, coding guidelines for outpatient and provider reporting of diagnoses will vary in a number of instances from those for inpatient diagnoses, recognizing that:

The Uniform Hospital Discharge Data Set (UHDDS) definition of principal diagnosis applies only to inpatients in acute, short-term, long-term care and psychiatric hospitals.

Coding guidelines for inconclusive diagnoses (probable, suspected, rule out, etc.) were developed for inpatient reporting and do not apply to outpatients.

A. Selection of first-listed condition

In the outpatient setting, the term first-listed diagnosis is used in lieu of principal diagnosis.

In determining the first-listed diagnosis the coding conventions of ICD-9-CM, as well as the general and disease specific guidelines take precedence over the outpatient guidelines.

Diagnoses often not established at the time of the initial encounter/visit. It may take two or more visits before the diagnosis is confirmed.

The most critical rule involves beginning the search for the correct code assignment through the Alphabetic Index. Never begin searching initially in the Tabular List as this will lead to coding errors.

1. Outpatient Surgery
   When a patient presents for outpatient surgery, code the reason for the surgery as the first-listed diagnosis (reason for the encounter), even if the surgery is not performed due to a contraindication.
2. Observation Stay
   When a patient is admitted for observation for a medical condition, assign a code for the medical condition as the first-listed diagnosis.

   When a patient presents for outpatient surgery and develops complications requiring admission to observation, code the reason for the surgery as the first reported diagnosis (reason for the encounter), followed by codes for the complications as secondary diagnoses.

B. Codes from 001.0 through V84.8

The appropriate code or codes from 001.0 through V84.8 must be used to identify diagnoses, symptoms, conditions, problems, complaints, or other reason(s) for the encounter/visit.

C. Accurate reporting of ICD-9-CM diagnosis codes

For accurate reporting of ICD-9-CM diagnosis codes, the documentation should describe the patient's condition, using terminology which includes specific diagnoses as well as symptoms, problems, or reasons for the encounter. There are ICD-9-CM codes to describe all of these.

D. Selection of codes 001.0 through 999.9

The selection of codes 001.0 through 999.9 will frequently be used to describe the reason for the encounter. These codes are from the section of ICD-9-CM for the classification of diseases and injuries (e.g. infectious and parasitic diseases; neoplasms; symptoms, signs, and ill-defined conditions, etc.).

E. Codes that describe symptoms and signs

Codes that describe symptoms and signs, as opposed to diagnoses, are acceptable for reporting purposes when a diagnosis has not been established (confirmed) by the provider. Chapter 16 of ICD-9-CM, Symptoms, Signs, and Ill-defined conditions (codes 780.0 - 799.9) contain many, but not all codes for symptoms.

F. Encounters for circumstances other than a disease or injury

ICD-9-CM provides codes to deal with encounters for circumstances other than a disease or injury. The Supplementary Classification of factors Influencing Health Status and Contact with Health Services (V01.0- V84.8) is provided to deal with occasions when circumstances other than a disease or injury are recorded as diagnosis or problems.

(a)

Figure 4.3 ICD-9-CM Guidelines for Coding and Reporting Outpatient Services

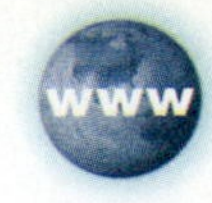

ICD-9-CM Official Guidelines

http://www.cdc.gov/nchs/data/icd9/icdguide.pdf

G. Level of Detail in Coding

1. ICD-9-CM codes with 3, 4, or 5 digits
   ICD-9-CM is composed of codes with either 3, 4, or 5 digits. Codes with three digits are included in ICD-9-CM as the heading of a category of codes that may be further subdivided by the use of fourth and/or fifth digits, which provide greater specificity.
2. Use of full number of digits required for a code.
   A three-digit code is to be used only if it is not further subdivided. Where fourth-digit subcategories and/or fifth-digit subclassifications are provided, they must be assigned. A code is invalid if it has no been coded to the full number of digits required for that code. See also discussion under Section I.b.3., General Coding Guidelines, Level of Detail in Coding.

H. ICD-9-CM code for the diagnosis, condition, problem, or other reason for encounter/visit

List first the ICD-9-CM code for the diagnosis, condition, problem, or other reason for encounter/visit shown in the medical record to be chiefly responsible for the services provided. List additional codes that describe any coexisting conditions. In some cases the first-listed diagnosis may be a symptom when a diagnosis has not been established (confirmed) by the physician.

I. "Probable", "suspected", "questionable", "rule out", or "working diagnosis"

Do not code diagnoses documented as "probable", "suspected," "questionable," "rule out," or "working diagnosis". Rather, code the condition(s) to the highest degree of certainty for that encounter/visit, such as symptoms, signs, abnormal test results, or other reason for the visit. Please note: This differs from the coding practices used by short-term, acute care, long-term care and psychiatric hospitals.

J. Chronic diseases

Chronic diseases treated on an ongoing basis may be coded and reported as many times as the patient receives treatment and care for the condition(s).

K. Code all documented conditions that coexist

Code all documented conditions that coexist at the time of the encounter/visit, and require or affect patient care treatment or management. Do not code conditions that were previously treated and no longer exist. However, history codes (V10-V19) may be used as secondary codes if the historical condition or family history has an impact on current care or influences treatment.

L. Patients receiving diagnostic services only

For patients receiving diagnostic services only during an encounter/visit, sequence first the diagnosis, condition, problem, or other reason for encounter/visit shown in the medical record to be chiefly responsible for the outpatient services provided during the encounter/visit. Codes for other diagnoses (e.g., chronic conditions) may be sequenced as additional diagnoses.

For outpatient encounters for diagnostic tests that have been interpreted by a physician, and the final report is available at the time of coding, code any confirmed or definitive diagnosis(es) documented in the interpretation. Do not code related signs and symptoms as additional diagnoses.

Please note: This differs from the coding practice in the hospital inpatient setting regarding abnormal findings on test results.

M. Patients receiving therapeutic services only

For patients receiving therapeutic services only during an encounter/visit, sequence first the diagnosis, condition, problem, or other reason for encounter/visit shown in the medical record to be chiefly responsible for the outpatient services provided during the encounter/visit. Codes for other diagnoses (e.g., chronic conditions) may be sequenced as additional diagnoses.

The only exception to this rule is that when the primary reason for the admission/encounter is chemotherapy, radiation therapy, or rehabilitation, the appropriate V code for the service is listed first, and the diagnosis or problem for which the service is being performed listed second.

N. Patients receiving preoperative evaluations only

For patients receiving preoperative evaluations only, sequence first a code from category V72.8, Other specified examinations, to describe the pre-op consultations. Assign a code for the condition to describe the reason for the surgery as an additional diagnosis. Code also any findings related to the pre-op evaluation.

O. Ambulatory surgery

For ambulatory surgery, code the diagnosis for which the surgery was performed. If the postoperative diagnosis is known to be different from the preoperative diagnosis at the time the diagnosis is confirmed, select the postoperative diagnosis for coding, since it is the most definitive.

P. Routine outpatient prenatal visits

For routine outpatient prenatal visits when no complications are present, codes V22.0, Supervision of normal first pregnancy, or V22.1, Supervision of other normal pregnancy, should be used as the principal diagnosis. These codes should not be used in conjunction with chapter 11 codes.

(b)

Figure 4.3 *(Continued)*

guidelines for what is to be coded and the order in which the codes should be listed. The key points from this section can be summarized as follows:

- Code the primary diagnosis first, followed by current coexisting conditions.
- Code to the highest level of certainty.
- Code to the highest level of specificity.

Code the Primary Diagnosis First, Followed by Current Coexisting Conditions

The ICD-9-CM code for the primary diagnosis is listed first.

EXAMPLE

Diagnostic Statement: Patient is an elderly female complaining of back pain. For the past five days, she has had signs of pyelonephritis, including urinary urgency, urinary incontinence, and back pain. Has had a little hematuria, but no past history of urinary difficulties. My diagnosis is pyelonephritis.

Primary Diagnosis: 590.80 Pyelonephritis

Additional codes are listed to describe all current documented coexisting conditions that affect patient treatment or require treatment during the encounter. Coexisting conditions may be related to the primary diagnosis, or they may involve a separate illness that the physician diagnoses and treats during the encounter.

EXAMPLE

Diagnostic Statement: Patient, a forty-five-year-old male, presents for complete physical examination for an insurance certification. During the examination, patient complains of occasional difficulty hearing; wax is removed from the left ear canal.

Primary Diagnosis: V70.3 Routine physical examination for insurance certification

Coexisting Condition: 380.4 Impacted cerumen

It is important to note that patients may have diseases or conditions that do not affect the encounter being coded. Some physicians add notes about previous conditions to provide an easy reference to a patient's history. Unless these conditions are directly involved with the patient's treatment, they are not considered in selecting codes. Also, conditions that were previously treated and no longer exist are not coded.

EXAMPLE

Chart Note: Mrs. Mackenzie, whose previous encounter was for her regularly scheduled blood pressure check, presents today with a new onset of psoriasis.

Primary Diagnosis: 696.1 Psoriasis, NOS

If the reason for the visit is a condition other than a disease or illness, the appropriate V code is used to code the encounter:

EXAMPLE

V72.3 Routine gynecological examination with Papanicolaou smear

Coding Acute versus Chronic Conditions

The reasons for patient encounters are often **acute** symptoms—generally, relatively sudden or severe problems. Acute conditions are coded with the specific code that is designated acute, if listed. Many patients, however, receive ongoing treatment for **chronic** conditions—those that continue over a long period of time or recur frequently. For example, a patient may need a regular gold injection for the management of rheumatoid arthritis. In such cases, the disease is coded and reported for as many times as the patient receives care for the condition.

In some cases, an encounter covers both an acute and a chronic condition. Some conditions do not have separate entries for both manifestations, so a single code applies. If both the acute and the chronic illnesses have codes, the acute code is listed first.

EXAMPLE

Acute Renal Failure 584.9

Chronic Renal Failure 585

Coding Late Effects

A **late effect** is a condition that remains after a patient's acute illness or injury has ended. Often called residual effects, some late effects happen soon after the disease is over, and others occur later. The diagnostic statement may say:

- Due to an old ... (for example, swelling due to old contusion of knee)
- Late ... (for example, nausea as a late effect of radiation sickness)
- Due to a previous ... (for example, abdominal mass due to a previous spleen injury)
- Traumatic (if not a current injury); including scarring or nonunion of a fracture (for example, malunion of fracture, left humerus)

In general, the main term *late* is followed by subterms that list the causes. Two codes are usually required. First reported is the code for the specific late effect (such as muscle soreness), followed by the code for the cause of the late effect (such as the late effect of rickets).

Code to the Highest Level of Certainty

If the physician has not established a diagnosis, the diagnosis codes that cover symptoms, signs, and ill-defined conditions are used. Inconclusive diagnoses, such as those preceded by "rule out," "suspected," or "probable," for example, are not coded. This rule—code only to the highest degree of certainty—exists because an unproven condition reported to a payer could prove damaging to the patient; such a statement could remain in others' records uncorrected. For example, if the statement "rule out aggressive breast carcinoma" is coded for cancer and a malignancy is not found, the patient could be denied medical insurance coverage because of the insurer's concern that the patient has cancer.

Coding Signs and Symptoms

A diagnosis is not always established at the first encounter. Follow-up visits may be required before the physician determines a primary diagnosis. During this process, although possible diagnoses may appear in a patient's medical record as the physician's work is progressing, these inconclusive diagnoses are not reported for reimbursement of service fees. Instead, the specific signs and symptoms are coded and reported. A *sign* is an objective indication that can be evaluated by the physician, such as weight loss. A *symptom* is a subjective statement by the patient that cannot be confirmed during an examination, such as pain. The following case provides an example of how symptoms and signs are coded:

EXAMPLE

Diagnostic Statement: Middle-aged male presents with abdominal pain and weight loss. He had to return home from vacation due to acute illness. He has not been eating well because of a vague upper- abdominal pain. He denies nausea, vomiting.

Billing Tip

Signs and Symptoms versus Rule-Outs

Do not code inconclusive rule-out diagnoses as if they exist; code symptoms, signs, or ill-defined conditions instead.

Billing Tip

Fifth-Digit Typographic Convention
Study the conventions in the ICD book you are using. Read and understand the publisher's convention for indicating the fifth-digit requirement, such as the use of a section mark, different color print, T, or ®.

He denies changes in bowel habit or blood in stool. Physical examination revealed no abdominal tenderness.

Primary Diagnosis: 789.06 Abdominal pain, epigastric region

Coexisting Condition: 783.2 Abnormal loss of weight

Coding the Reason for Surgery

Surgery is coded according to the diagnosis that is listed as the reason for the procedure. In some cases, the postoperative diagnosis is available and is different from the physician's primary diagnosis before the surgery. If so, the postoperative diagnosis is coded because it is the highest level of certainty available. For example, if an excisional biopsy is performed to evaluate mammographic breast lesions or a lump of unknown nature and the pathology results show a malignant neoplasm, the diagnosis code describing the site and nature of the neoplasm is used.

Code to the Highest Level of Specificity

A three-digit code is used only if a four-digit code is not provided in the ICD-9-CM. Likewise, a four-digit subcategory code is used only when no five-digit subclassification is listed. When a five-digit code is available, it must be used.

The more digits the code has, the more specific it becomes; the additional codes add to the clinical picture of the patient. Using the most specific code possible is referred to as coding to the highest level of specificity.

EXAMPLE

The category code 250 indicates a diagnosis of diabetes mellitus. Under this category, a fourth digit provides information about the cause or site, such as

250.1 Diabetes with ketoacidosis
250.2 Diabetes with hyperosmolarity
250.3 Diabetes with other coma
250.4 Diabetes with renal manifestations

Based on the medical record, a fifth digit must be selected and added to any of these four-digit codes according to which of these is documented:

0 Type II or unspecified type, not stated as uncontrolled
1 Type I, not stated as uncontrolled
2 Type II or unspecified type, uncontrolled
3 Type I, uncontrolled

If the patient is insulin-dependent, that is, routinely uses insulin, a V code V58.67 may be assigned to complete the clinical picture.

Overview of ICD-9-CM Chapters

In the following pages, each chapter of the ICD-9-CM is briefly introduced. Any special guidelines needed for accurate coding are described.

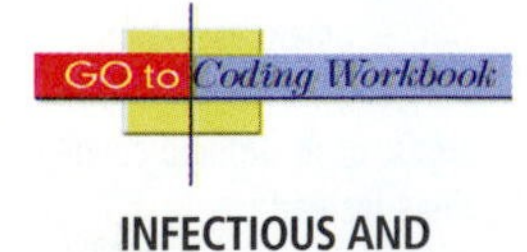

INFECTIOUS AND PARASITIC DISEASES

Infectious and Parasitic Diseases—Codes 001–139

Codes in Chapter 1 of the ICD-9-CM's Tabular List classify communicable infectious and parasitic diseases. Most categories describe a condition and the type of organism that causes it.

Thinking It Through — 4.5

Provide the diagnosis code(s) for the following cases, and explain the coding guideline that you applied to the case.

1. A thirty-six-year-old female patient presents to the physician's office for her yearly checkup. During the exam, the physician identifies a palpable, solitary lump in the left breast. The physician considers this significant and extends the exam to gather information for diagnosing this problem.

   ____

2. A forty-five-year-old male patient presents to the office complaining of headaches for the past twenty-four hours. Based on the examination, the physician orders an MRI to investigate a possible brain tumor.

   ____

3. An eighty-six-year-old female patient who has a chronic laryngeal ulcer presents for treatment of a painful episode.

   ____

4. A fifty-eight-year-old female patient has muscle weakness due to poliomyelitis in childhood.

   ____

5. A sixty-four-year-old male patient's diagnosis is degenerative osteoarthritis.

   ____

Neoplasms—Codes 140–239

Neoplasms are coded from Chapter 2 of the ICD-9-CM. Neoplasms, also called tumors, are growths that arise from normal tissue. Note that this category does not include a diagnosis statement with the word *mass*, which is a separate main term.

The Neoplasm Table

The Alphabetic Index contains the Neoplasm Table that points to codes for neoplasms. The table lists the anatomical location in the first column. The next six columns relate to the behavior of the neoplasm, described as

- One of three types of malignant tumor, each of which is progressive, rapid-growing, life-threatening, and made of cancerous cells:
  1. *Primary*: The neoplasm that is the encounter's main diagnosis is found at the site of origin.
  2. *Secondary*: The neoplasm that is the encounter's main diagnosis metastasized (spread) to an additional body site from the original location.
  3. *Carcinoma in situ*: The neoplasm is restricted to one site (a noninvasive type); this may also be referred to as *preinvasive cancer*.
- Benign—slow-growing, not life-threatening, made of normal or near-normal cells

- Uncertain behavior—not classifiable when the cells were examined
- Unspecified nature—no documentation of the nature of the neoplasm

As an example, the following entries are shown in the Neoplasm Table for a neoplasm of the colon:

In the Tabular List, neoplasms are listed in Chapter 2 under categories 140 through 239.

MALIGNANT						
	Primary	Secondary	Cancer in situ	Benign	Uncertain Behavior	Unspecified
Colon	154.0	197.5	230.4	211.4	235.2	239.0

M Codes

In the regular Alphabetic Index entries, the pointers for neoplasms also show morphology codes, known as M codes. M codes contain the letter M followed by four digits, a slash, and a final digit. M codes (listed in ICD-9-CM, Appendix A) are used by pathologists to report on and study the prevalence of various types of neoplasms. They are not used in physician practice (outpatient) coding. However, pathologists' reports help in selecting the correct code for a neoplasm. In the M code, the digit after the slash indicates the behavior of the neoplasm:

/0 Benign
/1 Uncertain whether benign or malignant/borderline malignant
/2 Carcinoma in situ: intraepithelial, noninfiltrating, or noninvasive
/3 Malignant, primary site
/6 Malignant, metastatic site, secondary site

These codes are related as follows to the Neoplasm Table and the Tabular List:

M CODE	NEOPLASM TABLE	TABULAR LIST
/0	Benign neoplasms	210–229
/1	Neoplasm of unspecified nature	239
	Neoplasms of uncertain behavior	235–238
/2	Carcinoma in situ	230–234
/3	Malignant neoplasm, stated or presumed to be primary	140–195 200–208
/6	Malignant neoplasms, stated or presumed to be secondary	196–198

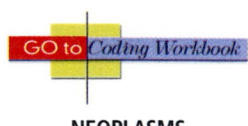

NEOPLASMS

For example, a pathologist's report might indicate the presence of an endometrioid adenofibroma. If it is benign, the M code is M8381/0, the equivalent of diagnosis code 220. If it is borderline malignant, the M code is M8381/1, and the diagnosis code is 236.2. If it is malignant, the M code is M8381/3, and the diagnosis code is 183.0.

In the case of a metastasized neoplasm, if the secondary site is the main reason for treatment, then the primary site is listed as a coexisting condition if it is still being treated. If the primary site is not documented, the code 199.1, malignant neoplasm without specification of site, other, is used. After the neoplasm is removed or is in remission, a V code for the personal history of malignant neoplasm is used.

Endocrine, Nutritional, and Metabolic Diseases, and Immunity Disorders—Codes 240–279

GO to *Coding Workbook*

ENDOCRINE, NUTRITIONAL, AND METABOLIC DISEASES AND IMMUNITY DISORDERS

Codes in Chapter 3 of the ICD-9-CM classify a variety of conditions. The most common disease in Chapter 3 is diabetes mellitus, which is a progressive disease of either type I or type II. Ninety percent of cases are type II.

Diseases of the Blood and Blood-Forming Organs—Codes 280–289

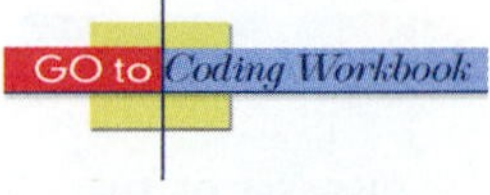

DISEASES OF THE BLOOD AND BLOOD-FORMING ORGANS

Codes in this brief ICD-9-CM chapter classify diseases of the blood and blood-forming organs, such as anemia and coagulation defects.

Mental Disorders—Codes 290–319

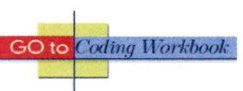

MENTAL DISORDERS

Codes in Chapter 5 of the ICD-9-CM classify the various types of mental disorders, including conditions of drug and alcohol dependency, Alzheimer's disease, schizophrenic disorders, and mood disturbances.

Most psychiatrists use the terminology found in the *Diagnostic and Statistical Manual of Mental Disorders (DSM)* for diagnoses, but the coding follows the ICD-9-CM. Appendix B of the ICD-9-CM contains a glossary of mental disorders. These psychiatric terms are used by physicians in diagnostic statements. This reference may be helpful in determining correct codes in the Mental Disorders chapter.

Diseases of the Nervous System and Sense Organs—Codes 320–389

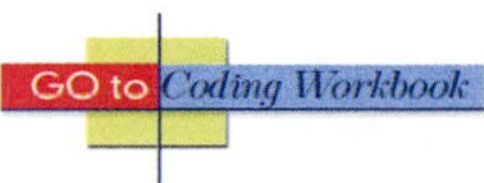

DISEASES OF THE NERVOUS SYSTEM AND SENSE ORGANS

Codes in Chapter 6 classify diseases of the central nervous system, the peripheral nervous system, the eye, and the ear.

Diseases of the Circulatory System—Codes 390–459

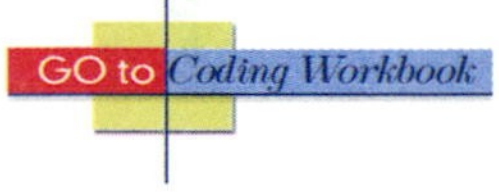

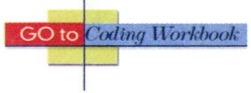

DISEASES OF THE CIRCULATORY SYSTEM

Because the circulatory system involves so many interrelated components, the disease process can create complex interrelated conditions. Many types of cardiovascular system disease, such as acute myocardial infarction (heart attack), require hospitalization of patients. The following introduction covers some frequently coded diagnoses. The notes and *code also* instructions in Chapter 7 of the Tabular List must be carefully observed to code circulatory diseases accurately.

Ischemic heart disease conditions—those caused by reduced blood flow to the heart—are coded under categories 410 through 414. Myocardial infarctions that are acute or have a documented duration of eight weeks or less are located in category 410. Chronic myocardial infarctions, or those that last longer than eight weeks, are coded to subcategory 414.8. An old or healed myocardial infarction without current symptoms is coded 412.

Other chronic ischemic heart diseases are coded under category 414. Coronary atherosclerosis, 414.0, requires a fifth digit for the type of artery involved and includes arteriosclerotic heart disease (ASHD), atherosclerotic heart disease, and other coronary conditions. A diagnosis of angina pectoris—an episode of chest pain from a temporary insufficiency of oxygen to the heart—is coded 413.9 unless it occurs only at night (413.0) or is diagnosed as Prinzmetal (angiospastic) angina (413.1).

Arteriosclerotic cardiovascular disease (ASCVD)—hardening of the arteries affecting the complete cardiovascular system—is coded 429.2. A second code for the arteriosclerosis, 440.9, is also needed for this diagnosis. Likewise, 440.9 is never the primary code when ASCVD is a diagnosis.

Hypertension is a diagnosis related to high (elevated) blood pressure. Almost all cases are due to unknown causes. This is called essential hypertension and is the primary diagnosis. In the few cases where the cause is known, the hypertension is called secondary, and its code is listed after the code for the cause.

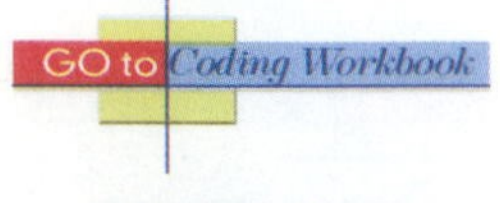

DISEASES OF THE RESPIRATORY SYSTEM

Diseases of the Respiratory System—Codes 460–519

Codes in Chapter 8 of the ICD-9-CM classify respiratory illnesses such as pneumonia, chronic obstructive pulmonary disease (COPD), and asthma. Pneumonia, a common respiratory infection, may be caused by one of a number of organisms. Many codes for pneumonia include the condition and the cause in a combination code, such as 480.2, pneumonia due to parainfluenza virus.

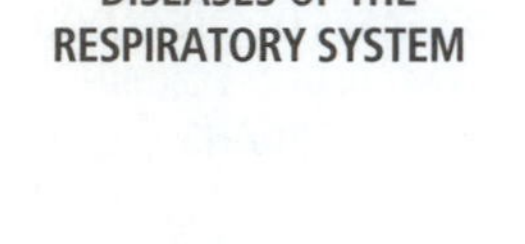

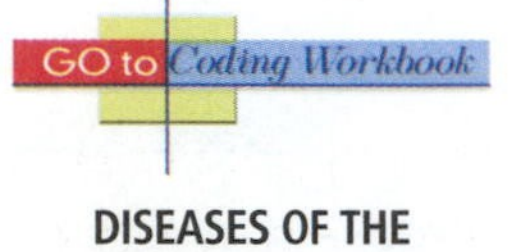

DISEASES OF THE DIGESTIVE SYSTEM

Diseases of the Digestive System—Codes 520–579

Codes in Chapter 9 of the ICD-9-CM classify diseases of the digestive system. Codes are listed according to anatomical location, beginning with the oral cavity and continuing through the intestines.

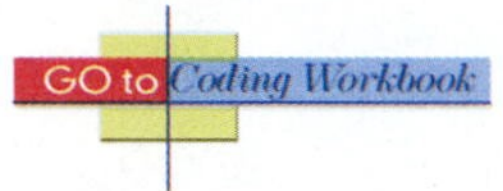

DISEASES OF THE GENITOURINARY SYSTEM

Diseases of the Genitourinary System—Codes 580–629

Codes in Chapter 10 of the ICD-9-CM classify diseases of the male and female genitourinary (GU) systems, such as infections of the genital tract, renal disease, conditions of the prostate, and problems with the cervix, vulva, and breast.

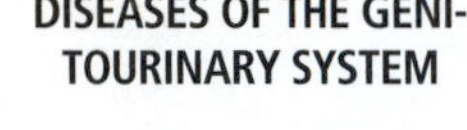

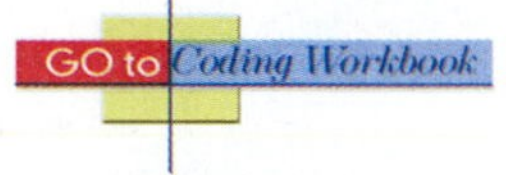

COMPLICATIONS OF PREGNANCY, CHILDBIRTH, AND THE PUERPERIUM

Complications of Pregnancy, Childbirth, and the Puerperium—Codes 630–677

Codes in Chapter 11 of the ICD-9-CM classify conditions that are involved with pregnancy, childbirth, and the puerperium (the six-week period following delivery). Many categories require a fifth digit that is based on when the complications occur (referred to as the episode of care): either before birth (antepartum), during birth, or after birth (postpartum).

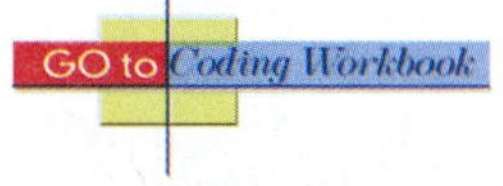

DISEASES OF THE SKIN AND SUBCUTANEOUS TISSUE

Diseases of the Skin and Subcutaneous Tissue—Codes 680–709

Codes in the ICD-9-CM's Chapter 12 classify skin infections, inflammations, and other diseases. Coders should be aware that an entire chapter or section may be subject to "Excludes" or "Includes" notes, based on the note's location. For example, the first section in this chapter (680–686) begins with a note excluding certain skin infections that are classified in Chapter 1.

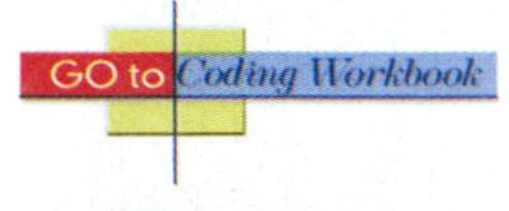

DISEASES OF THE MUSCULOSKELETAL SYSTEM AND CONNECTIVE TISSUE

Diseases of the Musculoskeletal System and Connective Tissue—Codes 710–739

Codes in Chapter 13 of the ICD-9-CM classify conditions of the bones and joints: arthropathies (joint disorders), dorsopathies (back disorders), rheumatism, and other diseases.

Congenital Anomalies—Codes 740–759

Codes in this brief ICD-9-CM Chapter 14 classify anomalies, malformations, and diseases that exist at birth. Unlike acquired disorders, congenital conditions are either hereditary or due to influencing factors during gestation.

Certain Conditions Originating in the Perinatal Period—Codes 760–779

Codes in Chapter 15 of the ICD-9-CM classify conditions of the fetus or the newborn infant, the neonate, up to twenty-eight days after birth. These codes are assigned only to conditions of the infant, not those of the mother.

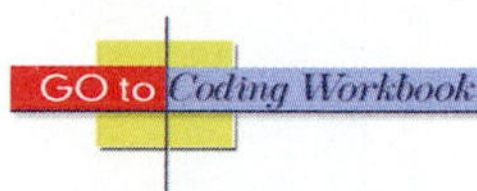

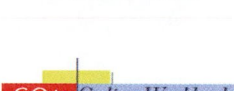

CONGENITAL ANOMALIES

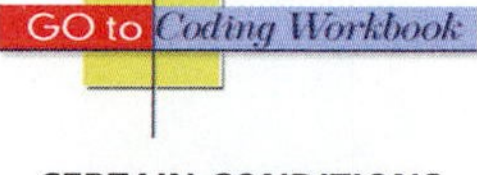

CERTAIN CONDITIONS ORIGINATING IN THE PERINATAL PERIOD

GO to *Coding Workbook*

SYMPTOMS, SIGNS, AND ILL-DEFINED CONDITIONS

Symptoms, Signs, and Ill-Defined Conditions—Codes 780–799

Codes in Chapter 16 of the ICD-9-CM classify patients' signs, symptoms, and ill-defined conditions for which a definitive diagnosis cannot be made. In physician practice coding, these codes are always used instead of coding rule-out, probable, or suspected conditions.

Injury and Poisoning—Codes 800–999

Codes in Chapter 17 of the ICD-9-CM classify injuries and wounds (fractures, dislocations, sprains, strains, internal injuries, and traumatic injuries), poisoning, and the late effects of injuries and poisoning. Often, E codes are also used to identify the cause of the injury or poisoning.

Fractures

Fractures are coded using categories 800 through 829. A fourth digit indicates whether the fracture is closed or open. When a fracture is closed, the broken bone does not pierce the skin. An open fracture involves breaking through the skin. If the fracture is not indicated as open or closed, it is coded as closed. A fifth digit is often used for the specific anatomical site. For example:

810 Fracture of clavicle

The following fifth-digit subclassification is for use with category 810:

0 unspecified part (Clavicle NOS)

1 sternal end of clavicle

2 shaft of clavicle

3 acromial end of clavicle

⑤ 810.0 Closed

⑤ 810.1 Open

When any of the following descriptions are used, a closed fracture is indicated:

Comminuted	Linear
Depressed	March
Elevated	Simple
Fissured	Slipped epiphysis
Greenstick	Spiral
Impacted	Unspecified

These descriptions indicate open fractures:

Compound
Infected
Missile
Puncture
With foreign body

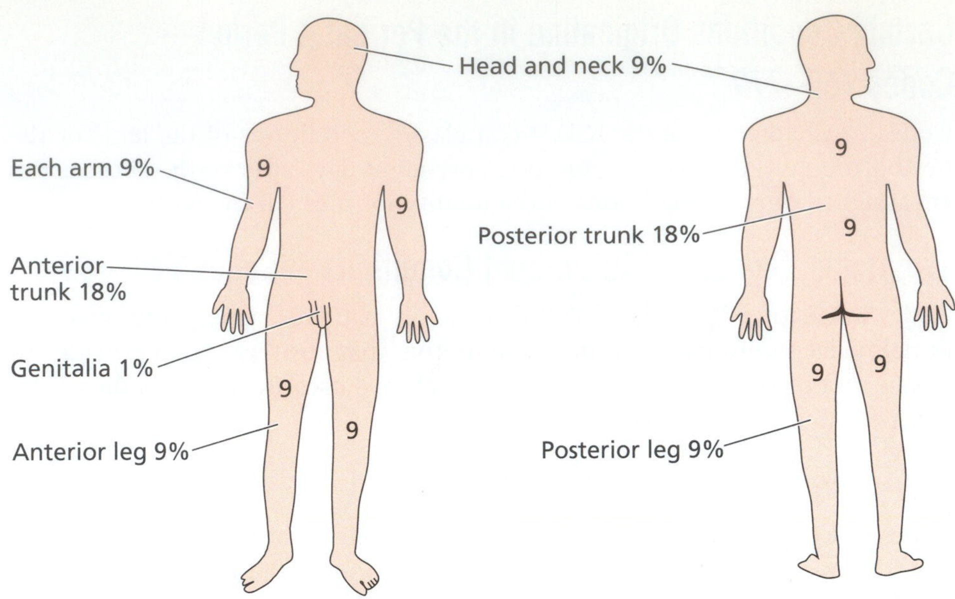

Figure 4.4 Coding Burns: The Rule of Nines

Burns

Burns are located in categories 940 through 949, where they are classified according to the cause, such as flames or radiation. They are grouped by severity and by how much of the body's surface is involved. Severity is rated as one of three degrees of burns:

1. *First-degree burn*: The epidermis (outer layer of skin) is damaged.
2. *Second-degree burn*: Both the epidermis and the dermis are damaged.
3. *Third-degree burn*: The most severe degree; the three layers of the skin—epidermis, dermis, and subcutaneous—are all damaged.

The total body surface area (TBSA) that is involved determines the extent of the burn for coding purposes (see Figure 4.4). When burns are coded according to extent (category 948), fourth-digit codes are used to show the percentage of TBSA for all of the burns. For third-degree burns, a fifth digit is also required to classify the percentage of third-degree burns:

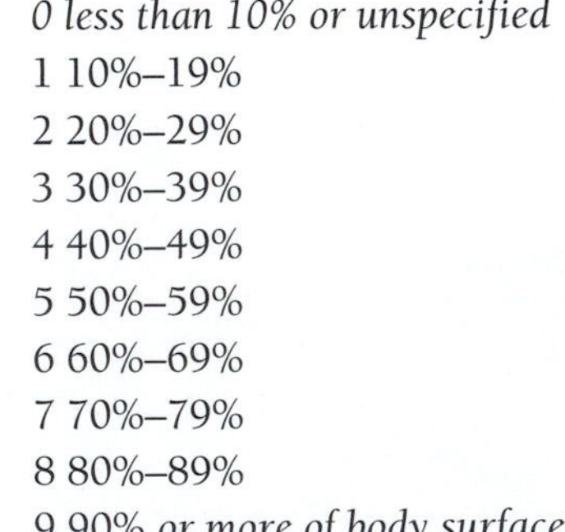

0 less than 10% or unspecified
1 10%–19%
2 20%–29%
3 30%–39%
4 40%–49%
5 50%–59%
6 60%–69%
7 70%–79%
8 80%–89%
9 *90% or more of body surface*

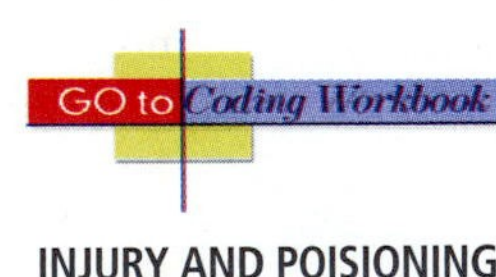

INJURY AND POISIONING

Review

Steps to Success

- ❒ Read this chapter and review the Key Terms and the Chapter Summary.
- ❒ Answer the Review Questions and Applying Your Knowledge in the Chapter Review.
- ❒ Access the chapter's websites and complete the Internet Activities to learn more about available professional resources.
- ❒ Complete the related chapter in the *Medical Insurance Workbook* to reinforce your understanding of medical coding for diagnoses.

Chapter Summary

1. The ICD-9-CM is the *Clinical Modification* of the World Health Organization's *International Classification of Diseases* used for diagnostic coding in the United States. ICD-9-CM codes are required under HIPAA for reporting patients' conditions on insurance claims and encounter forms. Codes are made up of three, four, or five numbers and a description.
2. Updates of ICD-9-CM codes, called the addenda, are issued twice a year. Medical practices must use the current codes for compliant coding and billing. Current codes are located on the NCHS website at http://www.cdc.gov/nchs/ICD9.htm
3. Two volumes of the ICD-9-CM are used in medical practices: the Tabular List (Volume 1) and the Alphabetic Index (Volume 2). The Alphabetic Index is used first in the process of finding a code. It contains an index of all the diseases that are classified in the Tabular List. These main terms may be followed by related subterms or supported by supplementary terms. The codes themselves are organized into seventeen chapters according to etiology or body system and are listed in numerical order in the Tabular List. A code category consists of a three-digit grouping of a single disease or a related condition. Subcategories have four digits to show the disease's etiology, site, or manifestation. Further clinical detail is supplied by fifth-digit subclassifications.
4. The conventions used in the ICD-9-CM must be observed to correctly select codes. Notes provide details about conditions that are either excluded or included under the code. The cross-reference *see* means that another main term is appropriate. A symbol is used to show a fifth-digit requirement. The abbreviation NOS (not otherwise specified or unspecified) indicates the code to use when a condition is not completely described. The abbreviation NEC (not elsewhere classified) indicates the code to use when the diagnosis does not match any other available code. Parentheses and brackets indicate supplementary terms. Colons and braces indicate that one or more words after the punctuation must appear in the diagnostic statement for the code to be applicable. Codes that are not used as primary appear in italics and are usually followed by instructions to code first underlying disease or use additional code.
5. V codes identify encounters for reasons other than illness or injury and are used for healthy patients receiving routine services, for therapeutic encounters, for a problem that is not currently affecting the patient's condition, and for preoperative evaluations.
6. E codes, which are never used as primary codes, classify the injuries resulting from various environmental events.

7. The three steps in the coding process are to (a) determine the reason for the encounter that is the patient's primary diagnosis, (b) locate the medical term in the Alphabetic Index, and (c) verify the code in the Tabular List.
8. The ICD-9-CM Official Guidelines for Coding and Reporting are located on the NCHS website at http://www.cdc.gov/nchs/icd9.htm.
9. Three key coding guidelines are to (a) code the primary diagnosis first, followed by current co-existing conditions, (b) code to the highest degree of certainty, never coding inconclusive, rule-out diagnoses, and (c) code to the highest level of specificity, using fifth digits or fourth digits when available.

Review Questions

Match the key terms with their definitions.

A. E code
B. unspecified
C. addenda
D. category
E. V code
F. manifestation
G. eponym
H. convention
I. main term
J. supplementary term

____ 1. Typographic technique or standard practice that provides visual guidelines for understanding printed material

____ 2. The medical term in boldfaced type that identifies a disease or condition in the Alphabetic Index

____ 3. An alphanumeric code used to identify the external cause of an injury or poisoning

____ 4. A nonessential word or phrase that helps define a diagnosis code

____ 5. Annual updates to the ICD-9-CM diagnostic coding system

____ 6. Refers to a code that should be used for an incompletely described condition

____ 7. An alphanumeric code used for an encounter that is not due to illness or injury

____ 8. A three-digit code that covers a single disease or related condition

____ 9. The characteristic signs or symptoms associated with a disease

____10. A condition or procedure that is named for the physician who discovered it

Decide whether each statement is true or false.

____ 1. In selecting correct diagnosis codes, the chapters of the Tabular List are first searched, and the code is then verified in the Alphabetic Index.

____ 2. Subcategories are four-digit diagnosis codes that define the etiology, site, or manifestation of a disease.

____ 3. In the Alphabetic Index, a *see* cross-reference must be followed.

____ 4. The etiology of a disease is the reason the patient presents for treatment.

____ 5. The fifth-digit requirement refers to the need to show a subclassification code for a particular diagnosis.

____ 6. A code that appears in italics is a secondary code and is not sequenced first.

____ 7. The coding instruction "use an additional code" means that supplying another code is optional.

____ 8. A patient has an appointment for a complaint of flulike symptoms. While the patient is in the office, the physician decides to conduct a complete physical examination. A V code is used as the primary diagnosis code for the encounter.

____ 9. When a diagnosis is being confirmed by tests or other procedures, only the patient's signs, symptoms, or vague condition are coded, not the possible or suspected disease.

____ 10. A patient's past, cured conditions have no applicability to the coding of current encounters except when late effects are noted.

Select the letter that best completes the statement or answers the question

____ 1. Outpatient coding is based on which volume or volumes of the ICD-9-CM?
A. Volume 1
B. Volumes 1 and 2
C. Volumes 1, 2, and 3
D. Volumes 2 and 3

____ 2. The medical terms in the Alphabetical Index are arranged by:
A. the condition or problem
B. the anatomical site
C. the etiology and the manifestation
D. the signs and symptoms

____ 3. An unintentional, harmful reaction to a correct dosage of a drug is called:
A. a late effect
B. a coexisting condition
C. an adverse effect
D. a manifestation

____ 4. A condition that remains or recurs after an acute illness has finished is called:
A. a late effect
B. a coexisting condition
C. an adverse effect
D. a manifestation

____ 5. A colon after a term in an *excludes* or *includes* note indicates that:
A. the term is not complete without one or more of the additional terms listed
B. the term requires a manifestation code
C. the synonyms, alternative wordings, or explanations that follow may appear in the diagnostic statement
D. the term requires a code for the underlying disease

____ 6. To code an encounter for chemotherapy, list the codes in the following order:
A. E code, condition code
B. condition code, E code
C. V code, condition code
D. condition code, V code

____ 7. The diagnostic statement "patient presents for removal of a cast" requires the use of which of the following types of codes?
A. E
B. V
C. R
D. M

____ 8. If a patient is treated for both an acute and a chronic condition, each of which has a separate code, how should the codes be listed?
A. V code, condition code
B. chronic code, acute code
C. acute code, V code
D. acute code, chronic code

____ 9. A late effect may be indicated in documentation by the use of the expression(s):
A. due to an old ... or due to a previous ...
B. malignant
C. missile, puncture, with foreign body
D. primary or secondary

____ 10. If a fracture is not documented as closed or open, it is coded as:
A. open
B. fissured
C. greenstick
D. closed

Answer the following questions.

1. List the three steps in the diagnostic coding process.

____

____

____

2. List three key coding guidelines for selecting correct diagnosis codes.

____

____

____

Applying Your Knowledge

Case 4.1 Coding Diagnoses

Supply the correct ICD-9-CM codes for the following diagnoses.

A. Brewer's infarct

B. conjunctivitis due to Reiter's disease

C. seasonal allergic rhinitis due to pollen

D. cardiac arrhythmia

E. backache

F. sebaceous cyst

G. breast disease, cystic

H. chronic cystitis

I. normal delivery

J. skin tags

K. acute myocarditis due to influenza

L. acute otitis media

M. endocarditis due to Q fever

N. influenza vaccination

O. vertigo

P. essential anemia

Q. muscle spasms

R. influenza with acute respiratory infection

S. pneumonia due to Streptococcus, Group B

T. menorrhagia

Case 4.2 Auditing Code Assignment

Audit the following cases to determine whether the correct codes have been reported in the correct order. If a coding mistake has been made, state the correct code and your reason for assigning it.

A

Chart note for Henry Blum, date of birth 11/4/53:

Examined patient on 12/6/2006. He was complaining of a facial rash. Examination revealed psoriasis and extensive seborrheic dermatitis over his upper eyebrows, nasolabial fold, and extending to the subnasal region.

The following codes were reported: 696.1, 690.1.

B

Physician's notes, 2/24/2005, patient George Kadar, DOB 10/11/1940:

Subjective: This sixty-year-old patient complains of voiding difficulties, primarily urinary incontinence. No complaints of urinary retention.

Objective: Rectal examination: enlarged prostate. Patient catheterized for residual urine of 200 cc. Urinalysis is essentially negative.

Assessment: Prostatic hypertrophy, benign.

Plan: Refer to urologist for cystoscopy.

The following code was reported: 600.0.

C

Patient: Gloria S. Diaz:

Subjective: This twenty-five-year-old female patient presents with pain in her left knee both when she moves it and when it is inactive. She denies previous trauma to this area but has had right-knee pain and arthritis in the past.

Objective: Examination revealed the left knee to be warm and slightly swollen compared to the right knee. Extension is 180 degrees; flexion is 90 degrees. Some tenderness in area.

Assessment: Left-knee pain probably due to chronic arthritis.

Plan: Daypro 600 mg 2-QD × 1 week; recheck in one week.

The following codes were reported: 719.48, 716.98.

Internet Activities

1. Access the website of the National Center for Health Statistics: http://www.cdc.gov/nchs/icd9.htm. Research current changes to the Official Guidelines. Preview the status of ICD-10-CM.
2. Access the website of CMS and research the topic ICD9 to locate the ICD-9-CM Provider & Diagnostic Codes Overview home page. Locate the most recent updates to ICD-9-CM (addendum).
3. Use a search engine to visit ICD lookup websites, and look up codes for diagnoses that you select. How easy were these websites to use?

Chapter 5

Procedural Coding: Introduction to CPT

CHAPTER OUTLINE

Current Procedurak Terminology, Fourth Edition (CPT)*

The Index

The Main Text

CPT Modifiers

The Appendixes

Coding Steps

Evaluation and Management Codes

Anesthesia Codes

Surgery Codes

Radiology Codes

Pathology and Laboratory Codes

Medicine Codes

Category II and III Codes

Learning Outcomes

After studying this chapter, you should be able to:

1. Discuss the purpose of the CPT code set.
2. Explain how to locate the periodic updates to CPT codes.
3. Describe the structure and content of the index and the main text in CPT.
4. Interpret the formats, conventions, and symbols used in CPT.
5. Describe the purpose and correct use of CPT modifiers.
6. List the three general steps for selecting correct CPT procedure codes.
7. Discuss the purpose, structure, and key guidelines for each of the six sections of CPT Category I codes.
8. Discuss the key components that are the basis for selection of CPT Evaluation and Management codes, and describe the steps for selecting correct codes.
9. Analyze procedural statements, apply appropriate physician practice coding guidelines, and assign correct CPT codes.

KEY TERMS

add-on code
ancillary services
bundling
Category I codes
Category II codes
Category III codes
consultation
Current Procedural Terminology (CPT)
descriptor
E/M codes
fragmented billing
global period
global surgery rule
key component
modifier
outpatient
panel
physical status modifier
primary procedure
professional component (PC)
secondary procedure
section guidelines
separate procedure
special reports
surgical package
technical component (TC)
unbundling
unlisted procedure

Procedure codes, like diagnosis codes, are an important part of the medical billing process. Standard procedure codes are used by physicians to report the medical, surgical, and diagnostic services they provide. These reported codes are used by payers to determine payments. Accurate procedural coding ensures that providers receive the maximum appropriate reimbursement.

Procedure codes are also used to establish guidelines for the delivery of the best possible care for patients. Medical researchers track various treatment plans for patients with similar diagnoses and evaluate patients' outcomes. The results are shared with physicians and payers so that best practices can be implemented. For example, this type of analysis has shown that a patient who has had a heart attack can reduce the risk of another attack by taking a class of drugs called beta blockers.

In the practice, physicians, medical coders, medical insurance specialists, or outside companies assign procedure codes. Medical insurance specialists verify the procedure codes and use them to report physicians' services to payers. This chapter provides a fundamental understanding of how to assign procedure codes so that medical insurance specialists can work effectively with claims. Knowledge of procedural coding—and of how to stay up-to-date—is the baseline for compliant billing.

CURRENT PROCEDURAL TERMINOLOGY, Fourth Edition (CPT)

HIPAA Tip

Mandated Code Set

CPT is the mandated code set for physician procedures and services under HIPAA Electronic Health Care Transactions and Code Sets.

The procedure codes for physicians' and other health care providers' services are selected from the *Current Procedural Terminology* data set, called **CPT**, which is owned and maintained by the American Medical Association (AMA).

History

CPT was first produced by the AMA in 1966. Its wide use began in 1983 when the Health Care Financing Administration (now named the Centers for Medicare and Medicaid, or CMS) decided that the CPT codes would be the standard for physician procedures paid by Medicare, Medicaid, and other government medical insurance programs.

CPT lists the procedures and services that are commonly performed by physicians across the country. There is also a need for codes for items that are used in medical practices but are not listed in CPT, like supplies and equipment. These codes are found in the Healthcare Common Procedure Coding System, referred to as HCPCS and pronounced hick-picks, which is covered in the next chapter of this text. Officially, CPT is the first part (called Level I) of HCPCS, and the supply codes are the second part (Level II). Most people, though, refer to the codes in the CPT book as *CPT codes* and the Level II codes as *HCPCS codes*.

HIPAA Tip

Mandated Use of Current Codes

Codes must be current as of the date of service.

Types of CPT Codes

There are three categories of CPT codes:

- Category I codes
- Category II codes
- Category III codes

Category I Codes

CPT **Category I** codes—which are the most numerous—have five digits (with no decimals). Each code has a **descriptor**, which is a brief explanation of the procedure:

99204	Office visit for evaluation and management of a new patient
00730	Anesthesia for procedures on upper posterior abdominal wall
24006	Arthrotomy of the elbow, with capsular excision for capsular release
70100	Radiologic examination of the mandible
80400	ACTH stimulation panel; for adrenal insufficiency
93000	Electrocardiogram, routine ECG with at least 12 leads; with interpretation and report

Although the codes are grouped into sections, such as Surgery, codes from all sections can be used by all types of physicians. For example, a family practitioner might use codes from the Surgery section to describe an office procedure such as the incision and drainage of an abscess.

Category II Codes

Category II codes are used to track performance measures for a medical goal such as reducing tobacco use. These codes are optional; they are not paid by insurance carriers. They help in the development of best practices for care and improve documentation. These codes have alphabetic characters for the fifth digit:

0002F	Tobacco use, smoking, assessed
0004F	Tobacco use cessation intervention, counseling

Category III Codes

Category III codes are temporary codes for emerging technology, services, and procedures. These codes also have alphabetic characters for the fifth digit:

0001T	Endovascular repair of infrarenal abdominal aortic aneurysm or dissection
0041T	Urinalysis infectious agent detection

A temporary code may become a permanent part of the regular codes if the service it identifies proves effective and is widely performed.

Organization and Format

The manual is made up of the main text—sections of codes—followed by appendixes and an index. The main text has the following six sections of Category I procedure codes:

- Evaluation and Management — Codes 99201–99499
- Anesthesia — Codes 00100–01999
- Surgery — Codes 10021–69990
- Radiology — Codes 70010–79999
- Pathology and Laboratory — Codes 80048–89356
- Medicine — Codes 90281–99602

Table 5.1 summarizes the types of codes, organization, and guidelines of these six main sections.

Updates

CPT is a proprietary code set, meaning that it is not available for free to the public. Instead, the information must be purchased, either in print or electronic format, from the AMA, which publishes the revised CPT codes.

During the year, practicing physicians, medical specialty societies, and state medical associations send their suggestions for revision to the AMA. This in-

TABLE 5.1 CPT Category I Code Sections

SECTION	DEFINITION OF CODES	STRUCTURE	KEY GUIDELINES
Evaluation and Management	Physicians' services that are performed to determine the best course for patient care	Organized by place and/or type of service	New/established patients; other definitions Unlisted services, special reports Selecting an E/M service level
Anesthesia	Anesthesia services by or supervised by a physician; includes general, regional, and local anesthesia	Organized by body site	Time-based Services covered (bundled) in codes Unlisted services/special reports Qualifying circumstances codes
Surgery	Surgical procedures performed by physicians	Organized by body system and then body site, followed by procedural groups	Surgical package definition Follow-up care definition Add-on codes Separate procedures Subsection notes Unlisted services/special reports Starred procedures
Radiology	Radiology services by or supervised by a physician	Organized by type of procedure followed by body site	Unlisted services/special reports Supervision and interpretation (professional and technical components)
Pathology and Laboratory	Pathology and laboratory services by physicians or by physician-supervised technicians	Organized by type of procedure	Complete procedure Panels Unlisted services/special reports
Medicine	Evaluation, therapeutic, and diagnostic procedures by or supervised by a physician	Organized by type of service or procedure	Subsection notes Multiple procedures reported separately Add-on codes Separate procedures Unlisted services/special reports

Thinking It Through — 5.1

Would you expect to locate codes for the following services or procedures in CPT? What range or series of codes would you investigate?

Service or Procedure Range or Series

1. Routine obstetric care including antepartum care, cesarean delivery, and postpartum care
2. Echocardiography
3. Radiologic examination, nasal bones, complete
4. Home visit for evaluation and management of an established patient
5. Drug test for amphetamines
6. Anesthesia for cardiac catheterization

CPT Updates

http://www.ama-assn.org/go/CPT

put is reviewed by the AMA's Editorial Panel, which includes physicians as well as representatives from the Health Insurance Association of America, CMS, the American Health Information Management Association (AHIMA), the American Hospital Association (AHA), and Blue Cross and Blue Shield. The panel decides what changes will be made in the annual revision of the printed reference book.

The annual changes for Category I codes are announced by the AMA on October 1 and are in effect for procedures and services provided after January 1 of the following year. The code books can be purchased in different formats, which range from a basic listing to an enhanced edition. The AMA also reports the new codes on its website.

Category II and III codes are prereleased on the AMA website and can be used on their implementation date even before they appear in the printed books.

Billing Tip

Updating Vaccine Codes and Category III Codes
Both vaccine product codes and Category III codes are released twice a year and have a six-month period for implementation. Offices billing these services should check for updates at the CPT website.

The Index

The assignment of a correct procedure code begins by reviewing the physician's statements in the patient's medical record to determine the service, procedure, or treatment that was performed. Then the index entry is located, which provides a pointer to the correct code range in the main text. Using the CPT index makes the process of selecting procedure codes more efficient. The index contains the descriptive terms that are listed in the sections of codes in the CPT.

Main Terms and Modifying Terms

The main terms in the index are printed in boldface type. There are five types of main terms:

1. The name of the procedure or service, such as echocardiography, extraction, and cast
2. The name of the organ or other anatomical site, such as stomach, wrist, and salivary gland

HIPAA Tip

Using the Current Codes

Practices must use new CPT codes on the date they are effective. There is no "grace period" or overlapping use of old and new codes. Keep codes on encounter forms and practice management programs up to date.

3. The name of the condition, such as abscess, wound, and postpartum care
4. A synonym or an eponym for the term, such as Noble Procedure, Ramstedt operation, and Fowler-Stephens orchiopexy
5. The abbreviation for the term, such as CAT scan and ECMO

Many terms are listed more than one way. For example, the kidney biopsy procedure is listed both as a procedure—Biopsy, kidney—and by the site—Kidney, biopsy.

A main term may be followed by subterms that further describe the entry. These additional indented terms help in the selection process. For example, the procedure repair of tennis elbow is located beneath *repair* under the main term *elbow* (see Figure 5.1).

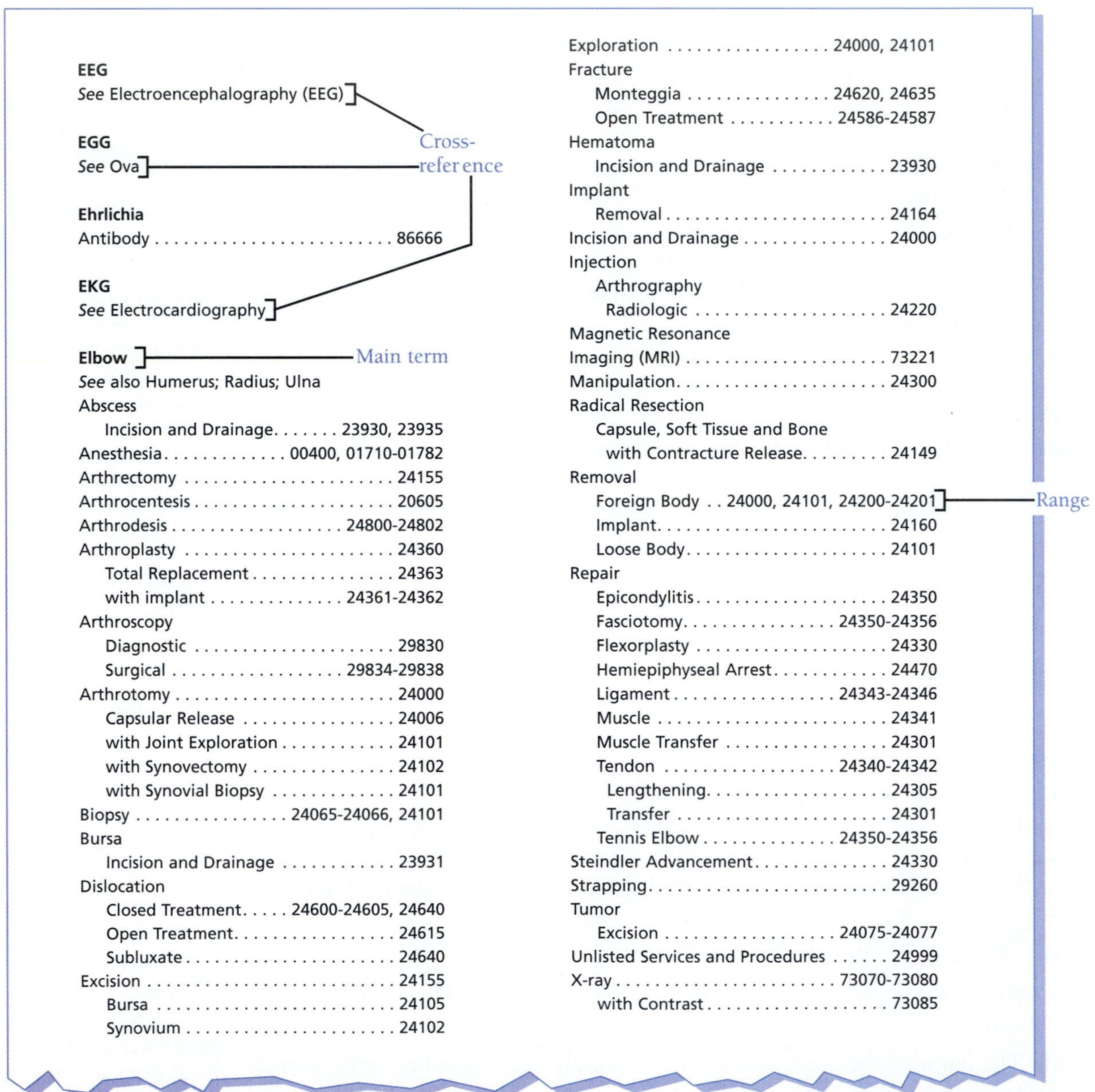

EEG
See Electroencephalography (EEG)

EGG
See Ova

Ehrlichia
Antibody 86666

EKG
See Electrocardiography

Elbow
See also Humerus; Radius; Ulna
Abscess
  Incision and Drainage. 23930, 23935
Anesthesia. 00400, 01710-01782
Arthrectomy 24155
Arthrocentesis 20605
Arthrodesis 24800-24802
Arthroplasty 24360
  Total Replacement 24363
  with implant 24361-24362
Arthroscopy
  Diagnostic 29830
  Surgical 29834-29838
Arthrotomy 24000
  Capsular Release 24006
  with Joint Exploration 24101
  with Synovectomy 24102
  with Synovial Biopsy 24101
Biopsy 24065-24066, 24101
Bursa
  Incision and Drainage 23931
Dislocation
  Closed Treatment. 24600-24605, 24640
  Open Treatment. 24615
  Subluxate 24640
Excision 24155
  Bursa 24105
  Synovium 24102
Exploration 24000, 24101
Fracture
  Monteggia 24620, 24635
  Open Treatment 24586-24587
Hematoma
  Incision and Drainage 23930
Implant
  Removal 24164
Incision and Drainage 24000
Injection
  Arthrography
    Radiologic 24220
Magnetic Resonance
Imaging (MRI) 73221
Manipulation. 24300
Radical Resection
  Capsule, Soft Tissue and Bone
    with Contracture Release. 24149
Removal
  Foreign Body . . 24000, 24101, 24200-24201
  Implant. 24160
  Loose Body. 24101
Repair
  Epicondylitis. 24350
  Fasciotomy. 24350-24356
  Flexorplasty 24330
  Hemiepiphyseal Arrest. 24470
  Ligament 24343-24346
  Muscle 24341
  Muscle Transfer 24301
  Tendon 24340-24342
    Lengthening. 24305
    Transfer 24301
  Tennis Elbow 24350-24356
Steindler Advancement. 24330
Strapping. 29260
Tumor
  Excision 24075-24077
Unlisted Services and Procedures 24999
X-ray 73070-73080
  with Contrast 73085

FIGURE 5.1 Example of Index Entries

Code Ranges

A range of codes is shown when more than one code applies to an entry. Two codes, either sequential or not, are separated by a comma:

Cervix
Biopsy. 57500, 57520

More than two sequential codes are separated by a hyphen:

Dislocation
Ankle
Closed Treatment 27840–27842

Cross-References and Convention

There are two types of cross-references:

1. *See* is a mandatory instruction. It tells the coder to refer to the term that follows it to find the code. It is used mainly for synonyms, eponyms, and abbreviations. For example, the cross-reference "See Electrocardiogram" follows EKG (see Figure 5.1).
2. *See also* tells the coder to look under the term that follows if the procedure is not listed below. For example, under *Elbow,* the cross-reference "See also Humerus; Radius; Ulna" points to those main terms if the entry is not located under *Elbow* (see Figure 5.1).

To save space, some connecting words are left out and must be assumed by the reader. For example:

Ear Cartilage
Graft
to face. 21235

should be read "graft of ear cartilage to face." The reader supplies the word *of*.

The Main Text

After the index is used to point to a possible code, the main text is read to verify the selection of the code (see Figure 5.2).

Each of the six sections of the main text lists procedure codes and descriptions under subsection headings. These headings group procedures or services, such as Therapeutic or Diagnostic Injections or Psychoanalysis; body systems, such as Digestive System; anatomical sites, such as Abdomen; and tests and examinations, such as Complete Blood Count (CBC). Following these headings are additional subgroups of procedures, systems, or sites. For example, Figure 5.2 illustrates the following structure, in which the body system appears as the subsection followed by a procedure subgroup:

Surgery Section <*The Section*>

Musculoskeletal System <*The Subsection*>

Endoscopy/Arthroscopy <*The Procedure Subgroup*>

The section, subsection, and code number range on a page are shown at the top of the page, making it easier to locate a code.

Billing Tip

Correct Coding Procedure
Never select a code based on only the index entry because the main text may have additional entries and important guidelines that alter the selection.

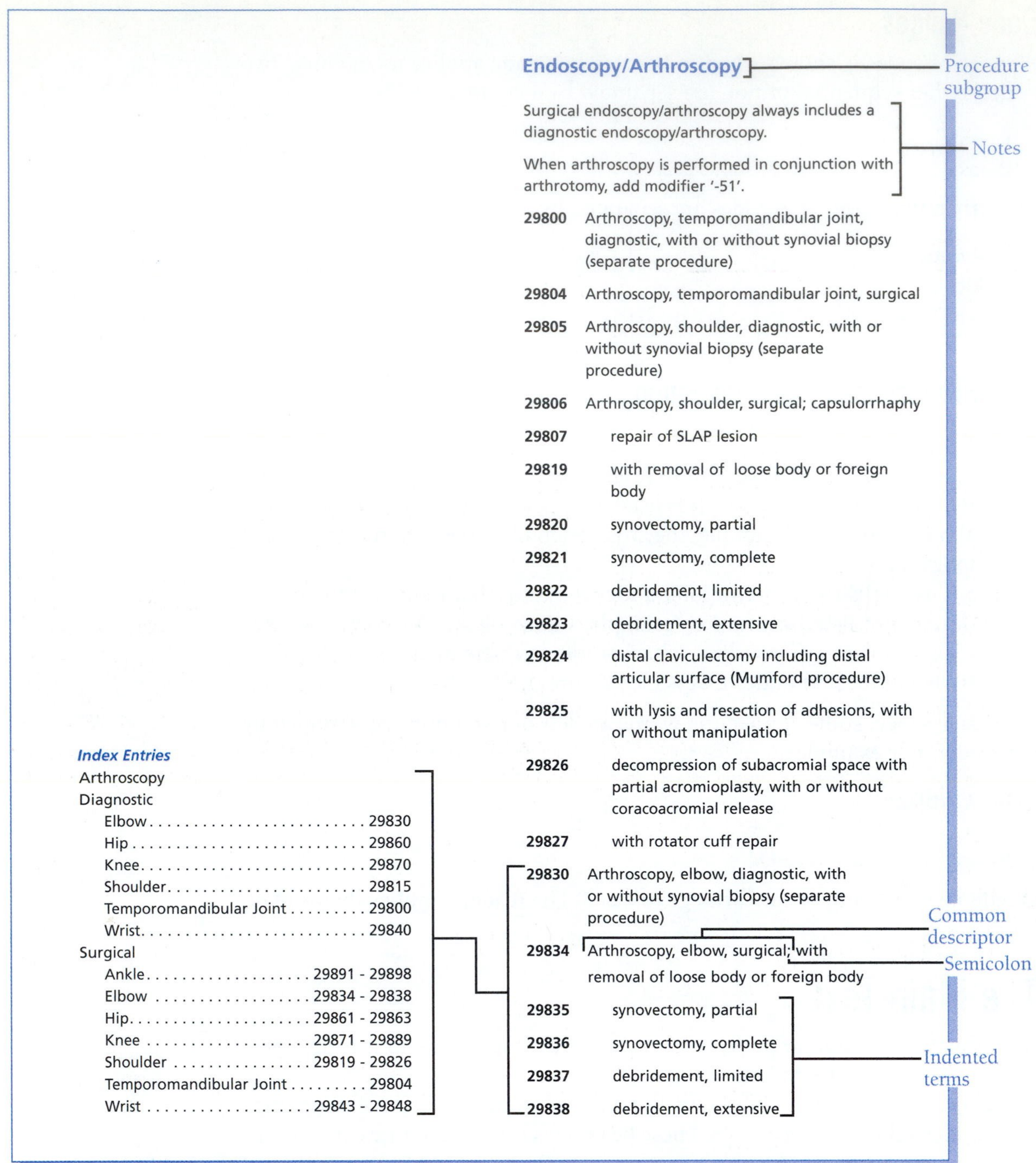

Endoscopy/Arthroscopy

Surgical endoscopy/arthroscopy always includes a diagnostic endoscopy/arthroscopy.

When arthroscopy is performed in conjunction with arthrotomy, add modifier '-51'.

29800 Arthroscopy, temporomandibular joint, diagnostic, with or without synovial biopsy (separate procedure)

29804 Arthroscopy, temporomandibular joint, surgical

29805 Arthroscopy, shoulder, diagnostic, with or without synovial biopsy (separate procedure)

29806 Arthroscopy, shoulder, surgical; capsulorrhaphy

29807 repair of SLAP lesion

29819 with removal of loose body or foreign body

29820 synovectomy, partial

29821 synovectomy, complete

29822 debridement, limited

29823 debridement, extensive

29824 distal claviculectomy including distal articular surface (Mumford procedure)

29825 with lysis and resection of adhesions, with or without manipulation

29826 decompression of subacromial space with partial acromioplasty, with or without coracoacromial release

29827 with rotator cuff repair

29830 Arthroscopy, elbow, diagnostic, with or without synovial biopsy (separate procedure)

29834 Arthroscopy, elbow, surgical; with removal of loose body or foreign body

29835 synovectomy, partial

29836 synovectomy, complete

29837 debridement, limited

29838 debridement, extensive

Index Entries

Arthroscopy
Diagnostic
- Elbow 29830
- Hip 29860
- Knee 29870
- Shoulder 29815
- Temporomandibular Joint 29800
- Wrist 29840

Surgical
- Ankle . . . . 29891 - 29898
- Elbow . . . . 29834 - 29838
- Hip . . . . 29861 - 29863
- Knee . . . . 29871 - 29889
- Shoulder . . . . 29819 - 29826
- Temporomandibular Joint 29804
- Wrist . . . . 29843 - 29848

FIGURE 5.2 Example of Code Listings from the Musculoskeletal System Subsection of the Surgery Section

Guidelines

Each section begins with **section guidelines** for the use of its codes. The guidelines cover definitions and items unique to the section. They also include special notes about the structure of the section or the rules for its use. The guidelines must be carefully studied and followed in order to correctly use the codes in the section. Some notes apply only to specific subsections. The guidelines list the subsections in which these notes occur, and the notes themselves begin those subsections (see Figure 5.2).

Unlisted Procedures

Most sections' guidelines give codes for **unlisted procedures**—those not completely described by any code in the section. For example, in the Evaluation and Management section, two unlisted codes are provided:

99429 Unlisted preventive medicine service

99499 Unlisted evaluation and management service

Unlisted procedure codes are used for new services or procedures that have not yet been assigned either Category I or III codes in CPT. When an unlisted code is reported to a payer, documentation of the procedure should accompany the claim. Often the operative report or a letter from the physician describing the procedure meets this need.

Special Reports

Some section guidelines suggest the use of **special reports** for rare or new procedures, especially unlisted procedures. These reports, which are mandatory, permit payers to assess the medical appropriateness of the procedures. The guidelines cover the information that should be in the report, such as a description of the nature, extent, and need for the procedure plus additional notes on the symptoms or findings.

Billing Tip

Unlisted Procedure Codes
Unlisted procedures require special reports which delay claims because they must be processed manually. Check with the payer to find out if a temporary code or Category III code has been assigned. If so, that code should be used. If not, use the unlisted code, and supply the payer-required documentation.

Format

Semicolons and Indentions

To save space in the book, CPT uses a semicolon and indentions when a common part of a main entry applies to entries that follow. For example, in the entries listed below, the procedure *partial laryngectomy (hemilaryngectomy)* is the common descriptor. This same descriptor applies to the four unique descriptors after the semicolon—*horizontal*, *laterovertical*, *anterovertical*, and *antero-latero-vertical*. Note that the common descriptor begins with a capital letter, but the unique descriptors after the semicolon do not. Also note that after the first listing, the second, third, and fourth descriptors are indented. Indenting visually reinforces the relationship between the entries and the common descriptor.

31370 Partial laryngectomy (hemilaryngectomy); horizontal

31375 laterovertical

31380 anterovertical

31382 antero-latero-vertical

This method shows the relationships among the entries without repeating the common word or words. Follow this case example in Figure 5.2:

Index Entry: Arthroscopy, Surgical. 29834–29838

Main Text: 29838 Arthroscopy, elbow, surgical; with debridement, extensive

Cross-References

Some codes and descriptors are followed by indented *see* or *use* entries in parentheses, which refer the coder to other codes. For example:

82239 Bile acids; total
82240 cholylglycine

(For bile pigments, urine, see 81000–81005)

Examples

Descriptors often contain clarifying examples in parentheses, sometimes with the abbreviation *e.g.* (meaning for example). These provide further descriptions, such as synonyms or examples, but they are not essential to the selection of the code. Here are examples:

87040 Culture, bacterial; blood, with isolation and presumptive identification of isolates (includes anaerobic culture, if appropriate)

50400 Pyeloplasty (Foley Y-pyeloplasty), plastic operation on renal pelvis, with or without plastic operation on ureter, nephropexy, nephrostomy, pyelostomy, or ureteral splinting; simple

50405 complicated (congenital kidney abnormality, secondary pyelosplasty, solitary kidney, calycoplasty)

Symbols for Changed Codes

These symbols have the following meanings when they appear next to CPT codes:

● A bullet (a black circle) indicates a new procedure code. The symbol appears next to the code only the year that it is added.

▲ A triangle indicates that the code's descriptor has changed. It, too, appears in only the year the descriptor is revised.

▶◀ Facing triangles (two triangles that face each other) enclose new or revised text other than the code's descriptor.

Symbol for Add-On Codes

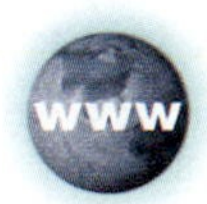

AMA Vaccine Code Updates

http://www.ama-assn.org/ama/pub/category/10902.html

A plus sign (+) next to a code in the main text indicates an **add-on code.** Add-on codes describe **secondary procedures** that are commonly carried out in addition to a **primary procedure.** Add-on codes usually use phrases such as *each additional* or *list separately in addition to the primary procedure* to show that they are never used as stand-alone codes. For example, the add-on code +15001 is used after the code for surgical preparation of a free skin graft site (15000) to provide a specific percentage or dimension of body area that was involved beyond the amount covered in the primary procedure.

Billing Tip

Vaccine Coding Prerelease

Stay up to date on approval status for vaccine codes with the thunderbolt symbol. These codes are prereleased every six months on the AMA website and can be used as soon as they appear.

Symbols for Conscious Sedation and for FDA Approval Pending

In CPT, the symbol ⊙ (a bullet inside a circle) next to a code means that conscious sedation is a part of the procedure that the surgeon performs. This means that for compliant coding, conscious sedation is not billed in addition to the code. Conscious sedation is a moderate, drug-induced depression of consciousness during which patients can respond to verbal commands. This type of sedation is typically used with procedures such as bronchoscopies.

Also used is the symbol ⚡ (a thunderbolt). This symbol is used with vaccine codes that have been submitted to the Federal Drug Administration (FDA) and are expected to be approved for use soon. The codes cannot be used until approved, at which point this symbol is removed.

CPT Modifiers

A CPT **modifier** is a two-digit number that may be attached to most five-digit procedure codes (see Table 5.2 on page 154). Modifiers are used to communi-

Thinking It Through — 5.2

1. **Find the following codes in the index of CPT. Underline the key term you used to find the code.**
   - **A.** Intracapsular lens extraction
   - **B.** Coombs test
   - **C.** X-ray of duodenum
   - **D.** Unlisted procedure, maxillofacial prosthetics
   - **E.** DTAP immunization
2. **Identify the symbol used to indicate a new procedure code, and list five new codes that appear in CPT.**
3. **Identify the symbol used to indicate a procedure that is usually done in addition to a primary procedure. Locate code 92981, and describe the unit of measure that is involved with this add-on code.**
4. **Identify the symbol that indicates that the code's description has been changed, and list five examples of codes with new or revised descriptors that appear in CPT.**
5. **Identify the symbols that enclose new or revised text other than the code's descriptor, and list five examples of codes with new or revised text that appear in CPT.**
6. **Identify the symbol next to a code that means that conscious sedation is a part of the procedure that the surgeon performs, and list five examples from CPT.**
7. **Identify the symbol next to a code that means that FDA approval is pending, and list one example from CPT's vaccines and toxoids code section (codes 90476–90749).**

cate special circumstances involved with procedures that have been performed. A modifier tells private and government payers that the physician considers the procedure to have been altered in some way. A modifier usually affects the normal level of reimbursement for the code to which it is attached.

For example, the modifier –76, Repeat Procedure by Same Physician, is used when the reporting physician repeats a procedure or service after doing the first one. A situation requiring this modifier to show the extra procedure might be:

> *Procedural Statement*: Physician performed a chest X-ray before placing a chest tube and then, after the chest tube was placed, performed a second chest X-ray to verify its position.
>
> *Code:* 71020–76 Radiologic examination, chest, two views, frontal and lateral; repeat procedure or service by same physician

The modifiers are listed in Appendix A of CPT. However, not all modifiers are available for use with every section's codes:

- Some modifiers apply only to certain sections. For example, the modifier –21, Prolonged Evaluation and Management Services, is used only with

TABLE 5.2 CPT Modifiers: Description and Common Use in Main Text Sections

Code	Description	E/M	Anesthesia	Surgery	Radiology	Pathology	Medicine
–21	Prolonged E/M Service	Yes	Never	Never	Never	Never	Never
–22	Unusual Procedural Service	Never	Yes	Yes	Yes	Yes	Yes
–23	Unusual Anesthesia	Never	Yes				Never
–24	Unrelated E/M Service by the Same Physician During a Postoperative Period	Yes	Never	Never	Never	Never	Never
–25	Significant, Separately Identifiable E/M Service by the Same Physician on the Same Day of the Procedure or Other Service	Yes	Never	Never	Never	Never	Never
–26	Professional Component	—	—	Yes	Yes	Yes	Yes
–32	Mandated Services	Yes	Yes	Yes	Yes	Yes	Yes
–47	Anesthesia by Surgeon	Never	Never	Yes	Never	Never	Never
–50	Bilateral Procedure	—	—	Yes	—	—	—
–51	Multiple Procedures	—	Yes	Yes	Yes	Never	Yes
–52	Reduced Services	Yes	—	Yes	Yes	Yes	Yes
–53	Discontinued Procedure	Never	Yes	Yes	Yes	Yes	Yes
–54	Surgical Care Only	—	—	Yes	—	—	—
–55	Postoperative Management Only	—	—	Yes	—	—	Yes
–56	Preoperative Management Only	—	—	Yes	—	—	Yes
–57	Decision for Surgery	Yes	—	—	—	—	Yes
–58	Staged or Related Procedure/Service by the Same Physician During the Postoperative Period	—	—	Yes	Yes	—	Yes
–59	Distinct Procedural Service	—	Yes	Yes	Yes	Yes	Yes
–62	Two Surgeons	Never	Never	Yes	Yes	Never	—
–63	Procedure Performed on Infants	—	—	Yes	Yes	—	Yes
–66	Surgical Team	Never	Never	Yes	Yes	Never	—
–76	Repeat Procedure by Same Physician	—	—	Yes	Yes	—	Yes
–77	Repeat Procedure by Another Physician	—	—	Yes	Yes	—	Yes
–78	Return to the Operating Room for a Related Procedure During the Postoperative Period	—	—	Yes	Yes	—	Yes
–79	Unrelated Procedure/Service by the Same Physician During the Postoperative Period	—	—	Yes	Yes	—	Yes
–80	Assistant Surgeon	Never	—	Yes	Yes	—	—
–81	Minimum Assistant Surgeon	Never	—	Yes	—	—	—
–82	Assistant Surgeon (When Qualified Resident Surgeon Not Available)	Never	—	Yes	—	—	—
–90	Reference (Outside) Laboratory	—	—	Yes	Yes	Yes	Yes
–91	Repeat Clinical Diagnostic Laboratory Test	—	—	Yes	Yes	Yes	Yes
–99	Multiple Modifiers	—	—	Yes	Yes	—	Yes

Source: CPT 2007
Key:
Yes = commonly used
— = not usually used with the codes in that section
Never = not used with the codes in that section

codes that are located in the Evaluation and Management section, as its descriptor implies.

- Add-on codes cannot be modified with –51, Multiple Procedures, because the add-on code is used to add increments to a primary procedure, so the need for multiple procedures is replaced by procedures added on.
- Codes that begin with ⦸ (a circle with a backslash) also cannot be modified with –51, Multiple Procedures.

What Do Modifiers Mean?

The use of a modifier means that a procedure was different from the description in CPT, but not in a way that changed the definition or required a different code. Modifiers are used mainly when:

- A procedure has two parts—a **technical component** (TC) performed by a technician, such as a radiologist, and a **professional component** (PC) that the physician performs, usually the interpretation and reporting of the results.
- A service or procedure has been performed more than once, by more than one physician, and/or in more than one location
- A service or procedure has been increased or reduced
- Only part of a procedure has been done
- A bilateral or multiple procedure has been performed
- Unusual difficulties occurred during the procedure

Billing Tip

Professional Component Modifier –26
The professional component modifier tells the payer that the physician did not perform all work, just the professional part, so only part of the fee is due. The other part of the fee, associated with the modifier –TC, is paid to the technician.

Assigning Modifiers

Modifiers are shown by adding a hyphen and the two-digit code to the CPT code. For example, a physician providing therapeutic radiology services in a hospital would report the modifier –26, Professional Component, as follows:

73090–26

This format means professional component only for an X-ray of the forearm. (In effect, it means that the physician who performed the service did not own the equipment used, so the fee is split between the physician and the equipment owner.)

Two or more modifiers may be used with one code to give the most accurate description possible. The use of two or more modifiers is shown by reporting –99, Multiple Modifiers, followed by the other modifiers, with the most essential modifier listed first.

Procedures: Multitrauma patient's extremely difficult surgery after a car accident; team surgery by orthopedic surgeon and neurosurgeon. The first surgical procedure carries these modifiers:

27236–99, –66, –51, –22

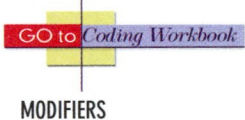

MODIFIERS

The Appendixes

The twelve appendixes contain information helpful to the coding process:

1. *Appendix A—Modifiers:* A complete listing of all modifiers used in CPT with descriptions and, in some cases, examples of usage
2. *Appendix B—Summary of Additions, Deletions, and Revisions:* A summary of the codes added, revised, and deleted in the current version

3. *Appendix C—Clinical Examples:* Case examples of the proper use of the codes in the Evaluation and Management section
4. *Appendix D—Summary of CPT Add-on Codes:* List of supplemental codes used for procedures that are commonly done in addition to the primary procedure
5. *Appendix E—Summary of CPT Codes Exempt from Modifier –51:* Codes to which the modifier showing multiple procedures cannot be attached because they already include a multiple descriptor
6. *Appendix F—Summary of CPT Codes Exempt from Modifier –63*
7. *Appendix G—Summary of CPT Codes Which Include Conscious Sedation*
8. *Appendix H—Alphabetic Index of Performance Measures by Clinical Condition or Topic*
9. *Appendix I—Genetic Testing Code Modifiers*
10. *Appendix J—Electrodiagnostic Medicine Listing of Sensory, Motor, and Mixed Nerves*
11. *Appendix K—Product Pending FDA Approval*
12. *Appendix L—Vascular Families*

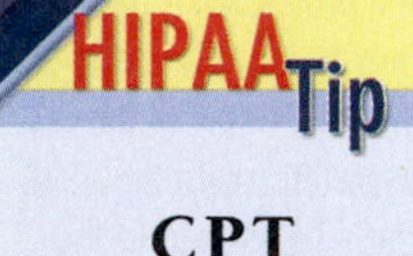

CPT Assistant

The American Medical Association's monthly publication CPT Assistant *is the authoritative guide to the correct use of CPT codes.*

Coding Steps

The correct process for reporting accurate procedure codes has three steps.

Step 1 Determine the Procedures and Services to Report

The first step is to review the documentation of the patient's visit and decide which procedures and/or services were performed. Then, based on knowledge of the CPT and of the payer's policies, a decision is made about which services can be charged and are to be reported.

Step 2 Identify the Correct Codes

The process for selecting correct codes is as follows:

1. The index is used to locate the main term for each procedure or service. If the term is not found, the organ or body site is looked up, and then the disease or injury. Further checking can be done to locate any synonyms, eponyms, or abbreviations associated with the main term. The entries under the main term are reviewed to see if any apply, and cross-references are checked.
2. If the main term cannot be located in the index, the medical insurance specialist reviews the main term selection with the physician for clarification. In some cases, there is a better or more common term that can be used.
3. The main text listing, including all section guidelines and notes for the particular subsection, is carefully reviewed to make the final code choice. Items that cannot be billed separately because they are covered under another, broader code are eliminated.
4. The codes to be reported for each day's services are ranked in order of highest to lowest rate of reimbursement. The actual order in which they were performed on a particular day is not important. For services on multiple dates, the earliest day is listed first, followed by subsequent dates of service. For example:

Date	*Procedure*	*Charge*
11/17/2008	**99204**	$202
11/20/2008	**43215**	$355
11/20/2008	**74235**	$75

Thinking It Through — 5.3

1. In CPT, what is the meaning of the symbol in front of code 93501?
2. Based on Appendix A of CPT, what modifiers would you assign in each of the following cases? Why?

CASE 1

Patient has recurrent cancer; surgeon performed a colectomy, which took forty-five minutes longer than the normal procedure due to dense adhesions from the patient's previous surgery.

CASE 2

Surgeon operating on an ingrown toenail administers a regional nerve block.

CASE 3

Patient was scheduled for a total diagnostic colonoscopy, but the patient went into respiratory distress during procedure; surgeon stopped the procedure.

CASE 4

Puncture aspiration of a cyst in the left breast and a cyst in the right breast.

CASE 5

A neurological surgeon and an orthopedic surgeon worked as cosurgeons.

Step 3 Determine the Need for Modifiers

The circumstances involved with the procedure or service may require the use of modifiers. The patient's diagnosis may affect this determination.

Evaluation And Management Codes

The codes in the Evaluation and Management section (**E/M codes**) cover physicians' services that are performed to determine the best course for patient care. The E/M codes are listed first in CPT because they are used so often by all types of physicians. Often called the cognitive codes, the E/M codes cover the complex process a physician uses to gather and analyze information about a patient's illness and to make decisions about the patient's condition and the best treatment or course of management. The actual treatments—such as surgical procedures and vaccines—are covered in the CPT sections that follow the E/M codes, such as the Surgery and Medicine sections.

Although CPT was first published in 1966, the Evaluation and Management section was not introduced until 1992. The E/M coding method came from a joint effort by CMS and the AMA to define ranges of services from simple to very complicated. Patients' conditions require different levels of information gathering, analysis, and decision making by physicians. For example, on the low end of a range might be a patient with a mild case of poison ivy. On the opposite end is a patient with a life-threatening condition. The E/M codes reflect these different levels. There are five codes to choose from for an office visit with a new patient, for example, and another five for office visits with established

Billing Tip

Assigning E/M Levels
In many practices, because of their complexity, physicians assign the E/M code levels and then medical coders or insurance specialists check them against documentation.

patients. A financial value (fee or prospective payment) is assigned by a payer to each code in a range. To justify the use of a higher-level code in the range—one that is tied to a higher value—the physician must perform and document specific clinical facts about the patient encounter.

Structure

Most codes in the E/M section are organized by the place of service, such as the office, the hospital, or a patient's home. A few (for example, consultations) are grouped by type of service. The subsections, detailed in Table 5.3, are as follows:

Office or Other Outpatient Services

Hospital Observation Services

Hospital Inpatient Services

Consultations

Emergency Department Services

Pediatric Patient Transport

Critical Care Services

Continuing Intensive Care Services

Nursing Facility Services

Domiciliary, Rest Home (e.g., Assisted Living Facility), or Home Care Plan Oversight Services

Home Services

Prolonged Services

Standby Services

Case Management Services

Care Plan Oversight Services

Preventive Medicine Service

Special/Other E/M Services

TABLE 5.3 E/M Code Organization by Type or Place of Service

Category/Subcategory	Code Numbers
Office or Other Outpatient Services	
New Patient	99201–99205
Established Patient	99211–99215
Hospital Observation Services	
Hospital Observation Discharge Services	99217
Initial Hospital Observation Services	99218–99220
Hospital Observation or Inpatient Care	
Services (Including Admission and Discharge Services)	99234–99236
Hospital Inpatient Services	
Initial Hospital Care	99221–99223
Subsequent Hospital Care	99231–99233
Hospital Discharge Services	99238–99239

TABLE 5.3 E/M Code Organization by Type or Place of Service (continued)	
Category/Subcategory	**Code Numbers**
Consultations	
Office Consultations	99241–99245
Initial Inpatient Consultations	99251–99255
Emergency Department Services	99281–99288
Pediatric Patient Transport	99289–99290
Critical Care Services	
Adult (over 24 months of age)	99291–99292
Pediatric	99293–99294
Neonatal	99295–99296
Continuing Intensive Services	99298–99300
Nursing Facility Services	
Initial Nursing Facility Care	99304–99306
Subsequent Nursing Facility Care	99307–99310
Nursing Facility Discharge Services	99315–99316
Other Nursing Facility Services	99318
Domiciliary, Rest Home or Custodial Care Services	
Established Patient	99334–99337
Domiciliary, Rest Home (e.g., Assisted Living Facility) or Home Care Plan Oversight Services	99339–99340
New Patient	99307–99310
Home Services	
New Patient	99341–99345
Established Patient	99347–99350
Prolonged Services	
With Direct Patient Contact	99354–99357
Without Direct Patient Contact	99358–99359
Standby Services	99360
Case Management Services	
Team Conferences	99361–99362
Telephone Calls	99371–99373
Care Plan Oversight Services	99374–99380
Preventive Medicine Services	
New Patient	99381–99387
Established Patient	99391–99397
Individual Counseling	99401–99404
Group Counseling	99411–99412
Other	99420–99429
Newborn Care	99431–99440
Special E/M Services	99450–99456
Other E/M Services	99499

A New or Established Patient?

Many subsections of E/M codes assign different code ranges for new patients and established patients. A new patient (NP) has not received any professional services from the physician (or from another physician of the same specialty in the same group practice) within the past three years. An established patient

Billing Tip

New and Established Patients
Be familiar with payers' guidelines on new and established patients, since some payers have special rules for deciding on the patient's status when the specialty group has subspecialties (for example, a hand surgeon in a surgery practice).

Billing Tip

Consults: Three Rs
Coders remember the three Rs of consults: request opinion, render service, report back.

Billing Tip

Consultation Requests and Reports
Consultation requests and reports must be written documents that are placed in the medical records. Under most managed care guidelines, the reports should be reviewed and initialed by the primary care physician, with documentation of follow-up plans.

(EP) has received professional services under those conditions (see Chapter 3, Figure 3.1, for a decision tree for determining patient status as NP or EP). The distinction is important because new patients typically require more effort by the physician and practice staff, who should therefore be paid more.

The term *any professional services* in the definitions of new and established patients means that the established category is used for a patient who had a face-to-face encounter with a physician. The same rule applies to a patient of a physician who moves to another group practice. If the patient then sees the physician (or another of the same specialty) in the new practice, the patient is established. In other words, the patient is new to the practice, but established to the provider.

A Consultation or A Referral?

To understand the subsection of E/M codes on consultations, review the difference between a consultation and a referral in coding terminology. A **consultation** occurs when a second physician, at the request of the patient's physician, examines the patient. The second physician usually focuses on a particular issue and reports a written opinion to the first physician. The physician providing a consultation ("consult") may perform a service for the patient but does not independently start a full course of treatment (although the consulting physician may recommend one) or take charge of the patient's care. Consultations require use of the E/M consultation codes (the range from 99241 to 99255).

On the other hand, when the patient is referred to another physician, either the total care or a specific portion of care is transferred to that provider (see Chapter 3, which describes the requirement by payers for referral authorization). The patient becomes a new patient of that doctor for the referred condition and may not return to the care of the referring physician until the completion of a course of treatment. Referrals require use of the regular office visit E/M service codes.

Although people sometimes use these terms to mean the same thing, a referral and a consultation are different. This distinction is important to medical insurance specialists because the amounts that can be charged for the two types of service are different. Under a referral, the PCP or other provider is sending the patient to another physician for specialized care. If the sending provider requests a consultation, this is asking for the opinion of another physician regarding the patient's care. The patient will be returned to the care of the original provider with the specialist's written consultation report containing an evaluation of the patient's condition and/or care.

Modifiers

A number of modifiers are commonly used with evaluation and management services:

–21 *Prolonged Evaluation and Management service:* Used when the services are greater than the highest level described for the code range.

–24 *Unrelated Evaluation and Management service by the same physician during a postoperative period:* Used when an E/M service that is not related to the reason for the surgery is provided within the postoperative time period included in the payer's reimbursement.

–25 *Significant, separately identifiable Evaluation and Management service by the same physician on the same day of the procedure or other service:* Used when the physician provides an E/M service in addition to another E/M service or a procedure on the same day. The E/M service to which the modifier is appended must be significant enough to report.

–32 *Mandated services:* Used when the procedure is required by a payer.

–52 *Reduced services:* Used when an E/M service is less extensive than the descriptor indicates.

–57 *Decision for surgery:* Used to indicate the visit at which the decision for surgery was made and the patient was counseled about risks and outcomes.

E/M Code Selection

To select the correct E/M code, eight steps are followed (see Figure 5.3).

Step 1. Determine the Category and Subcategory of Service Based on the Place of Service and the Patient's Status

The list of E/M categories—such as office visits, hospital services, and preventive medicine services—is used to locate the appropriate place or type of service in the index. In the main text of the selected category, the subcategory, such as new or established patient, is then chosen.

Documentation: initial hospital visit to established patient

Index: Hospital Services

Inpatient Services

Initial Care, New or Established Patient

Code Ranges: 99221–99223

For most types of service, from three to five codes are listed. To select an appropriate code from this range, consider three key components: (1) the history the

STEP 1	Determine the category and subcategory of service based on the place of service and the patient's status
STEP 2	Determine the extent of the history that is documented
STEP 3	Determine the extent of the examination that is documented
STEP 4	Determine the complexity of medical decision making that is documented
STEP 5	Analyze the requirements to report the service level
STEP 6	Verify the service level based on the nature of the presenting problem, time, counseling, and care coordination
STEP 7	Verify that the documentation is complete
STEP 8	Assign the code

FIGURE 5.3 Selecting an Evaluation and Management Code

physician documented, (2) the examination that was documented, and (3) the medical decisions the physician documented. (The exception to this guideline is selecting a code for counseling or coordination of care, where in some situations the amount of time the physician spends may be the only key component.)

Step 2. Determine the Extent of the History That Is Documented

History is the information the physician received by questioning the patient about the chief complaint and other signs or symptoms, about all or selected body systems, and about pertinent past history, family background, and other personal factors. (See Chapter 2, Figure 2.2, as an example of this documentation.)

The history is documented in the patient medical record as follows.

History of present illness (HPI) The history of the illness is a description of the development of the illness from the first sign or symptom that the patient experienced to the present time. These points about the illness or condition may be documented:

- Location (body area of the pain or symptom)
- Quality (type of pain or symptom, such as sudden or dull)
- Severity (degree of pain or symptom)
- Duration (how long the pain or symptom lasts and when it began)
- Timing (time of day the pain or symptom occurs)
- Context (any situation related to the pain or symptom, such as occurs after eating)
- Modifying factors (any factors that alter the pain or symptom)
- Associated signs and symptoms (things that also happen when the pain or symptom occurs)

Review of systems (ROS) The review of systems is an inventory of body systems. These systems are:

- Constitutional symptoms (such as fever or weight loss)
- Eyes
- Ears, nose, mouth, and throat
- Cardiovascular (CV)
- Respiratory
- Gastrointestinal (GI)
- Genitourinary (GU)
- Musculoskeletal
- Integumentary
- Neurological
- Psychiatric
- Endocrine
- Hematologic/lymphatic
- Allergic/immunologic

Past medical history (PMH) The past history of the patient's experiences with illnesses, injuries, and treatments contains data about other major illnesses and injuries, operations, and hospitalizations. It also covers current medications the patient is taking, allergies, immunization status, and diet.

Family history (FH) The family history reviews the medical events in the patient's family. It includes the health status or cause of death of parents, brothers and sisters, and children; specific diseases that are related to the patient's chief complaint or the patient's diagnosis; and the presence of any known hereditary diseases.

Social history (SH) The facts gathered in the social history, which depend on the patient's age, include marital status, employment, and other factors.

The histories documented after the HPI are sometimes referred to as PFSH, for past, family, and social history. This history is then categorized as one of four types on a scale from lesser to greater extent of amount of history obtained:

1. *Problem-focused:* Determining the patient's chief complaint and obtaining a brief history of the present illness
2. *Expanded problem-focused:* Determining the patient's chief complaint and obtaining a brief history of the present illness, plus a problem-pertinent system review of the particular body system that is involved
3. *Detailed:* Determining the chief complaint; obtaining an extended history of the present illness; reviewing both the problem-pertinent system and additional systems; and taking pertinent past, family, and/or social history
4. *Comprehensive:* Determining the chief complaint and taking an extended history of the present illness, a complete review of systems, and a complete past, family, and social history

Step 3. Determine the Extent of the Examination That Is Documented

The physician may examine a particular body area or organ system or may conduct a multisystem examination. The body areas are divided into the head and face; chest, including breasts and axilla; abdomen; genitalia, groin, and buttocks; back; and each extremity.

The organ systems that may be examined are the eyes; the ears, nose, mouth, and throat; cardiovascular; respiratory; gastrointestinal; genitourinary; musculoskeletal; skin; neurologic; psychiatric; and hematologic/lymphatic/immunologic.

The examination that the physician documents is categorized as one of four types on a scale from lesser to greater extent:

1. *Problem-focused:* A limited examination of the affected body area or system
2. *Expanded problem-focused:* A limited examination of the affected body area or system and other related areas
3. *Detailed:* An extended examination of the affected body area or system and other related areas
4. *Comprehensive:* A general multisystem examination or a complete examination of a single organ system

Step 4. Determine the Complexity of Medical Decision Making That Is Documented

The complexity of the medical decisions that the physician makes involves how many possible diagnoses or treatment options were considered; how much information (such as test results or previous records) was considered in analyzing the patient's problem; and how serious the illness is, meaning how much risk there is for significant complications, advanced illness, or death.

The decision-making process that the physician documents is categorized as one of four types on a scale from lesser to greater complexity:

1. *Straightforward:* Minimal diagnoses options, a minimal amount of data, and minimum risk
2. *Low complexity:* Limited diagnoses options, a low amount of data, and low risk

3. *Moderate complexity:* Multiple diagnoses options, a moderate amount of data, and moderate risk
4. *High complexity:* Extensive diagnoses options, an extensive amount of data, and high risk

Step 5. Analyze the Requirements to Report the Service Level

> **Billing Tip**
>
> **Three Key Components**
> This means that to select code 99203, the medical record must show that a detailed history and examination were taken and that medical decision-making was at least at the level of low complexity.

The descriptor for each E/M code explains the standards for its selection. For office visits and most other services to new patients and for initial care visits, all three of the **key components** must be documented. If there are two at a higher level and a third below that level, the standard is not met. This is stated in CPT as follows:

99203 Office or other outpatient visit for the evaluation and management of a new patient, which require these three key components:

- **a detailed history**
- **a detailed examination**
- **medical decision making of low complexity**

For most services for established patients and for subsequent care visits, two out of three of the key components must be met. For example:

> **Billing Tip**
>
> **Two of Three Key Components**
> This means that to select code 99213, the medical record must show that two out of the three factors are documented.

99213 Office or other outpatient visit for the evaluation and management of an established patient, which requires at least two of these three key components:

- **an expanded problem-focused history**
- **an expanded problem-focused examination**
- **medical decision making of low complexity**

Table 5.4 shows the type of decision tool many medical coders use to assign the correct E/M code for office visits with new and established patients.

Step 6. Verify the Service Level Based on the Nature of the Presenting Problem, Time, Counseling, and Care Coordination

> **Billing Tip**
>
> **The Time Factor**
> When a patient's visit is mainly about counseling and/or coordination of care regarding symptoms or illness, the length of time the physician spends is the controlling factor. If over 50 percent of the visit is spent counseling or coordinating care, time is the main factor. If an established patient's visit is thirty minutes, for example, and twenty minutes are spent counseling, the E/M code is 99214.

Nature of the Presenting Problem Many descriptors mention two additional components: (1) how severe the patient's condition is, referred to as the *nature of the presenting problem,* and (2) how much time the physician typically spends directly treating the patient. These factors, while not key components, help in selecting the correct E/M level. For example, the following wording appears in CPT after the 99214 code (office visit for the evaluation and management of an established patient):

Usually, the presenting problem(s) are of moderate to high severity. Physicians typically spend 25 minutes face-to-face with the patient and/or family.

The severity of the presenting problem helps determine medical necessity. Even if a physician documented comprehensive history and exam, with complex decision making, treating a minor problem like removal of uncomplicated sutures would not warrant a high E/M level.

Counseling Counseling is a discussion with a patient regarding areas such as diagnostic results, instructions for follow-up treatment, and patient education. It is mentioned as a typical part of each E/M service in the descriptor, but it is not required to be documented as a key component.

Care Coordination Coordination of care with other providers or agencies is also mentioned. When coordination of care is provided but the patient is not

TABLE 5.4 Evaluation and Management Code Selection Tool: Office Visits

	NEW PATIENTS					ESTABLISHED PATIENTS				
CPT Codes⇛	**99201 NP Level 1**	**99202 NP Level 2**	**99203 NP Level 3**	**99204 NP Level 4**	**99205 NP Level 5**	**99211 EP Level 1**	**99212 EP Level 2**	**99213 EP Level 3**	**99214 EP Level 4**	**99215 EP Level 5**
Key Components										
History:						*Minimal*				
Problem-focused	Y						Y			
Expanded Problem-focused		Y						Y		
Detailed			Y						Y	
Comprehensive				Y	Y					Y
Examination:						*Minimal*				
Problem-focused	Y						Y			
Expanded Problem-focused		Y						Y		
Detailed			Y						Y	
Comprehensive				Y	Y					Y
Medical Decision Making:						*Minimal*				
Straightforward	Y	Y					Y			
Low complexity			Y					Y		
Moderate complexity				Y					Y	
High complexity					Y					Y
NUMBER OF KEY COMPONENTS REQUIRED	**3**	**3**	**3**	**3**	**3**	**2**	**2**	**2**	**2**	**2**

present, codes from the case management and care plan oversight services subsections are reported.

Step 7. Verify That the Documentation Is Complete

The documentation must contain the record of the physician's work in enough detail to support the selected E/M code. The history, examination, and medical decision making must be sufficiently documented so that the medical necessity and appropriateness of the service could be determined by an independent auditor (see Chapter 7).

Step 8. Assign the Code

The code that has been selected is assigned. The need for any modifiers, based on the documentation of special circumstances, is also reviewed.

Reporting E/M Codes on Claims

Documentation Guidelines for Evaluation and Management

Two sets of guidelines for documenting evaluation and management codes have been published by CMS and the AMA: the 1995 Documentation Guidelines for Evaluation and Management Services and a 1997 version. CMS and most payers permit providers to use either the 1995 or the 1997 E/M guidelines. Table 5.5 on pages 166–167 shows the items that can be documented to satisfy the general multisystem examination requirements under the 1997 Documentation Guidelines, which are most commonly used. There are similar guidelines to Table 5.5 for each major medical specialty.

Billing Tip

Which Guidelines?
The medical practice should be clear about which set of guidelines, the 1995 or the 1997, it generally follows E/M coding and reporting.

TABLE 5.5 General Multi-System Examination

System/Body Area	Elements of Examination
Constitutional	• Measurement of any three of the following seven vital signs: 1) sitting or standing blood pressure 2) supine blood pressure, 3) pulse rate and regularity, 4) respiration, 5) temperature, 6) height, 7) weight (May be measured and recorded by ancillary staff) • General appearance of patient (eg, development, nutrition, body habitus, deformities, attention to grooming)
Eyes	• Inspection of conjunctivae and lids • Examination of pupils and irises (eg, reaction to light and accommodation, size and symmetry) • Opthalmoscopic examination of optic discs (eg, size, C/D ratio, appearance) and posterior segments (eg, vessel changes, exudates, hemorrhages)
Ears, Nose, Mouth and Throat	• External inspection of ears and nose (eg, overall appearance, scars, lesions, masses) • Otoscopic examination of external auditory canals and tympanic membranes • Assessment of hearing (eg, whispered voice, finger rub, tuning fork) • Inspection of nasal mucosa, septum and turbinates • Inspection of lips, teeth and gums • Examination of oropharynx: oral mucosa, salivary glands, hard and soft palates, tongue, tonsils and posterior pharynx
Neck	• Examination of neck (eg, masses, overall appearance, symmetry, tracheal position, crepitus) • Examination of thyroid (eg, enlargement, tenderness, mass)
Respiratory	• Assessment of respiratory effort (eg, intercostal retractions, use of accessory muscles, diaphragmatic movement) • Percussion of chest (eg, dullness, flatness, hyperresonance) • Palpation of chest (eg, tactile fremitus) • Auscultation of lungs (eg, breath sounds, adventitious sounds, rubs)
Cardiovascular	• Palpation of heart (eg, location, size, thrills) • Auscultation of heart with notation of abnormal sounds and murmurs Examination of: • carotid arteries (eg, pulse, amplitude, bruits) • abdominal aorta (eg, size, bruits) • femoral arteries (eg, pulse, amplitude, bruits) • pedal pulses (eg, pulse amplitude) • extremities for edema and/or varicosities
Chest (Breasts)	• Inspection of breasts (eg, symmetry, nipple discharge) • Palpation of breasts and axillae (eg, masses or lumps, tenderness)
Gastrointestinal (Abdomen)	• Examination of abdomen with notation of presence of masses or tenderness • Examination of liver and spleen • Examination for presence or absence of hernia • Examination (when indicated) of anus, perineum and rectum, including sphincter tone, presence of hemorrhoids, rectal masses • Obtain stool sample for occult blood text when indicated
Genitourinary	**Male:** • Examination of the scrotal contents (eg, hydrocele, spermatocele, tenderness of cord, testicular mass) • Examination of the penis • Digital rectal examination of prostate gland (eg, size, symmetry, nodularity, tenderness) **Female:** Pelvic examination (with or without specimen collection for smears and cultures) including • Examination of external genitalia (eg, general appearance, hair distribution, lesions) • Examination of urethra (eg, masses, tenderness, scarring) • Examination of bladder (eg, fullness, masses, tenderness) • Cervix (eg, general appearance, lesions, discharge) • Uterus (eg, size, contour, position, mobility, tenderness, consistency, descent or support) • Adnexa/parametria (eg, masses, tenderness, organomegaly, nodularity)

TABLE 5.5 General Multi-System Examination *(continued)*

System/Body Area	Elements of Examination
Lymphatic	Palpation of lymph nodes in **two or more** areas: • Neck • Axillae • Groin • Other
Musculoskeletal	• Examination of gait and station • Inspection and/or palpation of digits and nails (eg, clubbing, cyanosis, inflammatory conditions, petechiae, ischemia, infections, nodes) Examination of joints, bones and muscles of **one or more of the following six** areas: 1) head and neck; 2) spine, ribs and pelvis; 3) right upper extremity; 4) left upper extremity; 5) right lower extremity; and 6) left lower extremity. The examination of a given area includes: • Inspection and/or palpation with notation of presence of any misalignment, asymmetry, crepitation, defects, tenderness, masses, effusions • Assessment of range of motion with notation of any pain, crepitation or contracture • Assessment of stability with notation of any dislocation (luxation), subluxation or laxity • Assessment of muscle strength and tone (eg, flaccid, cog wheel, spastic) with notation of any atrophy or abnormal movements
Skin	• Inspection of skin and subcutaneous tissue (eg, rashes, lesions, ulcers) • Palpation of skin and subcutaneous tissue (eg, induration, subcutaneous nodules, tightening)
Neurologic	• Test cranial nerves with notation of any deficits • Examination of deep tendon reflexes with notation of pathological reflexes (eg, Babinski) • Examination of sensation (eg, by touch, pin, vibration, proprioception)
Psychiatric	• Description of patient's judgment and insight Brief assessment of mental status, including: • Orientation to time, place and person • Recent and remote memory • Mood and affect (eg, depression, anxiety, agitation)
	Content and Documentation Requirements
	Perform General Multi-System Examination
Level of Exam	**Perform and Document**
Problem Focused	**One to five** elements identified by a bullet.
Expanded Problem Focused	**At least six** elements identified by a bullet
Detailed	**At least two** elements identified by a bullet **from each of six areas/systems** or **at least 12** elements identified by a bullet **in two or more areas/systems.**
Comprehensive	**At least two** elements identified by a bullet **from each of nine areas/systems.**

Billing Tip

Modifier –25
During an annual physical examination, an illness or clinical sign of a condition may be found that requires the physician to conduct an additional evaluation. In this case, the preventive medicine service code is reported first, followed by the appropriate E/M code for the new problem, adding the –25 modifier, Significant, Separate E/M Service.

Thinking It Through — 5.4

1. In which category—problem-focused, expanded problem-focused, detailed, or comprehensive—would you place these statements concerning patient history? Why?

CASE A

Patient seen for follow-up of persistent sinus problems including pain, stuffiness, and greenish drainage over the past twenty days. She continues to have left-sided pain in the forehead and maxillary areas and feels that her symptoms are worse around dust. She gets drainage into her throat, which causes her to cough. Review of systems reveals no history of diabetes or asthma. She has thyroid problems for which she takes Synthroid®.

CASE B

Patient presents with a mild case of poison ivy on face and both hands contracted four days ago while gardening; has never been bothered by poison ivy before.

2. Using the office visit E/M codes, which code would you select for each of these cases?

CASE A

Chart note for established patient:

> S: **Patient returns for removal of stitches I placed about seven days ago. Reports normal itching around the wound area, but no pain or swelling.** ______________________
>
> O: **Wound at lateral aspect of the left eye looks well healed. Decision made to remove the 5-0 nylon sutures, which was done without difficulty.** ______________________
>
> A: **Laceration, healed.** ______________________
>
> P: **Patient advised to use vitamin E for scar prophylaxis.**
>
> ______________________

CASE B

Initial office evaluation by oncologist of a sixty-five-year-old female with sudden unexplained twenty-pound weight loss. Comprehensive history and examination performed.

CASE C

Office visit by established patient for regularly scheduled blood test to monitor long-term effects of Coumadin; nurse spends five minutes, reviews the test, confirms that the patient is feeling well, and states that no change in the dosage is necessary.

3. If a physician sees a patient in the hospital and the patient comes to the office for a follow-up visit, is the follow-up encounter coded for a new or established patient?

Office and Hospital Services

Office and other outpatient services are the most often reported E/M services. A patient is an **outpatient** unless admitted to a health care facility, such as a hospital or nursing home, for a twenty-four-hour period or longer.

- When a patient is evaluated and then admitted to a health care facility, the service is reported using the codes for initial hospital care (the range 99221–99223).
- The admitting physician uses the initial hospital care services codes. Only one provider can report these services; other physicians involved in the patient's care, such as a surgeon or radiologist, use other E/M service codes or other codes from appropriate sections.
- Codes for initial hospital observation case (99218–99220), initial hospital case (99221–99223), and initial inpatient consultations (99251–99255) should be reported by a physician only once for a patient admission.

Emergency Department Services An emergency department is hospital-based and is available to patients twenty-four hours a day. When emergency services are reported, whether the patient is new or established is not applicable. Time is not a factor in selecting the E/M service code. The code ranges are 99281 to 99288.

Preventive Medicine Services Preventive medicine services are used to report routine physical examinations in the absence of a patient complaint. These codes, in the range 99381 to 99429, are divided according to the age of the patient. Immunizations and other services, such as lab tests that are normal parts of an annual physical, are reported using the appropriate codes from the Medicine and the Pathology and Laboratory sections (see pages 177 through 180).

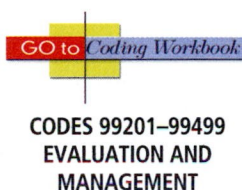

CODES 99201–99499 EVALUATION AND MANAGEMENT

Anesthesia Codes

The codes in the Anesthesia section are used to report anesthesia services performed or supervised by a physician. These services include general and regional anesthesia as well as supplementation of local anesthesia. Anesthesia codes each include the complete usual services of an anesthesiologist:

- Usual preoperative visits for evaluation and planning
- Care during the procedure, such as administering fluid or blood, placing monitoring devices or IV lines, laryngoscopy, interpreting lab data, and nerve stimulation
- Routine postoperative care

EXAMPLE

Anesthesiologist Report: Initial meeting with seven-year-old patient in good health, determined good candidate for required general anesthesia for tonsillectomy. Surgical procedure conducted April 4, 2008; patient in the supine position; administered general anesthesia via endotracheal tube. Routine monitoring during procedure. Following successful removal of the right and left tonsils, the patient was awakened and taken to the recovery room in satisfactory condition.

00170–P1 Anesthesia for intraoral procedures, including biopsy; not otherwise specified

(The modifier -P1 is discussed below.)

Postoperative critical care and pain management requested by the surgeon are not included and can be billed in addition to the main anesthesia code by the anesthesiologist.

Anesthesia codes are reimbursed according to time. The American Society of Anesthesiologists assigns a base unit value to each code. The anesthesiologist also records the amount of time spent with the patient during the procedure and adds this to the base value. Difficulties, such as a patient with severe systemic disease, also add to the value of the anesthesiologist's services.

Structure

The Anesthesia section's subsections are organized by body site. Under each subsection, the codes are arranged by procedures. For example, under the heading *Neck,* codes for procedures performed on various parts of the neck (the integumentary system; the esophagus, thyroid, larynx, trachea; and lymphatic system; and the major vessels) are listed. The body-site subsections are followed by two other subsections: (1) radiological procedures—that is, anesthesia services for patients receiving diagnostic or therapeutic radiology—and (2) other or unlisted procedures.

Modifiers

Two types of modifiers are used with anesthesia codes: (1) a modifier that describes the patient's health status and (2) the standard modifiers.

Physical Status Modifiers

Because the patient's health has a large effect on the level of difficulty of anesthesia services, anesthesia codes are assigned a **physical status modifier.** This modifier is added to the code. The patient's physical status is selected from this list:

P1 Normal, healthy patient
P2 Patient with mild systemic disease
P3 Patient with severe systemic disease
P4 Patient with severe systemic disease that is a constant threat to life
P5 Moribund patient who is not expected to survive without the operation
P6 Declared brain-dead patient whose organs are being removed for donation purposes

For example:

00320–P3 Anesthesia services provided to patient with severe diabetes for procedure on larynx

Billing Tip

Modifier –22
Many payers consider modifier –22 overused (abused). When it is used, the need for the increased service or procedure should be well documented.

Modifiers

The following standard modifiers are also commonly used with anesthesia codes:

–22 *Unusual procedural service:* Used with rare, unusual, or variable anesthesia services.

–23 *Unusual anesthesia service:* Used when the procedure normally requires either no anesthesia or local anesthesia but, because of unusual circumstances, general anesthesia is administered.

–32 *Mandated service:* Used when the procedure is required by a payer. For example, a PPO may require an independent evaluation of a patient before procedures are performed.

–51 *Multiple procedures:* Used to identify a second procedure or multiple procedures during the same operation.

–53 *Discontinued:* Used when the procedure is canceled after induction of anesthesia but before the incision is made. If the surgery is canceled after the evaluation of the patient, an E/M code is used rather than this modifier.

–59 *Distinct procedural service:* Used for a different encounter or procedure for the same patient on the same day; also used to describe the requirement for critical care and nonroutine pain management.

Note that modifier –37, Anesthesia by Surgeon, is used only during surgical procedures, not for services performed by anesthesiologists or anesthetists or supervised by surgeons.

For example, an anesthesia code with both types of modifiers appears as:

00320–P3–53	Anesthesia services provided to patient with severe diabetes for procedure on larynx; procedure discontinued because patient experienced a sudden drop in blood pressure

Add-On Codes for Qualifying Circumstances

Four add-on codes are used to indicate that the administration of the anesthesia involved important circumstances that had an effect on how it was performed. As add-on codes, these do not stand alone but always appear in addition to the primary procedure code. These four codes apply only to anesthesia and are described in the notes for the Anesthesia Section.

+99100 Anesthesia for patient of extreme age (under one year or over age seventy)

+99116 Anesthesia complicated by utilization of total body hypothermia

+99135 Anesthesia complicated by utilization of controlled hypotension

+99140 Anesthesia complicated by specified emergency conditions

Reporting Anesthesia Codes

Anesthesia services for Medicare patients and most other patients are reported using codes from the Anesthesia section. However, medical insurance specialists should be aware that some private payers require anesthesia services to be reported by procedure codes from the Surgery section rather than by codes from the Anesthesia section. The anesthesia modifier is added to the procedure code.

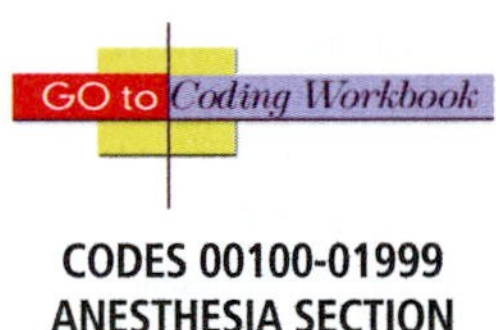

CODES 00100-01999
ANESTHESIA SECTION

Surgery Codes

The codes in the Surgery section are used for the many hundreds of surgical procedures performed by physicians. This is the largest procedure code section, with codes ranging from 10021 to 69990.

Surgical Package

Most surgical codes include all the usual services in addition to the operation itself:

- After the decision for surgery, one related E/M encounter on the date immediately before or on the date of the procedure
- The operation: preparing the patient for surgery, including injection of anesthesia by the surgeon (local infiltration, metacarpal/metatarsal/digital block, or topical anesthesia), and performing the operation, including normal additional procedures, such as debridement
- Immediate postoperative care, including dictating operative notes and talking with the family and other physicians
- Writing orders
- Evaluating the patient in the postanesthesia recovery area
- Typical postoperative follow-up care

A complete procedure includes the operation, the use of a local anesthetic, and postoperative care, all covered under a single code.

EXAMPLE

Procedural Statement: Procedure conducted two weeks ago in office to correct hallux valgus (bunions) on both feet; local nerve block administered, correction by simple exostectomy. Saw patient in office today for routine follow-up; complete healing.

Code: 28290–50 Bunion correction on both feet

In the Surgery section, the grouping of related work under a single procedure code is called a **surgical package** or **global surgery rule.** Government and private payers assign a fee to a surgical package code that reimburses all the services provided under it. The period of time that is covered for follow-up care is referred to as the **global period.** After the global period ends, additional services that are provided can be reported separately for additional payment. For most payers, there are two possible global preoperative periods—zero days and one day. Usually, there are three possible postoperative global periods: zero days, ten days, and ninety days.

Two types of services are not included in surgical package codes. These services are billed separately and are reimbursed in addition to the surgical package fee:

- Complications or recurrences that arise after therapeutic surgical procedures.
- Care for the condition for which a diagnostic surgical procedure is performed. Routine follow-up care included in the code refers only to care related to recovery from the diagnostic procedure itself, not the condition. For example, a diagnostic colonoscopy is performed to examine a growth in the patient's colon. An office visit after the surgery to evaluate the patient for chemotherapy because the tumor is cancerous is billed separately, not with code 99024 for a postoperative follow-up visit included in global service.

Compliance Guideline

The 1998 Women's Health and Cancer Rights Act requires all health plans that provide coverage for mastectomies to also provide coverage for associated treatments, such as breast reconstruction after surgery.

Separate Procedures

Some procedural code descriptors in the Surgery section are followed by the words *separate procedure* in parentheses. **Separate procedure** means that the procedure is usually done as an integral part of a surgical package—usually a larger procedure—but that in some situations it is not. If a separate procedure is performed alone or along with other procedures but for a separate purpose, it may be reported separately. For example:

42870 Excision or destruction lingual tonsil, any method (separate procedure)

Lingual tonsil excision is a separate procedure. It is usually a part of a routine tonsillectomy and so cannot be reported separately when a tonsillectomy is performed. When it is done independently, however, this code can be reported.

Structure

Most of the Surgery section's subsections are organized by body system and then divided by body site. Procedures are grouped next, under headings followed by specific procedures. For example:

Subsection:	DIGESTIVE SYSTEM
Site:	Lips
Heading—type of procedure:	Excision
Description—specific procedure:	**40490** Biopsy of lip

The exceptions to the usual subsection structure are the Laparoscopy/Hysteroscopy subsection, which groups those operative procedures, and the Maternity Care and Delivery subsection, organized by type of service, such as postpartum care.

Modifiers

A number of modifiers are commonly used to indicate special circumstances involved with surgical procedures.

–22 *Unusual procedural service:* Used with rare, unusual, or variable surgery services; requires documentation.

–26 *Professional component:* Used to report the professional components when a procedure has both professional and technical components.

–32 *Mandated service:* Used when the procedure is required by a payer or is a government, legislative, or regulatory requirement.

–47 *Anesthesia by surgeon:* Used when the surgeon (rather than an anesthesiologist) administers regional or general anesthesia (local/topical anesthesia is bundled in the surgical code).

–50 *Bilateral procedure:* Used when identical bilateral procedures were performed during the same operation, either through the same incision or on separate body parts, such as left and right bunion correction. Attach the bilateral modifier to the code for the first procedure to indicate that the procedure was done bilaterally. For example, to report a puncture aspiration of one cyst in each breast:

19100–50 Puncture aspiration of cyst of breast

–51 *Multiple procedures:* Used to identify a second procedure or multiple procedures during the same operation. The additional procedures are the same type and done to the same body system. Attach the modifier to the second procedure code. For example, to report two procedures, a bunionectomy on the great toe and, in the same session, correction of a hammertoe on the fourth toe:

28290 Hallux valgus (bunions) correction
28285–51 Hammertoe operation, one

–52 *Reduced services:* Used when a procedure is less extensive than described. The modifier is attached to the procedure code. It is not used to identify a reduced or a discounted fee. Instead, usually, the normal fee is listed, and the payer determines the amount of the reduction.

–53 *Discontinued procedure:* Used when the procedure is discontinued due to circumstances that threaten the patient's well-being—for example, surgery discontinued because the patient went into shock during the operation.

–54 *Surgical care only:* Added to the surgery code when the surgeon performs only the surgery itself, without preoperative or postoperative services. The fee will be reduced by the payer to reflect only that part of the surgical package.

–55 *Postoperative management only:* Added to the surgery code when the physician provides only the follow-up care in the global period after another physician has done the surgery. The fee will be reduced by the payer to reflect only that part of the surgical package.

–56 *Preoperative management only:* Added to the surgery code when the physician provides only preoperative care. The fee will be reduced by the payer to reflect only that part of the surgical package.

–58 *Staged or related procedure or service by the same physician during the postoperative period:* Used when the physician performs a postoperative procedure (1) as planned during the surgery to be done later, (2) that is more extensive than the original procedure, or (3) for therapy after diagnostic surgery.

–59 *Distinct procedural service:* Used for a different encounter or procedure for the same patient on the same day. A different patient encounter, an unrelated procedure, a different body site or system, or a separate incision or injury must be involved. The modifier may also be used to describe the requirement for critical care and nonroutine pain management. If a separate procedure is performed with other procedures, the –59 modifier is added to the separate code to show that it is a distinct, independent procedure, not part of a surgical package.

–62 *Two surgeons:* Used when a specific surgical procedure requires two surgeons, usually of different specialties; each appends the modifier to the surgical code. Usually each surgeon performs a distinct part of the procedure and dictates a separate operative report. If each surgeon reports different surgical procedure codes, the modifier is not used.

–63 *Procedure performed on infants:* Used when the patient is under twenty-four months of age.

–66 *Surgical team:* Used in very complex procedures that usually require the simultaneous services of physicians of different specialties. Usually used to report transplant-type procedures only.

–76 *Repeat procedure by same physician:* Used when a physician repeats a procedure performed earlier.

–77 *Repeat procedure by another physician:* Used when a physician repeats a procedure done by another physician.

–78 *Return to the operating room for a related procedure during the postoperative period:* Used when the patient develops a complication during the postoperative period that requires an additional procedure by the same physician.

–79 *Unrelated procedure or service by the same physician during the postoperative period:* Used when a second, unrelated surgical procedure is performed by the same physician during the postoperative period.

–80 *Assistant surgeon:* Used when a physician assists another during a surgical procedure. Each physician reports the services using the same code, but the assistant surgeon appends the modifier to the code.

–81 *Minimum assistant surgeon:* Used when an assistant surgeon assists another during only part of a surgical procedure.

–82 *Assistant surgeon (when qualified resident surgeon not available):* Used in teaching hospitals where residents usually assist with surgery but none was available during the reported procedure, so a surgeon performed the assistant's work.

–90 *Reference (outside) laboratory:* Used when laboratory procedures are done by someone other than the reporting physician.

–91 *Repeat clinical diagnostic laboratory test:* Used when laboratory procedures are repeated.

–99 *Multiple modifiers:* Used when more than one modifier is required; the –99 modifier is appended to the basic procedure, followed by the other modifiers in descending order.

Reporting Surgical Codes

Surgical package codes often are "bundled" by payers. **Bundling** is using a single payment for two or more related procedure codes. Bundled payment combinations are based on payers' judgment of the correct value for the physician's work. As an example of a bundled code, CPT 27370 codes an injection procedure for knee arthrography. If this code is billed, payers will not also pay for any of these codes on the same day of service:

20610 Injection of major joint

76000 Fluoroscopy (separate procedure)

76003 Fluoroscopic guidance

Because 27370 is bundled, neither 20610, 76000, nor 76003 should be billed with it; payment for each of these codes is already included in the payment rate.

When such services are billed, physicians must report the bundled code and not each of the other codes separately. Reporting anything that is included in the bundled code is considered **unbundling**, or **fragmented billing.** Doing so causes denied claims and may result in an audit.

Reporting Sequence

When payers reimburse multiple surgical procedures performed on the same day for the same patient, they pay the full amount of the first listed surgical procedure, but they often pay reduced percentages of the subsequent procedures. For maximum payment when multiple procedures are reported, the most complex or highest-level code—the procedure with the highest reimbursement value—should be listed first. The subsequent procedures are listed with the modifier –51 (indicating multiple procedures).

When warranted, to avoid reduced payment for multiple procedures, the modifier –59 is used to indicate distinct procedures rather than multiple procedures. This is usually done when the surgeon performs procedures on two different body

Thinking It Through — 5.5

1 Rank the following codes in order from highest to lowest reimbursement level, and explain your rationale.

44950–51

44950–59

44950–53

2 Compare and contrast the procedures that are included in bundled anesthesia codes and global surgical packages. What is the chief difference?

Billing Tip

Lesion Excision
The choice of the correct code for the surgical removal of a lesion depends on the pathology report. There are different code ranges for benign lesions and malignant lesions. Coders should wait for a pathology report before coding lesion excisions from the benign or malignant code ranges.

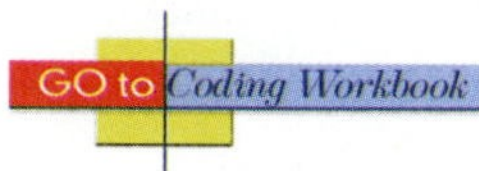

10021–69990
SURGERY SECTION

Billing Tip

Professional Component Requirement
Billing the professional component of a radiologic procedure requires a written interpretation from the physician. This documentation contains the patient's identifying information, the clinical indications for the procedure, the process followed, and the physician's impressions of the findings.

sites or organ systems, such as the excision of a lesion on the chest as well as the incision and drainage (I & D) of an abscess on the leg.

Bilateral Modifier

The bilateral modifier (–50) is attached to unilateral procedures that are done bilaterally. However, there are a few codes that are defined as bilateral procedures. For example:

32853 Lung transplant, double (bilateral sequential or en bloc)

The trend in annual updates is to replace bilateral codes with unilateral codes to which the –50 modifier is attached if needed.

Radiology Codes

The codes in the Radiology section are used to report radiological services performed by or supervised by a physician. Radiology procedures have two parts:

1. *The technical component:* The technologist, the equipment, and processing, including preinjection and postinjection services such as local anesthesia, placement of needle or catheter, and injection of contrast material
2. *The professional component:* The reading of the radiological examination and the written report of interpretation by the physician

Radiology codes follow the same types of guidelines as noted in the Surgery section. For example, some radiology codes are identified as separate procedure codes. These codes are usually part of a larger, more complex procedure and should not be reported as separate codes unless the procedure was done independently. Also, some codes are add-on codes, such as those covering additional vessels that are studied after the basic examination. These codes are used with the primary codes, not alone.

Unlisted Procedures and Special Reports

New procedures are common in the area of radiology services. There are codes for nearly twenty unlisted code areas, such as:

78299 Unlisted gastrointestinal procedure, diagnostic nuclear medicine

When unlisted codes are reported, a special report must be attached that defines the nature, extent, and need for the procedure and describes the time, effort, and equipment necessary to provide it.

Contrast Material

For some radiological procedures, the physician decides whether it is best to perform the procedure with or without contrast material, a substance administered in the patient's blood vessels that helps highlight the area under study. For example, computerized tomography (CT) and magnetic resonance imaging (MRI) provide different types of information about body parts and may be performed with or without contrast material. The term *with contrast* means only contrast materials given in the patient's veins or arteries. Contrast materials administered orally or rectally are coded as without contrast.

Structure and Modifiers

The diagnostic radiology, diagnostic ultrasound, and nuclear medicine subsections of the Radiology section are structured by type of procedure, followed by body sites and then specific procedures. For example:

Type:	Diagnostic Ultrasound
Body site:	Chest
Procedure:	Echography, chest, B-scan and/or real time with image documentation

The radiation oncology subsection is organized somewhat differently. The first group of codes covers the planning services oncologists perform to set up a patient's radiation therapy treatment for cancer.

The following modifiers are commonly used in the Radiology section: –22, –26, –32, –51, –52, –53, –58, –59, –62, –66, –76, –77, –78, –79, –80, –90, and –99. Table 5.2 on page 154 has a brief description of each modifier.

Billing Tip

Modifier –26

If the physician does not own the equipment used for the radiology procedure, the modifier –26 is appended to the code, such as:

76511–26 Ophthalmic biometry by ultrasound echography, A-Scan

Reporting Radiology Codes

Most radiology services are performed and billed by radiologists working in hospital or clinic settings. Medical practices usually do not have radiology equipment and instead refer patients to these specialists. In many cases, the radiologist performs both the technical and the professional components. Codes are selected based on body part, and the number/type of views.

GO to *Coding Workbook*

CODES 70010–79999 RADIOLOGY SECTION

Pathology and Laboratory Codes

The codes in the Pathology and Laboratory section cover services provided by physicians or by technicians under the supervision of physicians. A complete procedure includes:

- Ordering the test
- Taking and handling the sample
- Performing the actual test
- Analyzing and reporting on the test results.

Panels

Certain tests are customarily ordered together to detect particular diseases or malfunctioning organs. These related tests are grouped under laboratory

Billing Tip

Laboratory Work
Medicare does not permit a physician who does not perform the lab work to bill for it. However, other payers allow it. When the physician orders the lab test and then pays the lab (called the reference lab) for the service, the physician may then report that test. The modifier –90 is attached to the code for the lab test.

panels for reporting convenience. When a panel code is reported, all the listed tests must have been performed (otherwise, just the individual tests are billed). For example, the electrolyte panel requires these tests:

80051 Electrolyte panel
This panel must include the following:
Carbon dioxide (82374)
Chloride (82435)
Potassium (84132)
Sodium (84295)

Panels are bundled codes, so when a panel code is reported, no individual test within it may be additionally billed. Other tests that were performed outside that panel may be billed, of course.

Unlisted Procedures and Special Reports

New developments are frequent in pathology and laboratory services. There are codes for twelve unlisted code areas, such as:

86586 Unlisted antigen, each

Any unlisted code must be submitted with a special report that defines the nature, extent, and need for the procedure and describes the time, effort, and equipment necessary to provide it.

Structure and Modifiers

Procedures and services are listed in the Index under the following types of main terms:

- Name of the test, such as urinalysis, HIV, skin test
- Procedure, such as hormone assay
- Abbreviation, such as TLC screen
- Panel of tests, such as Complete Blood Count

The following modifiers are commonly used with pathology and laboratory codes: –22, –26, –32, –52, –53, –59, –90, and –91. Table 5.2 on page 154 has a brief description of each modifier.

Reporting Pathology and Laboratory Codes

List of Waived Tests and PPM Procedures
http://www.cms.hhs.gov/clia

Some medical practices have laboratory equipment and perform their own testing. In-office labs are guided by federal safety regulations from OSHA (the Occupational Safety and Health Administration), and the tests that can be performed are regulated by CLIA (the Clinical Laboratory Improvement Amendment of 1988). The CLIA certification program awards one of two levels of certification: (1) waived tests and provider-performed microscopy (PPM) procedures and (2) moderate- or high-complexity testing. The in-office lab with the first level can perform common tests, such as dipstick urinalysis and urine pregnancy, and PPM procedures such as nasal smears for eosinophils and pinworm exams.

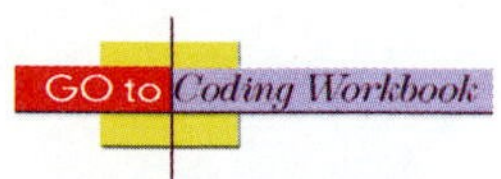

CODES 80048–89356 PATHOLOGY AND LABORATORY SECTION

If the medical practice does not have an in-office lab, the physician may either take the specimen, reporting this service only (for example, using code 36415 for venipuncture to obtain a blood sample), and send it to an outside lab for processing or refer the patient to an outside lab for the complete procedure.

Medicine Codes

The Medicine section contains the codes for the many types of evaluation, therapeutic, and diagnostic procedures that physicians perform. (Codes for the Evaluation and Management section described earlier in the chapter, 99201 to 99499, fall numerically at the end of this section, but they appear first in CPT because they are the most frequently used codes.) Medicine codes may be used for procedures and services done or supervised by a physician of any specialty. They include many procedures and services provided by family practice physicians, such as immunizations and injections. The services of many specialists, such as allergists, cardiologists, and psychiatrists, are also covered in the Medicine section. Some Medicine section codes are for **ancillary services** that are used to support diagnosis and treatment, like rehabilitation, occupational therapy, and nutrition therapy.

Codes from the Medicine section may be used with codes from any other section. Add-on codes and separate procedure codes are included in the Medicine section. Their use follows the guidelines described for previous sections. Unlisted procedure codes are provided for new procedures; a special report is required with unlisted codes.

Structure and Modifiers

The subsections are organized by type of service. Many subsections have notes containing usage guidelines and definitions. Some services, for example, have subcategories for new and established patients.

The following modifiers are commonly used with codes in the Medicine section: –22, –26, –32, –51, –52, –53, –55, –56, –57, –58, –59, –76, –77, –78, –79, –90, –91, and –99. Table 5.2 on page 154 has a brief description of each modifier.

Reporting Medicine Codes

- Some of the services in the Medicine section are considered Evaluation and Management services, even though they are not listed in the E/M section. For these codes, the –51 modifier, Multiple Procedures, may not be used. For example, if a physician makes a second, brief visit to a patient in the hospital and also provides psychoanalysis, these services are reported separately:

99231	Subsequent hospital care, problem focused/straightforward or low complexity decision making
90845	Psychoanalysis

- Immunizations require two codes, one for administering the immunization and the other for the particular vaccine or toxoid that is given. For example, when a patient receives a MMRV vaccine, these two codes are used:

90471	Immunization administration
90710	Measles, mumps, rubella, and varicella vaccine (MMRV), live, for subcutaneous use

- The descriptors for injection codes also require two codes, one for the injection and one for the substance that is injected (the exception is allergy shots, which have their own codes in the Allergy and Clinical Immunology subsection). For example, to report the intravenous administration of an anti-emetic:

90774	Therapeutic, prophylactic or diagnostic injection (specify substance or drug); intravenous push, single or initial substance/drug

Billing Tip

Immunizations and Office Visits
To report a patient's visit for just an immunization, some medical practices use E/M 99211 along with a code for the immunization. This is a misuse of the E/M code, which requires some significant, separate E/M service.

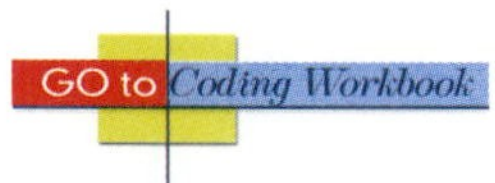

CODES 90281–99600 MEDICINE SECTION

Thinking It Through — 5.6

1. If a test for ferritin and a comprehensive metabolic panel are both performed, can both be reported?
2. Is it correct to report a comprehensive metabolic panel and an electrolyte panel for the same patient on the same day?
3. Which of these codes, 93000, 93005, or 93010, is used to report the technical component only of a routine ECG? Defend your decision.

Some commercial payers and Medicare use a HCPCS code, instead of CPT 99070, for the material that is injected, as covered in Chapter 6.

Category II and III Codes

The Category II code set contains supplemental tracking codes to help collect data regarding services, such as prenatal care and tobacco use cessation counseling, that are known to contribute to good patient care. Having codes available reduces the amount of administrative time needed to gather this data from documentation.

The use of these codes is optional and does not affect reimbursement. The codes are not required for correct coding and are not a substitute for Category I codes.

Category II codes are four digits followed by an alphabetical character. They are arranged according to the following categories:

- Composite Measures
- Patient Management
- Patient History
- Physical Examination
- Diagnostic Screening Processes or Results
- Therapeutic, Preventive or Other Interventions
- Follow-up or Other Outcomes
- Patient Safety

Billing Tip

Category II and III Code Updates
Category II and III codes are released twice a year, on January 1 and July 1.

Category II and III Updates
http://www.ama-assn.org/go/CPT

The Category III code set contains temporary codes for emerging technology, services, and procedures. If a Category III code is available for a new procedure, this code must be reported instead of a Category I unlisted code.

The codes in this section are not like CPT Category I codes, which require that the service or procedure be performed by many health care professionals in clinical practice in multiple locations and that FDA approval, as appropriate, has already been received. For these reasons, temporary codes for emerging technology, services, and procedures have been placed in a separate section of the CPT book. When a temporary service or procedure does meet these requirements, it is listed as a Category I code in the appropriate section of the main text.

Category III codes are four digits followed by an alphabetical character.

Note that modifiers can be used with Category III codes, but not with Category II codes.

Review

Steps to Success

- ❐ Read this chapter and review the Key Terms and the Chapter Summary.
- ❐ Answer the Review Questions and Applying Your Knowledge in the Chapter Review.
- ❐ Access the chapter's websites and complete the Internet Activities to learn more about available professional resources.
- ❐ Complete the related chapter in the *Medical Insurance Workbook* to reinforce your understanding of medical coding for procedures.

Chapter Summary

1. CPT, a publication of the American Medical Association, contains the most widely used system of codes for physicians' medical, diagnostic, and procedural services. CPT codes are required for reporting physician practice services on insurance claims and encounter forms. The codes have five digits and a description. Updated versions are released annually. Medical practices must use the current codes for proper billing and reimbursement.
2. Each year's CPT codes must be purchased from the American Medical Association, which also publishes changes online.
3. CPT contains six sections of Category I codes, Evaluation and Management, Anesthesia, Surgery, Radiology, Pathology and Laboratory, and Medicine, followed by the Category II and Category III codes, nine appendixes, and an index. The index is used first in the process of selecting a code; it contains alphabetic descriptive main terms and subterms for the procedures and services contained in the main text. The codes themselves are listed in the main text and are generally grouped by body system or site or by type of procedure.
4. Each coding section begins with section guidelines, which discuss definitions and rules for the use of codes, such as for unlisted codes, special reports, and notes for specific subsections. When a main entry has more than one code, a semicolon follows the common part of a descriptor in the main entry, and the unique descriptors that are related to the common description are indented below it. Seven symbols are used in the main text: (a) ● (a bullet or black circle) indicates a new procedure code; (b) ▲ (a triangle) indicates that the code's descriptor has changed; (c)▶◀ (facing triangles) enclose new or revised text other than the code's descriptor; (d) + (a plus sign) before a code indicates an add-on code that is used only along with other codes for primary procedures; (e) the symbol ⦿ next to a code means that conscious sedation is a part of the procedure that the surgeon performs; (f) a ⃠ indicates that the code cannot be modified with a –51 modifier; and (g) a ⚡ is used for codes for vaccines that are pending FDA approval.
5. A CPT modifier is a two-digit number that may be attached to most five-digit procedure codes to indicate that the procedure is different from the listed descriptor, but not in a way that changes the definition or requires a different code. Two or more modifiers may be used with one code to give the most accurate description possible.
6. The first step in selecting a procedure code is to determine the procedures and services to report by reviewing the documentation of the patient's visit. Next, after checking the coding system to use, CPT codes are located by finding the procedure in the index and verifying the code in the main text. The reporting order for the procedure codes places the code with the highest rate of reimbursement first. The final step is to determine whether modifiers are needed.

7. A summary of the six sections of Category I codes appears in Table 5.1 on page 146.
8. The key components for selecting Evaluation and Management codes are the extent of the history documented, the extent of the examination documented, and the complexity of the medical decision making. The steps for selecting correct E/M codes are to (a) determine the category and subcategory of service, (b) determine the extent of the history, (c) determine the extent of the examination, (d) determine the complexity of medical decision making, (e) analyze the requirements to report the service level, (f) verify the service level based on the nature of the presenting problem, time, counseling, and care coordination, (g) verify that the documentation is complete, and (h) assign the code.

Review Questions

Match the key terms with their definitions.

A. panel
B. professional component
C. separate procedure
D. Category III codes
E. global period
F. bundled code
G. Category II codes
H. add-on code
I. unlisted procedure
J. modifier

____ 1. The physician's skill, time, and expertise used in performing a procedure

____ 2. Temporary codes for emerging technology, services, and procedures

____ 3. Procedure code that groups related procedures under a single code

____ 4. A service that is not listed in CPT and requires a special report

____ 5. The inclusion of pre- and postoperative care for a specified period in the charges for a surgical procedure

____ 6. CPT codes that are used to track performance measures

____ 7. In CPT, a single code that groups laboratory tests that are frequently done together

____ 8. A procedure performed in addition to a primary procedure

____ 9. A secondary procedure that is performed with a primary procedure and that is indicated in CPT by a plus sign (+) next to the code

____10. A two-digit number indicating that special circumstances were involved with a procedure, such as a reduced service or a discontinued procedure

Decide whether each statement is true or false.

____ 1. In selecting correct procedure codes, the main text sections are first searched, and the code is then verified in the index.

____ 2. Category II codes are not reported for payment.

____ 3. In the CPT index, a *see* cross-reference must be followed.

____ 4. The section guidelines summarize the unlisted codes for the section.

____ 5. The phrases before the semicolon in a code descriptor define the unique entries; those after the semicolon are common.

____ 6. Descriptive entries in parentheses are not essential to code selection.

____ 7. A Category III code ends in a letter.

____ 8. Procedure codes are reported in order of increasing financial value for services performed on the same day.

____ 9. For new patients, two of the three key factors that are listed must be met.

____10. Because it is an evaluation of a patient, a consultation is coded using Evaluation and Management office services codes.

Select the letter that best completes the statement or answers the question.

____ 1. A new patient has not received services from the physician or from another physician of the same specialty in the same group practice for:
A. ninety days
B. one year
C. two years
D. three years

____ 2. When a physician asks a patient questions to obtain an inventory of constitutional symptoms and of the various body systems, the results are documented as the:
A. past medical history
B. family history
C. review of systems
D. comprehensive examination

____ 3. The abbreviation PFSH stands for:
A. past, family, and/or social history
B. patient, family, and/or systems history
C. past, family, and systems history
D. none of the above

____ 4. The examination that the physician conducts is categorized as:
A. straightforward, low complexity, moderate complexity, or high complexity
B. problem-focused, expanded problem-focused, detailed, or comprehensive
C. straightforward, problem-focused, detailed, or highly complex
D. low risk, moderate risk, or high risk

____ 5. The three key factors in selecting an Evaluation and Management code are:
A. time, severity of presenting problem, and history
B. history, examination, and time
C. past history, history of present illness, and chief complaint
D. history, examination, and medical decision making

____ 6. CPT code 99382 is an example of:
A. an emergency department service code
B. a preventive medicine service code
C. a consultation service code
D. a hospital observation code

____ 7. Anesthesia codes generally include:
A. preoperative evaluation and planning, normal care during the procedure, and routine care after the procedure
B. preparing the patient for the anesthetic, care during the procedure, postoperative care, and pain management as required by the surgeon
C. preoperative evaluation and planning, routine postoperative care, but not the administration of the anesthetic itself
D. all procedures that are ordered by the surgeon

____ 8. Surgery codes generally include:
A. all procedures done during the global period that comes before the surgery
B. preoperative evaluation and planning, the operation and normal additional procedures, and routine care after the procedure
C. all aspects of the operation, including preparing the patient for the surgery, performing the operation and normal additional procedures, as well as normal, uncomplicated follow-up
D. preoperative evaluation and planning, routine postoperative care, but not the operation itself

_____ 9. When a Surgery section code has a star next to it, the code descriptor covers:
   A. all procedures done during the global period that follows the surgery
   B. preoperative evaluation and planning, the operation and normal additional procedures, and routine care after the procedure
   C. the surgical procedure
   D. preoperative evaluation and planning, routine postoperative care, but not the surgical procedure

_____ 10. When a panel code from the Pathology and Laboratory section is reported:
   A. all the listed tests must have been performed
   B. 90 percent of the listed tests must have been performed
   C. 50 percent of the listed tests must have been performed
   D. all the listed tests must have been performed on the same day

Answer the following questions.

1. List the three steps in the procedural coding process.
2. List the three key components used to select E/M codes and the four levels each component has.

Applying Your Knowledge

Case 5.1 Coding Evaluation and Management Services

Supply the correct E/M CPT codes for the following procedures and services.

A. Office visit, new patient; detailed history and examination, low complexity medical decision making

B. Hospital visit, new patient; comprehensive history and examination, highly complex case

C. Office consultation for established patient; comprehensive history and examination, moderately complex medical decision making

D. Annual comprehensive physical examination for sixty-four-year-old new patient

E. Medical disability examination by treating physician

F. Hospital visit to previously admitted patient; expanded problem-focused history and examination, twenty-five minutes spent at bedside

G. Hospital emergency department call for established patient with cardiac infarction; detailed history and examination, moderately complex decision making

H. Third visit to established, stable patient in nursing facility, medical record and patient's status reviewed, no change made to medical plan

I. Home visit for new patient, straightforward case, problem-focused history and examination

J. Short telephone call to patient to report laboratory test results

Case 5.2 Coding Anesthesia and Surgery Procedures

Supply the correct CPT codes for the following procedures and services.

A. Anesthesia for vaginal delivery only

B. Anesthesia services for patient age seventy-six, healthy, for open procedure on wrist

C. Incision and drainage of infected wound after surgery

D. Destruction of flat wart

E. Closed treatment of acromioclavicular dislocation with manipulation

F. Complicated drainage of finger abscess

G. Paring of three skin lesions

H. Postpartum D & C

I. Excision of chest wall tumor including ribs

J. Transurethral electrosurgical resection of the prostate (TURP); patient has mild systemic disease; payer requires surgery codes

K. Amniocentesis, diagnostic

L. Ureterolithotomy on lower third of ureter

M. Tonsillectomy and adenoidectomy, patient age fifteen

N. Flexible sigmoidoscopy with specimen collection, separate procedure.

O. Kidner type procedure

P. Application of short leg splint

Q. Unilateral transorbital frontal sinusotomy

R. Puncture aspiration of three cysts in breast

S. Posterior arthrodesis for scoliosis patient, eleven vertebral segments

T. Routine obstetrical care, vaginal delivery

Case 5.3 Coding Radiology, Pathology and Laboratory, or Medicine Procedures

Supply the correct CPT codes for the following procedures and services.

A. Subcutaneous chemotherapy administration

B. Material (sterile tray) supplied by physician

C. Routine ECG with fifteen leads, with the physician providing only the interpretation and report of the test

D. CRH stimulation panel

E. Automated urinalysis for glucose, without microscopy

F. Aortography, thoracic, without serialography, radiological supervision and interpretation

G. Bone marrow smear interpretation

H. Physical therapy evaluation

I. Ingestion challenge test

J. Electrocorticogram at surgery, separate procedure

Case 5.4 Assigning Modifiers

A. What is the meaning of each of the modifiers used in the following case example? A multi-trauma patient had a bilateral knee procedure as part of team surgery following a motorcycle crash. The orthopedic surgeon also reconstructed the patient's pelvis and left wrist.

1. –99
2. –66
3. –51
4. –50

Supply the correct codes and modifiers for these cases.

B. A surgeon administers a regional Bier block and then monitors the patient and the block while repairing the flexor tendon of the forearm.

C. Primary care provider performs a frontal and lateral chest X-ray and observes a mass. The patient is sent to a pulmonologist, who, on the same day, repeats the frontal and lateral chest X-ray. How should the pulmonologist report the X-ray service?

D. A day after surgery for a knee replacement, the patient develops an infection in the surgical area and is returned to the operating room for debridement. Which modifier is attached to the second procedure?

Internet Activities

1. The American Academy of Professional Coders (AAPC) is a coding association that certifies medical coders and provides information on coding issues. Visit http://www.aapc.com, and list the specialty coding certifications that are available. Also review the online publication *The Added Edge* (under the *More* banner), and research recent coding articles.
2. Visit the website of the American Medical Association: http://www.ama-assn.org. Under the banner *CPT Codes and Resources,* read the information on the CPT process, and report on how new CPT codes are approved.
3. Medical societies such as the American Academy of Family Physicians also offer Internet tools to support their coding. Research this site at http://www.aafp/org, and locate this year's CPT code updates. Prepare a report on other information that you consider valuable from this website.

Chapter 6

Procedural Coding: Introduction to HCPCS

CHAPTER OUTLINE

Overview of HCPCS

Level II Codes

HCPCS Coding Procedures

HCPCS Billing Procedures

Learning Outcomes

After studying this chapter, you should be able to:

1. Discuss the purpose of the HCPCS code set.
2. Explain how to locate the periodic updates to HCPCS codes.
3. Describe the structure and content of the index, the Table of Drugs, and the main text in HCPCS.
4. Describe the purpose and correct use of HCPCS modifiers.
5. List the steps for assigning correct HCPCS codes and modifiers.
6. Discuss the tools used to verify billing rules for specific HCPCS codes.

Key Terms

CMS HCPCS Workgroup
Coverage Issues Manual (CIM)
durable medical equipment (DME)
durable medical equipment, prosthetics, orthotics, and supplies (DMEPOS)
Durable Medical Equipment Regional Carrier (DMERC)
Healthcare Common Procedure Coding System (HCPCS)
Level II
Level II modifiers
Medicare Carriers Manual (MCM)
permanent national codes
statistical analysis durable medical equipment regional carrier (SADMERC)
temporary national codes

The national codes for products, supplies, and those services not included in CPT are in the HCPCS Level II code set. HCPCS codes permit physician practices to bill for items provided to patients in Medicare, Medicaid, and many private payers' plans. Payers need to understand the medical necessity of these items for reimbursement, just as they do for CPT codes.

Overview of HCPCS

The **Healthcare Common Procedure Coding System,** referred to as HCPCS, was set up to give health care providers a coding system that describes specific products, supplies, and services that patients receive. HCPCS codes provide uniformity in medical services reporting and enable the collection of statistical data on medical procedures, products, and services. In the early 1980s, the use of HCPCS codes for claims was optional. With the implementation of the Health Insurance Portability and Accountability Act (HIPAA) of 1996, HCPCS has become mandatory for coding and billing.

HCPCS is technically made up of two sections of procedural codes. Level I, the CPT *(Current Procedural Terminology)* maintained by the American Medical Association (AMA), is covered in Chapter 5. The second section is the HCPCS **Level II** codes that identify supplies, products, and services not in Level I. The Centers for Medicare and Medicaid Services (CMS) is responsible for maintaining the HCPCS code set.

> **HIPAA Tip**
>
> **Level III Codes Phased Out**
>
> *Before December 31, 2003, HCPCS had a third level of codes. Level III consisted of local codes used by state Medicaid agencies, Medicare, and private payers, who determined the codes. HIPAA does not allow non-national codes, so the Level III codes have been*

Level II Codes

A Level II code is made up of five characters beginning with a letter followed by four numbers, such as J7630. The HCPCS Tabular List of codes has more than twenty sections, each of which covers a related group of items. For example, the E section covers **durable medical equipment (DME),** reusable medical equipment ordered by physicians for patients' use at home, such as walkers and wheelchairs. Durable medical equipment:

- Can withstand repeated use
- Is primarily and customarily used for a medical purpose
- Generally is not useful to a person in the absense of an illness or injury
- Is appropriate for use in the home

HCPCS Level II codes can be used in conjunction with the CPT codes on bills for patients and on claims for Medicare, Medicaid, and other payers. As with CPT codes, reporting HCPCS codes does not guarantee payment. Each payer's coverage and payment decisions apply. Also, decisions regarding the addition, deletion, and revision of HCPCS codes are made independent of the adjudication process.

> **HIPAA Tip**
>
> **Mandated Code Set**
>
> *HCPCS is the mandated code set for reporting supplies, orthotic and prosthetic devices, and durable medical equipment under HIPAA Electronic Health Care Transactions and Code Sets.*

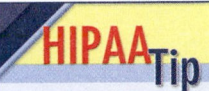

HCPCS Sections

HCPCS Level II Tabular List has the following sections:

A0000–A0999	Transport Services Including Ambulance
A4000–A8999	Medical and Surgical Supplies
A9000–A9999	Administrative, Miscellaneous, and Investigational
B4000–B9999	Enteral and Parenteral Therapy
C1000–C9999	C Codes (for use only under the hospital outpatient prospective payment system; not to be used to report other services; Updated quarterly by CMS)
D0000–D9999	Dental Procedures (copyrighted by the American Dental Association and not included in the general HCPCS coding text)
E0100–E9999	Durable Medical Equipment (DME)
G0000–G9999	Procedures/Professional Services (temporary) and Assigned by CMS (on temporary basis)
H0001–H1005	Alcohol and/or Drug Services
J0100–J8999	Drugs Other Than Chemotherapy
J9000–J9999	Chemotherapy Drugs
K0000–K9999	K Codes for Durable Medical Equipment (temporary codes assigned by CMS for the exclusive use of Durable Medical Equipment Regional Carriers)
L0100–L4999	Orthotic Procedures
L5000–L9999	Prosthetic Procedures
M0000–M0399	Medical Services
P0000–P2999	Pathology and Laboratory Services
Q0000–Q9999	Temporary Codes
R0000–R5999	Diagnostic Radiology Services
S0009–S9999	Temporary National Codes
T1000–T9999	National T Codes for State Medicaid Agencies (not valid for Medicare)
V0000–V2999	Vision Services
V5000–V5299	Hearing Services

Billing Tip

DMERCs
Medicare has four **Durable Medical Equipment Regional Carriers** or **DMERCs**, regional contracted carriers that process Medicare claims for durable medical equipment, prosthetics, orthotics, and supplies (DMEPOS).

Table 6.1 details these sections and provides examples of entries.

Permanent versus Temporary Codes

The **CMS HCPCS Workgroup** is a code advisory committee made up of representatives from CMS (Centers for Medicare and Medicaid Services) and other government agencies. Its role is to identify services for which new codes are needed. Temporary codes may later be given permanent status if they are widely used.

Table 6.1 HCPCS Level II Detailed Code Ranges and Examples

Section	Code Range	Example
Transportation services	A0000–A0999	A0300 Ambulance service; basic life support, nonemergency, all inclusive
Medical and surgical supplies	A4000–A7509	A4211 Supplies for self-administered injections
Administrative, miscellaneous and investigational	A9000–A9999	A9150 Nonprescription drugs
Enteral and parenteral therapy	B4000–B9999	B9000 Enteral nutrition infusion pump, without alarm
Pass-through items (outpatient prospective payment system)	C1079–C9716	C1731 Catheter, electrophysiology, diagnostic, other than 3D mapping, 20+ electrodes
Dental procedures	D0000–D9999	D0150 Comprehensive oral exam
Durable medical equipment (DME)	E0000–E9999	E0250 Hospital bed with side rails and mattress
Procedures and professional services	G0000–G9999	G0008 Administration of influenza virus vaccine
Alcohol and drug abuse treatment services	H0000–H9999	H0006 Alcohol and/or drug services; case management
Drugs administered other than oral method	J0000–J8999	J0120 Injection, tetracycline, up to 250 mg
Chemotherapy drugs	J9000–J9999	J9212 Injection, interferon alfacon-1, recombinant, 1 mcg
DME supplies	K0000–K9999	K0001 Standard wheelchair
Orthotic procedures	L0000–L4999	L1800 Knee orthosis (KO); elastic with stays
Prosthetic procedures	L5000–L9999	L5050 Ankle, symes; molded socket, SACH foot
Medical services	M0000–M9999	M0064 Brief office visit for the sole purpose of monitoring or changing drug prescriptions used to treat mental psychoneurotic and personality disorders
Laboratory and pathology	P0000–P9999	P3000 Screening Papanicolaou smear, cervical or vaginal, up to 3; by technician under physician supervision
Temporary codes	Q0000–Q0099	Q0035 Cardiokymography
Diagnostic radiology services	R0000–R5999	R0070 Transportation of portable X-ray equipment and personnel to home or nursing home, per trip to facility or location; one patient seen
Temporary national codes (non-Medicare)	S0000–S9999	S0187 Tamoxifen citrate, oral, 10 mg
National codes established for state Medicaid agency	T0000–T9999	T1001 Nursing assessment/evaluation
Vision services	V0000–V2999	V2020 Frames, purchases
Hearing services	V5000–V5999	V5364 Dysphagia screening

Source: HCPCS 2007

Billing Tip

Attachments for Claims with Miscellaneous Codes
Claims with miscellaneous codes are manually reviewed for medical necessity. Their use should be infrequent, because it may delay payment and increase chances of denied claims.

SADMERC Toll-free Helpline

(877) 735-1326

The helpline is operational between 9 A.M. and 4 P.M. (EST)

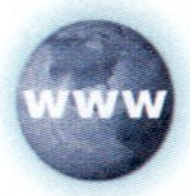

SADMERC product classification list of individual items and their code categories

http://www.palmettogba.com

Permanent Codes

The CMS HCPCS Workgroup maintains the **permanent national codes** that are available for use by all government and private payers. No code changes can be made unless all panel members agree. Advisers from private payers provide input to the Workgroup.

Some codes are *miscellaneous* or *not otherwise classified (NEC)* (as in ICD-9-CM codes). These codes are used by all payers to bill for items or services that do not have permanent national codes. Many of these codes become permanent national status in the updating process.

Before using a miscellaneous code on a claim form, the medical insurance specialist should check with the payer to determine whether there is a specific code that should instead be used. For Medicare claims sent to one of the DMERCs, the medical insurance specialist should check with the **statistical analysis durable medical equipment regional carrier** (SADMERC) under contract to CMS. The SADMERC is responsible for providing assistance in determining which HCPCS codes describe DMEPOS items for Medicare billing purposes.

Temporary Codes

The **temporary national codes** may also be used by all payers. When temporary codes become permanent national HCPCS Level II codes, the coding reference indicates the change.

- *C codes:* Valid only on Medicare claims and used specifically for the hospital outpatient prospective payment system
- *G codes:* For the professional component of services and procedures not found in the CPT
- *Q codes:* For drugs, medical equipment, and services that have not been given CPT codes and are not identifiable in the Level II codes, but are needed to process a billing claim
- *K codes:* Developed to assist DMERCs when no permanent national codes exist for the product or supply
- *S codes:* For private insurers to identify drugs, services, supplies, and procedures; used by the Medicaid program but not reimbursable under Medicare
- *H codes:* For state Medicaid agencies to identify mental health services (alcohol and drug treatment)
- *T codes:* For state Medicaid agencies when there are not permanent national codes; can be used for private insurers but not for Medicare

HCPCS Updates

HCPCS Level II is a public code set. Information about the codes and updates is located on the CMS HCPCS website. Many publishers also print easy-to-use HCPCS reference books.

HCPCS Level II permanent national codes are released on January 1 of each year and are reviewed continuously throughout the year. Any supplier or manufacturer can ask CMS to make changes. Requests must be submitted in writing and must describe the reason for the proposed changes. CMS must receive requests by January 3 of the current year for the changes to be considered for the next January 1 release. Revisions received after the deadline are considered for the next annual update.

Temporary national codes are updated quarterly. Once established, temporary codes are usually implemented within ninety days, so as to have time to inform physician practices and suppliers about them via bulletins and newsletters.

Thinking It Through — 6.1

Based on Table 6.1, in which section is each of the following HCPCS services located?

1. **Motorized wheelchair**
2. **Alcohol wipes, box**
3. **Recement crown**
4. **Ambulance waiting time**
5. **Contact lens, gas permeable**

The HCPCS website lists current HCPCS codes, has an alphabetical index of HCPCS codes by type of service or product, and also has an alphabetical table of drugs for which there are Level II codes. The newly established temporary codes and effective dates for their use are also posted to allow for quick dissemination of coding requests and decisions.

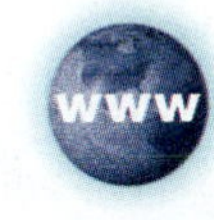

HCPCS Website

http://www.cms.hhs.gov/MedHCPCSGenInfo/

HCPCS Coding Procedures

To look up codes in the HCPCS Level II, follow the same coding conventions that are used to assign ICD-9-CM and CPT codes. When using the ICD-9-CM (covered in Chapter 4), the coder first uses the Alphabetic Index to locate the appropriate diagnosis, and then verifies the code selection using the Tabular List. Likewise for coding using the CPT, the Index—arranged alphabetically and located at the end of the text—is used to find the main term, which is then verified in the code sections that are arranged numerically.

Coding Steps

To assign HCPCS Level II codes, first look up the name of the supply or item in the index. The index is arranged alphabetically, with the main term in bold print followed by the HCPCS Level II code. Verify the code selection in the appropriate Tabular List section of the HCPCS Level II code book.

Assigning drug codes is made easier by the Table of Drugs in the HCPCS code book. It presents drugs in alphabetical order, followed by the dosage, the way the drug is administered (such as intravenously), and the HCPCS code.

Adenosine 6 mg	IV	J0150
Adenosine 30 mg	IV	J0152

Also to be checked are symbols next to some codes. Publishers use various symbols in HCPCS code books, but their meaning is always explained in the legend on the bottom of each page. The following example shows the symbols for new and revised codes used in one HCPCS code book:

New and Revised Text Characters

◀▶	**New**
⇦⇨	**Revised**
~~supply~~	**Deleted**

Compliance Guideline

Brand and Trade Names
To avoid the appearance of endorsing particular products, HCPCS does not use brand or trade names to describe products represented by codes.

Reporting Quantities

The coder should carefully review the description of quantities associated with HCPCS codes. Drug descriptions should be carefully checked to note the method of administration and the dosage. The selected code must match the dose and route that are documented in the medical record or on encounter form.

The administration methods common in offices include:

- *IV:* Intravenous injection
- *IM:* Intramuscular injection
- *IA:* Intraarterial injection
- *SC:* Subcutaneous injection
- *INH:* Inhalant
- *Oral:* Taken by mouth
- *Nasal Spray:* Sprayed into the nostril

The dosage is described in appropriate quantities, such as milligrams (mg) or milliliters (ml). For example, the listing for Prednisone is:

J7506 Prednisone, oral, per 5

If a patient's dosage is 10 mg, the code to report is:

J7506 X2

The HCPCS code is followed by the quantity 2. If the patient has been administered 12 mg, the unit indicator is 3.

Multiple units of other items are also reported by the HCPCS code followed by the units. Five surgical stockings would be coded as:

A4495 **X5**

HCPCS Modifiers

Like CPT, HCPCS Level II uses modifiers, called **Level II modifiers**, to provide additional information about services, supplies, and procedures. For example, a UE modifier is used when an item identified by a HCPCS code is used equipment, and a NU modifier is used for new equipment. HCPCS Level II modifiers are made up of either two letters or one letter and one number:

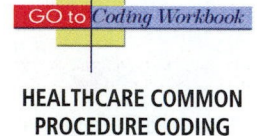

HEALTHCARE COMMON PROCEDURE CODING SYSTEM: LEVEL II CODES AND MODIFIERS

F5	Right hand, thumb
HS	Family/couple without client present

Payers may require the use of both Level II modifiers and CPT modifiers on claims. The modifiers in Table 6.2 are among the most prevalent.

HCPCS Billing Procedures

There are specific procedures to be followed for Medicare and Medicaid patients and for patients with private insurance. Some procedures require both a CPT code and a HCPCS code, such as reporting both the administration of an injection and the material that was injected.

Medicare and Medicaid Billing

When medical insurance specialists are processing claims for patients who have Medicaid or Medicare, they should consult HCPCS code books to iden-

Table 6.2 Selected HCPCS Level II (National) Modifiers

Modfier	Description
–CA	Procedure payable in the inpatient setting only when performed emergently on an outpatient who expires prior to admission
–E1	Upper left eyelid
–E2	Lower left eyelid
–E3	Upper right eyelid
–E4	Lower right eyelid
–FA	Left hand, thumb
–F1	Left hand, second digit
–F2	Left hand, third digit
–F3	Left hand, fourth digit
–F4	Left hand, fifth digit
–F5	Right hand, thumb
–F6	Right hand, second digit
–F7	Right hand, third digit
–F8	Right hand, fourth digit
–F9	Right hand, fifth digit
–GA	Waiver of liability statement on file
–GG	Performance and payment of a screening mammogram and diagnostic mammogram on the same patient, same day
–GY	Item or service statutorily excluded or does not meet the definition of any Medicare benefit
–GZ	Item or service expected to be denied as not reasonable and necessary
–LC	Left circumflex coronary artery
–LD	Left anterior descending coronary artery
–RC	Right coronary artery
–LT	Left side (identifies procedures performed on the left side of the body)
–RT	Right side (identifies procedures performed on the right side of the body)
–QM	Ambulance service provided under arrangement by a provider of services
–QN	Ambulance service furnished directly by a provider of services
–TA	Left foot, great toe
–T1	Left foot, second digit
–T2	Left foot, third digit
–T3	Left foot, fourth digit
–T4	Left foot, fifth digit
–T5	Right foot, great toe
–T6	Right foot, second digit
–T7	Right foot, third digit
–T8	Right foot, fourth digit
–T9	Right foot, fifth digit
–TC	Technical component

Source: HCPCS 2007

tify services reimbursable under HCPCS Level II. Symbols direct the biller or coder to Medicare billing rules that are reprinted in the appendixes of the HCPCS code books. For example, here are the symbols from one publication:

- ◆ **Not Covered by or Valid for Medicare**
- ✢ **Special Coverage Instructions Apply**
- ✻ **Carrier Discretion**

When the symbol for Special Coverage Instructions Apply appears, Medicare resources must be checked.

Billing Tip

HCPCS Anesthesia Modifiers

Medicare uses additional HCPCS modifiers for anesthesia services. These modifiers help clarify special situations when Medicare patient services are reported. For example, –AA is used when the anesthesiologist provides the anesthesia service directly instead of overseeing an assistant anesthetist.

Medicare Carriers Manual

The **Medicare Carriers Manual (MCM)** lists guidelines established by Medicare about coverage for HCPCS Level II services. A reference to this manual in a HCPCS code book includes the number of the section in which the relevant guidelines appear. For example:

✢J0205—Injection, Alglucerase, per 10 units

MCM 2049

Section 2049 in the MCM indicates that Alglucerase is used in chemotherapy and that self-administration is not covered by Medicare Part B unless a federal statute calls for such coverage.

> **Billing Tip**
>
> **Using the Medicare Carriers Manual**
> Consult the Medicare Carriers Manual when the descriptor of a HCPCS Level II code includes the MCM section number. For supplies billed on Medicare and Medicaid claims (see Chapters 10 and 11), the MCM provides important information that can make the difference between payer acceptance and rejection.

Coverage Issues Manual

The **Coverage Issues Manual (CIM)** is a collection of information about Medicare-qualified clinical trials, treatments, therapeutic interventions, diagnostic testing, durable medical equipment, therapies, and services. A reference to the CIM in a HCPCS code book looks like this:

✢E0310 Bed side rails, full length

CIM 60-18

The symbol in front of the number means that Special Coverage Instructions apply to this code. The listing 60-18 in the Coverage Issues Manual indicates that, for a claim to be accepted, a physician's prescription is needed and the hospital bed must be a medical necessity.

> **Billing Tip**
>
> **Keep HCPCS Updates**
> Retain HCPCS updates from private payers and keep them where they can be readily accessed when preparing claims.

Private Payer Billing

When commercial payers want participating practices to use HCPCS codes instead of the corresponding CPT codes, they inform the practices. For example, plans from the Blue Cross and Blue Shield Association send customers a monthly publication that outlines CPT and HCPCS changes, deletions, and additions as they relate to billing for services, procedures, and equipment.

Thinking It Through — 6.2

Using HCPCS Level II, assign the appropriate codes.

1. Ambulance service, basic life support, nonemergency transport
2. Breast pump, manual, any type
3. Zidovudine 10 mg
4. Laboratory certification, Wet mounts, including vaginal specimen
5. Hospital bed with mattress and side rails, totally electric

Review

Steps to Success

- ❒ Read this chapter and review the Key Terms and the Chapter Summary.
- ❒ Answer the Review Questions and Applying Your Knowledge in the Chapter Review.
- ❒ Access the chapter's websites and complete the Internet Activities to learn more about available professional resources.
- ❒ Complete the related chapter in the *Medical Insurance Workbook* to reinforce your understanding of medical coding using HCPCS.

Chapter Summary

1. The HCPCS code set is a coding system for specific products, supplies, and services that patients receive in the delivery of their care.
2. Annual updates to HCPCS codes are released on the CMS HCPCS website for use effective January 1 of each year, and annual HCPCS code books are published as a code reference. Interim updates for temporary codes are also found on the CMS HCPCS website.
3. The HCPCS index is arranged alphabetically, as is the Table of Drugs included in HCPCS code books. The main text is made up of sections of codes arranged numerically according to their initial letter, from Section A through Section V.
4. HCPCS modifiers are either two letters or a letter plus a number. Modifiers are used to clarify a HCPCS code by making it more specific.
5. Correct HCPCS coding follows the same general guidelines as ICD-9-CM and CPT coding. Begin by locating the item to be coded in the index (or the Table of Drugs), and then verify the probable code in the main sections. Assign appropriate modifiers.
6. Medicare billing rules for specific HCPCS codes are shown by references in the main sections next to the codes. The reference *MCM* means that a billing rule for that code's use must be looked up the appendix of the HCPCS code book containing the Medicare Carriers Manual or by checking the original source. The reference *CIM* likewise means that a billing rule must be checked in the Coverage Issues Manual.

Review Questions

Match the key terms with their definitions.

A. durable medical equipment (DME)
B. HCPCS
C. Medicare Carriers Manual (MCM)
D. permanent national codes
E. temporary national codes
F. Level II modifiers
G. Coverage Issues Manual (CIM)
H. CMS HCPCS Workgroup

____ 1. HCPCS Level II codes that are maintained for the use of all payers

____ 2. Reference containing guidelines established by Medicare related to covered services in HCPCS Level II

____ 3. HCPCS Level II codes that are used by individual payers for items not covered in permanent national codes

____ 4. Reference containing information related to Medicare-qualified clinical trials, treatments, therapeutic interventions, diagnostic testing, DME, therapies, and services

____ 5. Code set providing national codes for supplies, services, and products

____ 6. Reusable medical equipment for use in the home

____ 7. Two-character codes that are assigned to clarify Level II codes

____ 8. Government committee that maintains and advises on HCPCS Level II codes

Decide whether each statement is true or false.

____ 1. HCPCS Level II codes have six digits.

____ 2. HCPCS Level II codes are used only by hospitals.

____ 3. HIPAA mandates the use of HCPCS codes.

____ 4. CPT modifiers and HCPCS Level II modifiers are the same.

____ 5. HCPCS permanent national codes can be altered or deleted by a single payer alone.

____ 6. HCPCS permanent national codes are issued on January 1 of each year and must be used as of their effective date.

____ 7. HCPCS code books use symbols to show new, revised, and deleted codes and descriptors.

____ 8. Coding drugs involves paying attention to both the method of administration and the quantity administered.

____ 9. DME supplies are located in the K section of the main listing.

____ 10. Private payers are not permitted to use HCPCS codes; use is restricted to government programs.

Select the letter that best completes the statement or answers the question.

____ 1. Transportation services are HCPCS ______ codes.
A. A
B. B
C. C
D. D

____ 2. Vision and hearing services are HCPCS ______ codes.
A. D
B. E
C. H
D. V

____ 3. Temporary codes are HCPCS ______ codes.
A. D
B. Q
C. T
D. V

____ 4. Durable medical equipment (DME) codes are HCPCS ______ codes.
A. D
B. E
C. H
D. V

____ 5. Prosthetic procedures are HCPCS ______ codes.
A. D
B. E
C. H
D. L

____ 6. Temporary National Codes for private insurers to identify drugs, services, supplies, and procedures that are not reimbursable under Medicare are HCPCS _____ codes.
A. D
B. E
C. S
D. V

____ 7. Diagnostic radiology services are HCPCS _____ codes.
A. R
B. E
C. H
D. V

____ 8. Chemotherapy drugs are HCPCS _____ codes.
A. D
B. E
C. H
D. J

____ 9. Laboratory and pathology are HCPCS _____ codes.
A. D
B. E
C. P
D. V

____10. Dental codes are listed in HCPCS as _____ codes.
A. D
B. E
C. H
D. V

Define the following abbreviations:

1. MCM ______________________________
2. HCPCS ______________________________
3. DME ______________________________
4. CIM ______________________________
5. DMERC ______________________________
6. DMEPOS ______________________________

Applying Your Knowledge

Case 6.1 Assigning HCPCS Codes

Supply the correct HCPCS codes for the following.

A. Administration of hepatitis B vaccine __________

B. Each composite dressing, pad size more than 48 square inches, without adhesive border __________

C. Shoe lift, elevation, heel, tapered to metatarsals, per inch __________

D. Screening Papanicolaou smear, cervical or vaginal, up to 3 by technician under physician supervision __________

E. Hot water bottle __________

F. Half-length bedside rails __________

G. Injection of bevacizumab, 10 mg __________

H. Brachytherapy, source, palladium 103, per source __________

I. Enteral nutrition infusion pump, with alarm __________

J. Infusion of 1000 cc of normal saline solution __________

K. Prednisone acetate 1ml __________

L. Glucose test strips for dialysis __________

M. pHisoHex or Betadine solution __________

N. Distilled water used for nebulizer 100ml __________

O. Spring crutch, underarm __________

P. Walker heavy duty, multiple braking system __________

Q. Stationary infusion pump, parenteral __________

R. Assessment alcohol __________

S. Dacarbazine 400 mg __________

T. Miscellaneous, durable medical equipment __________

Case 6.2 Assigning HCPCS Modifiers

Supply the correct HCPCS modifiers for the following.

A. Left foot, great toe

B. Technical component

C. Waiver of liability statement on file

Case 6.3

The following e-mail announcement is on file in a medical practice that has many Medicare patients. One patient has recently had an encounter for a iloprost inhalation solution, 40 mcg.

> *Provider Types Affected*
>
> *Physicians, providers, and suppliers billing Medicare carriers, including Durable Medical Equipment Regional Carriers (DMERCs) or Fiscal Intermediaries (FIs) for iloprost inhalation solution.*
>
> *Provider Action Needed*
>
> *Effective July 1, 2005, for dates of service on or after July 1, 2005, HCPCS code Q4080, for iloprost inhalation solution, is being added to the HCPCS.*
>
> *Q4080 Iloprost, inhalation solution, administered through DME, 20 mcg*
>
> *Also, please note that while Medicare carriers and DMERCs will accept Q4080 to report iloprost inhalation solution, only Medicare DMERCs will make payment for Q4080.*
>
> *The official instruction issued to your carrier/DMERC/FI regarding this change may be found by going to http://www.cms.hhs.gov/manuals/transmittals/comm_date_dsc.asp. From that Web page, look for CR 3847 in the CR NUM column on the right, and then click on the file for that CR.*

A. What type of HCPCS code is being announced? ____________________

B. To be paid for the solution used during the patient's encounter, what entity should be billed?

____

C. What document number would the medical insurance specialist research on the CMS website for more information? ____________________

D. How would the code be entered on a claim form? ____________________

Internet Activities

1. Current HCPCS information is located on the CMS website. Visit this location: http://www.cms.hhs.gov/medhcpcsgeninfo/ Describe the types of information that are available.

Part 3 Claim Preparation

Chapter 7
Visit Charges and Compliant Billing

Chapter 8
Health Care Claim Preparation and Transmission

3

Chapter 7

Visit Charges and Compliant Billing

CHAPTER OUTLINE

Compliant Billing

Knowledge of Billing Rules

Compliance Errors

Strategies for Compliance

Audits

Comparing Physician Fees and Payer Fees

Payer Fee Schedules

Payment Methods

Learning Outcomes

After studying this chapter, you should be able to:

1. Explain the importance of properly linking diagnoses and procedures on health care claims.
2. Describe the use and format of Medicare's Correct Coding Initiative (CCI) edits.
3. Discuss types of coding and billing errors.
4. Explain major strategies that help ensure compliant billing.
5. Discuss the use of audit tools to verify code selection.
6. Describe the fee schedules that physicians create for their services.
7. Compare the usual, customary, and reasonable (UCR) and the resource-based relative value scale (RBRVS) methods of determining the fees that insurance carriers pay for providers' services.
8. Describe the steps used to calculate RBRVS payments under the Medicare Fee Schedule.
9. Identify the three methods most payers use to pay physicians.
10. Discuss the calculation of payments for participating and non-participating providers, and describe how balance billing regulations affect the charges that are due from patients.

Key Terms

advisory opinion
allowed charge
assumption coding
audit
balance billing
capitation rate (cap rate)
CCI column 1/column 2 code pair edit
CCI modifier indicator
CCI mutually exclusive code (MEC) edit
charge-based fee structure
code linkage
conversion factor
Correct Coding Initiative (CCI)
documentation template
downcoding
edits
excluded parties
external audit
geographic practice cost index (GPCI)
internal audit
job reference aid
Medicare Physician Fee Schedule (MPFS)
OIG Work Plan
professional courtesy
prospective audit
provider withhold
relative value scale (RVS)
relative value unit (RVU)
resource-based fee structure
resource-based relative value scale (RBRVS)
retrospective audit
truncated coding
upcoding
usual fee
usual, customary, and reasonable (UCR)
write off

Although physicians have the ultimate responsibility for proper documentation, correct coding, and compliance with billing regulations, medical insurance specialists help ensure maximum appropriate reimbursement by submitting correct, accurate health care claims. The process used to generate claims must comply with the rules imposed by federal and state laws as well as with payer requirements. Correct claims help reduce the chance of an investigation of the practice for fraud and the risk of liability if an investigation does occur.

Compliant Billing

In the medical billing process, after patients' encounters, physicians prepare and sign documentation of the visit. The next step is to post the medical codes and transactions of the patient's visit in the practice management program (PMP) and to prepare claims.

Correct claims report the connection between a billed service and a diagnosis. The diagnosis must support the billed service as necessary to treat or investigate the patient's condition. Payers analyze this connection, called **code linkage**, to decide if the charges are for medically necessary services. Figure 7.1 on page 206 shows a completed health care claim that correctly links the diagnosis and the procedure. Review the information on the lower left of the claim to see the diagnosis codes and the procedure codes. This chapter covers basic information about billing; Chapter 8 presents the mechanics of preparing and sending claims.

Compliance Guideline

Why Compliant Billing?
The possible consequences of billing incorrectly include:

- Denied claims
- Delays in processing claims and receiving payments
- Reduced payments
- Fines and other sanctions
- Loss of hospital privileges
- Exclusion from payers' programs
- Prison sentences
- Loss of the physician's license to practice medicine

Knowledge of Billing Rules

To prepare correct claims, it is important to know payers' billing rules that are stated in patients' medical insurance policies and in participation contracts. Because contracts change and rules are updated, medical insurance specialists also rely on payer bulletins, websites, and regular communications with payer representatives to keep up to date.

1500

HEALTH INSURANCE CLAIM FORM

APPROVED BY NATIONAL UNIFORM CLAIM COMMITTEE 08/05

MEDICARE NATIONWIDE
1000 HIGH ST
TOLEDO, OH 43601-0213

CARRIER

PICA | PICA

1. MEDICARE [X] (Medicare #) | MEDICAID [ ] (Medicaid #) | TRICARE CHAMPUS [ ] (Sponsor's SSN) | CHAMPVA [ ] (Member ID#) | GROUP HEALTH PLAN [ ] (SSN or ID) | FECA BLK LUNG [ ] (SSN) | OTHER [ ] (ID)

1a. INSURED'S I.D. NUMBER (For Program in Item 1): 302461884A

2. PATIENT'S NAME (Last Name, First Name, Middle Initial): HUANG ERIC

3. PATIENT'S BIRTH DATE MM DD YY: 03 13 1940 SEX M [X] F [ ]

4. INSURED'S NAME (Last Name, First Name, Middle Initial)

5. PATIENT'S ADDRESS (No., Street): 1109 BAUER ST

6. PATIENT RELATIONSHIP TO INSURED: Self [X] Spouse [ ] Child [ ] Other [ ]

7. INSURED'S ADDRESS (No., Street)

CITY: SHAKER HEIGHTS STATE: OH

8. PATIENT STATUS: Single [ ] Married [X] Other [ ]

CITY STATE

ZIP CODE: 44118 6789 TELEPHONE (Include Area Code): (555) 639 1787

Employed [ ] Full-Time Student [ ] Part-Time Student [ ]

ZIP CODE TELEPHONE (INCLUDE AREA CODE) ( )

9. OTHER INSURED'S NAME (Last Name, First Name, Middle Initial)

10. IS PATIENT'S CONDITION RELATED TO:

11. INSURED'S POLICY GROUP OR FECA NUMBER: NONE

a. OTHER INSURED'S POLICY OR GROUP NUMBER

a. EMPLOYMENT? (CURRENT OR PREVIOUS) [ ] YES [X] NO

a. INSURED'S DATE OF BIRTH MM DD YY SEX M [ ] F [ ]

b. OTHER INSURED'S DATE OF BIRTH MM DD YY SEX M [ ] F [ ]

b. AUTO ACCIDENT? [ ] YES [X] NO PLACE (State)

b. EMPLOYER'S NAME OR SCHOOL NAME

c. EMPLOYER'S NAME OR SCHOOL NAME

c. OTHER ACCIDENT? [ ] YES [X] NO

c. INSURANCE PLAN NAME OR PROGRAM NAME

d. INSURANCE PLAN NAME OR PROGRAM NAME

10d. RESERVED FOR LOCAL USE

d. IS THERE ANOTHER HEALTH BENEFIT PLAN? [ ] YES [ ] NO *If yes,* return to and complete item 9 a-d.

READ BACK OF FORM BEFORE COMPLETING & SIGNING THIS FORM.

12. PATIENT'S OR AUTHORIZED PERSON'S SIGNATURE I authorize the release of any medical or other information necessary to process this claim. I also request payment of government benefits either to myself or to the party who accepts assignment below.

SIGNED SIGNATURE ON FILE DATE

13. INSURED'S OR AUTHORIZED PERSON'S SIGNATURE I authorize payment of medical benefits to the undersigned physician or supplier for services described below.

SIGNED

PATIENT AND INSURED INFORMATION

14. DATE OF CURRENT: MM DD YY 10 09 2008 ◀ ILLNESS (First symptom) OR INJURY (Accident) OR PREGNANCY(LMP)

15. IF PATIENT HAS HAD SAME OR SIMILAR ILLNESS. GIVE FIRST DATE MM DD YY

16. DATES PATIENT UNABLE TO WORK IN CURRENT OCCUPATION FROM MM DD YY TO MM DD YY

17. NAME OF REFERRING PHYSICIAN OR OTHER SOURCE

17a.

17b. NPI

18. HOSPITALIZATION DATES RELATED TO CURRENT SERVICES FROM MM DD YY TO MM DD YY

19. RESERVED FOR LOCAL USE

20. OUTSIDE LAB? [ ] YES [X] NO $ CHARGES

21. DIAGNOSIS OR NATURE OF ILLNESS OR INJURY. (Relate Items 1,2,3 or 4 to Item 24e by Line)

1. 782 . 4 — Diagnosis code

2. ___ . ___

3. ___ . ___

4. ___ . ___

22. MEDICAID RESUBMISSION CODE ORIGINAL REF. NO.

23. PRIOR AUTHORIZATION NUMBER

	24. A. DATE(S) OF SERVICE From MM DD YY	To MM DD YY	B. PLACE OF SERVICE	C. EMG	D. PROCEDURES, SERVICES, OR SUPPLIES (Explain Unusual Circumstances) CPT/HCPCS MODIFIER	E. DIAGNOSIS POINTER	F. $ CHARGES	G. DAYS OR UNITS	H. EPSDT Family Plan	I. ID. QUAL.	J. RENDERING PROVIDER ID. #
1	10 09 2008	10 09 2008	11		99212 — Procedure	1	97 00	1		NPI	
2					Linkage					NPI	
3										NPI	
4										NPI	
5										NPI	
6										NPI	

25. FEDERAL TAX I.D. NUMBER: 16 1234567 SSN [ ] EIN [X]

26. PATIENT'S ACCOUNT NO.: HUANGER0

27. ACCEPT ASSIGNMENT? (For govt. claims, see back) [X] YES [ ] NO

28. TOTAL CHARGE: $ 97 00

29. AMOUNT PAID: $ 0 00

30. BALANCE DUE: $

31. SIGNATURE OF PHYSICIAN OR SUPPLIER INCLUDING DEGREES OR CREDENTIALS (I certify that the statements on the reverse apply to this bill and are made a part thereof.)

SIGNATURE ON FILE

SIGNED DATE

32. SERVICE FACILITY LOCATION INFORMATION: SAME

a. NPI b.

33. BILLING PROVIDER INFO & PHONE # ( )
CHRISTOPHER CONNOLLY MD
1400 WEST CENTER ST
TOLEDO OH 43601

a. NPI 1286927799 b.

PHYSICIAN OR SUPPLIER INFORMATION

NUCC Instruction Manual available at: www.nucc.org

FIGURE 7.1 Example of a Correct Health Care Claim Showing the Linkage Between the Diagnosis and the Billed Service

In this chapter, basic claim compliance is discussed. Chapters 9 through 13 cover the specific rules for these types of payers:

- Chapter 9 Private Payers/Blue Cross and Blue Shield
- Chapter 10 Medicare
- Chapter 11 Medicaid
- Chapter 12 TRICARE and CHAMPVA
- Chapter 13 Workers' Compensation and Disability

Medicare Regulations: The Correct Coding Initiative

The rules from the Centers for Medicare and Medicaid Services (CMS) about billing Medicare are published in the Federal Register and in CMS manuals such as the Medicare Carriers Manual and Coverage Issues Manual (see Chapter 6 and the CMS website). Especially important for billing is Medicare's national policy on correct coding, the Medicare National **Correct Coding Initiative (CCI).** CCI controls improper coding that would lead to inappropriate payment for Medicare claims. It has coding policies that are based on:

- Coding conventions in CPT
- Medicare's national and local coverage and payment policies
- National medical societies' coding guidelines
- Medicare's analysis of standard medical and surgical practice

Correct Coding Initiative Updates

http://www.cms.hhs.gov/physicians/cciedits/

CCI, updated every quarter, has many thousands of CPT code combinations called CCI **edits** that are used by computers in the Medicare system to check claims. The CCI edits are available on a CMS website, as shown in Figure 7.2 on page 208. CCI edits apply to claims that bill for more than one procedure performed on the same patient (Medicare beneficiary), on the same date of service, by the same performing provider. Claims are denied when codes reported together do not "pass" an edit.

Complete CCI Files: Medicare Claims Processing Manual (Publication 100-04), Chapter 23, Section 20.9

http://www.cms.hhs.gov/manuals/iom

CCI prevents billing two procedures that, according to Medicare, could not possibly have been performed together. Here are examples:

- Reporting the removal of an organ both through an open incision and with laparoscopy
- Reporting female- and male-specific codes for the same patient

CCI edits also test for unbundling. A claim should report a bundled procedure code instead of multiple codes that describe parts of the complete procedure. For example, since a single code is available to describe removal of the uterus, ovaries, and fallopian tubes, physicians should not use separate codes to report the removal of the uterus, ovaries, and fallopian tubes individually.

CCI requires physicians to report only the more extensive version of the procedure performed and disallows reporting of both extensive and limited procedures. For example, only a deep biopsy should be reported if both a deep biopsy and a superficial biopsy are performed at the same location.

Organization of the CCI Edits

CCI edits are organized into the following categories:

- Column 1/column 2 code pair edits
- Mutually exclusive code edits
- Modifier indicators

Column 1/Column 2 Code Pairs In the **CCI column 1/column 2 code pair edits**, two columns of codes are listed. Most often, the edit is based on one code being a component of the other. This means that the column 1 code includes all the services described by the column 2 code(s), so the column 2 code(s) cannot be billed together with the column 1 code for the same patient on the same day of service. Medicare pays for the column 1 code only; the column 2 code(s) are considered bundled into the column 1 code.

EXAMPLE:

Column 1	*Column 2*
27370	20610, 76000, 76003

Column1/Column 2 Edits

Column 1	Column 2	* = In existence prior to 1996	Effective Date	Deletion Date *=no data	Modifier 0=not allowed 1=allowed 9=not applicable
10021	19290		20020101	*	1
10021	36000		20021001	*	1
10021	36410		20021001	*	1
10021	37202		20021001	*	1
10021	62318		20021001	*	1
10021	62319		20021001	*	1
10021	64415		20021001	*	1
10021	64416		20030101	*	1
10021	64417		20021001	*	1
10021	64450		20021001	*	1
10021	64470		20021001	*	1
10021	64475		20021001	*	1
10021	76000		20030701	*	1
10021	76003		20030101	*	1
10021	76360		20030101	*	1
10021	76393		20030101	*	1
10021	76942		20030101	*	1

Mutually Exclusive Edits

Column 1	Column 2	* = In existence prior to 1996	Effective Date	Deletion Date *=no data	Modifier 0=not allowed 1=allowed 9=not applicable
11010	21240		19980101	*	1
11010	21242		19980101	*	1
11010	21243		19980101	*	1
11010	21244		19980101	*	1
11010	21245		19980101	*	1
11010	21246		19980101	*	1
11010	21247		19980101	*	1
11010	21248		19980101	*	1
11010	21249		19980101	*	1
11010	21255		19980101	*	1
11010	21256		19980101	*	1
11010	21260		19980101	*	1
11010	21261		19980101	*	1
11010	21263		19980101	*	1
11010	21267		19980101	*	1
11010	21268		19980101	*	1
11010	21270		19980101	*	1

FIGURE 7.2 Example of Medicare CCI Edits: Column 1/Column 2 Edits and Mutually Exclusive Edits

If 27370 is billed, neither 20610, 76000, nor 76003 should be billed with it, because the payment for each of these codes is already included in the column 1 code.

Mutually Exclusive Code Edits **CCI mutually exclusive code (MEC) edits** also list codes in two columns. According to CMS regulations, both services represented by these codes could not have reasonably been done during a single patient encounter, so they cannot be billed together. If the provider reports both codes from both columns for a patient on the same day, Medicare pays only the lower-paid code.

EXAMPLE

Column 1	*Column 2*
50021	49061, 50020

This means that a biller cannot report either 49061 or 50020 when reporting 50021.

Modifier Indicators In CPT coding, modifiers show particular circumstances related to a code on a claim. The **CCI modifier indicators** control modifier use to "break," or avoid, CCI edits. CCI modifier indicators appear next to items in both the CCI column 1/column 2 code pair list and the mutually exclusive code list. A CCI modifier indicator of 1 means that a CPT modifier *may* be used to bypass an edit (if the circumstances are appropriate). A CCI modifier indicator of 0 means that use of a CPT modifier will not change the edit, so the column 2 codes or mutually exclusive code edits will not be bypassed.

EXAMPLE
Flu vaccine code 90656 includes bundled flu vaccine codes 90655 and 90657–90660. It has a CCI indicator of 0. No modifier will be effective in bypassing these edits, so in every case only CPT 90656 will be paid.

Billing Tip

Resubmit Claims with Modifier Indicator of 9
If the CCI modifier indicator 9 appears on a claim denial, this means that the original edit was a mistake and is being withdrawn; resubmit it for payment if appropriate.

Other Government Regulations

Other government billing regulations are issued by the Office of Inspector General (OIG; see Chapter 2). Annually, as part of a Medicare Fraud and Abuse Initiative, the OIG announces the **OIG Work Plan** for the coming year. The Work Plan lists projects for sampling particular types of billing to determine whether there are problems. Practices study these initiatives and make sure their procedures comply with billing regulations. When regulations seem contradictory or unclear, the OIG issues **advisory opinions** on its OIG website. These opinions are legal advice only for the requesting parties, who, if they act according to the advice, cannot be investigated on the matter. However, they are good general guidelines for all practices to follow to avoid fraud and abuse.

The OIG website also has:

- Audit reports that summarize OIG findings after problems are investigated.
- The List of Excluded Individuals/Entities (LEIE), a database that provides information about **excluded parties**, as shown in Figure 7.3. If employees, physicians, or contractors have been found guilty of fraud, they may be

Billing Tip

Software for CCI Edits
Many vendors sell computer programs to check claims against the CCI edits before submitting them to Medicare. For example, one program identifies any mutually exclusive or column 1/column 2 codes and also indicates whether a modifier is required for payment.

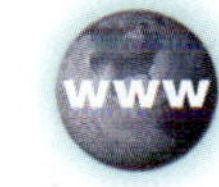

OIG Home Page
http://oig.hhs.gov

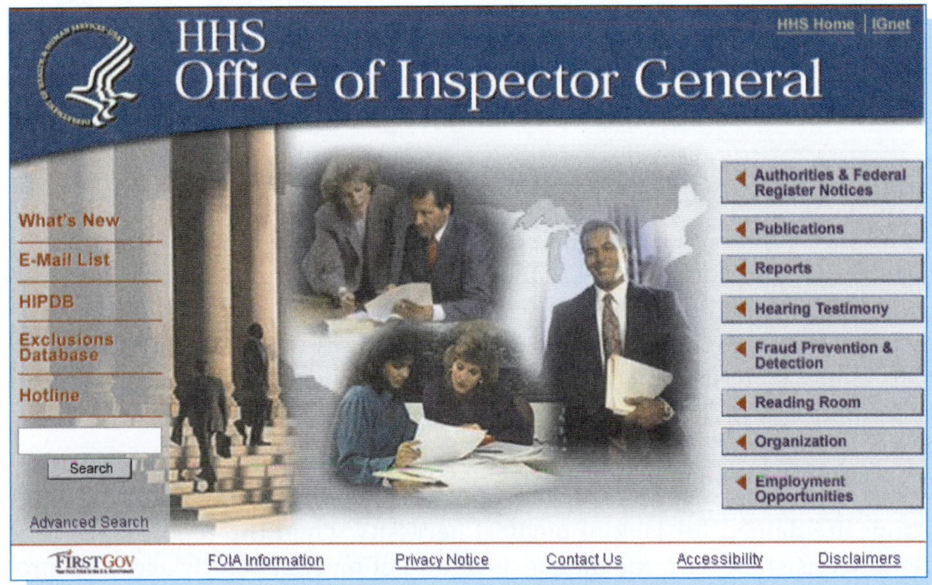

FIGURE 7.3 OIG Excluded Parties Website Home Page

Thinking it Through — 7.1

1. What type of code edit could be used for the following rule?

   Medicare Part B covers a screening Pap smear for women for the early detection of cervical cancer but will not pay for an E/M service for the patient on the same day.

2. An OIG fraud project found that during one month in a single state, there were 23,000 billings for an E/M service with the modifier –25 reported with one of these CPT-4 codes: 11055, 11056, 11057, and 11719, and with HCPCS code G0127 (trimming of dystrophic nails).

Look up the descriptors for the CPT codes. Do you think the procedures appear to be simple or complicated?

___

Why do you think that this billing combination continues to be under scrutiny by CMS?

___

excluded from work for government programs, and their names appear on the LEIE. An OIG exclusion has national scope and is important because knowingly hiring excluded people or companies is illegal.

Private Payer Regulations

CCI edits apply to Medicare claims only. Private payers, however, develop code edits similar to the CCI. Although private payers give information about payment policies in their contracts, handbooks, and bulletins, the exact code edits may not be released. At times, their claim-editing software does not follow CPT guidelines and bundles distinct procedures or does not accept properly used modifiers. In such cases, medical insurance specialists must follow up with the payer for clarification and possible appeal of denied claims (see Chapters 9 and 14).

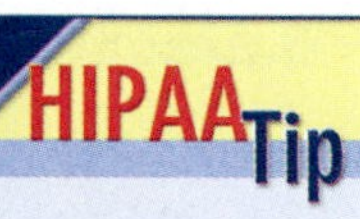

PHI and the Minimum Necessary Standard

PHI from the patient's medical record must be available for the payer to review if it is requested. Be sure to release only the minimum necessary information to answer the payer's questions.

Compliance Errors

Health care payers often base their decisions to pay or deny claims only on the diagnosis and procedure codes. The integrity of the request for payment rests on the accuracy and honesty of the coding and billing. Incorrect work may simply be an error, or it may represent a deliberate effort to obtain fraudulent payment. Some compliance errors are related to medical necessity; others are a result of incorrect code selection or billing practices.

Errors Relating to Code Linkage and Medical Necessity

Claims are denied for lack of medical necessity when the reported services are not consistent with the diagnosis or do not meet generally accepted professional medical standards of care. Each payer has its own list of medical necessity edits. In general, codes that support medical necessity meet these conditions:

- The CPT procedure codes match the ICD-9-CM diagnosis codes.

  EXAMPLE

  A procedure to drain an abscess of the external ear or auditory canal should be supported by a diagnosis of disorders of the external ear or an ear carbuncle or cyst.

- The procedures are not elective, experimental, or nonessential.

  EXAMPLE

  Cosmetic nasal surgery performed to improve a patient's appearance is typically excluded. However, a cosmetic procedure may be considered medically necessary when it is performed to repair an accidental injury or to improve the functioning of a malformed body member. A diagnosis of deviated septum, nasal obstruction, acquired facial deformity, or late effects of facial bone fracture supports medical necessity for cosmetic nasal surgery.

- The procedures are furnished at an appropriate level.

  EXAMPLE

  A high-level Evaluation and Management code for an office visit (such as 99204/99205 and 99214/99215) must be matched by a serious, complex condition such as a sudden, unexplained large loss of weight.

Errors Relating to the Coding Process

These coding problems may cause rejected claims:

- **Truncated coding**—using diagnosis codes that are not as specific as possible
- Mismatch between the gender or age of the patient and the selected code when the code involves selection for either criterion
- **Assumption coding**—reporting items or services that are not actually documented, but that the coder assumes were performed
- Altering documentation after services are reported
- Coding without proper documentation
- Reporting services provided by unlicensed or unqualified clinical personnel
- Coding a unilateral service twice instead of choosing the bilateral code
- Not satisfying the conditions of coverage for a particular service, such as the physician's direct supervision of a radiologist's work

Errors Relating to the Billing Process

A number of errors are related to the billing process. These are the most frequent errors:

- Billing noncovered services
- Billing overlimit services
- Unbundling
- Using an inappropriate modifier or no modifier when one is required
- Always assigning the same level of E/M service
- Billing a consultation instead of an office visit
- Billing invalid/outdated codes
- Either **upcoding**—using a procedure code that provides a higher reimbursement rate than the correct code—or **downcoding**—using a lower level code. Some physicians downcode to be "safe," especially E/M codes.
- Billing without proper signatures on file

Billing Tip

Query Physicians About Unspecified Diagnosis Codes

Unspecified diagnosis codes (often those that end in 0 or 9) indicate that a particular body site was not documented and are usually rejected by payers as being too vague to support medical necessity.

Billing Tip

Teamwork

When medical coding and billing are handled by separate departments or employees, they must work as a team to prepare correct claims. The medical insurance specialist contributes knowledge of the items that must be present for payment, and the medical coder presents the codes that are supported by the documentation.

Compliance Guideline

Fraudulent Code Changes

It is fraudulent to change a code for reimbursement purposes. Only the codes that are supported by the documentation, regardless of payer policy, should be reported.

Strategies for Compliance

Sending claims that generate payment at the highest appropriate level is a critical goal, but regulations can be unclear or can even conflict with each other. Compliant billing can be a difficult and complex assignment; the strategies discussed in this section are helpful.

Carefully Define Bundled Codes and Know Global Periods

To avoid unbundling, coders and medical insurance specialists must be clear on what individual procedures are contained in bundled codes and what the global periods are for surgical procedures (see Chapter 5). Many practices use Medicare's CCI list of bundling rules and global periods for deciding what is included in a procedure code; they inform their other payers that they are following this system of edits. If the payer has a unique set of edits, coders and billers need to have access to it.

Benchmark the Practice's E/M Codes with National Averages

Comparing the evaluation and management codes that the practice reports with national averages is a good way to monitor upcoding. Medical coding consulting firms as well as CMS and other payers have computer programs to profile average billing patterns for various types of codes. For example, reporting only the top two of a five-level E/M code range for new or established patient office visits would not fit a normal pattern and might appear fraudulent.

Use Modifiers Appropriately

CPT modifiers can eliminate any impression of duplicate billing or unbundling. Modifiers –25, –59, and –91 are especially important for compliant billing.

Modifier –25 : Significant, Separately Identifiable Evaluation and Management (E/M) Service by the Same Physician on the Same Day of the Procedure or Other Service

When a procedure is performed, the patient's condition may require the physician to perform an evaluation and management (E/M) service above and beyond the usual pre- and postoperative care associated with that procedure. In this case, modifier –25 is appended to the evaluation and management (E/M) code reported with the procedure code. The modifier –25 says that this was a significant, clearly separate E/M service by the same physician on the same day as the procedure. Note that a different diagnosis does not have to be involved.

EXAMPLE

An established patient is seen in a physician's office for a cough, runny nose, and sore throat that started five days ago. During examination, the patient also reports right and left earaches. The physician performs an expanded problem-focused history and examination with a medical decision making of low complexity. The physician also examines the patient's ear and performs earwax removal from the left and right ears. The patient is discharged home on antibiotics with the following diagnoses and procedures: common cold, impacted cerumen, and removal of impacted cerumen.

CPT codes on the claim are 99213–25 (covers office visit portion) and 69210 (covers removal of impacted cerumen).

Modifier –59: Distinct Procedural Service

Modifier –59 is used to indicate a procedure that was distinct or independent from other services performed on the same day. This may represent a different session or patient encounter, different procedure or surgery, different site or organ system, separate incision/excision, or separate injury (or area of injury in extensive injuries).

EXAMPLE

A physician performs a simple repair (2.5 centimeters in size) of a superficial wound to the right arm and also performs a partial thickness skin debridement of another site on the same arm.

CPT codes on the claim are 12001 (covers the repair of the superficial wound) and 11040–59 (covers skin debridement).

Modifier –91: Repeat Clinical Laboratory Test

Modifier –91 should be appended to a laboratory procedure or service to indicate a repeat test or procedure performed on the same day for patient management purposes. This modifier indicates that the physician or provider had to perform a repeat clinical diagnostic laboratory test that was distinct or separate from a lab panel or other lab services performed on the same day and that it was performed to obtain medically necessary subsequent reportable test values. This modifier should not be used to report repeat laboratory testing due to laboratory errors, quality control, or confirmation of results.

EXAMPLE

A patient undergoing chemotherapy for lung carcinoma has a CBC with automated platelet count performed prior to receiving chemotherapy. The patient has a very low platelet count and receives a platelet transfusion. The automated platelet count is repeated after the transfusion to determine that the platelet count is high enough for the patient to be sent home.

CPT codes on the claim are 85027 (covers automated CBC with automated platelet count) and 85049–91 (covers repeat automated platelet count).

In general, clarify coding and billing questions with physicians, and be sure that the physician adds any needed clarification to the documentation. Use the information from claims that are denied or paid at a lesser rate to modify procedures as needed.

Be Clear on Professional Courtesy and Discounts to Uninsured/Low-Income Patients

Professional Courtesy

Professional courtesy means that a physician has chosen to waive (not collect) the charges for services to other physicians and their families. Although this has been common practice in the past, many federal and state laws now prohibit professional courtesy. The routine waiver of deductibles and copays is unlawful because it results in false claims and violates antikickback rules.

Many physician practices study the OIG's *Compliance Program Guidance for Individual and Small Group Physician Practices* (see Chapter 2) and then consult with an attorney to clarify their professional courtesy arrangements. The resulting guidelines should be explained to the administrative staff in the practice's billing policies and procedures.

Billing Tips

Professional Courtesy

- Medicare and most private payers do not permit a physician to bill for the treatment of immediate family or household members.
- If professional courtesy *is* extended to a patient, no one is billed—neither the person receiving it nor the insurance carrier.

Billing Tip

Professional Courtesy and Other Discounts
Be aware of the practice's guidelines on professional courtesy and on discounts for uninsured/low-income patients for correct billing.

Billing Tip

Check the Documentation
Check the documentation to uncover billing information for frequently billed services. For example, if immunizations are often billed, make it standard procedure to research the quantity of the vaccine administered for correct billing.

Compliance Guideline

Compliant Tools
Encounter forms, job reference aids, and documentation templates should never link diagnoses and procedures. This could give the appearance of basing coding on reimbursement rather than on the patient's condition.

Discounts to Uninsured and Low-Income Patients

Many physician practices consider ability to pay when they bill patients. Under OIG guidelines, physicians may offer discounts to their uninsured and low-income patients. The practice's method for selecting people to receive discounts should be documented in the compliance plan and in its policies and procedures information.

Maintain Compliant Job Reference Aids and Documentation Templates

Many medical practices develop **job reference aids**, also known as cheat sheets, to help in the billing and coding process. These aids usually list the procedures and CPT codes that are most frequently billed by the practice. Some also list frequently used diagnoses with ICD codes.

Job reference aids can help select correct codes, but their use may also lead to questions about compliance. Are codes assigned by selecting those on the aid that are close to patients' conditions rather than by researching precise codes based on the documentation?

If these aids are used, these guidelines should be followed:

- Job reference aids should be dated, to be sure that current codes are in use, and reissued every year with updated codes.
- The job reference aid for CPT E/M codes must contain all the codes in a range. For example, if the E/M office visit codes are included, all ten codes should be listed (five levels each for both new and established patients).
- An aid for ICD-9-CM codes should be presented in one of two ways: (1) The aid should have only the ICD categories (three-digit numbers) to speed the code selection process, and the manual should be reviewed for the proper usage and highest degree of specificity. (2) If three-, four-, and five-digit codes are listed, the complete range should be shown, not one or two codes from the group. For example, if heartburn is to be listed, the complete range of symptoms involving the digestive system (787.0–787.99) should be shown, with the correct level of specificity shown as well.

Thinking it Through — 7.2

1. Medical necessity must be shown for emergency department visits for physicians' patients. If a four-year-old wakes at 3 A.M. with an earache and a temperature of 103°, in what order should the following diagnosis codes be listed to show the urgent reason for an emergency department visit with the child's pediatrician: 381.00, 780.6, 388.71?
2. The following diagnosis and procedure codes were rejected for payment. What is the probable reason for the payer's decision in each case?

   A. 881.1

   B. V50.3, 69090

   C. 054.79, 69145

   D. V70.0, 80050, 80053

Many practices also list CPT and ICD-9-CM codes on the office's encounter form. In some cases, these are the only codes listed; in others, these standard codes are shown next to the accounting codes the practice uses. Encounter forms, like job reference aids, must not preselect from various codes in a range. Instead, all the code possibilities should be listed so that it is clear that all have been considered before the code is checked on the encounter form.

Some physician practices have paper or electronic forms called **documentation templates** to assist physicians as they document examinations (see Chapter 2). The template prompts the physician to document the review of systems (ROS) that was done and to note medical necessity. Like other forms used in medical coding, these templates must be compliant and must clearly record the work done.

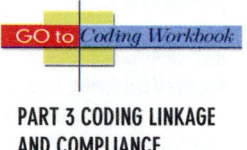

PART 3 CODING LINKAGE AND COMPLIANCE

Audits

Monitoring the coding and billing process for compliance is done either by the practice's compliance officer or by a staff member who is knowledgeable about coding and compliance regulations. The responsible person establishes a system for monitoring the process and performing regular compliance checks to ensure adherence to established policies and procedures.

An important compliance activity involves audits. An **audit** is a formal examination or review. An income tax audit is performed to find out if a person's or a firm's income or expenses were misreported. Similarly, compliance audits judge whether the practice's physicians and coding and billing staff comply with regulations for correct coding and billing.

An audit does not involve reviewing every claim and document. Instead, a representative sample of the whole is studied to reveal whether erroneous or fraudulent behavior exists. For instance, an auditor might make a random selection, such as a percentage of the claims for a particular date, or a targeted selection, such as all claims in a period that have a certain procedure code. If the auditor finds indications of a problem in the sample, more documents and more details are usually reviewed.

External Audits

In an **external audit**, private payers' or government investigators review selected records of a practice for compliance. Coding linkage, completeness of documentation, and adherence to documentation standards, such as the signing and dating of entries by the responsible health care professional, may all be studied. The accounting records are often reviewed as well.

Payers use computer programs of code edits to review claims before they are processed. This process is referred to as a prepayment audit. For example, the Medicare program performs computer checks before processing claims. Some prepayment audits check only to verify that documentation of the visit is on file, rather than investigating the details of the coding.

Audits conducted after payment has been made are called postpayment audits. Most payers conduct routine postpayment audits of physicians' practices to ensure that claims correctly reflect performed services, that services are billed accurately, and that the physicians and other health care providers who participate in the plan comply with the provisions of their contracts.

In a routine private-payer audit, the payer's auditor usually makes an appointment in advance and may conduct the review either in the practice's office or by taking copies of documents back to the payer's office. Often, the auditor requests

Compliance Guideline

Why Code Correctly?
According to a compliance officer who oversees physicians in three different hospitals and multiple practice sites in Northern California, correct coding is "good business practice, the most efficient and effective way to process a claim through successful payment, and reduces audit liability." [Available at HCPro's e-newsletter, Just Coding: http://www.justcoding.com/premium/content.cfm?content_id=51610}

Compliance Guideline

Importance of Documentation
According to CMS, E/M codes are the most frequently audited, because of continual findings of poor documentation. Some physicians even use lower codes than warranted to avoid an audit, but often their documentation does not justify even the lower code levels, so their actions reduce legitimate revenue and still do not protect them from investigation.

the complete medical records of selected plan members for a specified period. The claims information and documentation might include all office and progress notes, laboratory test results, referrals, X-rays, patient sign-in sheets, appointment books, and billing records. When problems are found, the investigation proceeds farther and may result in charges of fraud or abuse against the practice.

Internal Audits

To reduce the chance of an investigation or an external audit and to reduce potential liability when one occurs, most practices' compliance plans require **internal audits** to be conducted regularly by the medical practice staff or by a hired consultant. These audits are routine and are performed periodically without a reason to think that a compliance problem exists. They help the practice determine whether coding is being done appropriately and whether all performed services are being reported for maximum revenue. The goal is to uncover problems so that they can be corrected. They also help:

- Determine whether new procedures or treatments are correctly coded and documented
- Analyze the skills and knowledge of the personnel assigned to handle medical coding in the practice
- Locate areas where training or additional review of practice guidelines is needed
- Improve communications among the staff members involved with claims processing—medical coders, medical insurance specialists, and physicians

Internal audits are done either prospectively or retrospectively. A **prospective audit** (also called a concurrent audit), like a prepayment audit, is done before the claims are sent. Some practices audit a percentage of claims each day. Others audit claims for new or very complex procedures. These audits reduce the number of rejected or downcoded claims by verifying compliance before billing.

Retrospective audits are conducted after the claims have been sent and the remittance advice (RA) has been received. Auditing at this point in the process has two advantages: (1) The complete record, including the RA, is available, so the auditor knows which codes have been rejected or downcoded, and (2) there are usually more claims to sample. Retrospective audits are helpful in analyzing the explanations of rejected or reduced charges and making changes to the coding approach if needed.

Auditing Tools to Verify E/M Code Selection

As explained in Chapter 5, the key components for selecting evaluation and management codes are the extent of the history documented, the extent of the examination documented, and the complexity of the medical decision making. The 1995 and the 1997 versions of the CMS/AMA Documentation Guidelines for Evaluation and Management Services reduce the amount of subjectivity in making judgments about E/M codes, such as one person's opinion of what makes an examination extended. They do this by describing the specific items that may be documented for each of the three key E/M components. They also explain how many items are needed to place the E/M service at the appropriate level.

The documentation guidelines have precise number counts of these items, and these counts can be used to audit as well as to initially code services. The audit double-checks the selected code based on the documentation in the patient medical record. The auditor looks at the record and, usually using an auditing tool such as that shown in Figure 7.4, independently analyzes the

HISTORY

HPI (history of present illness) ❑ Location ❑ Severity ❑ Timing ❑ Modifying factors ❑ Quality ❑ Duration ❑ Context ❑ Associated signs and symptoms	Brief *1-3 elements*	Brief	Extended *≥ 4 elements or status of ≥ 3 chronic or inactive conditions*	Extended
ROS (review of systems) ❑ Constitutional (wt loss, etc) ❑ Ears, nose, mouth, throat ❑ GI ❑ GU ❑ Integumentary (skin, breast) ❑ Endo ❑ Hem/lymph ❑ Eyes ❑ Card/vasc ❑ Resp ❑ Musculo ❑ Neuro ❑ Psych ❑ All/imm ❑ "All others negative"	None	Pertinent to problem *1 system*	Extended *2-9 systems*	Complete *≥ 10 systems, or some systems with statement "all others negative"*
PFSH (past family and social history) ❑ Past medical history ❑ Family history ❑ Social history — Established/ Subsequent	None	None	One history area	Two or three history areas
No PFSH required: 99231-33, 99261-63, 99311-33 — New/Initial	None	None	One or two history area(s)	Three history areas
Circle the entry farthest to the right for each history area. To determine history level, draw a line down the column with the circle farthest to the left.	**PROBLEM FOCUSED**	**EXP. PROB. FOCUSED**	**DETAILED**	**COMPRE-HENSIVE**

EXAM

General Multi-system Exam		Single Organ System Exam
1-5 elements	PROBLEM FOCUSED	1-5 elements
≥6 elements	EXPANDED PROBLEM FOCUSED	≥6 elements
≥ 2 elements from 6 areas/systems OR ≥12 elements from at least 2 areas/systems	DETAILED	≥ 12 elements EXCEPT ≥9 elements for eye and psychiatric exams
≥2 elements from 9 areas/systems	COMPREHENSIVE	Perform and document all elements

COMPLEXITY

A

Number of Diagnoses or Treatment Options

Problems to Exam Physician	Number	X Points	= Result
Self-limited or minor (stable, improved or worsening)	Max = 2	1	
Est. problem (to examiner); stable, improved		1	
Est. problem (to examiner); worsening		2	
New problem (to examiner); no additional workup planned	Max = 1	3	
New prob. (to examiner); add. workup planned		4	
		TOTAL	

Bring total to line A in final Result for Complexity

B

Amount and/or Complexity of Data to Be Reviewed

Data to Be Reviewed	Points
Review and/or order of clinical lab tests	1
Review and/or order of tests in the radiology section of CPT	1
Review and/or order tests in the medicine section of CPT	1
Discussion of test results with performing physician	1
Decision to obtain old records and/or obtain history from someone other than patient	1
Review and summarization of old records and/or obtaining history from someone other than patient and/or discussion of case with another health care provider	2
Independent visualization of image, tracing or specimen itself (not simply review of report)	2
TOTAL	

Bring total to line B in final Result for Complexity

Draw a line down the column with 2 or 3 circles and circle decision making level OR Draw a line down the column with the center circle and circle the decision making level.

A	Number diagnoses or treatment options	≤1 Minimal	2 Limited	3 Multiple	≥4 Extensive
B	Amount and complexity of data	≤1 Minimal or low	2 Limited	3 Moderate	≥4 Extensive
C	Highest risk	Minimal	Low	Moderate	High
	Type of decision making	STRAIGHT-FORWARD	LOW COMPLEX.	MODERATE COMPLEX.	HIGH COMPLEX.

C

Risk of Complications and/or Morbidity or Mortality

Level of risk	Presenting Problem(s)	Diagnostic Procedure(s) Ordered	Management-Options Selected
MINIMAL	• One self-limited or minor problem, *e.g. cold, insect bite, tinea corporis*	• Laboratory tests requiring venipuncture • Chest xrays • EKG/EEG • Urinalysis • Ultrasound • KOH prep	• Rest • Gargles • Elastic bandages • Superficial dressings
LOW	• Two or more self-limited or minor problems • One stable chronic illness (*well-controlled hypertension or non-insulin dependent diabetes, cataract, BPH*) • Acute uncomplicated illness or injury (cystitis, allergic rhinitis, simple sprain)	• Physiological tests not under stress, *e.g. PFT* • Noncardiovascular imaging studies with contrast (*barium enema*) • Superficial needle biopsies • Clinical lab tests requiring arterial puncture • Skin biopsies	• Over-the-counter drugs • Minor surgery w/no identified risk factors • Physical therapy • Occupational therapy • IV fluids without additives
MODERATE	• One or more chronic illnesses with mild exacerbation, progression or side effects of tx • Two or more stable chronic illnesses • Undiagnosed new problem with uncertain prognosis (*breast lump*) • Acute illness with systemic symptoms (*pyelonephritis, pneumonia, colitis*) • Acute complicated injury (*head injury with brief loss of consciousness*)	• Physiologic tests under stress (*cardiac stress test, fetal contraction test*) • Diagnostic endoscopies with no identified risk factors • Deep needle or incisional bx • Cardiovascular imaging studies w/contrast and no identified risk factors (*arteriogram, cardiac cath*) • Obtain fluid from body cavity (*lumbar puncture, thoracentesis, culdocentesis*)	• Minor surgery with identified risk factors • Elective major surgery (open, percutaneous or endoscopic) with no identified risk factors • Prescription drug management • Therapeutic nuclear medicine • IV fluids w/additives • Closed tx of fracture or dislocation without manipulation
HIGH	• One or more chronic illnesses with severe exacerbation, progression or side effects of tx • Acute or chronic illnesses or injuries that may pose a threat to life or bodily function (*multiple trauma, acute MI, pulmonary embolus, severe respiratory distress, progressive severe rheumatoid arthritis, psychiatric illness with potential threat to self or others, peritonitis, acute renal failure*) • A sudden change in neurological status (*seizure, TIA, sensory loss*)	• Cardiovascular imaging studies with contrast with identified risk factors • Cardiac electrophysiological tests • Diagnostic endoscopies w/identified risk factor • Discography	• Elective major surgery (open, percutaneous or endoscopic) with identified risk factor • Emergency major surgery (open, percutaneous or endoscopic) • Parenteral controlled substances • Drug therapy requiring intensive monitoring for toxicity • Decision not to resuscitate or to de-escalate care because of poor prognosis

FIGURE 7.4 Example of Evaluation and Management Code Assignment Audit Form *(continued on next page)*

Transfer the history, exam and medical decision making results to the appropriate chart below and follow the specific instructions for that chart.

LEVEL OF SERVICE

OUTPATIENT, CONSULTS (OUTPATIENT, INPATIENT & CONFIRMATORY) AND ER

	New/Consults/ER					Established				
	If a column has 3 circles, draw a line down the column and circle the code OR find the column with the circle farthest to the left, draw a line down the column and circle the code.					If a column has 2 or 3 circles, draw a line down the column and circle the code OR draw a line down the column with the center circle and circle the code.				
History	PF	EPF	D ER: EPF	C ER: D	C	*Minimal problem that may*	PF	EPF	D	C
Examination	PF	EPF	D ER: EPF	C ER: D	C	*not require presence*	PF	EPF	D	C
Complexity of medical decision	SF	SF ER: L	L ER: M	M	H	*of physician*	SF	L	M	H
	99201 99241 99251 99281	99202 99242 99252 99282	99203 99243 99253 99283	99204 99244 99254 99284	99205 99245 99255 99285	99211	99212	99213	99214	99215

INPATIENT

	Initial Hospital/Observation			Subsequent Inpatient		
	If a column has 3 circles, draw a line down the column and circle the code OR find the column with the circle farthest to the left, draw a line down the column and circle the code.			If a column has 2 or 3 circles, draw a line down the column and circle the code OR draw a line down the column with the center circle and circle the code.		
History	D or C	C	C	PF interval	EPF interval	D interval
Examination	D or C	C	C	PF	EPF	D
Complexity of medical decision	SF/L	M	H	SF/L	M	H
	99221 99218 99234	99222 99219 99235	99223 99220 99236	99231	99232	99233

PF = Problem focused EPF = Expanded problem focused D = Detailed C = Comprehensive
SF = Straightforward L = Low M = Moderate H = High

TIME

If the physician documents total time and suggests that counseling or coordinating care dominates (more than 50%) the encounter, time may determine level of service. Documentation may refer to: prognosis, differential diagnosis, risks, benefits of treatment, instructions, compliance, risk reduction or discussion with another health care provider.

Does documentation reveal total time Time: Face-to-face in outpatient setting / Unit/floor in inpatient setting	❑ Yes	❑ No	If all answers are "yes," may select level based on time.
Does documentation describe the content of counseling or coordinating care	❑ Yes	❑ No	
Does documentation reveal that more than half of time was counseling or coordinating care	❑ Yes	❑ No	

FIGURE 7.4 Example of Evaluation and Management Code Assignment Audit Form *(continued)*

services that are documented. The auditor then compares the code that should be selected with the code that has been reported. When the resulting codes are not the same, the auditor has uncovered a possible problem in interpreting the documentation guidelines.

Many practices use this type of audit tool to help them conduct audits in a standard way. These tools are distributed to physicians and staff members to develop internal audits, not to make initial code selections. An experienced medical insurance specialist may be responsible for using the audit tool to monitor completed claims and to audit selected claims before they are released.

Auditing Example: Is It a Brief or Extended History of the Present Illness?

Selecting the Code

As part of selecting the correct E/M code, the coder (the physician or medical coder) determines the extent of history. The overall history is problem-focused, expanded problem-focused, detailed, or comprehensive. Part of determining this extent is based on the history of present illness (HPI). The HPI may include from none to eight factors in the patient's medical record:

- Location (where on the body the symptom is occurring)
- Quality (the character of the pain)
- Severity (the rank of the symptom or pain on a scale, such as 1 to 10)
- Duration (how long the symptom or pain has been present or how long it lasts when it occurs)
- Timing (when the symptom or pain occurs)
- Context (the situation that is associated with the pain or symptom, such as eating dairy products)
- Modifying factors (things done to make the pain or symptom change, such as using an ice pack for a headache)
- Associated signs and symptoms (other things that happen when this symptom or pain happens, such as "my chest pain makes me feel short of breath")

Depending on the count, the HPI is either brief or extended. A brief HPI has one to three of the elements. An extended HPI has at least four of the eight elements. The coder should make this judgment on the evidence in the patient's medical record, not on recollecting or making assumptions about what was actually done. Remember, if it is not documented, it did not happen.

Auditing the Code Selection

After the coding is done, the auditor examines the patient's medical record and analyzes the documentation. The HPI section at the top of Figure 7.4, which matches the Documentation Guidelines counts for HPI, is as follows:

HPI (history of present illness)				**Brief**	**Extended**
❑ Location	❑ Severity	❑ Timing	❑ Modifying factors	1–3 elements	4–8 elements
❑ Quality	❑ Duration	❑ Context	❑ Associated signs and symptoms		

Using this tool, the auditor checks off the appropriate items for HPI:

Patient's chief complaint: Right shoulder pain

History: The patient noted a sharp pain in the right shoulder about three days ago. The pain is worse when he lies on the arm.

Auditor's analysis: The HPI is extended; four elements are documented, as follows:

Location: Right shoulder

Quality: Sharp pain

Duration: Three days ago

Context: Worse when lies on arm

The auditor follows the form through all its elements to verify the overall selection of the evaluation and management code.

Thinking it Through — 7.3

Refer to Figure 7.4 on page 217 and read the instructions for Outpatient, Consults, and ER at the top and for the established patient section at the right. The instructions state: "If a column has 2 or 3 circles, draw a line down the column . . . and circle the code." In other words, for the established patient, it is not necessary to document the same level for all three components—history, examination, and decision making—to verify the code.

1. **Why is this the case?**
2. **What code is correct for an established patient with a PF (problem-focused) result in the History column, an EPF (expanded problem-focused) result in the Examination column, and a L (low) result in the Complexity of Medical Decision Making column?**

Comparing Physician Fees and Payer Fees

Patients often have questions like "How much will my insurance pay?" "How much will I owe?" "Why are these fees different from my previous doctor's fees?" Medical insurance specialists handle these questions based on their knowledge of the provider's current fees and their estimates of what patients' insurance plans will pay. Both to prepare compliant claims and to estimate what patients will owe, medical insurance specialists must be prepared to answer these key questions:

- What services are covered under the plan? Which services are not covered and therefore cannot be billed to the plan, but rather should be billed to the patient?
- What are the billing rules, fee schedules, and payment methods of the plan?
- In addition to noncovered services, what is the patient responsible for paying?

Sources for Physician Fee Schedules

Physicians establish a list of their **usual fees** for the procedures and services they frequently perform. Usual fees are defined as those that they charge to most of their patients most of the time under typical conditions. There are exceptions to the physician's fee schedule. For example, workers' compensation patients often must be charged according to a state-mandated fee schedule (see Chapter 13).

The typical ranges of physicians' fees nationwide are published in commercial databases. For example, Figure 7.5 shows the fees for a group of CPT codes from the surgical section. The first and second columns list the CPT codes and brief descriptions of the services. The third, fourth, and fifth columns show the following amounts:

- *Column 3:* Half (50 percent) of the reported fees were higher than this fee, and the other half were lower. This is called the *midpoint* of the range.
- *Column 4:* One-quarter (25 percent) of the fees were higher than this fee, and three-quarters (75 percent) were lower.
- *Column 5:* Ten percent of the fees were higher than this fee, and 90 percent were lower.

(1) CODE	(2) SHORT DESCRIPTION	(3) 50TH	(4) 75TH	(5) 90TH	(6) MFS	(7) RVU
APPLICATION OF CASTS AND STRAPPING						
29000	APPLICATION OF BODY CAST. HALO TYPE	478	617	753	151	4.12
29010	APPLY BODY CAST. RISSER JACKET	376	485	591	167	4.56
29015	APPLY BODY/HEAD CAST. RISSER JACKET	439	567	692	179	4.87
29020	APPLY BODY CAST, TURNBUCKLE JACKET	359	463	565	146	3.98
29025	APPLY BODY/HEAD CAST. TURNBUCKLE	384	496	605	113	3.09
29035	APPLY BODY CAST. SHOULDER TO HIPS	255	329	401	143	3.98
29040	APPLY BODY CAST. SHOULDER TO HIPS	339	438	534	160	4.36
29044	APPLY BODY CAST. SHOULDER TO HIPS	299	386	471	160	4.37
29046	APPLY BODY CAST. SHOULDER TO HIPS	324	419	511	176	4.80
29049	APPLY SHOULDER CAST. FIGURE-EIGHT	126	163	199	48	1.30
29055	APPLY SHOULDER CAST. SHOULDER SPICA	239	308	376	110	3.00
29058	APPLY SHOULDER CAST. VELPEAU	150	193	236	71	1.94
29065	APPLICATION OF LONG ARM CAST	122	157	191	63	1.73
29075	APPLICATION OF FOREARM CAST	95	121	147	52	1.42
29085	APPLICATION OF HAND/WRIST CAST	86	111	136	51	1.38
29105	APPLICATION OF LONG ARM SPLINT	82	106	129	51	1.38
29125	APPLY FOREARM SPLINT. STATIC	63	81	99	35	.96
29126	APPLY FOREARM SPLINT. DYNAMIC	109	140	171	43	1.17

FIGURE 7.5 Sample Physician Fee Database

For example, in Figure 7.5, CPT 29085, Application of hand/wrist cast, columns 3, 4, and 5 show the values $86, $111, and $136. This means that half of the reporting providers charged less than $86 for this service, and half charged more. Three-quarters of the reporting providers charged less than $111 for this service, and 25 percent charged more. Ninety percent of the reporting providers charged less than $136, while only 10 percent charged more. (The sixth and seventh columns contain Medicare data, which is discussed in the RBRVS section below. That section also describes reasonable fees.)

How Physician Fees Are Set and Managed

In every geographic area, there is a normal range of fees for commonly performed procedures. Different practices set their fees at some point along this range. They analyze the rates charged by other providers in the area, what government programs pay, and the payments of private carriers to develop their list of fees. Most try to set fees that are in line with patients' expectations so as to be competitive in attracting patients.

> **Billing Tip**
>
> **Setting Fees**
> **Most practices set their fees slightly above those paid by the highest reimbursing plan in which they participate.**

To keep track of whether the practice's fees are correctly set, reports from the practice management program are studied. These reports indicate the most frequently performed services (say, the top twenty procedures) and the providers' fees for them. This list is compared to the amounts that payers pay. If the providers' fees are always paid in full, the fees may be set too low—below payers' maximum allowable charges. If all fees are reduced by payers, the fees may be set too high. When the practice feels that fees are regularly too high or too low, the usual fee structure can be adjusted accordingly.

Medical insurance specialists update the practice's fee schedules when new codes are released. When new or altered CPT codes are among those the practice reports, the fees related to them must be updated, too. For example, if the definition of a surgical package changes, a surgeon's fees need to be altered to

Thinking it Through — 7.4

Based on Figure 7.5 on page 221:

1. Fifty percent of surveyed providers charged less than what amount for CPT 29044?
2. If four thousand providers were surveyed about their charges for CPT 29000, how many reported that they charged more than $617?

tie exactly to the revised elements of the package. Or a new procedure may need to be included. Providers may refer to the national databases or, more likely, review those databases and the Medicare rate of pay to establish the needed new fees.

Payer Fee Schedules

Payers, too, must establish the rates they pay providers. There are two main methods: charge-based and resource-based. **Charge-based fee structures** are based on the fees that providers of similar training and experience have charged for similar services. **Resource-based fee structures** are built by comparing three factors: (1) how difficult it is for the provider to do the procedure, (2) how much office overhead the procedure involves, and (3) the relative risk that the procedure presents to the patient and to the provider.

Usual, Customary, and Reasonable (UCR) Payment Structures

Payers that use a charge-based fee structure also analyze charges using one of the national databases. They create a schedule of **UCR (usual, customary, and reasonable)** fees by determining the percentage of the published fee ranges that they will pay. For example, a payer may decide to pay all surgical procedures reported in a specific geographical area at the midpoint of each range.

These UCR fees, for the most part, accurately reflect prevailing charges. However, fees may not be available for new or rare procedures. Lacking better information, a payer may set too low a fee for such procedures.

Relative Value Scale (RVS)

Another payment structure is called a **relative value scale (RVS).** Historically, the idea behind an RVS was that fees should reflect the relative difficulty of procedures. If most providers agreed that procedure A took more skill, effort, or time than procedure B, procedure A could be expected to have a higher fee than procedure B.

Although it is no longer used, the California Medical Association's *California Relative Value Studies*, published from 1956 to 1974, was the foundation for the RVS approach. Providers were interviewed to determine the amounts they had charged for each procedure. They were also asked how difficult each procedure was and how much risk the procedure presented to the patient and the provider. The results of the interviews were organized into a relative value scale.

In an RVS, each procedure in a group of related procedures is assigned a *relative value* in relation to a *base unit*. For example, if the base unit is 1 and these numbers are assigned—limited visual field examination 0.66; intermediate visual field examination 0.91; and extended visual field examination 1.33—the first two procedures are less difficult than the unit to which they are compared. The third procedure is more difficult. The relative value that is assigned is called the **relative value unit**, or **RVU**.

To calculate the price of each service, the relative value is multiplied by a **conversion factor**, which is a dollar amount that is assigned to the base unit. The conversion factor is increased or decreased each year so that it reflects changes in the cost of living index.

EXAMPLE

The year's conversion factor is $35.27.

The relative value of an extended visual field examination is 1.33.

This year's price for the extended visual field examination is $35.27 × 1.33 = $46.90.

The *California Relative Value Studies* eventually came under federal scrutiny and ceased to be published. It was accused of being a price-fixing book created by providers for providers. Despite the problems with this study, the relative value scale is a useful concept. Unlike providers, software companies and publishers are not restricted from gathering and publishing fee information, so the national fee databases they produce now list both UCR fees and a relative value for each procedure. Payers and providers may use the RVS factor in setting their fees.

Resource-Based Relative Value Scale (RBRVS)

The payment system used by Medicare is called the **resource-based relative value scale (RBRVS).** The RBRVS establishes relative value units for services. It replaces providers' consensus on fees—the historical charges—with a relative value that is based on resources—what each service really costs to provide.

There are three parts to an RBRVS fee:

1. *The nationally uniform RVU:* The relative value is based on three cost elements—the physician's work, the practice cost (overhead), and the cost of malpractice insurance. Another way of stating this is that every $1.00 of charge is made up of *x* cents for the physician's work, *x* cents for office expenses, and *x* cents for malpractice insurance. For example, the relative value for a simple office visit, such as to receive a flu shot, is much lower than the relative value for a complicated encounter such as the evaluation and management of uncontrolled diabetes in a patient. (Column 7 in Figure 7.5 lists the RVUs for procedures in column 1.)
2. *A geographic adjustment factor:* A geographic adjustment factor called the **geographic practice cost index (GPCI)** is a number that is used to multiply each relative value element so that it better reflects a geographical area's relative costs. For example, the cost of the provider's work is affected by average physician salaries in an area. The cost of the practice depends on things such as office rental prices and local taxes. Malpractice expense is also affected by where the work is done. The factor may either reduce or increase the relative values. For example, the GPCI lowers relative values in a rural area, where all costs of living are lower. A GPCI from a major city, where everything costs more, raises the relative values. In some states, a single GPCI applies; in others, different GPCIs are listed for large cities and for other areas.
3. *A nationally uniform conversion factor:* A uniform conversion factor is a dollar amount used to multiply the relative values to produce a payment

amount. It is used by Medicare to make adjustments according to changes in the cost of living index.

Note that when RBRVS fees are used, payments are considerably lower than when UCR fees are used. On average, according to a study done by the Medicare Payment Advisory Commission, a nonpartisan federal advisory panel, private health plans' fees are about 15 percent higher than Medicare fees. (For example, compare columns 3, 4, and 5 with column 6 in Figure 7.5.)

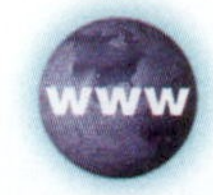

Medicare Fee Schedule

http://www.cms.hhs.gov/PhysicianFeeSched/

Medicare Physician Fee Schedule Updates

Each part of the RBRVS—the relative values, the GPCI, and the conversion factor—is updated each year by CMS. The year's **Medicare Physician Fee Schedule (MPFS)** is published by CMS in the *Federal Register* and is available on the CMS website.

Figure 7.6 shows the formula for calculating a Medicare payment. These steps are followed to apply the formula:

1. Determine the procedure code for the service.
2. Use the Medicare Fee Schedule to find the three RVUs—work, practice expense, and malpractice—for the procedure.
3. Use the Medicare GPCI list to find the three geographic practice cost indices (also for work, practice expense, and malpractice).
4. Multiply each RVU by its GPCI to calculate the adjusted value.
5. Add the three adjusted totals, and multiply the sum by the conversion factor to determine the payment.

Work RVU x Work GPCI = *W*
Practice-Expense RVU x Practice-Expense GPCI = *PE*
Malpractice RVU x Malpractice GPCI = *M*
Conversion Factor = *CF*

(*W* + *PE* + *M*) x *CF* = Payment

Example:

Work RVU = 6.39
Work GPCI = 0.998
6.39 x 0.998 = *W* = 6.37

Practice-Expense RVU = 5.87
Practice-Expense GPCI = 0.45
5.87 x 0.45 = *PE* = 2.64

Malpractice RVU = 1.20
Malpractice GPCI = 0.721
1.20 x 0.721 = *M* = 0.86

Conversion Factor = 34.54

(6.37 + 2.64 + 0.86) x 34.54 = $340.90 Payment

FIGURE 7.6 Medicare Physician Fee Schedule Formula

Thinking it Through — 7.5

Below are sample relative value units and geographic practice cost indices from a Medicare Fee Schedule. The conversion factor for this particular year is $34.7315.

Sample RVUs				
CPT/HCPCS	**Description**	**Work RVU**	**Practice Expense RVU**	**Malpractice Expense RVU**
33500	Repair heart vessel fistula	25.55	30.51	4.07
33502	Coronary artery correction	21.04	15.35	1.96
33503	Coronary artery graft	21.78	26	4.07
99203	OV new detailed	1.34	0.64	0.05
99204	OV new comprehensive	2.00	0.96	0.06

Sample GPCIs			
Locality	**Work GPCI**	**Practice Expense GPCI**	**Malpractice Expense GPCI**
San Francisco, CA	1.067	1.299	0.667
Manhattan, NY	1.093	1.353	1.654
Columbus, OH	0.990	0.939	1.074
Galveston, TX	0.988	0.970	1.386

Calculate the expected payments for:

1. **Office visit, new patient, detailed history/examination, low-complexity decision making, in Manhattan, NY ______**
2. **Coronary artery graft in San Francisco, CA ______**
3. **Repair heart vessel fistula in Columbus, OH ______**
4. **Coronary artery correction in Galveston, TX ______**

Payment Methods

In addition to setting various fee schedules, payers use one of three main methods to pay providers:

1. Allowed charges
2. Contracted fee schedule
3. Capitation

Allowed Charges

Many payers set an **allowed charge** for each procedure or service. This amount is the most the payer will pay any provider for that CPT code. Whether a provider actually receives the allowed charge depends on three things:

1. *The provider's usual charge for the procedure or service:* The usual charge on the physician's fee schedule may be higher than, equal to, or lower than the allowed charge.

2. *The provider's status in the particular plan or program*: The provider is either participating or nonparticipating (see Chapter 3). Participating (PAR) providers agree to accept allowed charges that are lower than their usual fees. In return, they are eligible for incentives, such as quicker payments of their claims and more patients.
3. *The payer's billing rules*: These rules govern whether the provider can bill a patient for the part of the charge that the payer does not cover.

Billing Tip

Allowed Charge: Other Terms
The allowed charge is also called a maximum allowable fee, maximum charge, allowed amount, allowed fee, or allowable charge.

When a payer has an allowed charge method, it never pays more than the allowed charge to a provider. If a provider's usual fee is higher, only the allowed charge is paid. If a provider's usual fee is lower, the payer reimburses that lower amount. The payer's payment is always the lower of the provider's charge or the allowed charge.

EXAMPLE
The payer's allowed charge for a new patient's evaluation and management (E/M) service (CPT 99204) is $160.

Provider A Usual Charge = $180	Payment = $160
Provider B Usual Charge = $140	Payment = $140

Whether a participating provider can bill the patient for the difference between a higher physician fee and a lower allowed charge—called **balance billing**—depends on the terms of the contract with the payer. Payers' rules may prohibit participating providers from balance billing the patient. Instead, the provider must **write off** the difference, meaning that the amount of the difference is subtracted from the patient's bill as an adjustment and never collected.

For example, Medicare-participating providers may not receive an amount greater than the Medicare allowed charge from the Medicare Physician Fee Schedule. Medicare is responsible for paying 80 percent of this allowed charge (after patients have met their annual deductibles; see Chapter 10). Patients are responsible for the other 20 percent.

EXAMPLE
A Medicare PAR provider has a usual charge of $200 for a diagnostic flexible sigmoidoscopy (CPT 45330), and the Medicare allowed charge is $84. The provider must write off the difference between the two amounts. The patient is responsible for 20 percent of the allowed charge, not of the provider's usual charge:

Provider's usual fee	$200.00
Medicare allowed charge	$ 84.00
Medicare pays 80%	$ 67.20
Patient pays 20%	$ 16.80

The total the provider can collect is $84. The provider must make an adjustment to the patient's account to write off the $116 difference between the usual fee and the allowed charge.

A provider who does not participate in a private plan can usually balance bill patients. In this situation, if the provider's usual charge is higher than the allowed charge, the patient must pay the difference. However, Medicare and other government-sponsored programs have different rules for nonparticipating providers, as explained in Chapters 10 through 12.

EXAMPLE
Payer policy: There is an allowed charge for each procedure. The plan provides a benefit of 100 percent of the provider's usual charges up to this maximum fee. Provider A is a participating provider; Provider B does not participate and can

balance bill. Both Provider A and Provider B perform abdominal hysterectomies (CPT 58150). The policy's allowed charge for this procedure is $2,880.

Provider A (PAR)	
Provider's usual charge	$3,100.00
Policy pays its allowed charge	$2,880.00
Provider writes off the difference between the usual charge and the allowed charge:	$ 220.00
Provider B (nonPAR)	
Provider's usual charge	$3,000.00
Policy pays its allowed charge	$2,880.00
Provider bills patient for the difference between the usual charge and the allowed charge; there is no write-off:	$ 120.00 ($3,000.00 – $2,880.00)

Coinsurance provisions in many private plans provide for patient cost-sharing. Rather than paying the provider the full allowed charge, for example, a plan may require the patient to pay 25 percent, while the plan pays 75 percent. In this case, if a provider's usual charges are higher than the plan's allowed charge, the patient owes more for a service from a nonparticipating provider than from a participating provider. The calculations are explained below.

EXAMPLE

Payer policy: A policy provides a benefit of 75 percent of the provider's usual charges, and there is a maximum allowed charge for each procedure. The patient is responsible for 25 percent of the maximum allowed charge. Balance billing is not permitted for plan participants.

Provider A is a participating provider, and Provider B is a nonparticipant in the plan. Provider A and Provider B both perform total abdominal hysterectomies (CPT 58150). The policy's allowed charge for this procedure is $2,880.00.

Provider A (PAR)	
Usual charge	$3,100.00
Policy pays 75% of its allowed charge	$2,160.00 (75% of $2,880.00)
Patient pays 25% of the allowed charge	$ 720.00 (25% of $2,880.00)
Provider writes off the difference between the usual charge and the allowed charge:	$ 220.00
Provider B (nonPAR)	
Usual charge	$3,000.00
Policy pays 75% of its allowed charge	$2,160.00 (75% of $2,880.00)
Patient pays for:	
(1) 25% of the allowed charge +	$ 720.00 (25% of $2,880.00)
(2) the difference between the usual charge and the allowed charge:	$ 120.00 ($3,000.00 – $2,880.00)
Patient pays $840.00 ($720.00 + $120.00)	
The provider has no write-off	

Thinking it Through — 7.6

A Medicare-participating surgeon in Galveston, TX, reports a normal charge of $6,282.00 to repair a heart vessel fistula. Using the Medicare Fee Schedule RVUs and GPCIs shown on page 225, calculate the following:

1 The allowed charge ______________________________

2 The provider's expected write-off______________________

Contracted Fee Schedule

Some payers, particularly those that contract directly with providers, establish fixed fee schedules with participating providers. They first decide what they will pay in particular geographical areas and then offer participation contracts with those fees to physician practices. If the practice chooses to join, it agrees by contract to accept the plan's fees for its member patients.

The plan's contract states the percentage of the charges, if any, its patients owe, and the percentage the payer covers. Participating providers can typically bill patients their usual charges for procedures and services that are not covered by the plan.

Capitation

The fixed prepayment for each plan member in a capitation contract (see Chapter 1), called the **capitation rate** or **cap rate**, is determined by the managed care organization that contracts with providers.

Setting the Cap Rate

To determine the cap rate, the plan first decides on the allowed charges for the contracted services and then analyzes the health-related characteristics of the plan's members. The plan calculates the number of times each age group and gender group of members is likely to use each of the covered services. For example, if the primary care provider (PCP) contract covers obstetrics and a large percentage of the group's members are young women who are likely to require services related to childbirth, the cap rate is higher than for a group of members containing a greater percentage of men or of women in their forties or fifties who are not as likely to require obstetrics services.

The plan's contract with the provider lists the services and procedures that are covered by the cap rate. For example, a typical contract with a primary care provider might include the following services:

Preventive care: well-child care, adult physical exams, gynecological exams, eye exams, and hearing exams

Counseling and telephone calls

Office visits

Medical care: medical care services such as therapeutic injections and immunizations, allergy immunotherapy, electrocardiograms, and pulmonary function tests

Local treatment of first-degree burns, application of dressings, suture removal, excision of small skin lesions, removal of foreign bodies or cerumen from external ear

TABLE 7.1 Example of a Capitation Schedule

Member Profile	Monthly Capitation Rate
0–2 Years, M/F	$30.10
2–4 Years, M/F	$ 8.15
5–19 Years, M/F	$ 7.56
20– 44 Years, M	$ 8.60
20–44 Years, F	$16.66
45–64 Years, M	$17.34
45–64 Years, F	$24.76
Over 65 Years, M, Non-Medicare	$24.22
Over 65 Years, F, Non-Medicare	$27.32
Over 65, M, Medicare Primary	$10.20
Over 65, F, Medicare Primary	$12.05

These services are covered in the per-member charge for each plan member who selects the PCP. This cap rate, usually a prepaid monthly payment (per member per month, or PMPM), may be a different rate for each category of plan member, as shown in Table 7.1, or an average rate. To set an average rate, the monthly capitation rate for each member profile is added, and the total is divided by the number of member profiles.

Noncovered services can be billed to patients using the provider's usual rate. Plans often require the provider to notify the patient in advance that a service is not covered and to state the fee for which the patient will be responsible.

Provider Withholds

Some managed care plans may also require a **provider withhold** from their participating providers. Under this provision of their contract with the provider, the plan withholds a percentage, such as 20 percent, from every payment to the provider. The amount withheld is supposed to be set aside in a fund to cover unanticipated medical expenses of the plan. At the close of a specified period, such as a year, the amount withheld is returned to the provider if the plan's financial goals have been achieved. Some plans pay back withholds depending on the overall goals of the plan, and some pay according to the individual provider's performance against goals.

Thinking it Through — 7.7

1 **In Table 7.1, which category of plan member does the plan consider likely to use the most medical services in a given period? The fewest services?**

2 **If the capitation schedule in Table 7.1 is used to calculate an average payment per patient, what is the average cap rate?**

Review

Steps to Success

- ❐ Read this chapter and review the Key Terms and the Chapter Summary.
- ❐ Answer the Review Questions and Applying Your Knowledge in the Chapter Review.
- ❐ Access the chapter's websites and complete the Internet Activities to learn more about available professional resources.
- ❐ Complete the related chapter in the *Medical Insurance Workbook* to reinforce your understanding of visit charges and compliant billing.

Chapter Summary

1. Diagnoses and procedures must be correctly linked on health care claims because payers analyze this connection to determine the medical necessity of the charges. Correct claims also comply with all applicable regulations and requirements. Codes should be appropriate and documented as well as compliant with each payer's rules.
2. The Medicare National Correct Coding Initiative (CCI) edits are computerized screenings designed to deny claims that do not comply with Medicare's rules on claims for more than one procedure performed on the same patient (Medicare beneficiary), on the same date of service, by the same performing provider. The three types of edits are: (a) column 1/column 2 pair codes, in which the first column's code includes any codes in the second column, which should not be billed separately; (b) mutually exclusive edits, which list code pairs that will not both be paid for the same date of service; and (c) modifier indicators, which note whether the appropriate use of a CPT modifier will allow the claim to bypass the edit.
3. Claims are rejected or downcoded because of (a) medical necessity errors, (b) coding errors, and (c) errors related to billing.
4. Major strategies to ensure compliant billing are to (a) carefully define bundled codes and know global periods, (b) benchmark the practice's E/M codes with national averages, (c) keep up to date through ongoing coding and billing education, (d) be clear on professional courtesy and discounts to uninsured/low-income patients, (e) maintain compliant job reference aids and documentation templates, and (f) audit the billing process.
5. Payer audits are routine external audits that are conducted to ensure practice compliance with coding and billing regulations. Prospective internal audits help the practice reduce the possibility that coding compliance errors will cause claims to be rejected or downcoded. Retrospective internal audits are used to analyze feedback from payers, identify problems, and address problems with additional training and better communication. E/M codes, because they are so frequently used, are an ongoing audit focus. Practices should conduct internal audits of their E/M claims using audit tools based on the joint CMS/AMA Documentation Guidelines for Evaluation and Management Services. This audit process highlights possible problems with the practice's interpretation of the guidelines or documentation approach.
6. Physicians set their fee schedules in relation to the fees that other providers charge for similar services.
7. Fee structures for providers' services are either charge-based or resource-based. Charge-based structures, such as UCR (usual, customary, and reasonable), are based on the fees that many providers have charged for similar services. Relative value scales (RVS) account for the relative difficulty of procedures by comparing the skill involved in each of a group of procedures. An RVS is charge-based if the charges that are attached to the relative values are based on histor-

ical fees. Resource-based relative value scales (RBRVS), such as the Medicare Physician Fee Schedule (MPFS), are built by comparing three cost factors: (a) how difficult it is for the provider to do the procedure, (b) how much office overhead the procedure involves, and (c) the relative risk that the procedure presents to the patient and the provider. Both charge-based and resource-based fee structures are affected by the geographical area in which the service is provided.

8. The following steps are used to calculate RBRVS payments under the MPFS: (a) determine the procedure code for the service; (b) use the MPFS to find the three RVUs—work, practice expense, and malpractice—for the procedure; (c) use the Medicare GPCI list to find the three geographic practice cost indices (also for work, practice expense, and malpractice); (d) multiply each RVU by its GPCI to calculate the adjusted value; (e) add the three adjusted totals, and multiply the sum by the annual conversion factor to determine the payment.

9. Most payers use one of three provider payment methods: allowed charges, contracted fee schedules, or capitation. When a maximum allowed charge is set by a payer for each service, a provider does not receive the difference from the payer if the provider's usual fee is greater. If the provider participates in the patient's plan, the difference is written off; if the provider does not participate, the plan's rules on balance billing determine whether the patient is responsible for the amount. Under a contracted fee schedule, the allowed charge for each service is all that the payer or the patient pays; no additional charges can be collected. Under capitation, the health care plan sets a capitation rate that pays for all contracted services to enrolled members for a given period.

10. Payments to participating providers are limited to the allowed charge. Some part of that amount is paid by the payer and some part by the patient according to the coinsurance provisions of the plan. Nonparticipating providers in most private plans (but not government-sponsored plans) can collect their usual fees, even when they are higher than the allowed charges, by receiving the specified part of an allowed charge from the payer and the rest of the allowed charge, plus the balance due resulting from a lower allowed charge and a higher usual charge, from the patient.

Review Questions

Match the key terms with their definitions.

A. edits
B. downcoding
C. capitation rate
D. usual fee
E. allowed charge
F. prospective audit
G. balance billing
H. write-off
I. conversion factor
J. OIG Work Plan

____ 1. Fee for a service or procedure that is charged by a provider for most patients under typical circumstances

____ 2. The maximum charge allowed by a payer for a specific service or procedure

____ 3. If the provider's usual fee is higher than the payer's allowed charge, the provider collects the difference from the insured, rather than writing it off

____ 4. The amount that a participating provider must deduct from a patient's account because of a contractual agreement to accept a payer's allowed charge

____ 5. The contractually set periodic prepayment amount to a provider for specified services to each enrolled plan member

____ 6. An internal audit conducted before claims are reported to payers

____ 7. A payer's review and reduction of a procedure code to a lower value than reported by the provider

____ 8. The OIG's annual list of planned projects under the Medicare Fraud and Abuse Initiative

____ 9. A computerized system used to screen claims

____ 10. Dollar amount used to multiply a relative value unit to arrive at a charge

Decide whether each statement is true or false.

____ 1. Resource-based fee structures are based on the procedure's difficulty, the practice expense it involves, and the risk it entails.

____ 2. The Medicare Fee Schedule is based on the UCR method of setting charges.

____ 3. The geographic practice cost index (GPCI) is used to adjust each of the cost elements when a Medicare charge is calculated.

____ 4. The Medicare Fee Schedule's conversion factor is set for a one-year period.

____ 5. If a provider's usual fee is higher than a payer's allowed charge, the higher of the two fees is paid.

____ 6. If a payer's allowed charge is higher than a provider's usual fee, the higher of the two fees is paid.

____ 7. If a payer does not permit a provider to balance bill a patient, the provider must write off the difference between the usual fee and the amount paid.

____ 8. Managed care capitation rates are based on the services that the group of members is likely to use.

____ 9. Under Medicare rules, no modifiers can be used with code combinations listed in the CCI.

____ 10. During an audit, all the claims from a particular period are usually examined.

Select the letter that best completes the statement or answers the question.

____ 1. The OIG Work Plan describes
   A. planned projects for investigating possible fraud in various billing areas
   B. legislative initiatives under HIPAA
   C. the FBI's investigations
   D. the current cases that are being prosecuted by the OIG's attorneys

____ 2. Under Medicare's code edits, mutually exclusive codes
   A. can be billed together if they are component codes
   B. can be billed together if they have a –1 modifier code attached
   C. cannot be billed together for the same patient on the same day
   D. cannot be billed more than once by a single provider on the same date of service

____ 3. Based on the RVU table on page 225, the smallest cost element in most Medicare RBRVS fees is
   A. malpractice expense
   B. practice expense
   C. work expense
   D. customary expense

____ 4. In calculations of RBRVS fees, the three relative value units are multiplied by
   A. their respective geographic practice cost indices
   B. the neutral budget factor
   C. the national conversion factor
   D. the UCR factor

____ 5. Medicare typically pays for what percentage of the allowed charge?
   A. 50 percent
   B. 60 percent
   C. 70 percent
   D. 80 percent

____ 6. If a participating provider's usual fee is $400 and the allowed amount is $350, what amount is written off?
A. zero
B. $25
C. $50
D. $75

____ 7. If a nonparticipating provider's usual fee is $400, the allowed amount is $350, and balance billing is permitted, what amount is written off?
A. zero
B. $25
C. $50
D. $75

____ 8. If a nonparticipating provider's usual fee is $400, the allowed amount is $350, and balance billing is not permitted, what amount is written off?
A. zero
B. $25
C. $50
D. $75

____ 9. The usual fees for excluded services are
A. written off
B. collected at the time of service
C. subtracted from the annual deductible
D. subject to balance billing rules

____10. An encounter form containing E/M codes should list
A. the most frequently billed codes
B. just blanks, so the correct E/M code can be entered
C. complete ranges of codes for each type or place of service listed
D. none of the above

Answer the following questions.

1. What is the formula for calculating a RBRVS charge using the Medicare Physician Fee Schedule?
2. Define the following abbreviations:

A. CCI ______________________________

B. GPCI ______________________________

C. MPFS ______________________________

D. UCR ______________________________

E. RVS ______________________________

F. RBRVS ______________________________

Applying Your Knowledge

Case 7.1 Auditing Linkage

A. Are the following procedure and diagnostic codes appropriately linked? If not, what is (are) the error(s)?

	CPT	ICD-9-CM	LINKED?
1.	76091	V76.12	
2.	99214	V54.8	
3.	57284	601.1, 041.1	
4.	96408	V58.1, 233.0	
5.	99203, 72040, 73600	824.2, 847.0, E888, E849.4	

B. A forty-year-old established female patient is having an annual checkup. During the examination, her physician identifies a lump in her left breast. The physician considers this a significant finding and performs the key components of a problem-focused E/M service. These four codes and modifier should be reported. In what order should they be listed?

CPT codes: 99212, 99396
ICD codes: V70.0, 611.72
Modifier: –25

Case 7.2 Calculating Expected Charges

Using the sample relative value units and GPCIs shown on page 225 and a conversion factor of $34.7315, calculate the expected charge for each of the following services:

A. CPT 99204 in Galveston, TX

B. CPT 33502 in Manhattan, NY

C. CPT 99203 in Columbus, OH

Case 7.3 Calculating Insurance Math

Dr. Mary Mandlebaum is a PAR provider in Medicare and in Mountville Health Plan, which has allowed charges for services and does not permit balance billing of plan members. She is not a PAR provider in the Ringdale Medical Plan. Based on the following table of charges, calculate the charges that the payer and the patient will pay in each of the situations. Show your calculations.

Service	CPT	Usual Charge	Mountville Health Plan Allowed Charge	Medicare Allowed Charge
Office/Outpatient Visit, New, Min.	99201	$54	$48	$43
Office/Outpatient Visit, New, Low	99202	$73	$65	$58
Office/Outpatient Visit, New, Mod.	99203	$100	$89	$80
Office/Outpatient Visit, New, Mod.	99204	$147	$129	$116
Office/Outpatient Visit, New, High	99205	$190	$168	$151
Office/Outpatient Visit, Est., Min.	99211	$29	$26	$22
Office/Outpatient Visit, Est., Low	99212	$44	$39	$35
Office/Outpatient Visit, Est., Mod.	99213	$60	$54	$48
Office/Outpatient Visit, Est., Mod.	99214	$87	$78	$70
Office/Outpatient Visit, Est., High	99215	$134	$119	$107
Rhythm ECG with Report	93040	$30	$36	$30
Breathing Capacity Test	94010	$83	$69	$58
DTAP Immunization	90700	$102	$87	$74

A. Insurance Plan: Mountville Health Plan; patient has met annual deductible of $250; 80–20 coinsurance

Services: CPT 99203, 90700

Payer Reimbursement: ____________ Patient Charge: ____________

B. Insurance Plan: Mountville Health Plan; patient has paid $125 toward an annual deductible of $500; 80–20 coinsurance

Services: CPT 99215, 93040, 94010

Payer Reimbursement: ____________ Patient Charge: ____________

C. Insurance Plan: Ringdale Medical Plan A; no deductible or coinsurance; copayment of $5/PAR; $25/NonPAR

Services: CPT 99212

Payer Reimbursement: ____________ Patient Charge: ____________

D. Insurance Plan: Ringdale Medical Plan B; patient has met annual deductible of $300; 80–20 coinsurance

Services: CPT 99215

Payer Reimbursement: ____________ Patient Charge: ____________

Insurance Plan: Medicare; annual deductible has been met by patient

Services: 99213, 93040

E. Payer Reimbursement: ____________ Patient Charge: ____________

Internet Activities

1. Explore the OIG website at http://oig.hhs.gov.

   a. Click "What's New." Select a recent audit, and prepare a report summarizing its major points.

   b. Using the search feature, locate a recent OIG Work Plan. Report on five points listed under "Medicare Physicians and Other Health Professionals."

2. At the CMS website, http://www.cms.hhs.gov/PhysicianFeeSched/, read and accept the CPT copyright notice, and then click start on the Medicare Physician Payment Systems page.

   After selecting Single HCPC Code and RVU, accept Default on the next screen. When prompted, enter 63012. View and record the description and RVU for the CPT code.

3. Visit the CMS website and search for information on this year's conversion factor for the Medicare Fee Schedule. Using this current factor, recalculate the math in the example that is shown in Figure 7.6 on page 224 to find the payment for this year.

Chapter 8

Health Care Claim Preparation and Transmission

CHAPTER OUTLINE

Introduction to Health Care Claims

Completing the CMS-1500 Claim

Completing the HIPAA 837 Claim

Clearinghouses and Claim Transmission

Learning Outcomes

After studying this chapter, you should be able to:

1. Discuss the content of the patient information section of the CMS-1500 claim.
2. Discuss the content of the physician or supplier information section of the CMS-1500 claim.
3. Describe use of a practice management program to prepare claims.
4. Compare required and situational data elements.
5. Identify the five sections of the HIPAA 837 claim transaction, and discuss the data elements that complete it.
6. Compare billing provider, pay-to provider, rendering provider, and referring/ordering provider.
7. Distinguish between a claim control number and a line item control number.
8. Discuss the role of clearinghouses in preparing HIPAA-compliant claims.
9. Explain how claim attachments and credit–debit information are handled.
10. Identify the three major methods of electronic claim transmission.

KeyTerms

- administrative code set
- billing provider
- claim attachment
- claim control number
- claim filing indicator code
- claim frequency code (claim submission reason code)
- claim scrubber
- clean claim
- CMS-1500
- CMS-1500 (08/05)
- data elements
- destination payer
- HIPAA X12 837 Health Care Claim or Equivalent Encounter Information
- HIPAA X12 276/277 Health Care Claim Status Inquiry/Response
- individual relationship code
- line item control number
- National Uniform Claim Committee (NUCC)
- other ID number
- outside laboratory
- pay-to provider
- place of service (POS) code
- qualifier
- rendering provider
- required data element
- responsible party
- service line information
- situational data element
- taxonomy code

Health care claims communicate critical data between providers and payers on behalf of patients. Claims are created by many different types of providers; in this chapter, the focus is on physician claims. Understanding the internal and EDI procedures used by the practice to prepare and transmit claims is important for success as a medical insurance specialist. Claim processing is a major task, and the numbers can be huge. For example, a forty-physician group practice with fifty-five thousand patients typically processes a thousand claims daily. Technology makes it possible to create, send, and track this volume of claims efficiently and effectively to ensure prompt payment to the practice.

Introduction to Health Care Claims

The HIPAA-mandated electronic transaction for claims is the **HIPAA X12 837 Health Care Claim or Equivalent Encounter Information**. This electronic transaction is usually called the "837 claim" or the "HIPAA claim." The electronic HIPAA claim is based on the **CMS-1500**, which is a paper claim form. The information on the electronic transaction and the paper form, with a few exceptions, is the same.

In the first section of this chapter, filling out a paper claim is introduced first as a way of understanding the data that claims generally require. Of course, the CMS-1500 is not usually filled out by transferring information directly from other office forms, like the patient information and encounter forms. Instead, claims are created when the medical insurance specialist uses a practice management program (PMP) that captures and organizes databases of claim information. The practice management program automates the process of creating correct claims, making it easy to update, correct, and manage the claim process.

The second section of the chapter explains terms and data items that the HIPAA 837 claim may contain in addition to the CMS-1500 information. Some of the data items relate to the capability of electronic claims to provide more detailed information than a paper claim can. Other items are needed to go with various types of information to help the receiver of the claim electronically sort the information.

Clearinghouses and transmission methods are covered in the third section of the chapter.As explained in Chapter 2, most practices use clearinghouses to take the PMP data and send payers correct claims. The methods of transmitting the HIPAA claim may affect some of the practice's claim procedures, but all methods require close and careful attention to security and protection of patients' protected health information (PHI).

Billing Tip

Knowledge of Claim Data

Medical insurance specialists become familiar with the information most often required on claims their practice prepares, so that they can efficiently research missing information and respond to payers' questions. Memorization is not required, but good thinking and organizational skills are.

Background

For many years, the CMS-1500 was the universal health claim accepted by most payers. The familiar red and black printed form was typed or computer-generated and mailed to payers. Sending paper claims became less common with the increased use of information technology (IT) in physician practices. HIPAA, with its emphasis on electronic transactions, has made the use of IT very common. HIPAA requires electronic transmission of claims, except for practices that have less than ten full-time or equivalent employees and never send any kind of electronic health care transactions (see Chapter 2). These excepted offices are the only providers that can still send paper claims. The HIPAA 837 claim sent electronically is mandated for all other physician practices.

HIPAA has changed the way things work on the payer side, too. Payers may not require providers to make changes or additions to the content of the HIPAA 837 claim. Further, they cannot refuse to accept the standard transaction or delay payment of any proper HIPAA transaction, claims included.

Billing Tip

Staying Up to Date with the CMS-1500

Check the NUCC website for updated instructions.

Claim Content

The **National Uniform Claim Committee** (NUCC), led by the American Medical Association, determines the content of both HIPAA 837 and CMS-1500 claims. The current CMS-1500 form, called the **CMS-1500 (08/05)**, was updated by the NUCC to allow spaces for the HIPAA-mandated National Provider Identifier (NPI). The 08/05 claim has fields for using both the NPI and other older identifying numbers called "legacy" numbers. This claim, mandated as of February 1, 2007, is the form covered in this chapter.

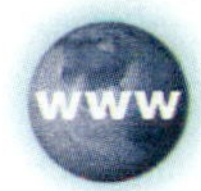

NUCC Home Page

http://www.nucc.org

Completing the CMS-1500 Claim

The CMS-1500 claim has a carrier block and thirty-three Item Numbers (INs), as shown in Figure 8.1 on page 240. The instructions for completing this claim are based on the NUCC publication *1500 Health Insurance Claim Form Reference Instruction Manual for 08/05 Version* available on the NUCC website.

Above the boxes, at the right, the Carrier Block is used for the insurance carrier's name and address. Item Numbers 1 through 13 refer to the patient and the patient's insurance coverage. This information is entered in the practice management program based on the patient information form and the patient insurance card. Item Numbers 14 through 33 contain information about the provider and the patient's condition, including the diagnoses, procedures, and charges. This information is entered from the encounter form and other documentation.

Billing Tip

Payer Instructions May Vary

The NUCC instructions do not address any particular payer. Best practice for paper claims is to check with each payer for specific information required on the form.

Patient Information

The items in the patient information section of the CMS-1500 identify the patient, the insured, and the health plan, and contain other case-related data and assignment of benefits/release information.

1500

HEALTH INSURANCE CLAIM FORM

APPROVED BY NATIONAL UNIFORM CLAIM COMMITTEE 08/05

PICA | PICA

1. MEDICARE (Medicare #) MEDICAID (Medicaid #) TRICARE CHAMPUS (Sponsor's SSN) CHAMPVA (Member ID#) GROUP HEALTH PLAN (SSN or ID) FECA BLK LUNG (SSN) OTHER (ID)

1a. INSURED'S I.D. NUMBER (For Program in Item 1)

2. PATIENT'S NAME (Last Name, First Name, Middle Initial)

3. PATIENT'S BIRTH DATE MM DD YY SEX M F

4. INSURED'S NAME (Last Name, First Name, Middle Initial)

5. PATIENT'S ADDRESS (No., Street)

6. PATIENT RELATIONSHIP TO INSURED Self Spouse Child Other

7. INSURED'S ADDRESS (No., Street)

CITY STATE

8. PATIENT STATUS Single Married Other

CITY STATE

ZIP CODE TELEPHONE (Include Area Code) ( )

Employed Full-Time Student Part-Time Student

ZIP CODE TELEPHONE (INCLUDE AREA CODE) ( )

9. OTHER INSURED'S NAME (Last Name, First Name, Middle Initial)

10. IS PATIENT'S CONDITION RELATED TO:

11. INSURED'S POLICY GROUP OR FECA NUMBER

a. OTHER INSURED'S POLICY OR GROUP NUMBER

a. EMPLOYMENT? (CURRENT OR PREVIOUS) YES NO

a. INSURED'S DATE OF BIRTH MM DD YY SEX M F

b. OTHER INSURED'S DATE OF BIRTH MM DD YY SEX M F

b. AUTO ACCIDENT? YES NO PLACE (State)

b. EMPLOYER'S NAME OR SCHOOL NAME

c. EMPLOYER'S NAME OR SCHOOL NAME

c. OTHER ACCIDENT? YES NO

c. INSURANCE PLAN NAME OR PROGRAM NAME

d. INSURANCE PLAN NAME OR PROGRAM NAME

10d. RESERVED FOR LOCAL USE

d. IS THERE ANOTHER HEALTH BENEFIT PLAN? YES NO *If yes*, return to and complete item 9 a-d.

READ BACK OF FORM BEFORE COMPLETING & SIGNING THIS FORM.

12. PATIENT'S OR AUTHORIZED PERSON'S SIGNATURE I authorize the release of any medical or other information necessary to process this claim. I also request payment of government benefits either to myself or to the party who accepts assignment below.

SIGNED DATE

13. INSURED'S OR AUTHORIZED PERSON'S SIGNATURE I authorize payment of medical benefits to the undersigned physician or supplier for services described below.

SIGNED

CARRIER

PATIENT AND INSURED INFORMATION

14. DATE OF CURRENT: MM DD YY ILLNESS (First symptom) OR INJURY (Accident) OR PREGNANCY(LMP)

15. IF PATIENT HAS HAD SAME OR SIMILAR ILLNESS. GIVE FIRST DATE MM DD YY

16. DATES PATIENT UNABLE TO WORK IN CURRENT OCCUPATION FROM MM DD YY TO MM DD YY

17. NAME OF REFERRING PHYSICIAN OR OTHER SOURCE

17a.

17b. NPI

18. HOSPITALIZATION DATES RELATED TO CURRENT SERVICES FROM MM DD YY TO MM DD YY

19. RESERVED FOR LOCAL USE

20. OUTSIDE LAB? YES NO $ CHARGES

21. DIAGNOSIS OR NATURE OF ILLNESS OR INJURY. (Relate Items 1,2,3 or 4 to Item 24e by Line)

1. ___ . ___

2. ___ . ___

3. ___ . ___

4. ___ . ___

22. MEDICAID RESUBMISSION CODE ORIGINAL REF. NO.

23. PRIOR AUTHORIZATION NUMBER

24. A. DATE(S) OF SERVICE From MM DD YY To MM DD YY	B. PLACE OF SERVICE	C. EMG	D. PROCEDURES, SERVICES, OR SUPPLIES (Explain Unusual Circumstances) CPT/HCPCS MODIFIER	E. DIAGNOSIS POINTER	F. $ CHARGES	G. DAYS OR UNITS	H. EPSDT Family Plan	I. ID. QUAL.	J. RENDERING PROVIDER ID. #
1								NPI	
2								NPI	
3								NPI	
4								NPI	
5								NPI	
6								NPI	

25. FEDERAL TAX I.D. NUMBER SSN EIN

26. PATIENT'S ACCOUNT NO.

27. ACCEPT ASSIGNMENT? (For govt. claims, see back) YES NO

28. TOTAL CHARGE $

29. AMOUNT PAID $

30. BALANCE DUE $

31. SIGNATURE OF PHYSICIAN OR SUPPLIER INCLUDING DEGREES OR CREDENTIALS (I certify that the statements on the reverse apply to this bill and are made a part thereof.)

SIGNED DATE

32.SERVICE FACILITY LOCATION INFORMATION

a. NPI b.

33. BILLING PROVIDER INFO & PHONE # ( )

a. NPI b.

PHYSICIAN OR SUPPLIER INFORMATION

NUCC Instruction Manual available at: www.nucc.org

FIGURE 8.1 CMS-1500 (08/05) Claim

Item Number 1: Type of Insurance

1. MEDICARE (Medicare #) MEDICAID (Medicaid #) TRICARE CHAMPUS (Sponsor's SSN) CHAMPVA (Member ID#) GROUP HEALTH PLAN (SSN or ID) FECA BLK LUNG (SSN) OTHER (ID)

Item Number 1 is used to indicate the type of insurance coverage. Five specific government programs are listed (Medicare, Medicaid, TRICARE/CHAMPUS, CHAMPVA, FECA Black Lung), as well as Group Health Plan and Other. If the patient has

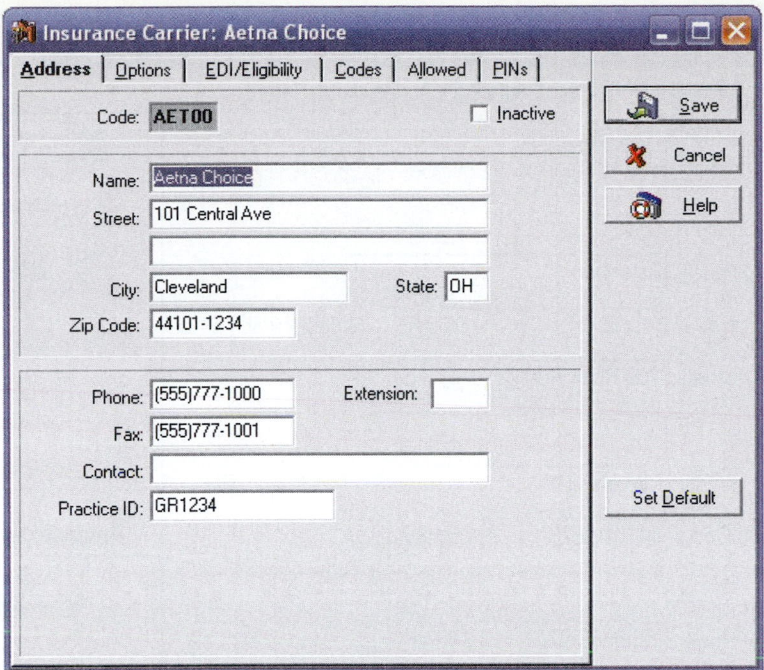

FIGURE 8.2 Example of Medisoft Screen for Payer Information

group contract insurance with a private payer, Group Health Plan is selected. The Other box indicates health insurance including HMOs, commercial insurance, automobile accident, liability, and workers' compensation. This information directs the claim to the correct program and may establish the primary payer.

Figure 8.2 shows a practice management screen used to record information about an insurance plan.

Item Number 1a: Insured's ID Number

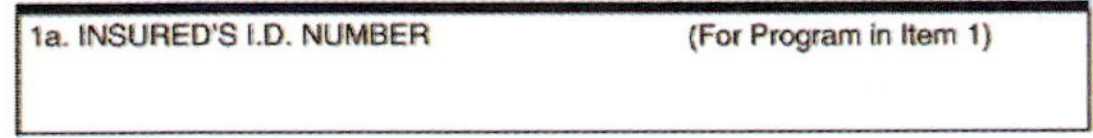

1a. INSURED'S I.D. NUMBER (For Program in Item 1)

The insured's ID number is the identification number of the person who holds the policy. Item Number 1a records the insurance identification number that appears on the insurance card of the person who holds the policy, who may or may not be the patient.

Item Number 2: Patient's Name

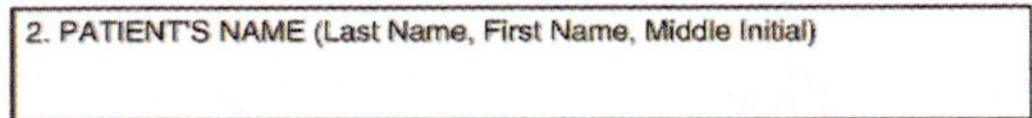

2. PATIENT'S NAME (Last Name, First Name, Middle Initial)

The patient's name is the name of the person who received the treatment or supplies, listed exactly as it appears on the insurance card. Do not change the spelling, even if the card is incorrect. The order in which the name should appear for most payers is last name, first name, and middle initial.

If the patient uses a last name suffix (e.g., Jr., Sr.) enter it after the last name and before the first name. Many claim forms are scanned into a payer's computerized claim system. Therefore, do not use punctuation other than a hyphen (-), which may be used in a hyphenated name.

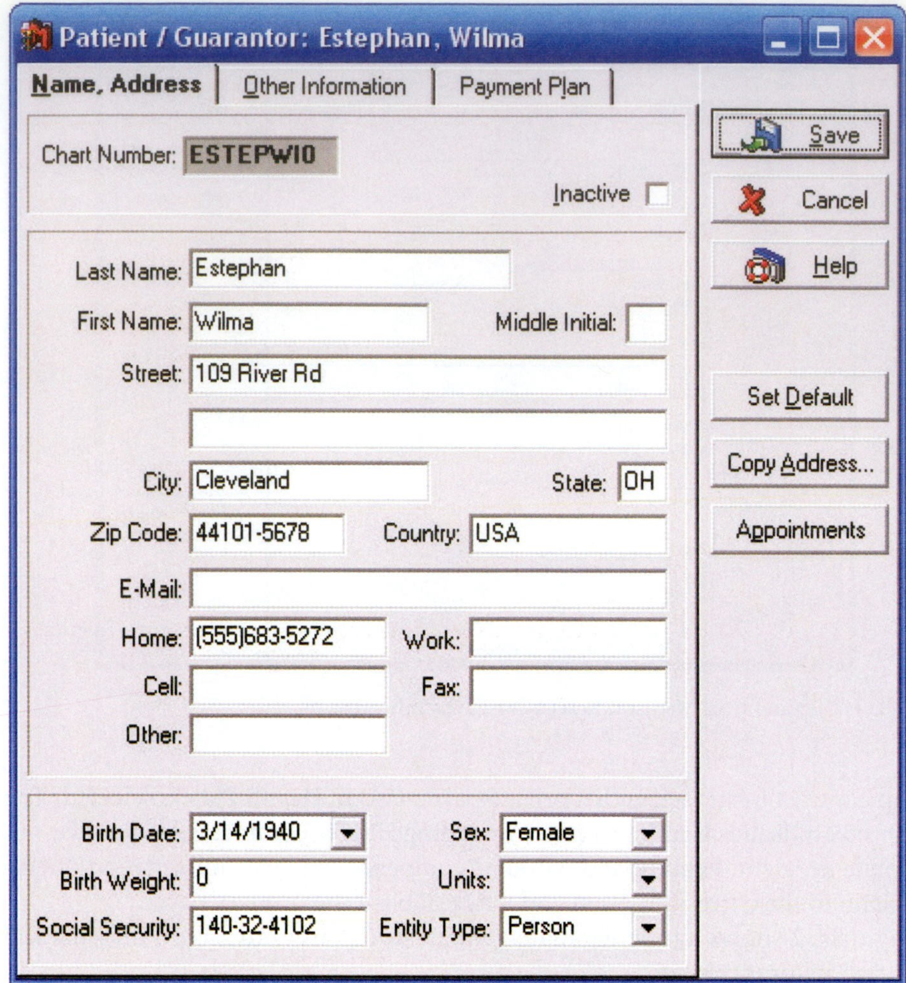

FIGURE 8.3 Example of Medisoft Screen for Patient Information

Figure 8.3 shows one of the patient/insured information screens from a practice management program.

Item Number 3: Patient's Birth Date/Sex

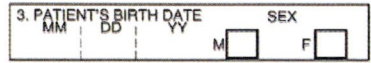

The patient's birth date and sex (gender) helps identify the patient by distinguishing among persons with similar names. Enter the patient's date of birth in eight-digit format (MM/DD/CCYY). Note that all four digits for the year are entered, even though the printed form indicates only two characters (YY). Use zeros before single digits. Enter an X in the correct box to indicate the sex of the patient.

Item Number 4: Insured's Name

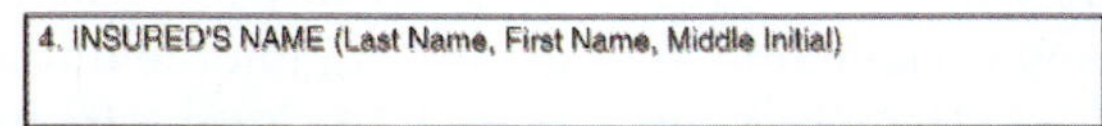

In IN 4, enter the full name of the person who holds the insurance policy (the insured), if not the patient. If the patient is a dependent, the insured may be a

spouse, parent, or other person. If the insured uses a last name suffix (e.g., Jr., Sr.) enter it after the last name and before the first name. Many claim forms are scanned into a payer's computerized claim system, so do not use punctuation other than a hyphen (-), which may be used in a hyphenated name.

Item Number 5: Patient's Address

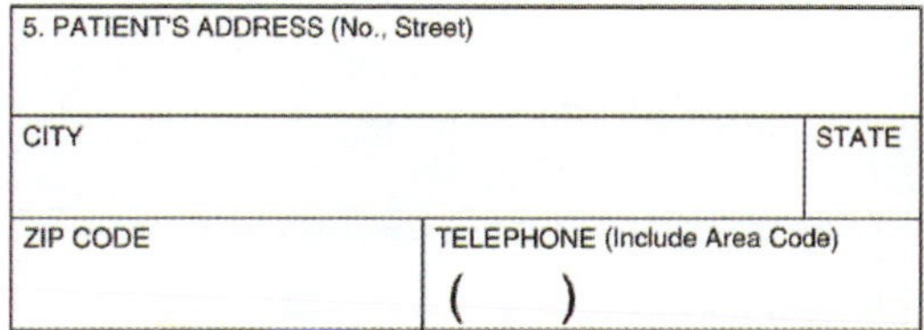

5. PATIENT'S ADDRESS (No., Street)

CITY | STATE

ZIP CODE | TELEPHONE (Include Area Code) ( )

Item Number 5 contains the patient's address and telephone number. The address includes the number and street, city, state, and Zip code. The first line is for the street address, the second line for the city and state, and the third line for the Zip code and phone number. Use the two-digit state abbreviation, and use the nine-digit Zip code if it is available.

Note that the patient's address refers to the patient's permanent residence. A temporary address or school address should not be used.

Item Number 6: Patient's Relationship to Insured

6. PATIENT RELATIONSHIP TO INSURED

Self ☐ Spouse ☐ Child ☐ Other ☐

In IN 6, enter the patient's relationship to the insured if FL 4 has been completed. Choosing self indicates that the insured is the patient. Spouse indicates that the patient is the husband or wife or qualified partner as defined by the insured's plan. Child means that the patient is the minor dependent as defined by the insured's plan. Other means that the patient is someone other than either self, spouse, or child. Other includes employee, ward, or dependent as defined by the insured's plan.

Item Number 7: Insured's Address

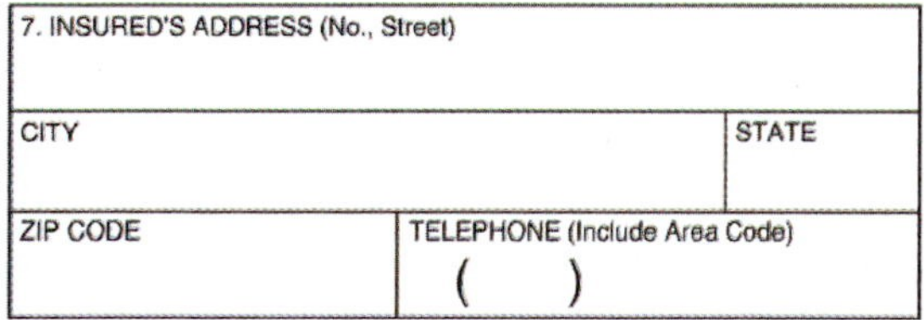

7. INSURED'S ADDRESS (No., Street)

CITY | STATE

ZIP CODE | TELEPHONE (Include Area Code) ( )

The insured's address refers to the insured's permanent residence, which may be different from the patient's address (IN 5). Enter the address and telephone number of the person who is listed in IN 4. For most payers, if the insured's address is the same as the patient's, enter SAME. This Item Number does not need to be completed if the patient is the insured person.

Item Number 8: Patient Status

8. PATIENT STATUS

Single ☐ Married ☐ Other ☐

Employed ☐ Full-Time Student ☐ Part-Time Student ☐

Enter an X in the box for the patient's marital status and for the patient's employment or student status. Choosing employed indicates that the patient has a job. Full-time student means that the patient is registered as a full-time student as defined by the postsecondary school or university. Part-time student means that the patient is registered as a part-time student as defined by the postsecondary school or university. This information is important for determination of liability and coordination of benefits (COB).

Item Number 9: Other Insured's Name

9. OTHER INSURED'S NAME (Last Name, First Name, Middle Initial)

If Item Number 11d is marked, complete Item Numbers 9 and 9a-d; otherwise, leave blank (or, for some payers, use SAME.). An entry in the other insured's name box indicates that there is a holder of another policy that may cover the patient. When additional group health coverage exists, enter the insured's name (the last name, first name, and middle initial of the enrollee in another health plan if it is different from that shown in IN 2).

Example: If a husband is covered by his employer's group policy and also by his wife's group health plan, enter the wife's name in IN 9.

Item Number 9a: Other Insured's Policy or Group Number

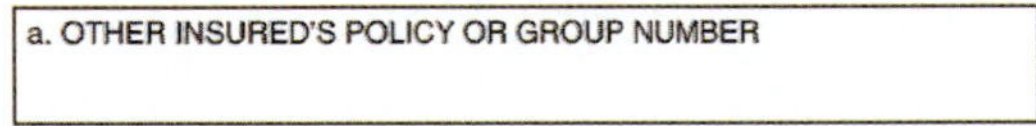
a. OTHER INSURED'S POLICY OR GROUP NUMBER

Enter the policy or group number of the other insurance plan.

Item Number 9b: Other Insured's Date of Birth

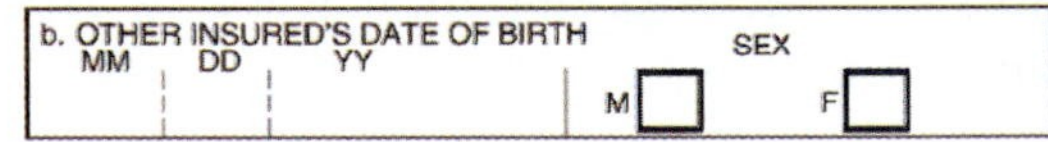
b. OTHER INSURED'S DATE OF BIRTH SEX
MM DD YY M F

Enter the eight-digit date of birth (MM/DD/CCYY) and the sex of the other insured as indicated in IN 9.

Item Number 9c Employer's Name or School Name

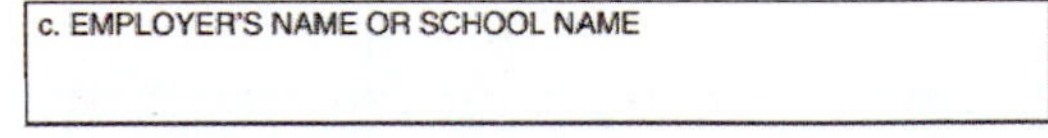
c. EMPLOYER'S NAME OR SCHOOL NAME

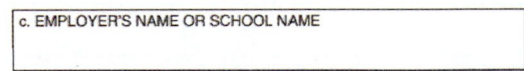

Enter the name of the other insured's employer or school. This box identifies the name of the employer or school attended by the other insured as indicated in IN 9.

Item Number 9d: Insurance Plan Name or Program Name

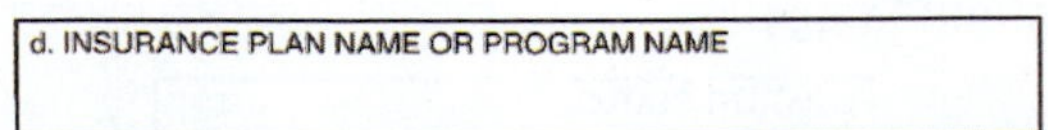
d. INSURANCE PLAN NAME OR PROGRAM NAME

Enter the other insured's insurance plan or program name. This box identifies the name of the plan or program of the other insured as indicated in IN 9.

Item Numbers 10a–10c: Is Patient Condition Related to:

10. IS PATIENT'S CONDITION RELATED TO:

a. EMPLOYMENT? (Current or Previous)

☐ YES ☐ NO

b. AUTO ACCIDENT? PLACE (State)

☐ YES ☐ NO

c. OTHER ACCIDENT?

☐ YES ☐ NO

This information indicates whether the patient's illness or injury is related to employment, auto accident, or other accident. Choosing employment (current or previous) indicates that the condition is related to the patient's job or workplace. Auto accident means that the condition is the result of an automobile accident. Other accident means that the condition is the result of any other type of accident.

When appropriate, enter an X in the correct box to indicate whether one or more of the services described in IN 24 are for a condition or injury that occurred on the job or as a result of an automobile or other accident. The state postal code must be shown if YES is checked in IN 10b for Auto Accident. Any item checked YES indicates that there may be other applicable insurance coverage that would be primary, such as automobile liability insurance. Primary insurance information must then be shown in IN 11.

Item Number 10d: Reserved for Local Use

10d. RESERVED FOR LOCAL USE

The content of IN 10d varies with the insurance plan. For example, some plans require the word *Attachment* in this Item Number if there is a paper attachment with the claim. Check instructions from the applicable public or private payer regarding the use of this field.

Item Number 11: Insured's Policy Group or FECA Number

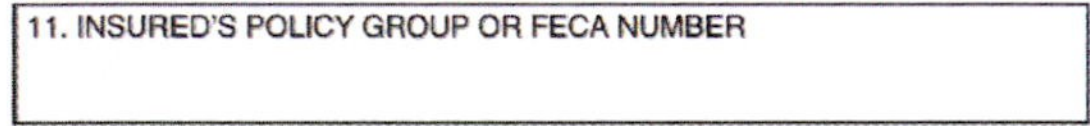

11. INSURED'S POLICY GROUP OR FECA NUMBER

Enter the insured's policy or group number as it appears on the insured's health care identification card. The insured's policy group or FECA number refers to the alphanumeric identifier for the health, auto, or other insurance plan coverage. For workers' compensation claims the workers' compensation carrier's alphanumeric identifier is used. The FECA (Federal Employees' Compensation Act) number is the nine-digit alphanumeric identifier assigned to a patient who is an employee of the federal government claiming work-related condition(s) under the Federal Employees Compensation Act (covered in Chapter 13).

Item Number 11a: Insured's Date of Birth/Sex

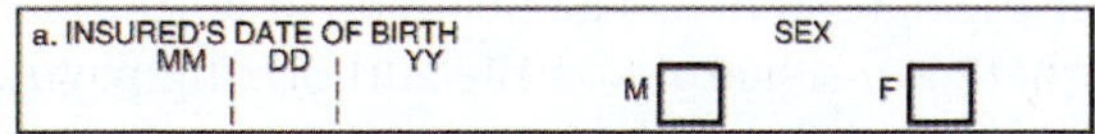

a. INSURED'S DATE OF BIRTH SEX
MM | DD | YY M ☐ F ☐

The insured's date of birth and sex (gender) refers to the birth date and gender of the insured when the insured and the patient are different individuals, as indicated in IN 1a. Enter the insured's eight-digit birth date (MM/DD/CCYY) and sex if different from IN 3 (patient's birth date and sex).

Item Number 11b: Employer's Name or School Name

b. EMPLOYER'S NAME OR SCHOOL NAME

Enter the name of the insured's employer or of the school attended by the insured indicated in IN 1a.

Item Number 11c: Insurance Plan Name or Program Name

c. INSURANCE PLAN NAME OR PROGRAM NAME

Enter the insurance plan or program name of the insured indicated in IN 1a. Note that some payers require the payer identification number of the primary insurer in this field.

Item Number 11d: Is There Another Health Benefit Plan?

d. IS THERE ANOTHER HEALTH BENEFIT PLAN?

☐ YES ☐ NO *If yes*, return to and complete item 9 a-d.

Select Yes if the patient is covered by additional insurance. If the answer is Yes, Item Numbers 9a through 9d must also be completed. If the patient does not have additional insurance, select No. If not known, leave blank.

Item Number 12: Patient's or Authorized Person's Signature

READ BACK OF FORM BEFORE COMPLETING & SIGNING THIS FORM.

12. PATIENT'S OR AUTHORIZED PERSON'S SIGNATURE I authorize the release of any medical or other information necessary to process this claim. I also request payment of government benefits either to myself or to the party who accepts assignment below.

SIGNED ______________________ DATE ______________

Enter "Signature on File," "SOF," or legal signature. When a legal signature is used, enter the date signed in six-digit format (MM/DD/YY) or eight-digit format (MM/DD/CCYY).

This entry mean that there is an authorization on file for the release of any medical or other information necessary to process and/or adjudicate the claim.

Compliance Guideline

Signature on File
If a release is required, make certain that the release on file is current (signed within the last twelve months) and that it covers the release of information pertaining to all the services listed on the claim before entering "Signature on File" or "SOF."

Item Number 13: Insured or Authorized Person's Signature

13. INSURED'S OR AUTHORIZED PERSON'S SIGNATURE I authorize payment of medical benefits to the undersigned physician or supplier for services described below.

SIGNED ______________________

Enter "Signature on File," "SOF," or the legal signature. When using the legal signature, enter the date signed. The insured's or authorized person's signature indicates that there is a signature on file authorizing payment of medical benefits directly to the provider of the services listed on the claim.

Thinking It Through 8.1

A sixty-one-year-old retired female patient is covered by her husband's insurance policy. Her husband is still working and receives health benefits through his employer.

1. What information belongs in IN 2 of the claim?
2. What information belongs in IN 4?
3. What information belongs in IN 11b?

Physician or Supplier Information

The items in this part of the CMS-1500 claim form identify the health care provider, describe the services performed, and give the payer additional information to process the claim.

It may be necessary to identify four different types of providers. It is common to have a physician practice as the **pay-to provider**—the entity that gets paid—plus a **rendering provider**—the doctor who provides care for the patient and is a member of the physician practice that gets the payment. Further, this physician practice may use a billing service or a clearinghouse to transmit claims, which is identified as a separate **billing provider**. (If the practice sends its own claims, it is both the pay-to provider and the billing provider.) Finally, another physician may have sent the patient, and needs to be identified as the referring or ordering physician.

Item Number 14: Date of Current Illness or Injury or Pregnancy

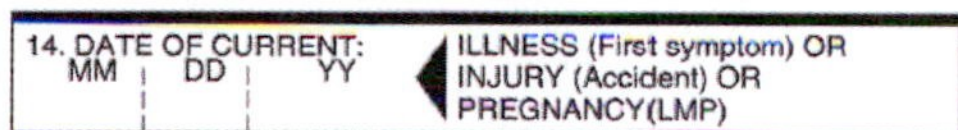

Enter the six-digit or eight-digit date for the first date of the present illness, injury, or pregnancy. For pregnancy, use the date of the last menstrual period (LMP) as the first date. This date refers to the first date of onset of illness, the actual date of injury, or the LMP for pregnancy.

Item Number 15: If Patient Has Had Same or Similar Illness

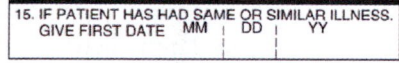

Enter the first date the patient had the same or a similar illness. Having had the same or a similar illness would indicate that the patient had a previously related condition. A previous pregnancy is not a similar illness. Leave blank if unknown.

Item Number 16: Dates Patient Unable to Work in Current Occupation

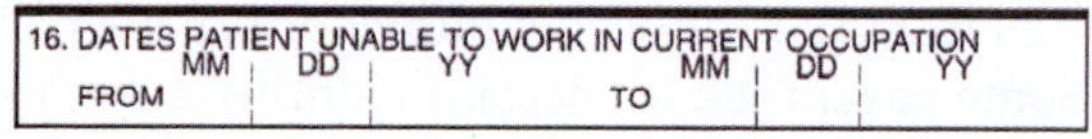

If the patient is employed and is unable to work in his or her current occupation, a six-digit or eight-digit date must be shown for the from–to dates that the patient is unable to work. An entry in this field may indicate employment-related insurance coverage.

Item Number 17: Name of Referring Physician or Other Source

17. NAME OF REFERRING PROVIDER OR OTHER SOURCE

The name of the referring or ordering provider is entered if the service or item was ordered or referred by a provider. The entry should have the name (first name, middle initial, last name) and credentials of the professional who referred or ordered the services or supplies on the claim.

Item Number 17a and 17b: ID Number of Referring Physician (split field)

17a.		
17b.	NPI	

Providers may have two types of ID numbers: a non-NPI ID and an NPI. The non-NPI ID number is called **other ID number** and refers to the payer-assigned unique identifier of the physician or other health care provider. The NPI number is the HIPAA National Provider Identifier number.

In IN 17a, the two parts of the other ID number are entered. The first part is a **qualifier**, which is a two-digit code indicating what the number represents. The second part is the number itself, which may be up to 17 characters long. Qualifiers are shown in Table 8.1. In IN 17b, the NPI Number is entered. For example:

17a.	1B	ABC1234567890
17b.	NPI	0123456789

Item Number 18: Hospitalization Dates Related to Current Services

18. HOSPITALIZATION DATES RELATED TO CURRENT SERVICES
FROM MM | DD | YY TO MM | DD | YY

The hospitalization dates related to current services refer to an inpatient stay and indicate the admission and discharge dates associated with the service(s) on the claim. If the services are needed because of a related hospitalization, enter the admission and discharge dates of that hospitalization in IN 18. For patients still hospitalized, the admission date is listed in the From box, and the To box is left blank.

Item Number 19: Reserved for Local Use

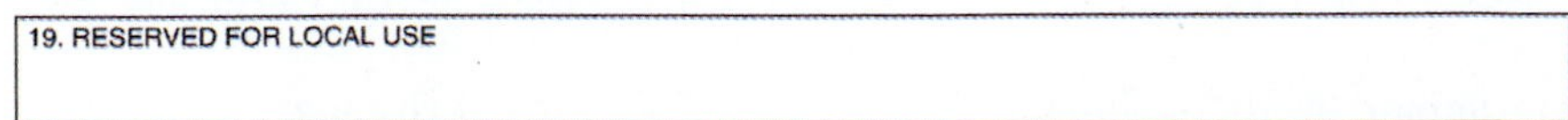
19. RESERVED FOR LOCAL USE

Refer to instructions from the applicable public or private payer regarding the use of this field. Some payers ask for certain identifiers in this field. (If identifiers are reported, the appropriate qualifiers describing the identifier should be used, as listed in Table 8.1). Medicare uses IN 19 to hold modifiers beyond the four that fit in IN 24D.

TABLE 8.1	Qualifiers for Other ID Numbers
Code	**Definition**
0B	State License Number
1B	Blue Shield Provider Number
1C	Medicare Provider Number
1D	Medicaid Provider Number
1G	Provider UPIN Number
1H	CHAMPUS Identification Number
EI	Employer's Identification Number
G2	Provider Commercial Number
LU	Location Number
N5	Provider Plan Network Identification Number
SY	Social Security Number (The Social Security number may not be used for Medicare.)
X5	State Industrial Accident Provider Number
ZZ	Provider Taxonomy

Item Number 20: Outside Lab? $Charges

20. OUTSIDE LAB?	$ CHARGES
☐ YES ☐ NO	

Outside lab? $Charges is used to show that services have been rendered by an independent provider, as indicated in IN 32, and to list the related costs.

Complete this item when the physician is billing for laboratory services, instead of the lab itself. Enter an X in Yes if the reported service was performed by an **outside laboratory**. If Yes is checked, enter the purchased price under charges. A yes response indicates that an entity other than the entity billing for the service performed the laboratory services. Checking No indicates that no purchased lab services are included on the claim. When Yes is chosen, IN 32 must be completed. When billing for multiple purchased lab services, each service should be submitted on a separate claim.

Item Number 21: Diagnosis or Nature of Illness or Injury (Relate Items 1, 2, 3, or 4 to Item 24e by Line)

21. DIAGNOSIS OR NATURE OF ILLNESS OR INJURY (Relate Items 1, 2, 3 or 4 to Item 24E by Line)	
1. ___ . ___	3. ___ . ___
2. ___ . ___	4. ___ . ___

ICD-9-CM codes that describe the patient's condition are entered in priority order. The code for the primary diagnosis is listed first. Additional codes for secondary diagnoses should be listed only when they are directly related to the services being provided (see Chapters 4 and 6). Each claim must list at least one code and may list up to four.

Billing Tip

Compliant Claims Require ICD-9-CM Codes
A claim that does not report at least one ICD-9-CM code will be denied.

Relate lines 1, 2, 3, 4 to the lines of service in IN 24e by line number. Do not provide narrative description in this box. The codes used should specify the highest level of detail possible, including the use of a fifth digit when appropriate.

Item Number 22: Medicaid Resubmission

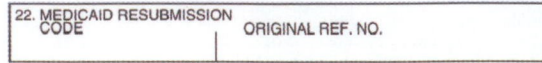

22. MEDICAID RESUBMISSION CODE | ORIGINAL REF. NO.

The Medicaid resubmission code refers to the number assigned by the destination payer or receiver to indicate a previously submitted claim or encounter. List the original reference number for resubmitted claims. Check instructions from the applicable public or private payer regarding the use of this field. This Item Number is left blank for all claims except those for Medicaid plans that require a resubmission number and the original claim reference number.

Item Number 23: Prior Authorization Number

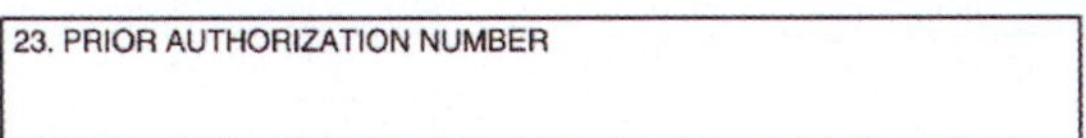

23. PRIOR AUTHORIZATION NUMBER

Some procedures and diagnostic tests require preauthorization. If required, enter the preauthorization number assigned by the payer.

Section 24

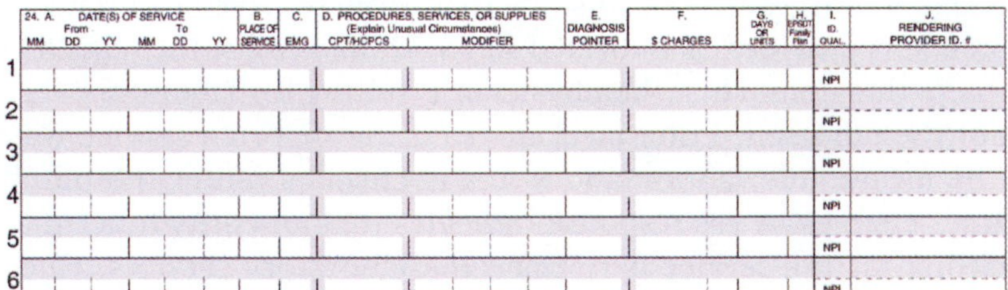

	24. A. DATE(S) OF SERVICE From MM	DD	YY	To MM	DD	YY	B. PLACE OF SERVICE	C. EMG	D. PROCEDURES, SERVICES, OR SUPPLIES (Explain Unusual Circumstances) CPT/HCPCS	MODIFIER	E. DIAGNOSIS POINTER	F. $ CHARGES	G. DAYS OR UNITS	H. EPSDT Family Plan	I. ID. QUAL.	J. RENDERING PROVIDER ID. #
1															NPI	
2															NPI	
3															NPI	
4															NPI	
5															NPI	
6															NPI	

Section 24 of the claim reports the **service line information**—that is, the procedures—performed for the patient. Each item of service line information has a procedure code and a charge, with additional information as detailed below. Figure 8.4 shows a practice management screen used to record service line information.

The six service lines in section 24, which contains INs 24A through 24J, have been divided horizontally to hold both the NPI and a proprietary identifier and to permit the submission of supplemental information to support the billed service. For example, when billing HCPCS codes for products such as drugs, durable medical equipment, or supplies, the payer may require supplemental information using these indicators and codes:

- N4 indicator and the National Drug Codes (NDC)
- VP indicator and Health Industry Business Communications Council (HIBCC) or OZ indicator and Global Trade Item Number (GTIN), formerly Universal Product Codes (UPC)
- Anesthesia duration: in hours and/or minutes and start and end times

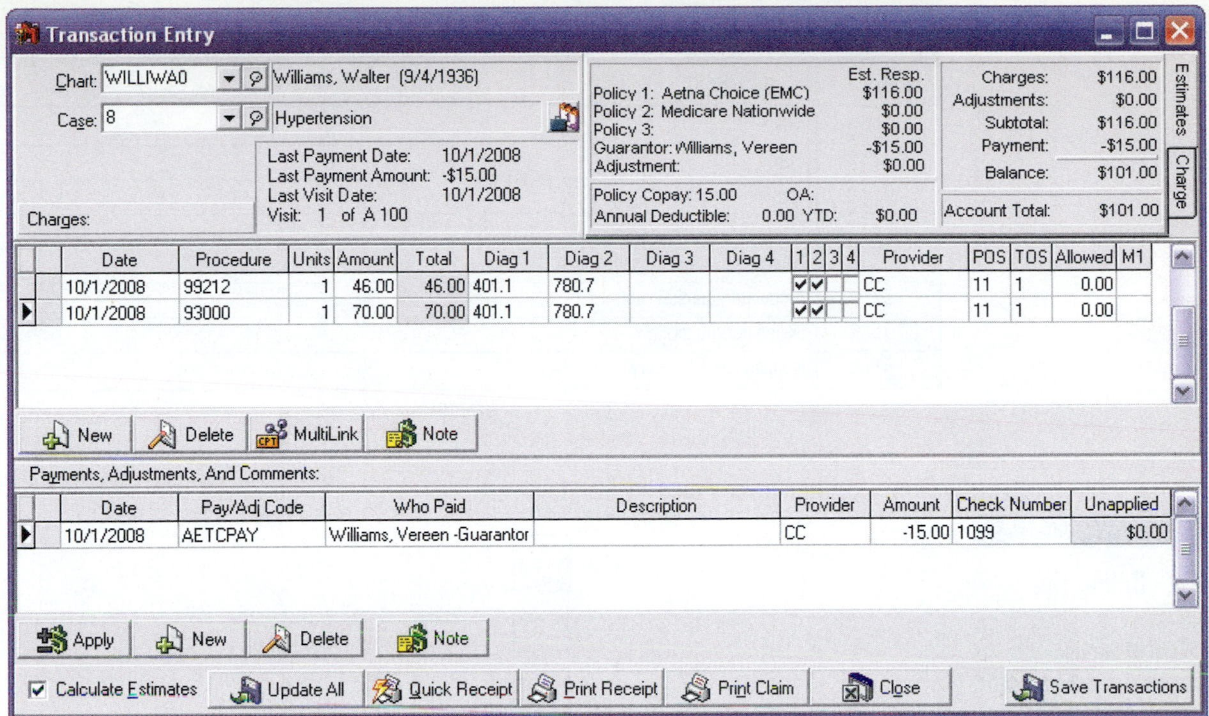

FIGURE 8.4 Example of Medisoft Screen for Service Line Information

This information is to be placed in the upper shaded section of INs 24C through 24H.

> **Billing Tip**
>
> **Correct Use of Section 24**
>
> The top portions of the six service lines are shaded. The shading is not intended to allow the billing of twelve lines of service.

Item Number 24A: Dates of Service

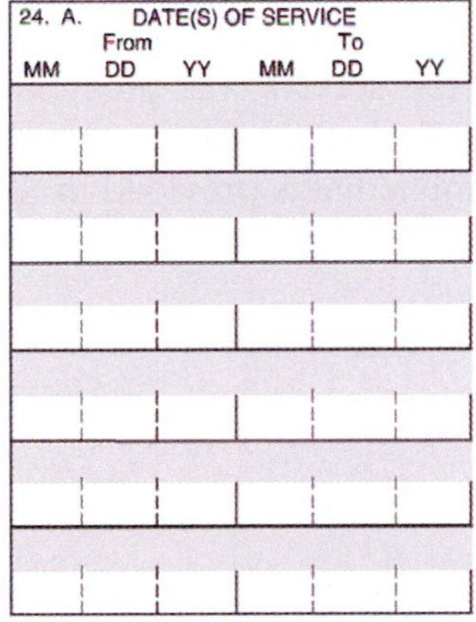

Date(s) of service indicate the actual month, day, and year the service was provided. Grouping services refers to a charge for a series of identical services without listing each date of service.

Enter the from and to date(s) of service. If there is only one date of service, enter that date under From, and leave To blank or reenter the From date. When grouping services, the place of service, procedure code, charges, and individual provider for each line must be identical for that service line. Grouping is allowed only for services on consecutive days. The number of days must correspond to the number of units in IN 24G.

TABLE 8.2 Selected Place of Service Codes

Code	Definition
11	Office
12	Home
21	Inpatient hospital
22	Outpatient hospital
23	Emergency room—hospital
24	Ambulatory surgical center
31	Skilled nursing facility
81	Independent laboratory

Item Number 24B: Place of Service

B. PLACE OF SERVICE

> **Billing Tip**
>
> **Place of Service**
> Payers may authorize different payments for different locations. Higher payments may be made for physician office services, and lower payments for services in ambulatory surgical centers (ASC) and hospital outpatient departments. When a service is performed in an ASC or outpatient department, check to determine whether it falls under the category of an office service.

In 24B, enter the appropriate two-digit code from the place of service code list for each item used or service performed. A **place of service (POS) code** describes the location where the service was provided. The POS code is also called the facility type code. Table 8.2 (above) shows typical codes for physician practice claims. A complete list is provided in Appendix B.

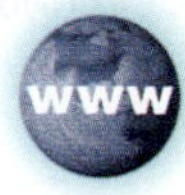

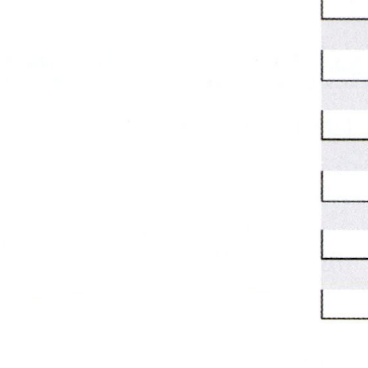

POS Codes
http://www.cms.hhs.gov/PlaceofServiceCodes

Item Number 24C: EMG

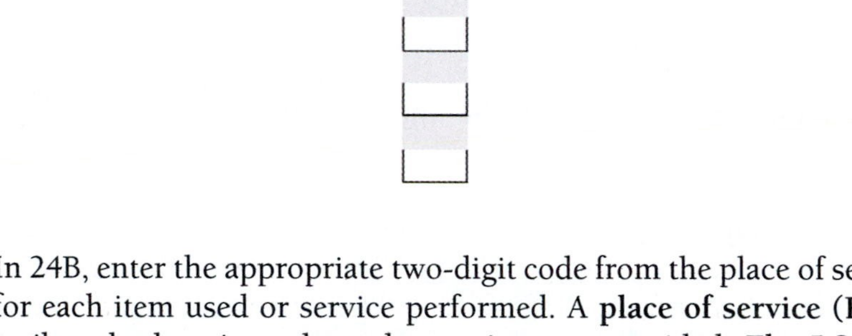

> **Billing Tip**
>
> **IN 24C**
> In the past, this Item Number was Type of Service, which is no longer used. Type of service codes have been eliminated from the CMS-1500 08/05 claim.

Item Number 24C is EMG, for emergency indicator, as defined by federal or state regulations or programs, payer contracts, or HIPAA claim rules. Generally, an emergency situation is one in which the patient requires immediate medical intervention as a result of severe, life-threatening, or potentially disabling conditions. Check with the payer to determine whether the emergency indicator is necessary. If required, enter "Y" for yes or "N" for no in the bottom unshaded portion of the field.

Item Number 24D: Procedures, Services, or Supplies

D. PROCEDURES, SERVICES, OR SUPPLIES (Explain Unusual Circumstances) CPT/HCPCS	MODIFIER			

Enter the CPT or HCPCS codes and modifiers (if applicable) in effect on the date of service. Just the specific procedure codes are entered; not the descriptors. State-defined procedure and supply codes are needed for workers' compensation claims.

> **Billing Tip**
>
> **Unlisted Procedure Code**
> When reporting an unlisted procedure code (see Chapter 5), include a narrative description in IN 19 if a coherent description can be given within the confines of that box. Otherwise, an attachment must be submitted with the claim.

Item Number 24E: Diagnosis Pointer

E. DIAGNOSIS POINTER

The diagnosis pointer refers to the line number from IN 21 that provides the link between diagnosis and treatment. In IN 24E, enter the diagnosis code reference number (pointer) as shown in IN 21 to relate the date of service and the procedures performed to the primary diagnosis. When multiple services are performed, the primary reference number for each service should be listed. Do not enter ICD-9-CM diagnosis codes in 24E.

> **Billing Tip**
>
> **How Many Pointers?**
> According to the NUCC manual, up to four diagnosis pointers can be listed per service line.

Item Number 24F: $ Charges

F.
$ CHARGES

Billing Tip

Billing for Capitated Visits
If the claim is to report an encounter under a MCO capitation contract, a value of zero may be used.

Item Number 24F lists the total billed charges for each service line in IN 24D. A charge for each service line must be reported. If the claim reports an encounter with no charge, such as a capitated visit, a value of zero may be used.

The numbers should be entered without dollar signs, decimals, or commas. Enter 00 in the cents area if the amount is a whole number (for example, 32.00). If the services are for multiple days or units, the number of days or units must be multiplied by the charge to determine the entry in IN 24F. This is done automatically when a practice management program is used to create the claim.

Item Number 24G: Days or Units

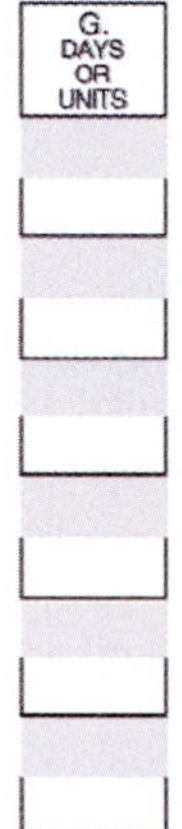

Enter the number of days or units for the service line. This field is most commonly used for multiple visits, units of supplies, anesthesia units or minutes, or oxygen volume. If only one service is performed, the numeral 1 must be entered.

> The drug Prednisone (see Chapter 6, page 194) for oral administration is reported per 5-mg units. If the patient receives 10 mg, the HCPCS code J7506 (FL 24F) is followed by "2" in IN 24G.

When payers require the NDC to support billing HCPCS codes for drugs and the defined NDC units and HCPCS units are not the same, enter the applicable NDC-related units in the upper shaded portion of this field.

When payers require anesthesia time information, convert hours into minutes, and continue the description in the upper shaded portion of this field as needed.

Item Number 24H: EPSDT Family Plan

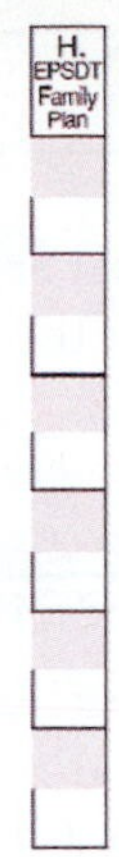
H.
EPSDT
Family
Plan

The Item Number for EPSDT Family Plan refers to certain services that may be covered under some state Medicaid plans (see Chapter 11). In the bottom unshaded portion of the field, enter the correct alpha referral code if the service is related to early and periodic screening, diagnosis, and treatment (EPSDT).

Item Number 24I: ID Qualifier

I. ID. QUAL.	J. RENDERING PROVIDER ID. #
NPI	
NPI	
NPI	
NPI	
NPI	
NPI	

Item Number 24I works together with IN 24J. These boxes are used to enter an ID number for the rendering provider—the individual who is providing the service. (Note that the numbers are needed only if the rendering provider is not the same as the billing provider shown in IN 33.) If the number is an NPI, it goes in IN 24J in the unshaded area next to the 24I label NPI. If the number is a non-NPI (other ID number), the qualifier identifying the type of number goes in IN 24I next to the number in 24J. Refer to Table 8.1 on page 249 for the common qualifiers.

Notes:

- Even though the NPI is to be fully implemented in 2008, it is assumed that there will always be providers who do not have NPIs and whose non-NPI identifiers need to be reported on claim forms.
- INs 24I, 24J, and 24K were formerly EMG (now located in IN 24C), and COB/Local Use (both now deleted).

Item Number 25: Federal Tax ID Number

25. FEDERAL TAX I.D. NUMBER SSN EIN

Enter the physician's or supplier's Social Security number or Employer Identification Number (EIN) in IN 25. Mark the appropriate box (SSN or EIN).

Item Number 26: Patient's Account No.

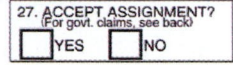

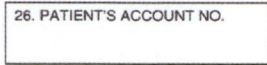
26. PATIENT'S ACCOUNT NO.

Enter the patient account number used by the practice's accounting system. This information is used primarily to help identify patients and post payments when working with remittance advices.

Item Number 27: Accept Assignment?

27. ACCEPT ASSIGNMENT? (For govt. claims, see back) YES NO

Enter a capital X in the correct box. Yes means that the provider agrees to accept assignment under the terms of Medicare. Other payers may require this entry, too, to show participation.

Item Number 28: Total Charge

28. TOTAL CHARGE $

Item Number 28 lists the total of all charges in Item Number 24F, lines 1 through 6. Do not use dollar signs or commas. If the claim is to be submitted on paper and there are more services to be billed, put *continued* here, and put the total charge on the last claim form page.

Item Number 29: Amount Paid

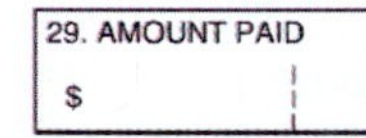
29. AMOUNT PAID $

Enter the amount of the patient payment that is applied to the *covered* services listed on this claim in IN 29. If there is also payment from another insurance carrier, include this amount. If no payment was made, enter none or 0.00.

Item Number 30: Balance Due

30. BALANCE DUE $

Check with the applicable public or private payer regarding the use of this field. Generally, for fee-for-service, subtract the amount in IN 29 from the amount in IN 28, and enter the balance in IN 30. Do not use dollar signs or commas.

Billing Tip

What Does Amount Paid Include?
The amount paid does not include payment for non-covered charges, deductibles, previous claims, or primary payers.

Item Number 31: Signature of Physician or Supplier Including Degrees or Credentials

31. SIGNATURE OF PHYSICIAN OR SUPPLIER INCLUDING DEGREES OR CREDENTIALS
(I certify that the statements on the reverse apply to this bill and are made a part thereof.)

SIGNED DATE

Enter the legal signature and credentials of the provider or supplier (or representative), "Signature on File," or "SOF." Enter the date the form was signed.

Item Number 32: Service Facility Location Information

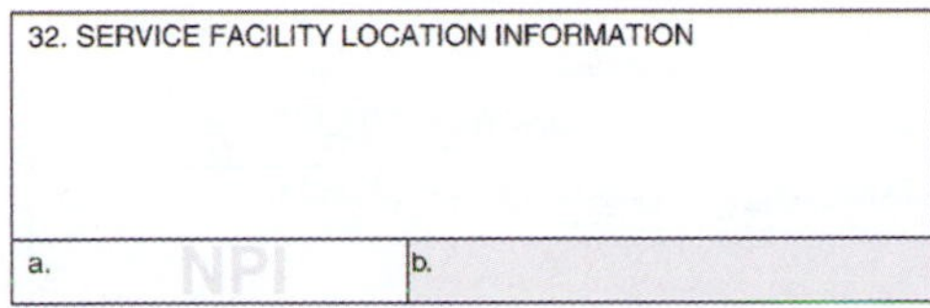
32. SERVICE FACILITY LOCATION INFORMATION

a. NPI | b.

If the place of service is other than the physician's office or the patient's home, enter the name, address, city, state, and Zip code of the location where the services were rendered. Otherwise enter SAME.

Physicians who are billing for purchased diagnostic tests or radiology services must identify the supplier's name, address, Zip code, and NPI in IN 32a. Enter the payer-assigned identifying non-NPI number of the service facility in IN 32b with its qualifier (see Table 8.1 on page 249).

Billing Tip

Address for Service Facility
Do not use a post office (PO) box in the service facility address.

Item Number 33: Billing Provider Information

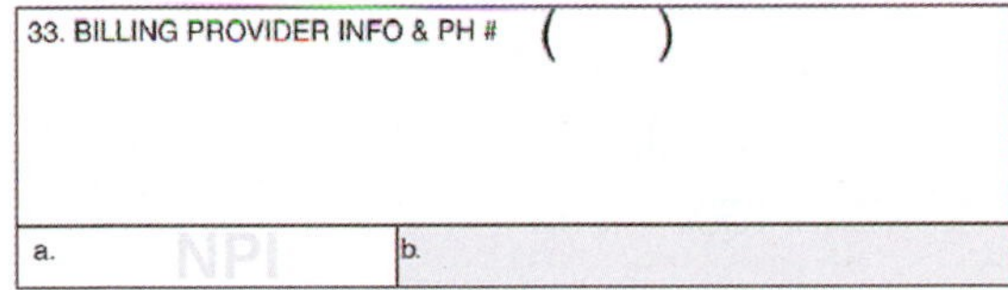
33. BILLING PROVIDER INFO & PH # ( )

a. NPI | b.

Enter the provider's billing name, address, Zip code, phone number, NPI, non-NPI number, and appropriate qualifier. The NPI should be placed in IN 33a. Enter the identifying non-NPI number and its qualifier in IN 33b.

A Note on Taxonomy Codes

Item Number 17a may be completed with a **taxonomy code**. A taxonomy code is a ten-digit number that stands for a physician's medical specialty. The type of specialty may affect the physician's pay, usually because of the payer's contract with the physician. For example, nuclear medicine is usually a higher-paid specialty than internal medicine. An internist who is also certified in nuclear medicine would report the nuclear medicine taxonomy code when billing for that service and use the internal medicine taxonomy code when reporting internal medicine claims.

Most practice management programs store taxonomy-code databases (see Figure 8.5 on page 258). Appendix A provides a list of medical specialities and their taxonomy codes.

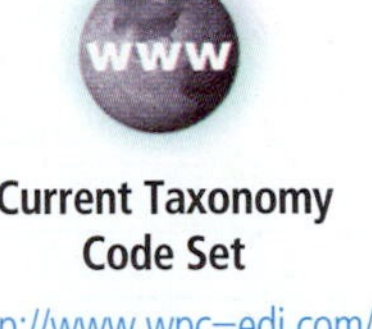

Current Taxonomy Code Set
http://www.wpc=edi.com/codes/taxonomy

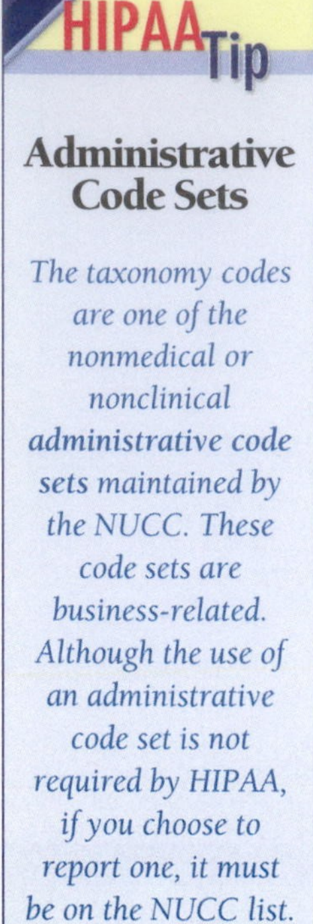

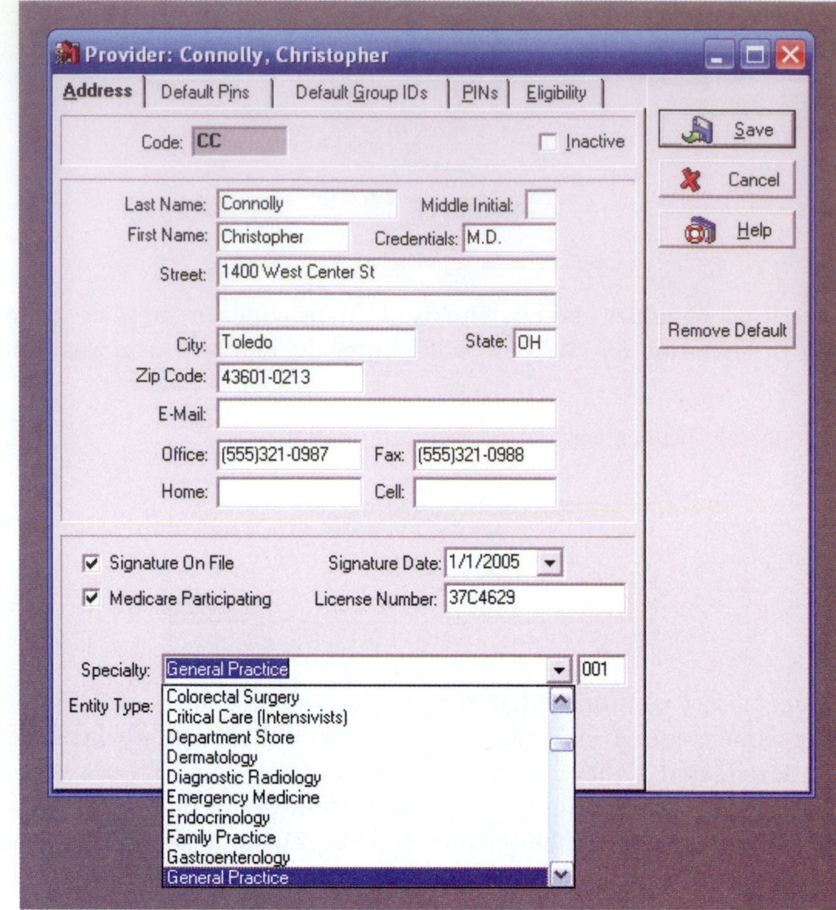

FIGURE 8.5 Example of Medisoft Screen for Taxonomy Code Selection

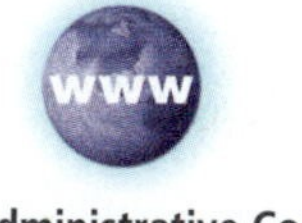

All Administrative Code Sets for HIPAA Transactions

http://www.wpc-edi.com/codes/codes/Codes.asp

Summary of Claim Information

Table 8.3 summarizes the information that is generally required for correct completion of the CMS-1500 claim.

TABLE 8.3 CMS-1500 Claim Completion

Item Number	Content
1	**Medicare, Medicaid, TRICARE/CHAMPUS, CHAMPVA, FECA Black Lung, Group Health Plan, or Other**: Enter t he type of insurance.
1a	**Insured's ID Number**: The insurance identification number that appears on the insurance card of the policyholder.
2	**Patient's Name**: As it appears on the insurance card.
3	**Patient's Birth Date/Sex**: Date of birth in eight-digit format; appropriate selection for male or female.
4	**Insured's Name**: The full name of the person who holds the insurance policy (the insured) if not the patient. If the patient is a dependent, the insured may be a spouse, parent, or other person.
5	**Patient's Address**: Address includes the number and street, city, state, Zip code, and telephone number.
6	**Patient's Relationship to Insured**: Self, spouse, child, or other. Self means that the patient is the policyholder.
7	**Insured's Address**: Address and telephone number of the insured person listed in IN 4 if not the same as the patient's address.
8	**Patient Status**: Marital status and employment status—employed, full-time student, or part-time student.

TABLE 8.3 CMS-1500 Claim Completion *continued*

Item Number	Content
9	**Other Insured's Name**: If there is additional insurance coverage, the insured's name.
9a	**Other Insured's Policy or Group Number**: The policy or group number of the other insurance plan.
9b	**Other Insured's Date of Birth**: Date of birth and sex of the other insured.
9c	**Employer's Name or School Name**: Other insured's employer or school.
9d	**Insurance Plan Name or Program Name**: Other insured's insurance plan or program name.
10a–10c	**Is Patient Condition Related to**: To indicate whether the patient's condition is the result of a work injury, an automobile accident, or another type of accident.
10d	**Reserved for Local Use**: Varies with the insurance plan.
11	**Insured's Policy Group or FECA Number**: As it appears on the insurance identification card.
11a	**Insured's Date of Birth/Sex**: The insured's date of birth and sex if the patient is not the insured.
11b	**Employer's Name or School Name**: Insured's employer or school.
11c	**Insurance Plan Name or Program Name**: Of the insured.
11d	**Is There Another Health Benefit Plan?** Yes if the patient is covered by additional insurance. If yes, IN 9a–9d must also be completed.
12	**Patient's or Authorized Person's Signature**: 12 Enter "Signature on File," "SOF," or a legal signature per practice policy.
13	**Insured or Authorized Person's Signature**: Enter "Signature on File," "SOF," or a legal signature to indicate that there is a signature on file assigning benefits to the provider.
14	**Date of Current Illness or Injury or Pregnancy**: The date that symptoms first began for the current illness, injury, or pregnancy. For pregnancy, enter the date of the patient's last menstrual period (LMP).
15	**If Patient Has Had Same or Similar Illness**: Date when the patient first consulted the provider for treatment of the same or a similar condition.
16	**Dates Patient Unable to Work in Current Occupation**: Dates the patient has been unable to work.
17	**Name of Referring Physician or Other Source**: Name of the physician or other source who referred the patient to the billing provider.
17a,b	**ID Number of Referring Physician**: Identifying number(s) for the referring physician.
18	**Hospitalization Dates Related to Current Services**: If the services provided are needed because of a related hospitalization, the admission and discharge dates are entered. For patients still hospitalized, the admission date is listed in the From box, and the To box is left blank.
19	**Reserved for Local Use**
20	**Outside Lab? $Charges**: Completed if billing for outside lab services.
21	**Diagnosis or Nature of Illness or Injury**: ICD-9-CM codes in priority order.
22	**Medicaid Resubmission**: Medicaid-specific.
23	**Prior Authorization Number**: If required by payer, report the assigned number.
24A	**Dates of Service**: Date(s) service was provided.
24B	**Place of Service**: A place of service (POS) code describes the location at which the service was provided.
24C	**EMG**: Payer-specific code.
24D	**Procedures, Services, or Supplies**: CPT and HCPCS codes and applicable modifiers for services provided.
24E	**Diagnosis Pointer**: Using the numbers (1, 2, 3, 4) listed to the left of the diagnosis codes in IN 21, enter the diagnosis for each service listed in IN 24D.
24F	**$ Charges**: For each service listed in IN 24D, enter charges without dollar signs and decimals.
24G	**Days or Units**: The number or days or units.
24H	**EPSDT Family Plan**: Medicaid-specific.
24I and 24J	**ID Qualifier** and **ID Numbers**.
25	**Federal Tax ID Number**: Physician's or supplier's Social Security number or Employer Identification Number (EIN).
26	**Patient's Account No.:** Patient account number used by the practice's accounting system.
27	**Accept Assignment?** If the physician accepts Medicare assignment, select Yes.
28	**Total Charge**: Total of all charges in IN 24F.
29	**Amount Paid**: Amount of the payments received for the services listed on this claim.
30	**Balance Due**: May be payer-specific; generally balance resulting from subtracting the amount in IN 29 from the amount in IN 28.
31	**Signature of Physician or Supplier Including Degrees or Credentials**: Provider's or supplier's signature, the date of the signature, and the provider's credentials (such as MD).
32	**Service Facility Location Information**: Complete if IN 20 is completed with the name, address, and ID numbers of place of service.
33	**Billing Provider Information**: Billing office name, address, Zip Code, and ID numbers.

Billing Tip

Follow Payer Guidelines
Always check with the payer for the claim to ensure correct completion.

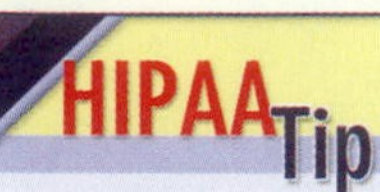

Physician Claims: The 837 P

The HIPAA transaction for electronic claims generated by physicians is called the HIPAA 837 P, with P standing for professional services. The hospital version of the claim is called 847 I, with I meaning

HIPAA Tip

X12 837 Health Care Claims or Equivalent Encounter Information/ Coordination of Benefits

The HIPAA Health Care Claims or Equivalent Encounter Information/ Coordination of Benefits transaction is also called the X12 837. It is used to send a claim to both the primary payer and a secondary payer.

Thinking It Through 8.2

1. A patient who had a minor automobile accident was treated in the emergency room and released. What place of service code is reported?
2. A supplier of durable medical equipment has a non-NPI number of A5FT for a Blue Cross and Blue Shield claim. What non-NPI qualifier should be reported?
3. If a physician practice uses a billing service to prepare and transmit its health care claims, which entity is the pay-to provider and which the billing provider?

Completing The HIPAA 837 Claim

Most of the information reported on the CMS-1500 is also used on the HIPAA 837 claim. Table 8.4 shows a comparison. When the HIPAA 837 electronic transaction was mandated, vendors upgraded their PMPs to reflect new requirements. PMP vendors are responsible for (1) keeping their software products up to date, (2) receiving certification from HIPAA testing vendors that their software can accommodate HIPAA-mandated transactions, and (3) training office personnel in the use of new features.

Most PMPs are set up to automatically supply the various items of information electronic claims need. Some different terms are in use with the HIPAA claim, though, and a few additional information items must be relayed to the payer. This section covers those items as it presents the basic organization of the HIPAA 837 claim. When working for physician practices, medical insurance specialists and billers learn the particular elements they need to supply as they process claims.

Claim Organization

The HIPAA 837 claim contains many **data elements**. Examples of data elements are a patient's first name, middle name or initial, and last name. Although these data elements are essentially the same as those used to complete a CMS-1500, they are organized in a different way. This organization is efficient for electronic transmission, rather than for use on a paper form.

The elements are transmitted in the five major sections, or levels, of the claim:

1. Provider
2. Subscriber (guarantor/insured/policyholder) and patient (the subscriber or another person)
3. Payer
4. Claim details
5. Services

The levels are set up as a hierarchy, with the provider at the top, so that when the claim is sent electronically, the only data elements that have to be sent are those that do not repeat previous data. For example, when the provider is sending a batch of claims, provider data is sent once for all of them. If the subscriber and the patient are the same, then the patient data is not needed. But if the subscriber and the patient are different people, information about both is transmitted.

There are four types of data elements:

1. *Required (R) data elements*: For **required data elements**, the provider must supply the data element on every claim, and payers must accept the data element.
2. *Required if applicable (RIA) data elements*: These **situational data elements** are conditional on specific situations. For example, if the insured differs from the patient, the insured's name must be entered.
3. *Not required unless specified under contract (NRUC)*: These elements are required only when they are part of a contract between a provider and a payer or when they are specified by state or federal legislation or regulations.
4. *Not required (NR)*: These elements are not required for submission and/or receipt of a claim or encounter.

Table 8.5 on pages 272–273 summarizes all the data elements that can be reported. Review this table after you have read this section.

Provider Information

Like the CMS-1500, the HIPAA 837 claim requires data on these types of providers, as applicable:

- Billing provider
- Pay-to provider
- Rendering provider
- Referring provider

For each provider, an NPI number and possibly non-NPI numbers with the qualifiers shown in Table 8.1 on page 249 are reported.

Subscriber Information

The HIPAA 837 uses the term subscriber for the insurance policyholder or guarantor, meaning the same as *insured* on the CMS-1500 claim. The subscriber may be the patient or someone else. If the subscriber and patient are not the same person, data elements about the patient are also required. The name and address of any **responsible party**—the entity or person other than the subscriber or patient who has financial responsibility for the bill—is reported if applicable.

Claim Filing Indicator Code

A **claim filing indicator code** is an administrative code used to identify the type of health plan, such as a PPO. One of the claim filing indicator codes shown in Table 8.6 on page 264 is reported. These codes are valid until a National Payer ID system is made into law.

Relationship of Patient to Subscriber

The HIPAA 837 claim allows for a more detailed description of the relationship of the patient to the subscriber. When the patient and the subscriber are not the same person, an **individual relationship code** is required to specify the patient's relationship to the subscriber. The current list of choices is shown in Table 8.7 on page 265.

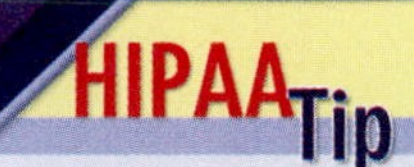

Verifying and Updating Information About Subscribers and Patients

The HIPAA Eligibility for a Health Plan transaction (the provider's inquiry and the payer's response) is used to verify insurance coverage and eligibility for benefits, as noted in Chapter 3. If that transaction turns up new or different information, the changes are correctly posted in the practice management

HIPAA Tip

HIPAA National Plan Identifier

Under HIPAA, the Department of Health and Human Services must adopt a standard health plan identifier system. Each plan's number will be its National Payer ID. The number is also called the National Health Plan ID.

TABLE 8.4 Crosswalk of the CMS 1500 (08/05) to the HIPAA 837P

CMS Item Number		837 Data Element
Carrier Block	Name and Address of Payer	
1	Insurance Plan/Program	Claim Filing Indicator
1a	Insured's ID Number	Subscriber Primary Identifier
2	Patient Last Name	Patient Last Name
	Patient First Name	Patient First Name
	Patient Middle Name	Patient Middle Initial
		Patient Name Suffix
3	Patient Birth Date	Patient Birth Date
	Sex	Patient Gender code
4	Insured Last Name	Subscriber Last Name
	Insured First Name	Subscriber First Name
	Insured Middle Initial	Subscriber Middle Name
		Subscriber Name Suffix
5	Patient's Address	Patient Address Lines 1, 2
	City	Patient City Name
	State	Patient State Code
	Zip Code	Patient Zip Code
	Telephone	NOT USED
6	Patient Relationship to Insured: Self, Spouse, Child, Other	Code for Patient's Relationship to Subscriber
7	Insured's Address	Subscriber Address Lines 1, 2
	City	Subscriber City Name
	State	Subscriber State Code
	Zip Code	Subscriber Zip Code
	Telephone	NOT USED
8	Patient Status	NOT USED
9	Other Insured Last Name	Other Subscriber Last Name
	Other Insured First Name	Other Subscriber First Name
	Other Insured Middle Initial	Other Subscriber Middle Name
		Other Subscriber Name Suffix
9a	Other Insured Policy or Group number	Other Subscriber Primary Identification
9b	Other Insured Date of Birth	Other Insured Date of Birth
	Sex	Other Insured Gender code
9c	Employer's Name or School Name	NOT USED
9d	Insurance Plan Name or Program Name	Other Payer Organization Name
10	Is Patient's Condition Related To:	Related causes information
10a	Employment (current or previous)	Related causes code
10b	Auto Accident	Related causes code
10b	Place (state)	Auto accident state or province code
10c	Other Accident	Related causes code
11	Insured Policy Group or FECA number	
11a	Insured Date of Birth	Subscriber Date of Birth
	Sex	Subscriber Gender code
11b	Employer's name or school name	NOT USED
11c	Insurance plan name or program name	Payer Name
11d	Is there another health benefit plan	Entity identifier code

TABLE 8.4 Crosswalk of the CMS 1500 (08/05) to the HIPAA 837P *continued*

CMS Item Number		837 Data Element
12	Patient's or authorized person's signature (and date)	Release of Information Code
		Patient signature source code
13	Insured's or authorized person's signature	Benefits assignment Certification indicator
14	Date of Current: Illness, Injury, Pregnancy (LMP)	Initial treatment date
		Accident/LMP Date
		Last menstrual period
15	If patient has had same or similar illness, give first date	Similar Illness or Symptom Date
16	Dates patient unable to work in current occupation From/To	Disability From/To Dates
17	Name of Referring Provider or Other Source	Referring Provider Last Name/First Name or Organization
17a/b	ID/NPI of referring physician	Referring Provider NPI
18	Hospitalization dates related to current services From/To	Admission Date/Discharge Date
19	Reserved for local use	
20	Outside Lab? $ Charges	
21	Diagnosis or nature of illness or injury, ICD-9-CM Codes 1 through 4	ICD-9-CM Codes 1 through 8
22	Medicaid resubmission code/Ref. No.	NOT USED
23	Prior Authorization Number	Prior Authorization Number
24A	Dates of Service (From/To MM DD YY)	Order date
24B	Place of Service (Code)	Place of Service Code
24C	EMG	Emergency Indicator
24D	Procedures, services, or supplies CPT/HCPCS and Modifiers	Procedure Codes/Modifiers
24E	Diagnosis Pointers	Diagnosis Code Pointers
24F	$ Charges	Line Item Charge Amount
24G	Days or units	Service Unit Count
24H	EPSDT/Family Plan	Special Program Indicator
24I	ID Qualifier	Identification Code Qualifier
24J	Rendering Provider ID#	NPI/NonNPI ID No.
25	Federal Tax ID Number	Pay-to Provider ID Code and Qualifier
26	Patient's Account No.	Patient Account Number
27	Accept Assignment?	Medicare Assignment Code
28	Total Charge	Total Claim Charge Amount
29	Amount Paid	Patient Paid Amount
30	Balance Due	NOT USED
31	Signature of Physician or supplier (Signed)/Date	NOT USED
32	Service Facility Location Information	Laboratory or Facility Information
33	Billing Provider Info & PH#, NPI/ID (If Not Same as Rendering Provider)	Billing Provider Last/First or Organizational Name, Address, NPI/NonNPI ID (If Not Same as Rendering Provider)

Billing Tip

NR Data Elements
In the category of not required are a number of Item Numbers from the CMS-1500 that are not needed on the HIPAA 837 claim. Following is a partial list:

- Patient's/insured telephone number(s)
- Patient's employment or student status
- Insured's marital status and gender
- Employer's or school name
- Balance due
- Physician's signature

Billing Tip

Rejection of Claims Missing Required Elements
Under HIPAA, failure to transmit required data elements can cause a claim to be rejected by the payer.

Compliance Guideline

Correct Code Sets
The correct medical code sets are those valid at the time the health care is provided. The correct administrative code sets are those valid at the time the transaction—such as the claim—is started.

Billing Tip

Billing Provider Name and Telephone Number
Note that a billing provider contact name and telephone number are required data elements.

TABLE 8.6 Claim Filing Indicator Codes

Code	Definition
09	Self-pay
10	Central certification
11	Other nonfederal programs
12	Preferred provider organization (PPO)
13	Point of service (POS)
14	Exclusive provider organization (EPO)
15	Indemnity insurance
16	Health maintenance organization (HMO) Medicare risk plan
AM	Automobile medical
BL	Blue Cross and Blue Shield
CH	CHAMPUS (TRICARE)
CI	Commercial insurance company
DS	Disability
HM	Health maintenance organization
LI	Liability
LM	Liability medical
MB	Medicare Part B
MC	Medicaid
OF	Other federal program
TV	Title V
VA	Department of Veteran's Affairs plan
WC	Workers' compensation health claim
ZZ	Unknown

Billing Tip

Patient Relationship to Insured
Patient information forms and electronic medical records should record the relationship of the patient to the insured according to HIPAA categories, so that this data can be included on the HIPAA 837 claim.

Billing Tip

Patient Address
The patient's address is a required data element, so, "Unknown" should be entered if the address is not known.

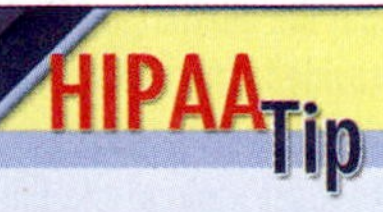

Coordination of Benefits

The 837 claim transaction is also used to send data elements regarding coordination of benefits to other payers on the claim.

Other Data Elements

These situational data elements are required if another payer is known to potentially be involved in paying the claim:

- Other Subscriber Birth Date
- Other Subscriber Gender Code (F [female], M [male], or U [unknown])
- Other Subscriber Address

Patient-specific information may be reported in certain circumstances, such as:

- Patient Death Date (required when the patient is known to be deceased and the provider knows the date on which the patient died)
- Weight
- Pregnancy Indicator Code (Y [yes] required for a pregnant patient when mandated by law)

Payer Information

This section contains information about the payer to whom the claim is going to be sent, called the **destination payer**. A payer responsibility sequence number code identifies whether the insurance carrier is the primary (P), secondary (S), or tertiary (T) payer. This code is used when more than one insurance plan is responsible for payment. The T code is used for the payer

TABLE 8.7 Relationship Codes

Code	Definition
01	Spouse
04	Grandfather or grandmother
05	Grandson or granddaughter
07	Nephew or niece
09	Adopted child
10	Foster child
15	Ward
17	Stepson or stepdaughter
19	Child
20	Employee
21	Unknown
22	Handicapped dependent
23	Sponsored dependent
24	Dependent of a minor dependent
29	Significant other
32	Mother
33	Father
34	Other adult
36	Emancipated minor
39	Organ donor
40	Cadaver donor
41	Injured plaintiff
43	Child where insured has no financial responsibility
53	Life partner
G8	Other relationship

of last resort, such as Medicaid (see Chapter 11 for an explanation of "payer of last resort").

Claim Information

The claim information section reports information related to the particular claim. For example, if the patient's visit is the result of an accident, a description of the accident is included. Data elements about the rendering provider—if not the same as the billing provider or the pay-to provider—are supplied. If another provider referred the patient for care, the claim includes data elements about the referring physician or primary care physician (PCP).

Claim Control Number

A **claim control number**, unique for each claim, is assigned by the sender. The maximum number of characters is twenty. The claim control number will appear on payments that come from payers (see Chapter 14), so it is important for tracking purposes.

Billing Tip

Assigning a Claim Control Number
Although sometimes called the patient account number, the claim control number should not be the same as the practice's account number for the patient. It may, however, incorporate the account number. For example, if the account number is A1234, a three-digit number might be added for each claim, beginning with A1234001.

Billing Tip

Mammography Claims
The mammography certification number is required when mammography services are rendered by a certified mammography provider.

Claim Frequency Code

The **claim frequency code**, also called the **claim submission reason code**, for physician practice claims indicates whether this claim is one of the following:

Code	Definition
1	*Original claim*: The initial claim sent for the patient on the date of service for the procedure
7	*Replacement of prior claim*: Used if an original claim is being replaced with a new claim
8	*Void/cancel of prior claim*: Used to completely eliminate a submitted claim

The first claim is always a 1. Payers do not usually allow for corrections to be sent after a claim has been submitted; instead, an entire new claim is transmitted. However, some payers cannot process a claim with the frequency code 7 (replace a submitted claim). In this situation, submit a void/cancel of prior claim (frequency code 8) to cancel the original incorrect claim, and then submit a new, correct claim.

When a claim is replaced, the original claim number (Claim Original Reference Number) is reported.

Billing Tip

Podiatric, Physical Therapy, and Occupational Therapy Claims
The last-seen date must be reported when (1) a claim involves an independent physical therapist's or occupational therapist's services or a physician's services involving routine foot care, and (2) the timing and/or frequency of visits affects payment for services.

Billing Tip

Accident Claims
If the reported services are a result of an accident, the claim allows entries for the date and time of the accident; whether it is an auto accident, an accident caused by another party, an employment-related accident, or another type of accident; and the state or country in which the accident occurred.

HIPAA Tip

PHI On Attachments

A payer should receive only data needed to process the claim in question. If an attachment has PHI related to another patient, those data must be marked over or deleted. Information about other dates of service or conditions not pertinent to the claim should also be crossed through or deleted.

Diagnosis Codes

The HIPAA 837 permits up to eight ICD-9-CM codes to be reported. The order of entry is not regulated. Each diagnosis code must be directly related to the patient's treatment. Up to four of these codes can be linked to each procedure code that is reported.

Claim Note

A claim note may be used when a statement needs to be included, such as to satisfy a state requirement or to provide details about a patient's medical treatment that are not reported elsewhere in the claim.

Service Line Information

The HIPAA 837 has the same elements as the CMS-1500 at the service line level. Different information for a particular service line, such as a prior authorization number that applies only to that service, can be supplied at the service line level.

Diagnosis Code Pointers

A total of four diagnosis codes can be linked to each service line procedure. At least one diagnosis code must be linked to the procedure code. Codes two, three, and four may also be linked, in declining level of importance regarding the patient's treatment, to the service line.

Line Item Control Number

A line item control number is a unique number assigned to each service line by the sender. Like the claim control number, it is used to track payments from the insurance carrier, but for a particular service rather than for the entire claim.

Claim Attachments

A **claim attachment** is additional data in printed or electronic format sent to support a claim. Examples include lab results, specialty consultation notes, and discharge notes. A HIPAA transaction standard for electronic health care claim attachments is under development. When it is adopted, payers will be required to accept all attachments that are submitted by providers according to the standard. Until then, health plans can require providers to submit claim attachments in the format they specify.

Credit–Debit Information

Most practices accept credit or debit cards for payment. (Note that this payment option is currently prohibited for some federal health plans such as Medicaid and TRICARE.) A credit or debit card may be used to arrange for paying the patient or subscriber portion of a claim when that amount is not known at the time of service. In this case, the card owner authorizes payment via a consent form for a future charge up to a maximum amount, allowing the provider to bill the credit card after the claim has been adjudicated and the amount due from the patient is known. When this option is used, the amount charged to the card is reported to its owner once billed.

Billing Tip

Specialty Claim Service Line Information
Claims for various payers require additional data elements. These include Medicare claims (Chapter 10), EPSDT/Medicaid claims (Chapter 11), and workers' compensation and disability claims (Chapter 13).

Clearinghouses And Claim Transmission

Claims are prepared for transmission after all required data elements have been posted to the practice management software program. The data elements that are transmitted are not seen physically, as they would be on a paper form. Instead, these elements are in a computer file. The typical flow of a claim ready for transmission is shown in Figure 8.6 on page 268. Note that in some cases both the sender and the receiver have clearinghouses, so the provider's clearinghouse transmits to the payer's clearinghouse.

Checking Claims

An important step comes before claim transmittal—checking the claim. Most PMPs provide a way for the medical insurance specialist to review claims for accuracy and to create a record of claims that are about to be sent. For example, Medisoft has a claim editing function. (See Figure 8.7 on page 269, which shows the screen that medical insurance specialists use to check and edit a claim.)

HIPAA Tip

X12 276/277 Health Care Claim Status Inquiry/Response

The HIPAA X12 276/277 Health Care Claim Status Inquiry/Response transaction is the electronic format used by practices to ask payers about the status of claims. It has two parts: an inquiry and a response. It is also called the X12 276/277. The number 276 refers to the inquiry transaction, and 277 refers to the response that the payer returns.

Thinking It Through 8.3

1. **A retiree is covered by his wife's insurance policy. His wife is still working and receives health benefits through her employer, which has a PPO plan.**
   - **A.** What code describes the spouse's relationship to the subscriber?
   - **B.** What claim filing indicator code is reported?
   - **C.** What claim filing indicator code is likely to be used if the insurance is TRICARE?
2. **What type of code would show whether a claim is the original claim, a replacement, or being cancelled?**

Billing Tip

Functional Acknowledgement 997
The EDI term for the acknowledgement of a file transmission is the 997. This is not a standard HIPAA transaction, but is used with the HIPAA transaction to report that it has been received by the payer.

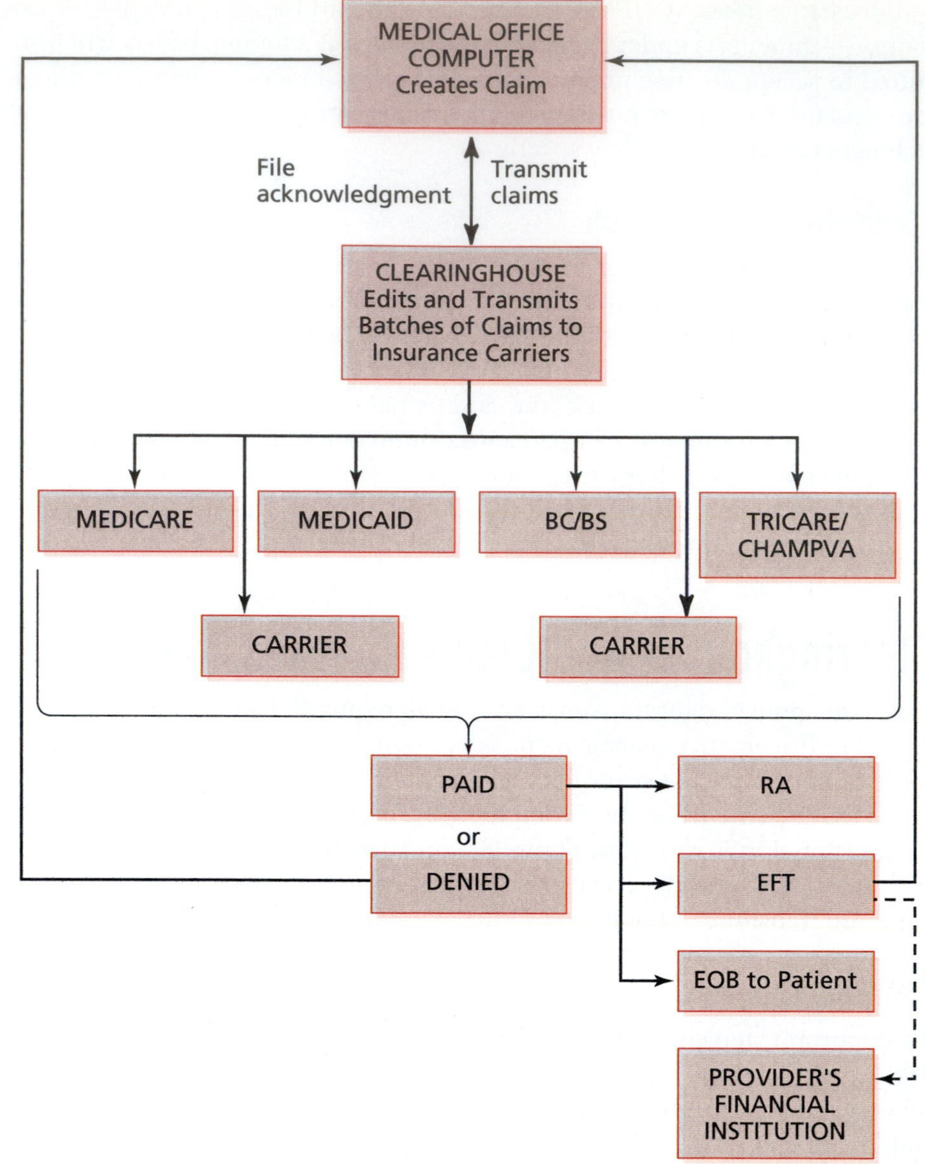

FIGURE 8.6 Claim Flow Using a Clearinghouse

Compliance Guideline

Disclosing Information for Payment Purposes
Under HIPAA, covered entities such as physician practices may disclose patients' PHI for payment purposes. For example, a provider may disclose a patient's name to a financial institution in order to cash a check or to a clearinghouse to initiate electronic transactions.

Transmitting Claims

Practices handle transmission of electronic claims—which may be called electronic media claims, or EMC—in a variety of ways. By far the most common method is to hire outside vendors—clearinghouses—to handle this task. The outside vendor is a business associate under HIPAA (see Chapter 2) that must follow the practice's guidelines to ensure that patients' PHI remains secure and private.

There are three major methods of transmitting claims electronically: direct transmission to the payer, clearinghouse use, and direct data entry.

Transmit Claims Directly

In the direct transmission approach, providers and payers exchange transactions directly without using a clearinghouse. To do this requires special technology. The provider must supply all the HIPAA data elements and follow specific EDI formatting rules.

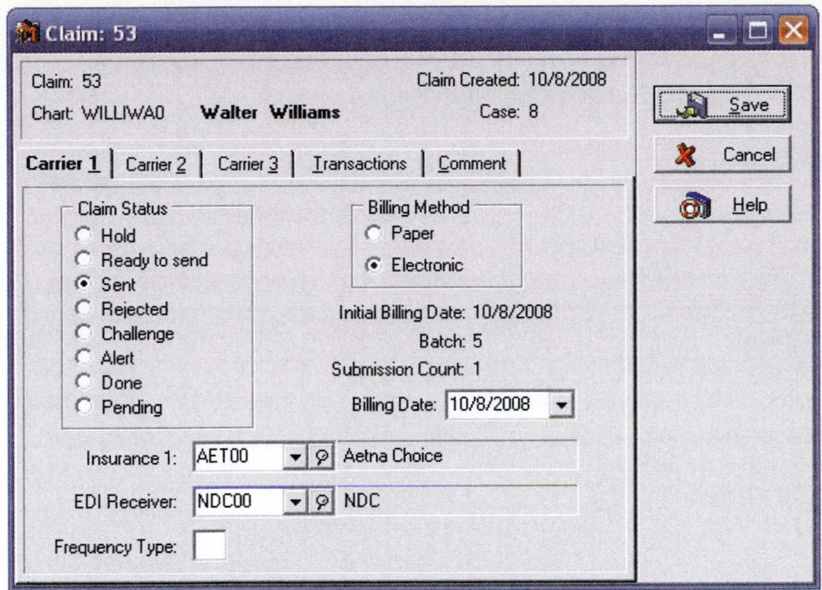

FIGURE 8.7 Example of Medisoft Claim Edit Screen

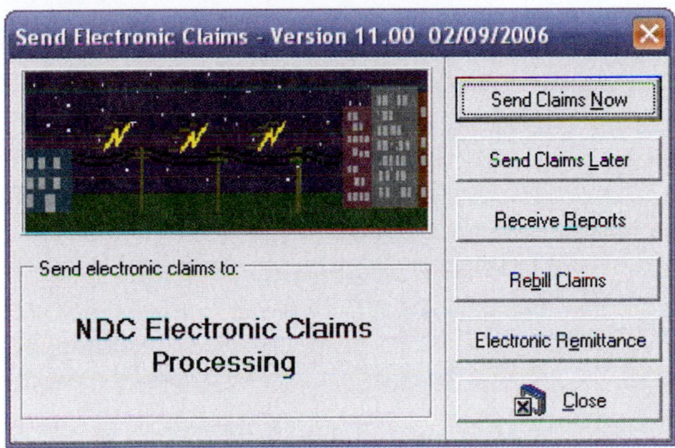

FIGURE 8.8 Example of Medisoft Screen for Claim Transmission

Use a Clearinghouse

The majority of providers use clearinghouses to send and receive data in correct EDI format (see Figure 8.8). Under HIPAA, clearinghouses can accept nonstandard formats and translate them into the standard format. Clearinghouses must receive all required data elements from providers; they cannot create or modify data content. After a PMP-created file is sent, the clearinghouse correlates, or "maps," the content of each Item Number or data element to the HIPAA 837 transaction based on the payer's instructions.

A practice may choose to use a clearinghouse to transmit all claims, or it may use a combination of direct transmission and a clearinghouse. For example, it may send claims directly to Medicare, Medicaid, and a few other major commercial payers and use a clearinghouse to send claims to other payers.

When the PMP has sent the claims, a verification report such as that shown in Figure 8.9 on page 270 provides a summary of what was sent. Later, the receiver will send back an electronic response showing that the transmission was received (see Chapter 14).

Billing Tip

Clearinghouses
There are many electronic claims and transaction processing firms in the health care industry. Two of the largest are NDC Health and Emdeon. Other firms include Navicure, ProxyMed, Medifax-EDI, MedUnite, and Electronic Network Systems.

Valley Associates, P.C.

EMC Verification

EMC Batch Verification Report

Filename: C:\MediData\MI\EMC\ndcreq.dat
Chart Number Range: ALL
Date Created Range: ALL

Billing Code Range: ALL
Provider: ALL
Insurance Carrier Range: ALL

Claim#	Chart#	Patient Name	Policy#	Group#	Referring Provider	Facility
	Date From	Proc. Code	Modifiers	Pos Tos Units	Diagnoses	Amount

Provider: Christopher Connolly (CC)

Claim#	Chart#	Patient Name	Policy#	Group#	Referring Provider	Facility
53	WILLIWA0	Walter Williams	ABC103562239	BDC1001	Not Found	Not Found

Primary Carrier: Aetna Choice (AET00)
Diagnoses: 1: 401.1 Benign Essential Hypertension
2: 780.7 Fatigue

Date From	Proc. Code	Modifiers	Pos	Tos	Units	Diagnoses	Amount
10/01/2008	99212		11	1	1	Diagnosis: 1, 2	$46.00
10/01/2008	93000		11	1	1	Diagnosis: 1, 2	$70.00
						Claim 53 Total:	$116.00

Claim#	Chart#	Patient Name	Policy#	Group#	Referring Provider	Facility
52	PEREZCA0	Carmen Perez	140603312X		Not Found	Not Found

Primary Carrier: Cigna HMO Plus (CIG00)
Diagnoses: 1: 493.00 Extrinsic Asthma

Date From	Proc. Code	Modifiers	Pos	Tos	Units	Diagnoses	Amount
10/01/2008	99213		11	1	1	Diagnosis: 1	$62.00
						Claim 52 Total:	$62.00

Claim#	Chart#	Patient Name	Policy#	Group#	Referring Provider	Facility
48	PORCEJE0	Jennifer Porcelli	7123408080X	G0119	Not Found	Not Found

Primary Carrier: Oxford Freedom (OXF00)
Diagnoses: 1: 465.9 Upper Respiratory Infection

Date From	Proc. Code	Modifiers	Pos	Tos	Units	Diagnoses	Amount
10/13/2008	99212		11	1	1	Diagnosis: 1	$46.00
10/13/2008	87081		11	1	1	Diagnosis: 1	$30.00
						Claim 48 Total:	$76.00

Provider Christopher Connolly (CC) Total: $254.00

Total Transaction(s): 5
Total Claim(s): 3

Batch Total: $254.00

FIGURE 8.9 Example of Medisoft EMC Verification Report

Use Direct Data Entry (DDE)

Some payers offer online direct data entry (DDE) to providers. DDE involves using an Internet-based service into which employees key the standard data elements. Although the data elements must meet the HIPAA standards regarding content, they do not have to be formatted for standard EDI. Instead, they are loaded directly into the health plans' computers.

Clean Claims

Although health care claims require many data elements and are complex, it is often the simple errors that keep practices from generating **clean claims**—that is, claims that are accepted for adjudication by payers. Following are common errors:

- Missing or incomplete service facility name, address, and identification for services rendered outside the office or home. This includes invalid Zip codes or state abbreviations.
- Missing Medicare assignment indicator or benefits assignment indicator.
- Invalid provider identifier (when present) for rendering provider, referring provider, or others.
- Missing part of the name or the identifier of the referring provider.
- Missing or invalid patient birth date.
- Missing payer name and/or payer identifier, required for both primary and secondary payers.
- Incomplete other payer information. This is required in all secondary claims and all primary claims that will involve a secondary payer.
- Invalid procedure codes.

Billing Tip

"Dropping to Paper"
"Dropping to paper" describes a situation in which a CMS-1500 paper claim needs to be printed and sent to a payer. Some practices, for instance, have a policy of doing this when a claim has been transmitted electronically twice but receipt is not acknowledged.

Data Entry Tips

Following are tips for entering data:

- Do not use prefixes for people's names, such as Mr., Ms., or Dr.
- Unless required by a particular insurance carrier, do not use special characters such as dashes, hyphens, commas, or apostrophes.
- Use only valid data in all fields; avoid words such as *same*.
- Do not use a dash, space, or special character in a Zip code field.
- Do not use hyphens, dashes, spaces, special characters, or parentheses in telephone numbers.
- Most billing programs or claim transmission programs automatically reformat data such as dates as required by the claim format.

Check with payers for exceptions to these guidelines.

Billing Tip

Editing
Editing software programs called claim scrubbers make sure that all required fields are filled, make sure that only valid codes are used, and perform other checks. Some providers use clearinghouses for editing, and others use claim scrubbers in their billing department before they send claims.

Table 8.5 HIPAA Claim Data Elements

PROVIDER, SUBSCRIBER, PATIENT, PAYER

Billing Provider

- Last or Organization Name
  - First Name
  - Middle Name
  - Name Suffix
- Primary Identifier: NPI
- Address 1
- Address 2
- City Name
- State/Province Code
- Zip Code
- Country Code
- Secondary Identifiers, such as State License Number
- Contact Name
- Communication Numbers
  - Telephone Number
  - Fax
  - E-mail
  - Telephone Extension
- Taxonomy Code
- Currency Code

Pay-to Provider

- Last or Organization Name
  - First Name
  - Middle Name
  - Name Suffix
- Primary Identifier: NPI
- Address 1
- Address 2
- City Name
- State/Province Code
- Zip Code
- Country Code
- Secondary Identifiers, such as State License Number
- Taxonomy Code

Subscriber

- Insured Group or Policy Number
- Group or Plan Name
- Insurance Type Code
- Claim Filing Indicator Code
- Last Name
- First Name
- Middle Name
- Name Suffix
- Primary Identifier
  - Member Identification Number
  - National Individual Identifier
  - IHS/CHS Tribe Residency Code
- Secondary Identifiers
  - HIS Health Record Number
  - Insurance Policy Number
  - SSN
- Patient's Relationship to Subscriber
- Other Subscriber Information
- Birth Date
- Gender Code
- Address Line 1
- Address Line 2
- City Name
- State/Province Code
- Zip Code
- Country Code

Patient

- Last Name
- First Name
- Middle Name
- Name Suffix
- Primary Identifier
  - Member ID Number
  - National Individual Identifier
- Address 1
- Address 2
- City Name
- State/Province Code
- Zip Code
- Country Code
- Birth Date
- Gender Code
- Secondary Identifiers
  - IHS Health Record Number
  - Insurance Policy Number
  - SSN
- Death Date
- Weight
- Pregnancy Indicator

Responsible Party

- Last or Organization Name
- First Name
- Middle Name
- Suffix Name
- Address 1
- Address 2
- City Name
- State/Province Code
- Zip Code
- Country Code

Payer

- Payer Responsibility Sequence Number Code
- Organization Name
- Primary Identifier
  - Payer ID
  - National Plan ID
- Address 1
- Address 2
- City Name
- State/Province Code
- Zip Code
- Secondary Identifiers
  - Claim Office Number
  - NAIC Code
  - TIN
- Assignment of Benefits
- Release of Information Code
- Patient Signature Source Code
- Referral Number
- Prior Authorization Number

Table 8.5 HIPAA Claim Data Elements *continued*

CLAIM

Claim Level

Claim Control Number (Patient Account Number)
Total Submitted Charges
Place of Service Code
Claim Frequency Code
Provider Signature on File
Medicare Assignment Code
Participation Agreement
Delay Reason Code
Onset of Current Symptoms or Illness Date
Similar Illness/Symptom Onset Date
Last Menstrual Period Date
Admission Date
Discharge Date
Patient Amount Paid
Claim Original Reference Number
Investigational Device Exemption Number
Medical Record Number
Note Reference Code
Claim Note
Diagnosis Code 1–8
Accident Claims
- Accident Cause
  - Auto Accident
  - Another Party Responsible
  - Employment Related
  - Other Accident
- Auto Accident State/Province Code
- Auto Accident Country Code
- Accident Date
- Accident Hour

Rendering Provider

Last or Organization Name
First Name
Middle Name
Name Suffix
Primary Identifier: NPI
Taxonomy Code
Secondary Identifiers

Referring/PCP Providers

Last or Organization Name
First Name
Middle Name
Name Suffix
Primary Identifier: NPI
Taxonomy Code
Secondary Identifiers
Proc

Service Facility Location

Type Code
Last or Organization Name
Primary Identifier: NPI
Address 1
Address 2
City Name
State/Province Code
Zip Code
Country Code
Secondary Identifiers

SERVICE LINE INFORMATION

Procedure Type Code
Procedure Code
Modifiers 1–4
Line Item Charge Amount
Units of Service/Anesthesia Minutes
Place of Service Code
Diagnosis Code Pointers 1–4
Emergency Indicator
Copay Status Code
Service Date Begun
Service Date End
Shipped Date
Onset Date
Similar Illness or Symptom Date
Referral/Prior Authorization Number
Line Item Control Number
Ambulatory Patient Group
Sales Tax Amount
Postage Claimed Amount
Line Note Text
Rendering/Referring/PCP Provider at the Service Line Level
Service Facility Location at the Service Line Level

Review

Steps to Success

- ❒ Read this chapter and review the Key Terms and the Chapter Summary.
- ❒ Answer the Review Questions and Applying Your Knowledge in the Chapter Review.
- ❒ Access the chapter's websites and complete the Internet Activities to learn more about available professional resources.
- ❒ Complete the related chapter in the *Medical Insurance Workbook* to reinforce your understanding of health care claim preparation and transmission.

Chapter Summary

1. The upper portion of the CMS-1500 claim form (Item Numbers 1–13) lists demographic information about the patient and specific information about the patient's insurance coverage.
2. The lower portion of the CMS-1500 claim form (Item Numbers 14–33) contains information about the provider or supplier and the patient's condition, including the diagnoses, procedures, and charges.
3. The information needed to complete claims is gathered from the practice management program's databases. First, data about the patient, guarantor (subscriber), insurance coverage, and demographics are entered based on the patient information form, insurance card, and payer verification data. After the patient's visit, the transactions—the charges and payments—are entered as detailed on the encounter form. The PMP combines the elements from its relevant databases and prepares the claim that has been specified, either the HIPAA claim (837) or a paper claim (CMS-1500 08/05). Any missing elements and information are added during the claim editing process.
4. Required data elements must be provided on the claim and accepted by a payer; situational elements must be provided under certain conditions.
5. The HIPAA 837 claim transaction has five major sections: (a) provider, (b) subscriber/patient, (c) payer, (d) claim information, and (e) services. Most of the information from the practice management program that is gathered for CMS-1500 claims is included on the HIPAA 837. Additional data elements include claim filing indicator code, individual relationship code, claim control number, claim submission reason code, and line item control number.
6. The billing provider is the entity that is transmitting the claim to the payer, usually a billing service or a clearinghouse. The pay-to provider receives the payment from the insurance carrier. A rendering provider is a physician who provides the patient's treatment but is not the pay-to provider. A referring/ordering provider has sent the patient for treatment.
7. A claim control number is a unique number given to each claim to track the claim's payments. A line item control number is another unique number assigned to each service line. Like the claim control number, it is used to track payments from the insurance carrier, but for a particular service rather than for the entire claim.
8. Clearinghouses, which are business associates of covered entities under HIPAA and must therefore adhere to proper practices for privacy and security of PHI, help providers and payers communicate using HIPAA transactions. They take nonstandard EDI communications and convert them to HIPAA-standard communications.
9. Claim attachments may be electronic or paper. A claim attachment number is assigned, and the type of attachment is reported with a code. Patient credit–debit information for future payment of the amount due after the carrier pays can also be reported using the health care claim transaction.

10. Three methods for claim transmittal are (a) direct transmission, in which the claim is sent by EDI directly to the payer's computer system, (b) via a clearinghouse that transmits the data file to the payer in correct format, and (c) direct data entry, in which the provider keys data elements directly into the payer's computer system, rather than transmitting them via EDI.

Review Questions

Match the key terms with their definitions.

A. billing provider	____ 1. Unique number assigned by the sender to a claim
B. claim control number	____ 2. Unique number assigned by the sender to each service line on a claim
C. destination payer	____ 3. Software used to check claims
D. line item control number	____ 4. Stands for the type of provider specialty
	____ 5. Entity providing patient care for this claim if other than the billing/pay-to provider
E. pay-to provider	____ 6. Entity that is to receive payment for the claim
F. POS code	____ 7. Stands for the type of facility in which services reported on the claim were provided
G. claim scrubber	____ 8. Insurance carrier that is to receive the claim
H. rendering provider	____ 9. Entity that is sending the claim to the payer
I. subscriber	____ 10. The insurance policyholder or guarantor for the claim
J. taxonomy code	

Decide whether each statement is true or false.

____ 1. When a claim is created, the medical insurance specialist enters information about the charges and payments for a patient's visit.

____ 2. The five major sections of the HIPAA claim are provider, patient, payer, history, and services.

____ 3. Some data elements are always required on a claim, such as the patient's full name, address, date of birth, and gender.

____ 4. The billing provider and the rendering provider are usually the same person or organization.

____ 5. If the services reported on a claim involve a preauthorization, the preauthorization number should be reported.

____ 6. Claim control number, place of service code, and total submitted charges are data elements reported in the claim-level section of the HIPAA claim.

____ 7. Neither diagnosis codes nor procedure codes are required data elements.

____ 8. Claim attachments can be submitted in paper or electronic form.

____ 9. HIPAA standards require the use of NPIs for providers, when available.

____ 10. Many items of information are common to CMS-1500 and HIPAA 837 claims.

Select the letter that best completes the statement or answers the question.

____ 1. The NPI is used to report the ____ on a claim.
   A. provider identifier
   B. patient identifier
   C. payer identifier
   D. employer identifier

_____ 2. On HIPAA claims, a required data element
   A. is optional
   B. must be supplied
   C. is entered in capital letters
   D. none of the above

_____ 3. The HIPAA X12 276/277 Health Care Claim Status Inquiry/Response transaction is used to
   A. transmit claims
   B. transmit claim attachments
   C. ask about the status of claims that have been transmitted
   D. transmit paper claims

_____ 4. How many diagnosis code pointers can be assigned to a procedure code?
   A. one
   B. two
   C. three
   D. four

_____ 5. The content of claims and the taxonomy codes are set by
   A. HIPAA
   B. NUCC
   C. ICD-9-CM
   D. CPT/HCPCS

_____ 6. The number of the HIPAA claim transaction is
   A. CMS-1500
   B. HCFA-1500
   C. X12 837
   D. X12 834

_____ 7. If a physician practice sends claims directly to a payer, which of these entities is *not* additionally reported?
   A. referring provider
   B. rendering provider
   C. billing provider
   D. pay-to provider

_____ 8. The POS code for a military treatment facility is
   A. 12
   B. 26
   C. 42
   D. 72

_____ 9. Which of the following may be the same person as the patient?
   A. referring provider
   B. subscriber
   C. pay-to provider
   D. destination payer

_____ 10. Which of the following is *not* a commonly used transmission method for HIPAA claims?
   A. fax
   B. direct data entry
   C. direct transmission
   D. clearinghouse

Answer following questions.

1. List the five major sections of the HIPAA claim.
   A. ______________________________
   B. ______________________________
   C. ______________________________
   D. ______________________________
   E. ______________________________
2. Define these abbreviations:
   A. EMG ______________________________
   B. POS ______________________________
   C. NUCC ______________________________
   D. DDE ______________________________

Applying Your Knowledge

Case 8.1 Calculating Insurance Math

In order to complete the service line information on claims when units of measure are involved, insurance math is required. For example, this is the HCPCS description for an injection of the drug Eloxatin:

J9263 oxaliplatain, 0.5 mg

If the physician provided 50-mg infusion of the drug, instead of an injection, the service line is

J9263 X100

to report a unit of 50 (100 × .05 mg = 50). What is the unit reported for service line information if a 150-mg infusion is provided?

Abstracting Insurance Information

In the cases that follow, you play the role of a medical insurance specialist who is preparing HIPAA claims for transmission. Assume that you are working with the practice's PMP to enter the transactions. The information you enter is based on the patient information form and the encounter form.

- Claim control numbers are created by adding the eight-digit date to the patient account number, as in PORCEJE0-01012008.
- A copayment of $15 is collected from each Oxford PPO patient at the time of the visit. A copayment of $10 is collected for Oxford HMO.

Note: For these case studies, do not subtract the copayment from the charges; the payer's allowed fees have already been reduced by the amount of the copayment.

- The practice uses NDC as its clearinghouse to transmit claims.
- The necessary data for the payer and the clearinghouse are stored in the program's databases.

Provider Information

Practice Name	Valley Associates, PC
Address	1400 West Center Street Toledo, OH 43601-0213
Employer ID Number	16-1234567
National Provider Identifier	876-039-9261
Oxford PPO Provider Number	1011
Oxford HMO Provider Number	2567
Physician Name	Christopher M. Connolly, MD
Medicare	Accepts Assignment
Physician Signature	On File

Answer the questions that follow each case.

Case 8.2 From the Patient Information Form:

Name	Jennifer Porcelli
Sex	Female
Birth Date	07/05/1965
Address	310 Sussex Turnpike Shaker Heights, OH 44118-2345
Employer	24/7 Inc.
SSN	712-34-0808
Insurance Policy Group Number	G0119
Insurance Plan/ Program Name	Oxford Freedom PPO
Member ID	712340808X
Assignment of Benefits	Y
Signature on File	Y
Encounter Form	See page 279.

Questions

A. What is the name of the pay-to provider?

B. List the pay-to provider's primary and other (non-NPI) identification number/qualifier for this claim.

C. Are the subscriber and the patient the same person?

D. What copayment is collected?

E. What amount is being billed on the claim?

VALLEY ASSOCIATES, PC

Christopher M. Connolly, MD - Internal Medicine
555-967-0303
FED I.D. #16-1234567

PATIENT NAME	APPT. DATE/TIME
Porcelli, Jennifer	10/6/2008 12:30 pm
PATIENT NO.	**DX**
PORCEJE0	1. 465.9 upper respiratory infection 2. 3. 4.

DESCRIPTION	✓	CPT	FEE	DESCRIPTION	✓	CPT	FEE
OFFICE VISITS				**PROCEDURES**			
New Patient				Diagnostic Anoscopy		46600	
LI Problem Focused		99201		ECG Complete		93000	
LII Expanded		99202		I&D, Abscess		10060	
LIII Detailed		99203		Pap Smear		88150	
LIV Comp./Mod.		99204		Removal of Cerumen		69210	
LV Comp./High		99205		Removal 1 Lesion		17000	
Established Patient				Removal 2-14 Lesions		17003	
LI Minimum		99211		Removal 15+ Lesions		17004	
LII Problem Focused	✓	99212	46	Rhythm ECG w/Report		93040	
LIII Expanded		99213		Rhythm ECG w/Tracing		93041	
LIV Detailed		99214		Sigmoidoscopy, diag.		45330	
LV Comp./High		99215					
				LABORATORY			
PREVENTIVE VISIT				Bacteria Culture		87081	
New Patient				Fungal Culture		87101	
Age 12-17		99384		Glucose Finger Stick		82948	
Age 18-39		99385		Lipid Panel		80061	
Age 40-64		99386		Specimen Handling		99000	
Age 65+		99387		Stool/Occult Blood		82270	
Established Patient				Tine Test		85008	
Age 12-17		99394		Tuberculin PPD		85590	
Age 18-39		99395		Urinalysis		81000	
Age 40-64		99396		Venipuncture		36415	
Age 65+		99397					
				INJECTION/IMMUN.			
CONSULTATION: OFFICE/OP				Immun. Admin.		90471	
Requested By:				Ea. Add'l.		90472	
LI Problem Focused		99241		Hepatitis A Immun		90632	
LII Expanded		99242		Hepatitis B Immun		90746	
LIII Detailed		99243		Influenza Immun		90659	
LIV Comp./Mod.		99244		Pneumovax		90732	
LV Comp./High		99245					
				TOTAL FEES			

Encounter Form for Case 8.2

Case 8.3 From the Patient Information Form:

Name	Kalpesh Shah
Sex	M
Birth Date	01/21/1998
SSN	330-42-7928
Assignment of Benefits	Y
Signature on File	Y

Primary Insurance

Insured	Raj Shah
Patient Relationship to Insured	Son
Insured's Birth Date	02/16/1970
Insured's Sex	M
Insured's Address	1433 Third Avenue Cleveland, OH 44101-1234
Insured's Employer	Cleveland Savings Bank
Insured's SSN	330-21-1209
Insurance Policy Group Number	G0904
Insurance Plan/ Program Name	Oxford Freedom PPO
Member ID	3302112090X
Encounter Form	See page 281

Questions

A. Are the subscriber and the patient the same person?

B. What is the code for the patient's relationship to the insured?

C. What is the claim filing indicator code?

D. What amount is being billed on the claim?

E. What claim control number would you assign to the claim?

VALLEY ASSOCIATES, PC
Christopher M. Connolly, MD - Internal Medicine
555-967-0303
FED I.D. #16-1234567

PATIENT NAME	APPT. DATE/TIME
Shah, Kalpesh	10/6/2008 3:30 pm
PATIENT NO.	**DX**
SHAHKAL0	1. 380.4 cerumen in ear 2. 3. 4.

DESCRIPTION	✓	CPT	FEE	DESCRIPTION	✓	CPT	FEE
OFFICE VISITS				**PROCEDURES**			
New Patient				Diagnostic Anoscopy		46600	
LI Problem Focused		99201		ECG Complete		93000	
LII Expanded		99202		I&D, Abscess		10060	
LIII Detailed		99203		Pap Smear		88150	
LIV Comp./Mod.		99204		Removal of Cerumen	✓	69210	63
LV Comp./High		99205		Removal 1 Lesion		17000	
Established Patient				Removal 2-14 Lesions		17003	
LI Minimum	✓	99211	30	Removal 15+ Lesions		17004	
LII Problem Focused		99212		Rhythm ECG w/Report		93040	
LIII Expanded		99213		Rhythm ECG w/Tracing		93041	
LIV Detailed		99214		Sigmoidoscopy, diag.		45330	
LV Comp./High		99215					
				LABORATORY			
PREVENTIVE VISIT				Bacteria Culture		87081	
New Patient				Fungal Culture		87101	
Age 12-17		99384		Glucose Finger Stick		82948	
Age 18-39		99385		Lipid Panel		80061	
Age 40-64		99386		Specimen Handling		99000	
Age 65+		99387		Stool/Occult Blood		82270	
Established Patient				Tine Test		85008	
Age 12-17		99394		Tuberculin PPD		85590	
Age 18-39		99395		Urinalysis		81000	
Age 40-64		99396		Venipuncture		36415	
Age 65+		99397					
				INJECTION/IMMUN.			
CONSULTATION: OFFICE/OP				Immun. Admin.		90471	
Requested By:				Ea. Add'l.		90472	
LI Problem Focused		99241		Hepatitis A Immun		90632	
LII Expanded		99242		Hepatitis B Immun		90746	
LIII Detailed		99243		Influenza Immun		90659	
LIV Comp./Mod.		99244		Pneumovax		90732	
LV Comp./High		99245					
				TOTAL FEES			

Encounter Form for Case 8.3

Case 8.4 From the Patient Information Form:

Name	Josephine Smith
Sex	F
Birth Date	05/04/1977
SSN	610-32-7842
Address	9 Brook Rd. Alliance, OH 44601-1812
Employer	Central Ohio Oil
Referring Provider	Dr. Mark Abelman, MD, Family Medicine
Insurance Policy Group Number	G0404
Insurance Plan/ Program Name	Oxford Choice HMO
Member ID	610327842X
Assignment of Benefits	Y
Signature on File	Y
Encounter Form	See page 283.

Questions

A. List the pay-to provider's primary and other (nonNPI) identification number/qualifier for this claim.

B. What amount is being billed on the claim?

C. What two data elements should be reported since a referral is involved?

D. What claim control number would you assign to the claim?

E. What claim filing indicator code would you assign?

VALLEY ASSOCIATES, PC
Christopher M. Connolly, MD - Internal Medicine
555-967-0303
FED I.D. #16-1234567

PATIENT NAME	APPT. DATE/TIME
Smith, Josephine	10/10/2008 1:00 pm
PATIENT NO.	**DX**
SMITHJO0	1. 401.1 benign essential hypertension 2. 3. 4.

DESCRIPTION	✓	CPT	FEE	DESCRIPTION	✓	CPT	FEE
OFFICE VISITS				**PROCEDURES**			
New Patient				Diagnostic Anoscopy		46600	
LI Problem Focused		99201		ECG Complete	✓	93000	70
LII Expanded		99202		I&D, Abscess		10060	
LIII Detailed		99203		Pap Smear		88150	
LIV Comp./Mod.		99204		Removal of Cerumen		69210	
LV Comp./High		99205		Removal 1 Lesion		17000	
Established Patient				Removal 2-14 Lesions		17003	
LI Minimum		99211		Removal 15+ Lesions		17004	
LII Problem Focused		99212		Rhythm ECG w/Report		93040	
LIII Expanded	✓	99213	62	Rhythm ECG w/Tracing		93041	
LIV Detailed		99214		Sigmoidoscopy, diag.		45330	
LV Comp./High		99215					
				LABORATORY			
PREVENTIVE VISIT				Bacteria Culture		87081	
New Patient				Fungal Culture		87101	
Age 12-17		99384		Glucose Finger Stick		82948	
Age 18-39		99385		Lipid Panel		80061	
Age 40-64		99386		Specimen Handling		99000	
Age 65+		99387		Stool/Occult Blood		82270	
Established Patient				Tine Test		85008	
Age 12-17		99394		Tuberculin PPD		85590	
Age 18-39		99395		Urinalysis		81000	
Age 40-64		99396		Venipuncture		36415	
Age 65+		99397					
				INJECTION/IMMUN.			
CONSULTATION: OFFICE/OP				Immun. Admin.		90471	
Requested By:				Ea. Add'l.		90472	
LI Problem Focused		99241		Hepatitis A Immun		90632	
LII Expanded		99242		Hepatitis B Immun		90746	
LIII Detailed		99243		Influenza Immun		90659	
LIV Comp./Mod.		99244		Pneumovax		90732	
LV Comp./High		99245					
				TOTAL FEES			

Encounter Form for Case 8.4

Internet Activities

1. Visit the website of the National Uniform Claim Committee (NUCC) to locate information on taxonomy codes.
2. The Washington Publishing Company is a designated publishing company specializing in distributing EDI information from organizations that develop, maintain, and implement EDI standards. Use a search engine such as Google or Yahoo to locate the WPC website and briefly review the X12 837 Professional Implementation Guidelines and Addenda.

Part 4 Payers

Chapter 9
Private Payers/Blue Cross and Blue Shield

Chapter 10
Medicare

Chapter 11
Medicaid

Chapter 12
TRICARE and CHAMPVA

Chapter 13
Workers' Compensation and Disability

Chapter 9

Private Payers/Blue Cross and Blue Shield

CHAPTER OUTLINE

Private Insurance

Features of Group Health Plans

Types of Private Payer Plans

Consumer-Driven Health Plans

Major Private Payers and the Blue Cross and Blue Shield Association

Participation Contracts

Interpreting Compensation and Billing Guidelines

Private Payer Billing Management and Claim Completion

Capitation Management

Learning Outcomes

After studying this chapter, you should be able to:

1. Compare employer-sponsored and self-funded health plans.
2. Describe the major features of group health plans regarding eligibility, portability, and required coverage.
3. Discuss provider payment under preferred provider organizations, health maintenance organizations, point-of-service plans, and indemnity plans.
4. Describe the two components of consumer-driven health plans and their effect on cash flow.
5. Compare and contrast health reimbursement accounts, health savings accounts, and flexible spending accounts.
6. List the five main parts of participation contracts and describe their purpose.
7. Describe the information needed to collect copayments and bill for surgical procedures under contracted plans.
8. Discuss the use of plan summary grids.
9. Describe the steps in the medical billing process that ensure correct preparation of private payer claims.
10. Discuss the key points in managing billing for capitated services.

Key Terms

administrative services only (ASO)
BlueCard
Blue Cross and Blue Shield Association (BCBS)
carve out
Consolidated Omnibus Budget Reconciliation Act (COBRA)
credentialing
creditable coverage
discounted fee-for-service
elective surgery
Employee Retirement Income Security Act of 1974 (ERISA)
episode of care (EOC) option
family deductible
Federal Employees Health Benefits (FEHB) program
Flexible Blue
flexible savings account (FSA)
formulary
group health plan (GHP)
health reimbursement account (HRA)
health savings account (HSA)
high-deductible health plan (HDHP)
home plan
host plan
independent practice association (IPA)
individual deductible
individual health plan (IHP)
late enrollee
maximum benefit limit
monthly enrollment list
open enrollment period
pay-for-performance (P4P)
plan summary grid
precertification
repricer
rider
Section 125 cafeteria plan
silent PPOs
stop-loss provision
subcapitation
Summary Plan Description (SPD)
third-party claims administrator (TPAs)
tiered network
utilization review
utilization review organization (URO)
waiting period

Medical insurance specialists must become knowledgeable about the billing rules of the private plans that insure their patients, especially how they affect coverage of services and financial responsibility. This chapter covers procedures for billing under the leading types of managed care plans. Also covered are plans with funding options controlled by patients, which are emerging as a popular insurance model. Because these consumer-driven health plans have high deductibles due before benefits start, patients need to understand what their bills will be, and medical insurance specialists need to know how to collect these amounts. In every case, a clear financial policy that describes patients' financial obligations is increasingly important for medical practices.

Private Insurance

People who are not covered by entitlement programs such as government-sponsored health insurance are usually covered by private insurance. Many employers offer their employees the opportunity to become covered under employee health care benefit plans (see Figure 9.1 on page 288). Sponsorship of medical insurance is an important benefit to employees, and it also gives employers federal income tax advantages.

Employer-Sponsored Medical Insurance

Many employees have medical insurance coverage under **group health plans (GHP)** that their employers buy from insurance companies. Human resources departments manage these health care benefits, negotiating with health plans and then selecting a number of products to offer employees. Both basic plans and riders are offered. **Riders**, also called options, may be purchased by employees to add coverage such as vision and dental services. Another popular rider is for complementary health care, covering treatments such as chiropractic/manual manipulation, acupuncture, massage therapy, dietetic counseling, and vitamin and minerals.

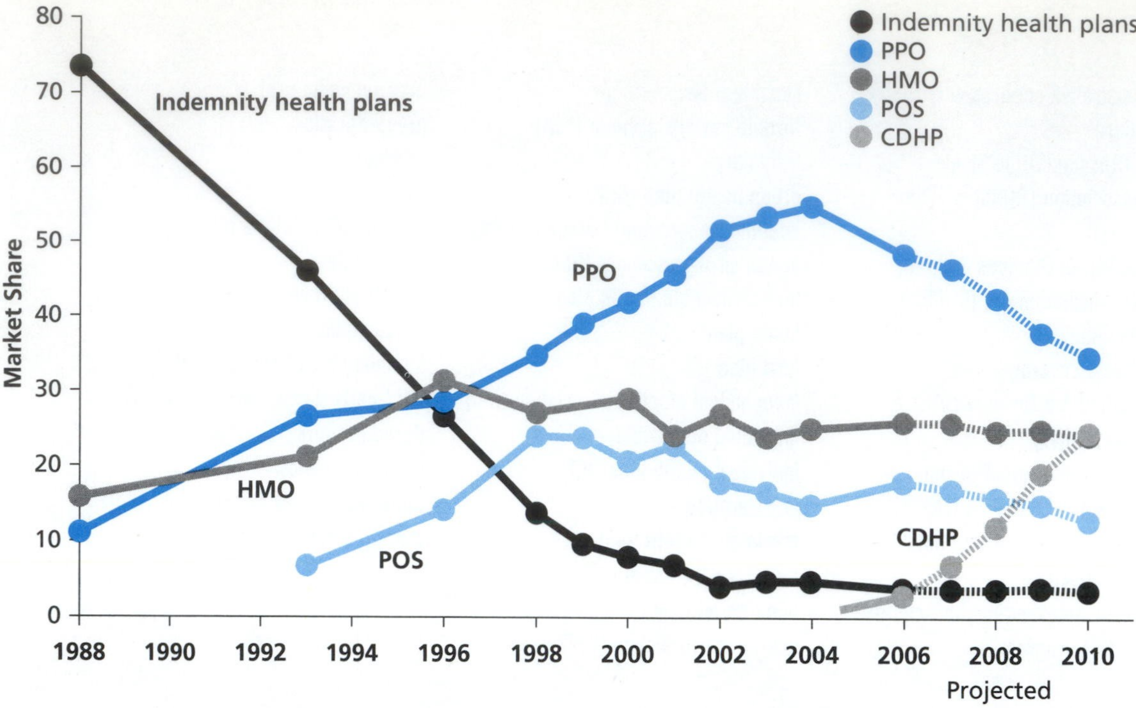

FIGURE 9.1 Medical Group Plans Offered by Payer

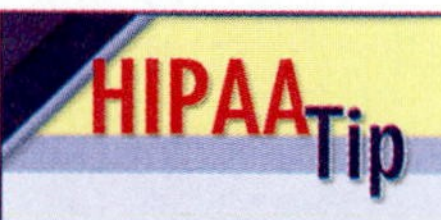

Group Health Plan Regulation

Employer-sponsored group health plans must follow federal and state laws that mandate coverage of specific benefits or treatments and access to care. When a state law is more restrictive than the related federal law, the state law is followed.

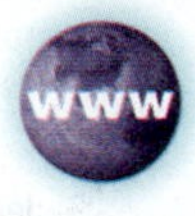

FEHB

http://www.opm.gov/insure/health

Employers may **carve out** certain benefits—that is, change standard coverage or providers—during negotiations to reduce the price. An employer may:

- Omit a specific benefit, such as coverage of prescription drugs.
- Use a different network of providers for a certain type of care, such as negotiating with a local practice network for mental health coverage.
- Hire a pharmacy benefit manager (PBM) to operate the prescription drug benefit more inexpensively. (Because PBMs do this work for many employers, they represent a large group of buyers and can negotiate favorable prices with pharmaceutical companies for each employer.)

During specified periods (usually once a year) called **open enrollment periods**, the employee chooses a particular set of benefits for the coming benefit period (see Figure 9.2). The employer provides tools (often web-based) and information to help employees match their personal and family needs with the best-priced plans. Employees can customize the policies by choosing to accept various levels of premiums, deductibles, and other costs.

Federal Employees Health Benefits Program

The largest employer-sponsored health program in the United States is the **Federal Employees Health Benefits (FEHB) program**, which covers more than 8 million federal employees, retirees, and their families through more than 250 health plans from a number of carriers. FEHB is administered by the federal government's Office of Personnel Management (OPM), which receives and deposits premiums and remits payments to the carriers. Each carrier is responsible for furnishing identification cards and benefits brochures to enrollees, adjudicating claims, and maintaining records.

DECISION #1
Deductible
A ☐ $300
B ☐ $600
C ☐ $900
D ☐ $1,500
E ☐ $2,500

DECISION #2
Coinsurance*/out-of-pocket limit
A ☐ 80% / $2,200
B ☐ 80% / $4,400
C ☐ 70% / $5,000
D ☐ 60% / $5,000
E ☐ 70% / $10,000

DECISION #3
Prescription-drug access
A ☐ No formulary
B ☐ Formulary

DECISION #4
Medical access
A ☐ Broad network
B ☐ Select network

*for in-network coverage

FIGURE 9.2 Example of Selecting Benefits During Open Enrollment

Self-funded Health Plans

To save money, some large employers cover the costs of employee medical benefits themselves rather than buying insurance from other companies. They create self-funded (or –insured) health plans that do not pay premiums to an insurance carrier or a managed care organization. Instead, self-funded health plans "insure themselves" and assume the risk of paying directly for medical services, setting aside funds with which to pay benefits. The employer establishes the benefit levels and the plan types offered to employees. Self-funded health plans may set up their own provider networks or, more often, lease a managed care organization's networks. They may also buy other types of insurance—like a vision package—instead of insuring the benefit themselves.

In contrast to employer-sponsored "fully insured plans," which are regulated by state laws, self-funded health plans are regulated by the federal **Employee Retirement Income Security Act of 1974 (ERISA)**. ERISA is run by the federal Department of Labor's Pension and Welfare Benefits Administration (EBSA). Self-funded plan members receive a **Summary Plan Description (SPD)** from the plan that describes their benefits and legal rights.

Self-funded health plans often hire **third-party claims administrators (TPAs)** to handle tasks like collecting premiums, keeping lists of members up to date, and processing and paying claims. Often an insurance carrier or managed care organization works as the TPA under an **administrative services only (ASO)** contract.

Individual Health Plans

Individual health plans (IHP) can be purchased. Almost 10 percent of people with private health insurance have individual plans. People often elect to enroll in individual plans, although coverage is expensive, in order to continue their health insurance between jobs. Purchasers also include self-employed entrepreneurs, students, recent college graduates, and early retirees. Individual insurance plans usually have basic benefits without the riders or additional features associated with group health plans.

HIPAA Tip

• ***TPAs Are Business Associates*** *Third-party claims administrators are business associates of health plans and must satisfy the normal privacy and security requirements during health care transactions.*

• ***Group Health Plans and PHI*** *Both employer-sponsored health plans and self-funded health plans are group health plans (GHP) under HIPAA and must follow HIPAA rules.*

Billing Tip

Timely Payments
Group health plans must follow states' Clean Claims Act and/or Prompt Payment Act and pay claims they accept for processing on a timely basis. ERISA (self-funded) plans are obligated by the federal Department of Labor to follow similar rules.

Features of Group Health Plans

A common way that employers organize employees' choices of plans is by creating a tax structure called a **Section 125 cafeteria plan** (the word *cafeteria* implies that employees may choose from a wide array of options). Under income tax law, the employer can collect an employee's insurance cost through a pretax payroll deduction, and that money is excluded from the income the employee has to pay taxes on. (When a policyholder pays premiums any other way, the policyholder generally pays income tax on that money and can deduct the cost only if the entire year's medical expenses are greater than 7.5 percent of his or her income.)

Eligibility for Benefits

The group health plan specifies the rules for eligibility and the process of enrolling and disenrolling members. Rules cover employment status, such a full-time, part-time, disabled, and laid-off or terminated employees, as well as the conditions for enrolling dependents.

Waiting Period

Many plans have a **waiting period**, an amount of time that must pass before a newly hired employee or a dependent is eligible to enroll. The waiting period is the time between the date of hire and the date the insurance becomes effective.

Late Enrollees

The plan may impose different eligibility rules on a **late enrollee**, an individual who enrolls in a plan at a time other than the earliest possible enrollment date or a special enrollment date. For example, special enrollment may occur when a person becomes a new dependent through marriage.

Premiums and Deductibles

As explained in Chapter 1, most plans require annual premiums. Although employers used to pay the total premiums as a benefit for employees, currently they pay an average of 80 percent of the cost.

Many health plans also have a deductible that is due per time period. Noncovered services under the plan that the patient must pay out-of-pocket do not count toward satisfying a deductible. Some plans require an **individual deductible** that must be met for each person—whether the policyholder or a covered dependent—who has an encounter. Others have a **family deductible** that can be met by the combined payments of any covered members of the insured's family.

Benefit Limits

Plans often have a **maximim benefit limit** (also called a lifetime limit), a monetary amount after which benefits end, and may also impose a condition-specific lifetime limit. For example, the plan may have a $500,000 lifetime limit on all benefits covered under the plan for any policyholder and a $2,000 limit on benefits provided for a specific health condition of an individual policyholder. Some plans may also have an annual benefit limit that restricts the amount payable in a given year.

Tiered Networks

Tiered networks reimburse more for providers who are considered of highest quality and cost-effectiveness by the plan. The aim of tiered networks is to steer patients toward the best providers (under the plan's performance measurements). Tiered networks are common for prescription drug coverage, where medications in the plan's drug **formulary**, a list of approved drugs, have smaller copayments than do nonformulary drugs.

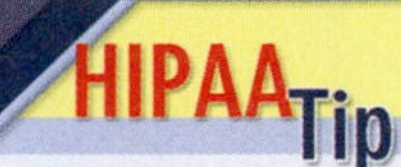

State Law and Preexisting Condition Exclusions

The six-month look-back period and the length of the preexisting condition limitation extension period are shortened under the laws of some states.

Portability and Required Coverage

A number of regulations govern group health coverage in situations such as changing jobs, pregnancy, and certain illnesses.

COBRA

The **Consolidated Omnibus Budget Reconciliation Act (COBRA)** (1985; amended 1986) gives an employee who is leaving a job the right to continue health coverage under the employers' plan for a limited time at his or her own expense. COBRA participants usually pay more than do active employees, since the employer usually pays part of the premium for an active employee, while a COBRA participant generally pays the entire premium. However, COBRA is ordinarily less expensive than individual health coverage.

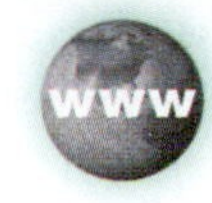

COBRA Information

http://www.dol.gov/ebsa

HIPAA

HIPAA (1996) adds more rules to COBRA to help people with preexisting conditions when they are newly employed. For cost control, many private plans limit or exclude coverage of patients' previous illnesses or conditions. HIPAA regulates these exclusions. Plans can "look back" into the patient's medical history for a period of six months to find conditions that they will exclude, but they cannot look back for a longer period. Also, the preexisting condition limitation cannot last more than twelve months after the effective date of coverage (eighteen months for late enrollees).

The patient's previous **creditable coverage** also must be taken into account when an employee joins a new plan. Creditable coverage is health insurance under a group health plan, health insurance, or the Medicaid program known as SCHIP (see Chapter 11). Note that medical discount cards are not insurance and do not qualify as creditable coverage.

If the patient was previously covered by medical insurance, that plan had to supply a certificate of coverage when the patient's coverage ended. The patient gives this document to the new plan, because having previous coverage can reduce the length of limitation the plan can put in the person's new insurance policy. Under the standard calculation method, the patient receives credit for previous coverage that occurred without a break of sixty-three days or more. (Any coverage occurring before a break in coverage of sixty-three days or more is not credited against a preexisting condition exclusion period.)

HIPAA Tip

Pregnancy and Childbirth Rules

A preexisting condition exclusion cannot be applied to pregnancy or to a newborn, adopted child, or child placed for adoption if the child is covered under a group health plan within thirty days after birth, adoption, or placement for adoption.

Other Federally Guaranteed Insurance Provisions

Three other federal laws govern private insurance coverage:

- The Newborns' and Mothers' Health Protection Act provides protections for mothers and their newborn children relating to the length of hospital stays after childbirth. Unless state law says otherwise, plans cannot restrict benefits for a hospital stay for childbirth to less than forty-eight hours following

Thinking it Through — 9.1

1. If a GHP has a ninety-day waiting period, on what day does health coverage become effective?
2. In terms of enrollment in a health plan, what is the status of an infant born to a subscriber in the plan?
3. A patient pays for a cosmetic procedure that is not medically necessary under the terms of the plan. Does this payment count towards the deductible?
4. Why is it important to verify a patient's eligibility for benefits? Can you think of events, like job-status change, that might affect coverage?

Billing Tip

PPOs
About half of all consumers with health insurance are enrolled in a PPO.

a vaginal delivery or ninety-six hours following delivery by cesarean section. Plans are permitted to require preauthorization for the hospitalization.

- The Women's Health and Cancer Rights Act provides protections for individuals who elect breast reconstruction after a mastectomy. Plans must cover all stages of breast reconstruction, procedures on the other breast to produce a symmetrical appearance, prostheses, and treatment of physical complications of the mastectomy, including lymphodema. State laws may be more restrictive than this act and may require a minimum length of hospitalization after the procedure.
- The Mental Health Parity Act provides for parity (equality) with medical/surgical benefits when plans set lifetime or annual dollar limits on mental health benefits (except for substance abuse or chemical dependency).

Types of Private Payer Plans

Preferred provider organizations (PPOs) are the most popular type of private plan, followed by health maintenance organizations (HMOs), especially the point-of-service (POS) variety. Few employees choose indemnity plans because they would have to pay more. Consumer-driven health plans (CDHP) that combine a high-deductible health plan with a funding option of some type are rapidly growing in popularity among both employers and employees. Table 9.1 reviews private payer plan types that were introduced in Chapter 1. Figure 9.3 on page 294 presents typical features of a popular PPO plan.

Billing Tip

Private Payers
Private payers do not necessarily operate under the same regulations as government-sponsored programs. Each payer's rules and interpretations may vary. The definitions of basic terms (for example, the age range for neonate) differ, as do preauthorization requirements. Research each payer's rules for correct billing and reimbursement.

Preferred Provider Organizations

Physicians, hospitals and clinics, and pharmacies contract with the PPO plan to provide care to its insured people. These medical providers accept the PPO plan's fee schedule and guidelines for its managed medical care. PPOs generally pay participating providers based on a discount from their physician fee schedules, called **discounted fee-for-service**.

Under a PPO, the patient pays an annual premium and often a deductible. A PPO plan may offer either a low deductible with a higher premium or a high deductible with a lower premium. Insured members pay a copayment at the time of each medical service. Each person may also have a yearly deductible to pay out of pocket. Coinsurance is often charged for in-network providers.

TABLE 9.1 Types of Private Payer Plans	
Plan Type	**Participating Provider Payment Method**
Preferred Provider Organization (PPO)	Discounted Fee-for-Service
Staff Health Maintenance Organization (HMO)	Salary
Group HMO	Salary or Contracted Cap Rate
Independent Practice Association (IPA)	PCP: Contracted Cap Rate Specialist: Fee-for-Service
Point-of-Service (POS) Plan	PCPs: Contracted Cap Rate Referred Providers: Contracted Cap Rate or Discounted Fee-for-Service
Indemnity	Fee-for-Service
Consumer-Driven Health Plan (Combined High-Deductible Health Plan and Funding Option)	Up to Deductible: Payment by Patient After Deductible: Discounted Fee-for-Service

A patient may see an out-of-network doctor without a referral or preauthorization, but the deductible for out-of-network services may be higher and the percentage the plan will pay may be lower. In other words, the patient will be responsible for a greater part of the fee, as illustrated by the "in-network" versus "out-of-network" columns in Figure 9.3 (on page 294). This encourages people insured by PPOs to use in-network physicians, other medical providers, and hospitals.

Health Maintenance Organizations

A health maintenance organization (HMO) is licensed by the state. For its lower costs, the HMO has the most stringent guidelines and the narrowest choice of providers. Its members are assigned to primary care physicians and must use network providers to be covered, except in emergencies. In an *open-panel HMO*, any physician who meets the HMO's standards of care may join the HMO as a provider. These physicians usually operate from their own offices and also see non-HMO patients. In a *closed-panel HMO*, the physicians are either HMO employees or belong to a group that has a contract with the HMO.

Health maintenance organizations were originally designed to cover all basic services for an annual premium and visit copayments. This arrangement is called "first-dollar coverage" because no deductible is required and patients do not make out-of-pocket payments. Because of expenses, however, HMOs may now apply deductibles to family coverage, and employer-sponsored HMOs are also beginning to replace copayments with coinsurance for some benefits.

HMOs have traditionally emphasized preventive and wellness services as well as disease management. Figure 9.4 on page 295 lists the programs that are often included in these plans. (Note that PPOs also often include many of these services.)

An HMO is organized around a business model. The model is based on how the terms of the agreement connect the provider and the plan. In all, however, enrollees must see HMO providers in order to be covered.

Staff Model

In a staff HMO, physicians are employed by the organization. All the premiums and other revenues come to the HMO, which in turn pays the physicians' salaries. For medical care, patients visit clinics and health centers owned by the HMO.

Standard Benefits

This is a preferred provider organization (PPO) plan. That means members can receive the highest level of benefits when they use any of the more than 5,000 physicians and other health care professionals in this network. When members receive covered in-network services, they simply pay a copayment. Members can also receive care from providers that are not part of the network, however benefits are often lower and covered claims are subject to deductible, coinsurance and charges above the maximum allowable amount. Referrals are not needed from a Primary Care Physician to receive care from a specialist.

PREVENTIVE CARE	In-Network	Out-of-Network
Well child care		
Birth through 12 years	OV Copayment	Deductible & Coinsurance
All others	OV Copayment	Deductible & Coinsurance
Periodic, routine health examinations	OV Copayment	Deductible & Coinsurance
Routine eye exams	OV Copayment	Deductible & Coinsurance
Routine OB/GYN visits	OV Copayment	Deductible & Coinsurance
Mammography	No Charge	Deductible & Coinsurance
Hearing Screening	OV Copayment	Deductible & Coinsurance
MEDICAL CARE	**In-Network**	**Out-of-Network**
PCP office visits	OV Copayment	Deductible & Coinsurance
Specialist office visits	OV Copayment	Deductible & Coinsurance
Outpatient mental health & substance abuse – *prior authorization required*	OV Copayment	Deductible & Coinsurance
Maternity care – *initial visit subject to copayment, no charge thereafter*	OV Copayment	Deductible & Coinsurance
Diagnostic lab, x-ray and testing	No Charge	Deductible & Coinsurance
High-cost outpatient diagnostics – *prior authorization required. The following are subject to copayment: MRI, MRA, CAT, CTA, PET, SPECT scans*	No Charge OR $200 Copayment	Deductible & Coinsurance Deductible & Coinsurance
Allergy Services		
Office visits/testing	OV Copayment	Deductible & Coinsurance
Injections – *80 visits in 3 years*	$25 Copayment	Deductible & Coinsurance
HOSPITAL CARE – Prior authorization required	**In-Network**	**Out-of-Network**
Semi-private room *(General/Medical/Surgical/Maternity)*	HSP Copayment	Deductible & Coinsurance
Skilled nursing facility – *up to 120 days per calendar year*	HSP Copayment	Deductible & Coinsurance
Rehabilitative services – *up to 60 days per calendar year*	No Charge	Deductible & Coinsurance
Outpatient surgery – *in a hospital or surgi-center*	OS Copayment	Deductible & Coinsurance
EMERGENCY CARE	**In-Network**	**Out-of-Network**
Walk-in centers	OV Copayment	Deductible & Coinsurance
Urgent care centers – *at participating centers only*	UR Copayment	Not Covered
Emergency care – *copayment waived if admitted*	ER Copayment	ER Copayment
Ambulance	No Charge	No Charge
OTHER HEALTH CARE	**In-Network**	**Out-of-Network**
Outpatient rehabilitative services – *30 visit maximum for PT, OT, and ST per year. 20 visit maximum for Chiro. per year.*	OV Copayment	Deductible & Coinsurance
Durable medical equipment/Prosthetic devices – *Unlimited maximum per calendar year*	No Charge OR 20%	Deductible & Coinsurance
Infertility Services (diagnosis and treatment)	Not Covered	Not Covered
Home Health Care	No Charge	$50 Deductible & 20% Coinsurance

KEY: Office Visit (OV) Copayment; Hospital (HSP) Copayment; Emergency Room (ER) Copayment; Outpatient Surgery (OS) Copayment; Urgent Care (UR) Copayment

PREVENTIVE CARE SCHEDULES

Well Child Care (including immunizations)
- 6 exams, birth to age 1
- 6 exams, ages 1 – 5
- 1 exam every 2 years, ages 6 – 10
- 1 exam every year, ages 11 – 21

Adult Exams
- 1 exam every 5 years, ages 22 – 29
- 1 exam every 3 years, ages 30 – 39
- 1 exam every 2 years, ages 40 – 49
- 1 exam every year, ages 50+

Mammography
- 1 baseline screening, ages 35 – 39
- 1 screening per year, ages 40+

Vision Exams
- 1 exam every 2 calendar years

Hearing Exams
- 1 exam per calendar year

OB/GYN Exams
- 1 exam per calendar year

FIGURE 9.3 Example of Range of PPO Benefits for a Popular Plan

Group (Network) Model

A group (network) HMO contracts with more than one physician group. In some plans, HMO members receive medical services in HMO-owned facilities from providers who work only for that HMO. In others, members visit the providers' facilities, and the providers can also treat nonmember patients.

The practices under contract are paid a per member per month (PMPM) capitated rate for each subscriber assigned to them for primary care services.

Complete preventive or screening program:	Wellness and health promotion program:
Colorectal cancer screening for ages 50+ • Reminders issued • FOBT (fecal occult blood test) • DCBE (double contrast barium enema) • Sigmoidoscopy • Colonoscopy Prostate cancer screening for ages 50+ Cervical cancer screening for ages 21+ • Reminders issued • Thin prep test • Auto prep test • Papnet test Breast cancer screening • Reminders issued • Mammography Diabetes screening for ages 46+ Osteoporosis screening Back care and injury prevention Nutrition counseling HIV/AIDS prevention counseling Hearing tests for newborns; seniors	Chronic disease self-management programs 24-hour nurse phone line Prenatal care education Menopause management Alcohol dependency counseling Violence prevention counseling Access to a fitness center Stress reduction program Health-risk appraisal Care manager services to caregivers of enrollees **Disease management and chronic care programs for:** Congestive heart failure Coronary artery disease Diabetes Asthma High-risk pregnancy Depression

FIGURE 9.4 Typical Preventive, Wellness, and Disease Management Services of HMO and POS Plans

Practices may hire other providers to handle certain services, such as laboratory tests. The other providers work under a **subcapitation** agreement (a PMPM that covers their services) or an **episode of care (EOC) option**, which is a flat fee for all services for a particular treatment. For example, an EOC fee is established for coronary bypass surgery or hip replacement surgery; the fixed rate per patient includes preoperative and postoperative treatment as well as the surgery itself. If complications arise, additional fees are usually paid.

Compliance Guideline

Termination of Patients
HMOs and POSs regulate a primary care physician's decision to terminate a relationship with a patient. The PCP must first ask the payer for permission to do so, and must then send a certified letter to the patient, who must sign and return it. The PCP must provide emergency care until the patient has a new PCP.

Independent Practice Association Model

An **independent practice association (IPA)** type of HMO is an association formed by physicians with separately owned practices who contract together to provide care for HMO members. An HMO pays negotiated fees for medical services to the IPA. The IPA in turn pays its physician members, either by a capitated rate or a fee. Providers may join more than one IPA and usually also see nonmember patients.

Point-of-Service (POS) Plans

A point-of-service (POS) plan is a hybrid of HMO and PPO networks. Members may choose from a primary or secondary network. The primary network is HMO-like, and the secondary network is often a PPO network. Like HMOs, POS plans charge an annual premium and a copayment for office visits. Monthly premiums are slightly higher than for HMOs but offer the benefit of some coverage for visits to nonnetwork physicians for specialty care. A POS may be structured as a tiered plan, for example, with different rates for specially designated providers, regular participating providers, and out-of-network providers.

Billing Tip

POS: Two Meanings
POS for claims means place of service; POS relating to health plans means point of service.

Indemnity Plans

Indemnity plans require premium, deductible, and coinsurance payments. They typically cover 70 to 80 percent of costs for covered benefits after

Billing Tip

Comparing Participation
Figure 9.5 shows participation in HMOs, PPOs, and capitated plans by medical specialty.

deductibles are met. Some plans are structured with high deductibles, such as $5,000 to $10,000, in order to offer policyholders a relatively less expensive premium. Many have some managed care features, as payers compete for employers' contracts and try to control costs.

Consumer-Driven Health Plans

Consumer-driven (or consumer-directed) health plans (CDHPs) combine two components: (1) a high-deductible health plan and (2) one or more tax-preferred savings accounts that the patient (the "consumer") directs. The two plans work together: The high-deductible health plan covers catastrophic losses, while the savings account pays out-of-pocket or noncovered expenses.

CDHPs empower consumers to manage their use of health care services and products. Experts in the health care industry believe that people who pay medical expenses themselves will be more careful about how their dollars are spent. CDHPs eliminate most copayment coverage and shift responsibility for managing the dollars in the savings accounts to individuals. Therefore, people will research medical issues and make informed choices. For the CDHP approach to work, then, consumers must be able to find accurate health care information. Companies (and health plans) meet this need by providing explanations of common medical conditions and treatments. Companies also have web-based tools to compare cost estimates for in-network or out-of-network visits and for drug prices. CDHPs encourage people to seek routine well-care benefits.

The High-Deductible Health Plan

The first part of a CDHP is a **high-deductible health plan (HDHP)**, usually a PPO. The annual deductible is over $1,000. Many of the plan's covered preventive care services, as well as coverage for accidents, disability, dental care, vision care, and long-term care, are not subject to this deductible.

The Funding Options

Three types of CDHP funding options (Table 9.2) may be combined with high-deductible health plans to form consumer-driven health plans.

TABLE 9.2 Comparisons of CDHP Funding Options

HEALTH REIMBURSEMENT ACCOUNT	HEALTH SAVINGS ACCOUNT
Contributions from employer	Contributions from individual (regardless of employment status), employer, or both
Rollovers allowed within employer-set limits	Unused funds roll over indefinitely
Portability allowed under employer's rules	Funds are portable (job change; retirement)
Tax-deductible deposits	Tax-deductible deposits
Tax-free withdrawals for qualified expenses	Tax-free withdrawals for qualified expenses
	Tax-free interest can be earned
FLEXIBLE SAVINGS ACCOUNT	
Contributions from employer and/or employee	
Unused funds revert to employer	
No portability	
Tax-advantaged deposits	
Tax-free withdrawals for qualified expenses	

	Percentage of physicians participating in:		
	HMOs	PPOs	Capitation
Allergists/Allergy immunologists	89	96	19
Cardiologists	69	85	34
Dermatologists	62	87	9
Endocrinologists	78	86	22
FPs	74	82	46
Gastroenterologists	76	87	26
GPs	51	72	48
General surgeons	76	92	15
Hematologists	86	86	40
Infectious disease specialists	76	81	30
Internists	76	86	51
Nephrologists	76	80	59
Neurosurgeons	70	83	15
Ob/gyns	81	86	22
Ophthalmologists	75	83	22
Orthopedic surgeons	74	84	13
Pediatricians	86	90	58
Plastic surgeons	50	60	10
Psychiatrists	51	55	7
Pulmonologists	79	88	23
Rheumatologists	73	87	20
Thoracic surgeons	80	76	37
Urologists	79	84	26
All Primary Care	77	85	47
All Respondents	75	84	37

FIGURE 9.5 Comparison of Physician Participation by Plan Type and Medical Specialty

Health Reimbursement Accounts

A **health reimbursement account (HRA)** is a medical reimbursement plan set up and funded by an employer. HRAs are usually offered to employees with health plans that have high deductibles. Employees may submit claims to the HRA to be paid back for out-of-pocket medical expenses. For example, an employee may pay a health plan deductible, copayments, coinsurance, and any medical expenses not covered by the group health plan and may then request reimbursement from the HRA. If the employer authorizes this approach, funds in the account that are left at the end of the benefit period can roll over to the next year's HRA.

Health Savings Accounts

The most popular and fastest growing type of account is the **health savings account (HSA)**, which was first established in 2004. Health savings accounts, too, are designed to pay for qualified medical expenses of individuals who have high-deductible health plans (HDHP) and are under age sixty-five.

The Medicare Prescription Drug, Improvement, and Modernization Act of 2003 added a section to the Internal Revenue Service (IRS) tax code to permit HSAs. An HSA is a savings account created by an individual. Employers that wish to encourage employees to set up HSAs offer a qualified high-deductible health plan to go with it. Both employee and employer can contribute to the HSA. The maximum amount that can be saved each year is set by the IRS. The

IRS also sets the maximum out-of-pocket spending under HSA-compatible high-deductible health plans.

The HSA money can be held in an account by an employer, a bank, or a health plan. This holder is referred to as a "custodian" for the account. The federal government decides the limits on the amount of the contribution that is tax-sheltered, just as it does for IRAs.

HSAs do not have to be used up at the end of a year. Instead, the account can roll over from year to year and be taken along by an employee who changes jobs or retires. HSAs can earn tax-free interest and can be used for nonmedical purposes after age sixty-five.

Flexible Savings (Spending) Accounts

Some companies offer **flexible savings accounts (FSAs)** that augment employees' other health insurance coverage. Employees have the option of putting pretax dollars from their salaries in the FSA; they can then use the fund to pay for certain medical and dependent care expenses. The permitted expenses include cost-sharing (deductibles, copayments, coinsurance), medical expenses that are not covered under the regular insurance plan (such as routine physical examinations, eyeglasses, and many over-the-counter medical supplies), and child care. Employers may contribute to each employee's account.

The FSA may be used in one of two ways. In some companies, the employee has to file a claim with the plan after paying a bill. For example, the employee may submit a receipt from a drugstore for a prescription or an Explanation of Benefits (EOB) from the health plan that shows that the patient, not the plan, paid the bill. In the other way, the company gives the employee a credit or debit card to use to pay the bills as they occur, and the employee is responsible for keeping records that prove that the expenses were in the "permitted" category.

The disadvantage of an FSA as compared with an HSA is that unused dollars go back to the employer under the "use it or lose it" rule at the end of the year. Employees must try to predict their year's expenses to avoid either overfunding or underfunding the account. For this reason, HSAs are growing in popularity.

Billing Under Consumer-Driven Health Plans

Consumer-driven health plans reduce providers' cash flow because visit copayments are being replaced by high deductibles that are not collected until after claims are paid. As more employer-sponsored plan members are covered under CDHPs, physician reimbursement up to the amount of the deductible will come from the patient's funding option and, if there is not enough money there, out of pocket. CDHP payment works as follows:

- The group health plan establishes a funding option (HRA, HSA, FSA, or some combination) designed to help pay out-of-pocket medical expenses.
- The patient uses the money in the account to pay for qualified medical services.
- The total deductible must be met before any benefits are paid by the HDHP.
- Once the deductible is met, the HDHP covers a portion of the benefits according to the policy. The funding option can also be used to pay the uncovered portion.

Following is an example of payments under a CDHP with a HSA fund of $1,000 and a deductible of $1,000. The HDHP has a 80-20 coinsurance. The plan pays the visit charges as billed.

Office visits for the patient:

First visit charge	$150	$150 paid from HSA (leaving a balance in the fund of $850)
Second visit charge	$450	$450 paid from HSA (leaving a balance in the fund of $400)
Third visit charge	$600	$400 paid from HSA (emptying the HSA fund)
		$160 paid by the HDHP (the balance of $200 on the charge X 80%)
		$40 coinsurance to be paid by the patient (the balance of $200 X 20%)

For medical practices, the best situation is an integrated CDHP in which the same plan runs both the HDHP and the funding options. This approach helps reduce paperwork and speed payment. For example, if an HSA is run by the same payer as the HDHP, a claim for charges is sent to the payer. The payer's RA/EOB states what the plan and the patient are each responsible for paying. If payment is due from the patient's HSA, that amount is withdrawn and paid to the provider. If the patient's deductible has been met, the plan pays its obligation.

Another popular payment method is a credit or a debit card provided by the plan. The patient can use it to pay for health-related expenses up to the amount in the fund. The cards may be preloaded with the member's coverage and copayment data.

Educating patients about their financial responsibility before they leave encounters, extending credit wisely, and improving collections are all key to avoiding uncollectible accounts under CDHPs.

Billing Tip

CDHP Enrollment
Most enrollees in consumer-driven health care are in plans that build on insurance carriers' existing provider network and negotiated rates.

Major Private Payers and the Blue Cross and Blue Shield Association

A small number of large insurance companies dominate the national market and offer employers all types of health plans, including self-funded plans. Local or regional payers are often affiliated with a national plan or with the Blue Cross and Blue Shield Association. Some carriers offer health insurance to individuals and to small business. The law in a few states, such as Maryland, requires major insurance carriers to provide limited health plans that can be afforded by small businesses.

Private payers supply complete insurance services, such as:

- Contracting with employers and with individuals to provide insurance benefits
- Setting up physician, hospital, and pharmacy networks
- Establishing fees
- Processing claims
- Managing the insurance risk

Many large insurers own specialty companies that have insurance products in related areas. They may handle behavioral health, dental, vision, and life insurance. Many also work as federal government contractors for Medicare and Medicaid programs and handle prescription management divisions.

Major Payers and Accrediting Groups

The major national payers are listed below. Note that the Blue Cross and Blue Shield Association (BCBS), which has both for-profit and nonprofit members, is not a payer; it is an association of more than forty payers. Its national scope, however, means that knowing about its programs is important for all medical insurance specialists.

- *WellPoint, Inc.:* WellPoint is the nation's largest health insurer in terms of enrollment. It is also the largest owner of Blue Cross and Blue Shield plans, serving as the Blue Cross licensee in California and the Blue Cross and Blue Shield licensee in Georgia, Missouri, and Wisconsin as well as serving Colorado, Connecticut, Indiana, Kentucky, Maine, Nevada, New Hampshire, Ohio, and Virginia under Anthem Blue Cross and Blue Shield (see the discussion of the Blue Cross and Blue Shield Association below).
- *UnitedHealth Group:* UnitedHealth Group is the second-largest health insurer and runs plans under its UnitedHealthcare subsidiary. It owns other major regional insurers, such as Oxford Health Plans.
- *Aetna:* With more than 14 million members, Aetna has a full range of products, including health care, dental, pharmacy, group life, behavioral health, disability and long-term care benefits. The company has a nationwide network of more than 700,000 health care professionals, including over 418,000 primary care and specialist doctors and over 4,000 hospitals.
- *CIGNA Health Care:* CIGNA is a large health insurer with strong enrollment in the Northeast and the West.
- *Kaiser Permanente*: The largest nonprofit HMO, Kaiser Permanente is a prepaid group practice that offers both health care services and insurance in one package. It runs physician groups, hospitals, and health plans in western, midwestern, and southeastern states plus Washington, D.C.
- *Health Net:* Health Net operates health plans in the West and Northeast and has group, individual, Medicare, Medicaid, and TRICARE programs.
- *Humana Inc.:* Humana is particularly strong in the South and Southeast. It offers both traditional and consumer-driven products. Humana handles TRICARE operations in the Southeast.
- *Coventry:* Coventry Health Care is a national managed health care company based in Bethesda, Maryland operating health plans, insurance companies, network rental / managed care services companies, and workers' compensation services companies. It provides a full range of risk and fee-based managed care products and services.

Outside agencies accredit and rate private payers. The major accrediting organizations are summarized in Table 9.3. Payers are also monitored by industry groups such as the National Association of Insurance Commissioners.

Billing Tip

Pay for Performance
BCBS is often a leader in efforts to improve health care. One example is pay-for-performance (P4P) programs that have financial incentives like bonuses for excellence in such performance measures as the NCQA HEDIS rating.

Blue Cross and Blue Shield Association

Founded in the 1930s to provide low-cost medical insurance, the **Blue Cross and Blue Shield Association (BCBS)** is a national organization of independent companies called Member Plans that insure more than 90 million people. About 50 percent of the plan subscribers (policyholders) join PPOs; 23 percent are in indemnity plans; 19 percent are in HMOs; and 8 percent are in point-of-service plans. BCBS has one investor-owned company, WellPoint, and a number of nonprofit companies. All offer a full range of health plans, including consumer-driven health plans, to individuals, small and large employer groups, senior citizens, federal government employees, and others. In addition

TABLE 9.3 Plan Accrediting Organizations

- *National Committee for Quality Assurance (NCQA):* An independent nonprofit organization, NCQA is the leader in accrediting HMOs and PPOs. Working with the health care industry, NCQA developed a group of performance measures called HEDIS (Health Plan Employer Data and Information Set). HEDIS provides employers and consumers with information about each plan's effectiveness in preventing and treating disease, about policyholders' access to care, about documentation, and about members' satisfaction with care. NCQA's guidelines on the process by which plans select physicians and hospitals to join their networks, called **credentialing**, include performance measures. NCQA requires plans to review the credentials of all providers in their plans every two years to ensure that the providers continue to meet appropriate standards of professional competence.
- *Utilization Review Accreditation Commission (URAC):* URAC, also known as the American Accreditation Healthcare Commission, is another leading accrediting group. Like NCQA, it is a nonprofit organization that establishes standards for managed health care plans. URAC has accreditation programs addressing both the security and privacy of health information as required by HIPAA.
- *Joint Commission on Accreditation of Healthcare Organizations (JCAHO):* JCAHO (often called the Joint Commission) sets and monitors standards for many types of patient care. JCAHO is made up of members from the American College of Surgeons, the American College of Physicians, the American Medical Association, the American Hospital Association, and the American Dental Association. JCAHO verifies compliance with accreditation standards for hospitals, long-term care facilities, psychiatric facilities, home health agencies, ambulatory care facilities, and pathology and clinical laboratory services. JCAHO works with NCQA and the American Medical Accreditation Program to coordinate the measurement of the quality of health care across the entire health care system.
- *American Medical Accreditation Program (AMAP):* AMAP helps alleviate the pressures facing physicians, health plans, and hospitals by reducing cost and administrative effort while simultaneously documenting quality. As a comprehensive program, AMAP measures and evaluates individual physicians against national standards, criteria, and peer performance in five areas: credentials, personal qualifications, environment of care, clinical performance, and patient care.
- *Accreditation Association for Ambulatory Health Care, Inc.(AAAHC):* AAAHC has accredited managed care organizations for more than twenty years. Its program emphasizes an assessment of clinical records, enrollee and provider satisfaction, provider qualifications, utilization of resources, and quality of care.

to major medical and hospital insurance, the "Blues" also have freestanding dental, vision, mental health, prescription, and hearing plans.

Subscriber Identification Card

Since BCBS offers local and national programs through many individual plans, Blue Cross and Blue Shield subscriber identification cards are used to determine the type of plan a person is covered by (see Figure 9.6 on page 302). Most BCBS cards list the following information:

Plan name

Type of plan

Subscriber name

Subscriber identification number (the subscriber's Social Security number has been replaced with a unique ID)

Effective date of coverage

BCBS plan codes and coverage codes

Participation in reciprocity plan with other BCBS plans

Copayments, coinsurance, and deductible amounts

Information about additional coverage, such as prescription medication and mental health care

Information about preauthorization requirements

Claim submission address

Contact phone numbers

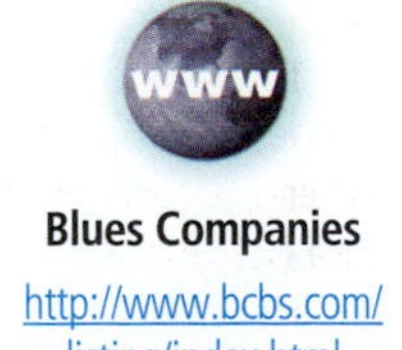

Blues Companies

http://www.bcbs.com/listing/index.html

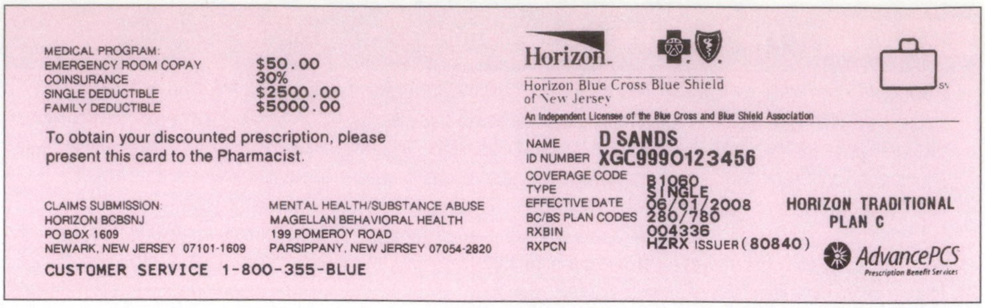

MEDICAL PROGRAM:
EMERGENCY ROOM COPAY $50.00
COINSURANCE 30%
SINGLE DEDUCTIBLE $2500.00
FAMILY DEDUCTIBLE $5000.00

To obtain your discounted prescription, please present this card to the Pharmacist.

CLAIMS SUBMISSION:
HORIZON BCBSNJ
PO BOX 1609
NEWARK, NEW JERSEY 07101-1609

MENTAL HEALTH/SUBSTANCE ABUSE
MAGELLAN BEHAVIORAL HEALTH
199 POMEROY ROAD
PARSIPPANY, NEW JERSEY 07054-2820

CUSTOMER SERVICE 1-800-355-BLUE

Horizon.

Horizon Blue Cross Blue Shield of New Jersey

An Independent Licensee of the Blue Cross and Blue Shield Association

NAME D SANDS
ID NUMBER XGC9990123456
COVERAGE CODE B1060
TYPE SINGLE
EFFECTIVE DATE 06/01/2008
BC/BS PLAN CODES 280/780
RXBIN 004336
RXPCN HZRX ISSUER(80840)

HORIZON TRADITIONAL PLAN C

AdvancePCS
Prescription Benefit Services

Front

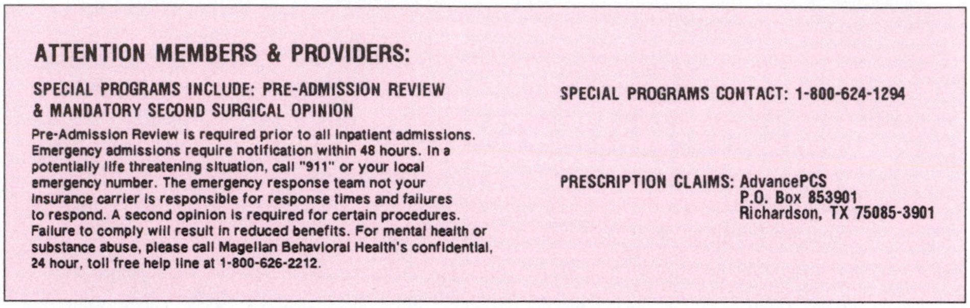

ATTENTION MEMBERS & PROVIDERS:

SPECIAL PROGRAMS INCLUDE: PRE-ADMISSION REVIEW & MANDATORY SECOND SURGICAL OPINION

Pre-Admission Review is required prior to all inpatient admissions. Emergency admissions require notification within 48 hours. In a potentially life threatening situation, call "911" or your local emergency number. The emergency response team not your insurance carrier is responsible for response times and failures to respond. A second opinion is required for certain procedures. Failure to comply will result in reduced benefits. For mental health or substance abuse, please call Magellan Behavioral Health's confidential, 24 hour, toll free help line at 1-800-626-2212.

SPECIAL PROGRAMS CONTACT: 1-800-624-1294

PRESCRIPTION CLAIMS: AdvancePCS
P.O. Box 853901
Richardson, TX 75085-3901

Back

FIGURE 9.6 Blue Cross and Blue Shield Subscriber Card.

Types of Plans

An indemnity BCBS plan has an individual and family deductible and a coinsurance payment. Individual annual deductibles may range from as little as $100 to as much as $2,500 or more. The family deductible is usually twice the amount of the individual deductible. Once the deductible has been met, the plan pays a percentage of the charges, usually 70, 80, or 90 percent, until an annual maximum out-of-pocket amount has been reached. After that, the plan pays 100 percent of approved charges until the end of the benefit year. At the beginning of the new benefit year, the out-of-pocket amount resets, and 100 percent reimbursement does not occur until the out-of-pocket maximum for the new year has been met. Once the cap has been met, charges by nonparticipating providers are paid at 100 percent of the allowed amount. If the charges exceed the allowed amount, the patient must pay the balance to the provider, even though the annual cap has been met.

> **Billing Tip**
>
> **BCBS Participation**
> Participating providers in BCBS plans are often called member physicians.

BCBS plans also offer many types of managed care programs, including the following:

- *HMO:* A patient must choose a primary care physician who is in the BCBS network. HMO has an Away From Home Care® Program that provides emergency room coverage if the subscriber needs care when traveling. Many Blue Cross and Blue Shield plans also have a Guest Membership through the Away From Home Care Program. A Guest Membership is a courtesy enrollment for members who are temporarily residing outside of their home HMO service area for at least ninety days.
- *POS:* Members of a POS plan may receive treatment from a provider in the network, or they may choose to see a provider outside the network and pay a higher fee. Depending on the particular plan, a patient may or may not have a primary care provider.

- *PPO:* Physicians and other health care providers sign participation contracts with BCBS agreeing to accept reduced fees in exchange for membership in the network. As network members, providers are listed in a provider directory and receive referrals from other network members. PPO subscribers have the PPO℠ on their Blue ID cards. A patient may choose to see a network provider or, for higher fees, a nonnetwork provider.

BlueCard Program

The **BlueCard** program is a nationwide program that makes it easy for patients to receive treatment when outside their local service area and also makes it easy for a provider to receive payment when treating patients enrolled in plans outside the provider's service area. The program links participating providers and independent BCBS plans throughout the nation with a single electronic claim processing and reimbursement system. It works as follows:

1. A subscriber who requires medical care while traveling outside the service area presents the subscriber ID card to a BCBS participating provider.
2. The provider verifies the subscriber's membership and benefit coverage by calling the BlueCard eligibility number. Only the required copayment can be collected; the provider cannot ask the patient to pay any other fees.
3. After providing treatment, the provider submits the claim to the local BCBS plan in his or her service area, which is referred to as the **host plan**.
4. The host plan sends the claim via modem to the patient's **home plan** (the plan in effect when the patient is at home), which processes the claim and sends it back to the host plan.
5. The host plan pays the provider according to local payment methods, and the home plan sends the remittance advice. For example, if a subscriber from New Jersey requires treatment while traveling in Delaware, the provider in Delaware can treat the patient, file the claim, and collect payment from the Delaware plan.

Flexible Blue Plan

Blue Cross and Blue Shield companies also offer a consumer-driven health plan called **Flexible Blue**. This plan combines a comprehensive PPO plan with either an HSA, an HRA, or a FSA. Also part of the CDHP are online decision-support resources.

Thinking it Through — 9.2

1. Given the many different insurance plans with which medical insurance specialists work, what do you think are the most important items of information that should be available about a plan?
2. Review the PPO plan benefits shown in Figure 9.3 on page 294. How would you summarize the rules for in-network versus out-of-network preventive care? Medical care? Is preauthorization needed for in-network hospital care?

Participation Contracts

Providers, like employers and employees, must evaluate health plans. They judge which plans to participate in based primarily on the financial arrangements that are offered. Because managed care organizations are the predominant health care delivery systems, most medical practices have a number of contracts with plans in their area. Figure 9.7 shows the notice of participation posted in an orthopedic specialty.

Contract Provisions

When a participation contract is being considered by a practice's contract evaluation team, an experienced medical insurance specialist may be asked to assist. The team is usually led by a practice manager or by a committee of physicians; an outside attorney typically reviews the contract as well. The

Welcome to Newton Major Orthopedic Associates, P.C.

In order to make your visit as pleasant as possible, we have compiled a list of the most commonly asked questions regarding insurance and billing in this office.

With which insurance plans does NMOA participate?

Aetna/US Healthcare Plans
CIGNA
Blue Choice PPO: POS, PPO, Prestige, Select
Focus Workers Compensation PPO
Health Care Value Management, Inc.
Health Choice
Health Direct
Kaiser Permanente
Medicare
Medicaid
MedSpan
MD Health Plan
Oxford Health Plan
Physician Health Services
Prudential Healthcare
POS Plan
Wellcare

What can I expect if NMOA participates with my insurance?

We will file a claim with your insurance company for any charges. Your insurance may require you to pay a copay at the time of services. You are responsible for any deductibles and non-covered services. You may need to obtain a referral from your primary care physician. Failure to obtain a referral may result in rescheduling of your appointment until you can obtain one.

What can I expect if NMOA does not participate with my insurance?

Payment is expected at the time of service. You will receive a statement within two weeks. Use it to file a claim. As a courtesy, NMOA will submit any surgery claims to your insurance carrier, but you are responsible for payment.

FIGURE 9.7 Example of Practice Participation List

managed care organization's business history, accreditation standing, and licensure status are reviewed.

The major question to be answered is whether participation in the plan is a good financial opportunity. All plans pay less than the physicians' fees schedules, so there is less revenue for each procedure. Some plans pay fees that are very low, and even gaining many more patients who have this plan may not make it profitable. The evaluation team checks the fees the plan pays for the CPT codes that the practice's providers most often bill. If the plan reduces payment for these services too much, the evaluation team may decide not to join, even though participation would bring more patients.

Other aspects of the plan, such as its medical necessity guidelines, are also considered. Some physicians do not accept certain plans because, in their view, complying with the plans' health care protocols will limit their professional medical judgment in treating patients.

The main parts of participation contracts are the following:

- Introductory section (often called "recitals" and "definitions")
- Contract purpose and covered medical services
- Physician's responsibilities
- Managed care plan obligations
- Compensation and billing guidelines

Introductory Section

The introductory section is important because it lists the names of the contracting parties and defines the terms used in the contract. Often, the contract mentions that the provider's manual is part of the agreement and is to be referred to for specific points. The section also states the ways the plan may use participating physicians' names. Some plans wish to provide lists of participating physicians to plan members. Other plans, however, want to use the providers' names in newspaper, radio, or television advertisements.

This section also specifically indicates who the payer is, such as "First Health Plan, a federally qualified health maintenance organization," or "Golden Gate Insurance Company, a stock company." Payer information must be noted so that claims are sent to the correct organization. For example, although a self-funded health plan may create the plan, a third-party administrator (TPA) may be responsible for processing and paying claims.

Contract Purpose and Covered Medical Services

Since MCOs offer multiple products—HMO, PPO, POS, CDHP, and fee-for-service options—a contract may be for one or several of these products. The contract should state the type of plan and the medical services to be provided to its members. In addition to office visits and preventive medical services, which are usual, obstetrician-gynecologist, behavioral health, physical and occupational therapy, emergency and urgent care, and diagnostic laboratory services may be covered.

Under a capitation plan, the exact covered services (with a list of CPTs) included in the cap rate should appear (see Chapter 7). For example, when a provider gives a patient an MMR (measles, mumps, and rubella virus) vaccine, two fees are involved: one for giving the injection (called the administration of the immunization) and a second for the dosage of the vaccine itself. Under a capitated primary care contract, the covered medical services provisions state whether both the fee for injecting vaccines and the cost of injectable materials are included in the cap rate, or just the immunization administration.

Physician's Responsibilities

The physician's responsibilities under the plan include the following:

- *Covered services*: The contract should stipulate the services that the provider must offer to plan members.
- *Acceptance of plan members*: The contract states whether providers must see all plan members who wish to use their services or some percentage or specific number of members. For example, capitated plans often require primary care physicians to accept at least a certain number of patients who are enrolled in the plan. If treating this number of patients means that the plan's enrollees will make up a large part of the practice, providers must decide whether the plan's payment structure is high enough before agreeing to participate.
- *Referrals*: This part of the contract states whether providers must refer patients to other participating providers only. It also covers the conditions under which the referral rules do not apply, such as in an emergency.
- *Preauthorization*: If the provider is responsible for securing preauthorization for the patient, as is the case in most HMOs, this is stated.
- *Quality assurance/utilization review:* Providers typically must agree to allow access to certain records for the payer's quality assurance and utilization review (QA/UR) activities. **Utilization review** refers to the payer's process for determining medical necessity—whether the review is conducted before or after the services are provided.
- *Other provisions*: Providers' credentials, health plan protocols, HIPAA Privacy policies, record retention, and other guidelines from the payer's medical review program are covered.

Billing Tip

Withdrawing from a Contract
Most participation contracts require physicians to notify patients if the physicians withdraw from the patients' managed care organization.

Managed Care Plan Obligations

Managed care plan obligations include the following:

- *Identification of enrolled patients:* The plan's method of identifying enrolled patients should be specified. Usually, this is with an identification card like the one shown in Figure 9.8. In this example, the provider network, the schedule of benefits, the office visit copayment, the name of the policyholder, the group, the type of contract, the patient's identification number, and the patient's dependents are listed.
- *Payments:* A claim turnaround time is specified in the contract. This tells how long it will take for a physician to be paid for services.
- *Other compensation:* This indicates whether any incentives, bonuses, and withholds apply (see Chapter 7).
- *Protection against loss:* If the provider is assuming financial risk for the cost of care, as happens under capitation, the contract should have a **stop-loss provision**. This clause limits the provider's costs if there is an unexpectedly high use of services. For example, a cap rate might be based on a typical E/M service pattern, with most patients requiring midlevel service and few needing low or high levels. If a large number of patients require comprehensive histories and examinations with complex medical decision making during one month, or if one patient had multiple visits, the cap rate would not be adequate pay. Stop-loss provisions state a dollar amount over which the provider will be repaid.

Under plans in which providers must refer patients to other participating providers only, the providers' compliance is evaluated by the plan, and incentives or bonuses may be tied to how well a provider observes the referral rules. For this reason, a stated obligation of the plan should be to provide and regularly update the list of participating providers, so that providers are sure they are referring their patients correctly.

PHYSICIANS
HEALTH SERVICE

NETWORK: 003 SCHEDULE: C77 OFC: $15
SUBSCRIBER: GEORGE HERKER
GROUP: POS
CONTRACT: CHARTER POS
RIDERS: P, CM, C2, PS

IDENTIFICATION
100329712 For Pharmacy Questions 877-747-9378

BILLING CODE	NAME
01	GEORGE A.
02	MARY B.
03	ANDREW E.
04	PETER E.

AdvanceRx

Front

Physicians Health Services

PLEASE BE SURE TO CARRY THIS CARD AND PRESENT IT AT THE TIME OF SERVICE
If you have questions, call PHS Customer Relations at (800) 555-1000
E-mail Address: member@phs.com Internet Address: http://www.phs.com

MEMBERS: Medical Services provided by a non-PHS physician will be subject to deductibles and coinsurance. Please refer to your plan documents to determine what services are covered and/or may require prior authorization.
EMERGENCIES: You are covered for emergencies worldwide. If the situation is life-threatening, go to the nearest hospital or call 911. If not life-threatening, but urgent, attempt to contact your PHS physician first. If you are away from home and are admitted to an out-of-area hospital, call PHS as soon as possible at (800) 555-1000.

To submit billing, complete a current, original HCFA 1500 or UB92. Include the PHS ID# and the member's two-digit billing code which appear on the front of this card.

Mail Claims To: PHS Claims Dept., P.O. Box 981, Randall CT 06691-0981
For electronic claims submission information call the Claims EDI Dept at (800) 555-1001
This Card Does Not Guarantee Coverage

Back

FIGURE 9.8 Example of an Insurance Card for a POS Plan

Compensation and Billing Guidelines

The compensation and billing guidelines cover fees, billing requirements, claim filing deadlines, patients' financial responsibilities, and balance-billing rules. The rules for collecting patients' payments are described, as are how to coordinate benefits when another plan is primary.

> **Billing Tip**
>
> **List All NPIs**
> The contract should list the NPIs (National Provider Identifiers) of all practitioners who will bill under it, not only the NPI for the practice itself.

Interpreting Compensation and Billing Guidelines

Participation contracts other than for capitated plans often state the basis for the payer's allowed amounts. A payer may base allowed amounts on a percentage of the Medicare Physician Fee Schedule (MPFS) or a discounted fee-for-service arrangement.

> **Billing Tip**
>
> **When the MPFS Is the Base**
> If a payer's fee schedule is based on the Medicare Physician Fee Schedule, the contract should state which year's MPFS is going to be used.

Compiling Billing Data

Practices generally bill out from their normal fee schedules, rather than billing the contracted fees, even if they are known. Writing off the differences between

Thinking it Through — 9.3

In what section of a participation contract is each of the following phrases located?

1. Physician has accurately completed the Participating Physician Credentialing Application that accompanies this agreement and has been accepted by the Plan. Physician shall promptly notify Plan of any change in this information, including any change in its principal place of business, within seven days of such change.

   ____

2. "Members" means enrollees or enrolled dependents covered by a Plan benefit agreement.

   ____

3. Physician agrees to accept the Plan fee schedule or physician's billed charges, whichever is less, as payment in full for all medical services provided to members.

   ____

4. Physician agrees to allow review and duplication of any data free of charge and other records maintained on members which relate to this agreement.

   ____

5. Plan agrees to provide current identification cards for members.

   ____

6. Plan shall deduct any copayments and deductible amounts required by the Plan benefit agreement from the allowed payment due Physician under this agreement.

   ____

7. Plan intends, by entering into this agreement, to make available quality health care to Plan members by contracting with Physician. Physician intends to provide such care in a cost-effective manner.

   ____

Billing Tip

Increasing Covered Services
Keep a record of services that were not paid over a year's billing period. This record provides a basis for negotiating a revised contract in order to cover more services.

normal fees and payments under the participation contract is done when the RA/EOB is processed (see Chapters 14 and 15). Billing this way permits the practice to track how much revenue is lost by participating in a particular contract, which is valuable information for future contract negotiations.

Physician's Fee Schedule for CPT 99211	$25
Contract Fee for PAR Providers for CPT 99211	$18
Loss of Revenue per Visit for CPT 99211	$7
Service Performed × 500 Visits Annually	
Annual Lost Revenue for This CPT Code	$3,500

A record can be kept of lost revenue per each commonly billed CPT code. To negotiate higher fees, a practice may compare the difference in payer accounts over a year for its commonly billed procedures and use this comparison when negotiating contract renewal.

Getting Billing Information

Private payers have traditionally been reluctant to tell providers what their fee schedules, code edits, and other billing practices are. However, a group of state medical societies considered these business practices to be unfair. This group sued the largest private payers in a class-action suit alleging that the payers had conspired to delay, downcode, and deny provider claims for more than a decade. The suit never came to court, though, because each of the sued companies settled out of court before its trial began.

These settlements by each payer promise to fix many billing problems. The following lists representative issues and resolutions under the settlements:

- Payers will provide fee schedule amounts for at least two hundred CPT codes.
- Payers will list all services requiring precertification.
- Payers will follow consistent bundling edits and will publish significant edits (those that cause more than five hundred denials and payment reductions) as well as the code combinations that will not be paid even with modifiers –25 or –59.
- Surgical global periods will not be longer than Medicare's.
- Payers will not automatically downcode, reduce, or reassign E/M services except to change an established visit code to a new visit code.
- Payers will process clean claims within thirty days (paper claims) or fifteen days (electronic claims).

Billing for No-Shows

The contract determines whether a participating provider can charge a patient for a product used to set up a procedure when the patient cancels. Often, a physician may bill only for a rendered service, not for a service that is not delivered, including cancellations and no-shows. In nonparticipating situations, have patients agree in writing to pay before scheduling procedures. Follow the practice's financial policy for billing for no-shows or cancellations.

Collecting Copayments

Payers vary as to the copayment(s) required. Some plans require a copayment only when an E/M service is provided, and others require it when the patient visits an office for any procedure or service. Copayment amounts may also vary according to the service performed. Some plans have different copayment amounts for office visits, emergency room visits, ambulance services, and preventive services. When two services, such as an E/M service and a billable procedure, are performed on the same date of service, either one or two copayments may be required, again depending on the payer.

Another variable in collecting copayments involves primary and secondary plans. Medical insurance specialists should verify whether a copayment is to be collected under the secondary plan. Usually it is not, unless the primary plan does not cover the service or if the member is satisfying a deductible for the primary plan.

The payer's rules about copayment calculations also need to be understood. Most plans require the patient's copayment to be subtracted from the amount

Billing Tip

Payment for New Procedures
Payment policy for a new procedure may be announced by a payer. If the practice performs this procedure, it should notify its other PAR plans that this procedure will be reported for payment in the future and should request their allowed charge and any other regulations for payment.

Billing Tip

Prompt-Payment Discounts
Payers may offer prompt payment in return for larger-than-contracted fees. Acceptance of these offers for expedited review and payment is a matter of practice policy.

Compliance Guideline

Avoid Price Fixing
Office of Inspector General (OIG) rules prohibit practices from discussing pricing and rates with other practices.

Compliance Guideline

Collect Copays
The practice is obligated to follow payer copayment guidelines. Routinely waiving copays and deductibles may be fraudulent under participation contracts. This should be stated in the financial policy that patients are given.

due to the provider from the payer. This treats the copayment like a deductible or coinsurance payment. The contract (or provider's manual) states the policy in terms such as "All member copayments, deductibles, and coinsurance apply." (The word *apply* means that they should be taken into account when the payer calculates the balance due to the provider.)

The plan is a PPO that pays 75 percent of the provider's usual charge. A $5 copayment is due, and the copayment is applied toward the provider payment.

Provider's usual charge	$100.00
Payer allowed fee ($100 × 75%)	$ 75.00
Patient copay subtracted	–$ 5.00
Payer pays	$ 70.00
Provider collects a total of	$ 75.00

Note that a few plans, though, do not deduct the patient's copayment from the usual charge. Instead, the plan has a lower allowed fee for the service, so often the provider collects the same amount in the end. For example:

The plan is a PPO that pays 70 percent of the provider's usual charge. A $5 copayment is due to the provider as well.

Provider's usual charge	$100.00
Payer allowed fee ($100 × 70%)	$ 70.00
Patient copay collected	$ 5.00
Payer pays	$ 70.00
Provider collects a total of	$ 75.00

Both approaches are acceptable. The rules must be clear to the medical insurance specialist for correct calculations of the expected payment from the payer.

Billing Tip

State Prohibition of Silent PPOs

At least eight states (California, Illinois, Louisiana, Minnesota, North Carolina, Oklahoma, and Wisconsin) prohibit silent PPOs, and state insurance commissions in other states may be considering such laws.

Avoiding Silent PPOs

Silent PPOs—also called *network-sharing agreements*—occur when a managed care organization leases its PPO provider network list to another entity, such as a smaller PPO, so the other entity can take advantage of the discounts negotiated by the original PPO. This can cause a practice to accept a PAR payment for a service to a patient who is not enrolled in a plan it participates in. In most cases, the physician is led to believe that the discount is legitimate. Most experts recommend trying to negotiate a phrase in participation contracts stating that the MCO cannot lease any terms of the agreement—including the physician's discounted services—or assign benefits to another payer.

Billing Tip

The Term Precertification

Precertification ("precert") is another term for preauthorization. It is usually applied to hospital admissions and outpatient surgery. Both terms have the same meaning.

Billing Surgical Procedures

Most managed care plans have rules for authorizing emergency surgical procedures and elective surgery. Emergency surgery usually must be approved within a specified period, such as forty-eight hours, after admission was required. **Elective surgery** is a procedure that can be scheduled ahead of time, but which may be medically necessary. It usually requires preauthorization during a specified period before the service is performed. The preauthorization requirement is usually shown on the patient's insurance card (see Figure 9.9). The practice must send a completed preauthorization form or online application for review in advance of the admission. Figure 9.10 on page 312 shows an example of a precertification form.

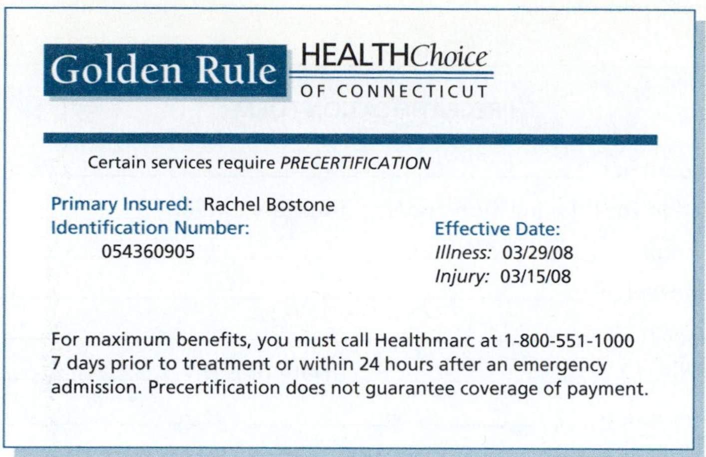

Front

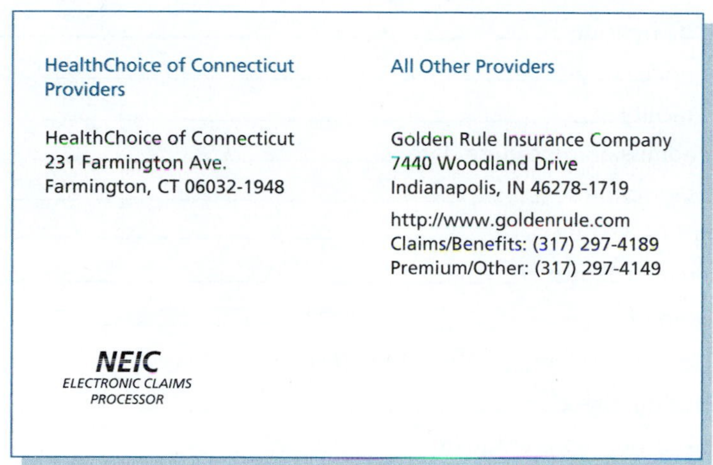

Back

FIGURE 9.9 Example of an Insurance Card Showing Precertification Requirement

Some elective surgical procedures are done on an inpatient basis, so the patient is admitted to the hospital; others are done on an outpatient basis. The following are common outpatient surgeries:

- Abdominal hernia
- Bunionectomy
- Carpal tunnel
- Destruction of cutaneous vascular proliferative lesions
- Knee arthroscopy
- Otoplasty
- Sclerotherapy

For a major course of treatment, such as surgery, chemotherapy, and radiation for a patient with cancer, many private payers use the services of a **utilization review organization (URO)**. The URO is hired by the payer to evaluate the medical necessity of planned procedures. When a provider (or a patient) requests preauthorization for a treatment plan, the URO issues a report of its findings. As shown in Figure 9.11 on page 313, the patient and provider are both notified of the results. If the planned services are not covered, the patient should agree to pay for them before the treatment begins.

Billing Tip

Out-of-Network Services
Many plans require preauthorization for out-of-network services even though they are covered under the plan.

PRECERTIFICATION FORM

Insurance carrier ______________________________

Certification for [ ] admission and/or [ ] surgery and/or [ ] ______________

Patient name ______________________________

Street address ______________________________

City/state/zip ______________________________

Telephone ______________ Date of birth ______________

Subscriber name ______________________________

Employer ______________________________

Member no. ______________ Group no. ______________

Admitting physician ______________________________

Provider no. ______________________________

Hospital/facility ______________________________

Planned admission/procedure date ______________________________

Diagnosis/symptoms ______________________________

Treatment/procedure ______________________________

Estimated length of stay ______________________________

Complicating factors ______________________________

Second opinion required [ ] Yes [ ] No If yes, [ ] Obtained

Corroborating physician ______________________________

Insurance carrier representative ______________________________

Approval [ ] Yes [ ] No If yes, certification no. ______________

If no, resason(s) for denial ______________________________

FIGURE 9.10 Precertification Form for Hospital Admission or Surgery

Private Payer Billing Management and Claim Completion

Organizing job aids, such as the plan summary grid described below, and following the steps of the billing process will provide answers to these essential questions:

- What services are covered under the plan? What conditions establish medical necessity for these services? Are these correctly coded and linked?
- Which services are not covered?
- What are the billing rules—the bundling and global periods—of the plan?
- What is the patient responsible for paying at the time of the encounter and after adjudication?

Case number: G631000
Procedure: Axillary node dissection

Dear Patient:

As you may know, ABC is a utilization review company that contracts with insurance companies, managed care organizations, and self-insured groups to review the health care services provided to people covered under their medical plans and to make recommendations regarding the medical necessity and efficiency of these health care services. ABC is not an insurer, and does not make eligibility, benefit, or coverage decisions.

We have received information about the procedure scheduled for 08/12/2009 at Downtown Hospital. Based on review of this information, we find this outpatient procedure to be medically necessary and efficient.

If the treatment plan is changed, or if admission to the hospital is necessary, please contact your insurance company immediately.

ABC's recommendation is not a decision regarding payment of a particular claim. Your medical plan payer is responsible for making final payment and eligibility decisions. Any questions about a claim, deductible, or copayment should be directed to your medical plan.

Sincerely,

ABC Reviewer
Medical Care Coordinator

cc: George Ballister, M.D.
Downtown Hospital

FIGURE 9.11 Example of Letter from Utilization Review Organization

Plan Summary Grids

Medical insurance specialists organize each plan's benefit and payment information for easy access. For each participation contract, a **plan summary grid** should be prepared or updated. The grid summarizes key items from the contract, such as the payers' names and plans, patient financial responsibility (copayments; which services are subject to deductibles), referral and preauthorization requirements, covered and noncovered services, billing information, and participating labs. Some offices use a form like the one shown in Figure 9.12 on page 314.

Other key information includes:

- The major code edits for bundled procedures and services
- The global follow-up times for major and minor surgical procedures

PAYER NAME____
PLAN NAME ____
PLAN TYPE (PPO, HMO, FFS, OTHER)_____________________
PAYER WEBSITE ______________________________________

PARTICIPATION CONTRACT ACTIVE DATE?_____________
Provider Customer Service Phone Contact to check benefits, eligibility, claim status, request verification _________________________
Correspondence, Claim Appeals, and Reconsiderations to: __________________

REQUIRED FACILITIES AND PREAUTHORIZATION FOR: YES NO
Referrals: In Network ____
Out-of-Network____
Imaging:
CT Scans ____________________
MRA Scans ____________________
MRI Scans __________________
Nuclear Cardiology Studies ___________
PET Scans __________________
Other __________________

Participating Labs ____
Hospital Admission ____
Known Excluded Services ___________________________________

PATIENT FINANCIAL RESPONSIBILITY
Copayments: Office Visit__________
Well care, age birth to ____ Amount: _________
Well care, age _______ to _______ Amount: _________
Labs covered in Office _________
Outside Labs_______________
Deductible
No _____Yes ____ Amount________ Collect Before or After Service?_______
CDHP Plan?
No _____Yes ____ Amount________ Collect Before or After Service?_______
Coinsurance
No _____Yes ____ Amount________ Collect Before or After Service?_______
Excluded Services Collect Before or After Service?_______

CLAIMS
Electronic Payer ID: ______________
Paper Claims to:

Timely Filing: ____________________________

FIGURE 9.12 Plan Summary Grid

Billing Tip

Consult Versus Referral
Plans often have forms that misuse the terms refer and consult. A consultation occurs when a physician, at the request of another physician, examines the patient and reports an opinion to the requestor. Under a referral, care (a portion or all) is transferred to another physician. However, a plan's referral form may in fact be the correct one to use when consultation is required. This usage should be clarified with the plan.

HIPAA Tip

278 Referral and Authorization

The HIPAA 278 Referral and Authorization is the electronic format used to obtain approval for preauthorizations and referrals.

- The policies for multiple procedure reimbursement (whether the payer fully reimburses multiple procedures performed on the same date of service or pays fully for the first service only and pays the rest at a reduced percentage)
- Verification procedures
- Documentation requirements, such as special reports for unlisted procedure codes or the name of the serum, the dosage, and the route of administration for immunizations
- Appeal procedures

The practice management program (PMP) is also updated with each payer's name and contact information, the plan type, and payment information.

Medical Billing Process

The first seven steps of the standard medical billing process (see Chapter 1) are followed to complete correct claims and transmit them to private payers. Study the steps below. (The last three steps of the process for private payers, covering adjudication and RA/EOB, appeals, patient billing and collections, are covered in Chapters 14 and 15.)

Step 1 Preregister Patients

The general guidelines apply to the preregistration process for private health plan patients: Collect and enter basic demographic and insurance information.

Step 2 Establish Financial Responsibility for Visit

The initial information for a new patient's plan is taken from the patient's information form (PIF). Changes in insurance coverage for established patients are noted on an update to the patient information form.

Verify Insurance Eligibility Based on the copies of insurance cards, contact the payer to double-check that the patient is eligible for services. Be sure to accurately enter the patient's name and ID number as it appears on the card.

The payer ID and logo on the insurance card identify the payer. If the card lists multiple PPOs and is not clear, contact the payer to select the correct payer for that patient. If the provider is a primary care physician and the plan requires registration of a PCP, the insurance card often lists the correct provider's name.

Check Coverage Depending on the type of practice, coverage for some of the following services may be specifically verified:

- Office visits
- Lab coverage (note that many managed care organizations specify which laboratory must be used for tests)
- Diagnostic X-rays
- Pap smear coverage
- Coverage of psychiatric visits, including the number of visits covered and the coinsurance for each
- Physical or occupational therapy
- Durable medical equipment (DME)
- Foot care

A patient with a self-funded health plan may have an ID card with a familiar plan to which claims should be sent. But that plan is handling the claims processing only; it is not providing the insurance. Do not assume that the patient's coverage is the same as it is for members of that health plan. Locate the actual name of the self-insured plan to verify eligibility and check benefits (for example, Lehigh Portland Cement or Tufts).

Coordinate Benefits Next, determine the primary plan for the patient, following the guidelines on page 91. Under coordination of benefits provisions, if the patient has signed an assignment of benefits statement, the provider is responsible for reporting any additional insurance coverage to the primary payer. Review the PIF to determine whether the patient has secondary or supplemental coverage that should be reported on the primary payer's claim.

Meet Preauthorization/Referral Requirements Additionally, check for and meet the payer's preauthorization and/or referral requirements. Referrals and preauthorizations are examples of the provider's contractual requirement to give

Billing Tip

Lab Requirements
Practices should post a notice to patients stating that if patients do not tell them about their plans' lab requirements and the specimen is sent to the wrong lab, the practice is not responsible for the costs.

HIPAA Tip

270/271 Eligibility for Benefits Transaction

The HIPAA 270/271 Eligibility for a Health Plan transaction (the inquiry from the provider and the response from the payer) is the electronic format used to verify benefits.

the plan notice of services performed. In most cases, payers require data that support clinical necessity if a required preauthorization was not obtained according to plan guidelines.

Notes on Nonparticipation When poviders do not participate in patients' plans, patients are told this before the encounters and are notified about their responsibility for payment. Many practices collect either a deposit or a full payment from the patient in advance in this situation. If the patient has out-of-network benefits and the practice chooses to bill the plan on the patient's behalf, the rate of pay is often uncertain. Most payers have a **repricer**, a company that works for the plan and sets the discounts for out-of-network visits. The practice may go along with the repricer's discounts to avoid further negotiations over a small sum. The problem, though, is that payment is often sent to the beneficiary rather than to the practice, which then has to try to collect. When the patient's plan is billed, the patient should assign benefits to avoid this problem. Check the practice's financial policy for guidance on this point. State laws may also apply.

Step 3 Check In Patients

Be sure that the correct copayment has been collected from the patient for the planned service. For example, if the plan summary grid for the patient's plan lists an office visit copay and that is the nature of the encounter, collect the copay and post it to the patient's account.

Step 4 Check Out Patients

Based on the encounter information, update the practice management program to reflect the appropriate diagnoses, services, and charges. Analyze the patient's financial responsibility, according to the practice's financial policy, for:

- Deductibles, especially in consumer-driven health plans
- Payment for noncovered services
- Balance due from previous encounters

Apply collected payments to the patient's account and provide a receipt for payment.

Step 5 Review Coding Compliance

Verify that the diagnosis and procedure codes are current as of the date of service. Check that the codes are properly linked and documented, showing the medical necessity for the services.

Step 6 Check Billing Compliance

Using the plan summary grid, verify that all charges planned for the claim are billable.

Billing Tip

Payer Instructions May Vary
The NUCC instructions do not address any particular payer. Best practice for paper claims is to check with each payer for specific information required on the form.

Step 7 Prepare and Transmit Claims

Participating providers submit claims to payers on behalf of patients; nonparticipating providers may elect to do this as well. Private payer claims are completed using either the HIPAA 837 claim or the CMS-1500 paper claim. CMS-1500 general completion guidelines are described in Table 9.4 and shown in Figure 9.13 on page 319. Claims must be submitted according to the plan's guidelines for timely filing. The filing deadline is based on the date of service on the claim, not the sent or received date.

TABLE 9.4 Private Payer CMS-1500 (08/05) Claim Completion

Item Number	Content
1	Indicate Group if the patient is covered by an employer-sponsored plan; check Other if the patient is covered by an individual health plan.
1a	Enter the insurance identification number that appears on the patient's insurance card.
2	Record the patient's name *exactly* as it appears on the insurance card, entering it in last name, first name, middle initial order. Do not use any punctuation or abbreviations.
3	Enter the patient's date of birth in eight-digit format; make the appropriate selection for male or female.
4	If the insured and the patient are not the same person, enter the name of the person who holds the insurance policy (the insured/subscriber), in last name, first name, and middle initial order.
5	Enter the patient's mailing address, including the number and street, city, state, ZIP code, and the home telephone number.
6	Select the appropriate box for the relationship.
7	If IN 4 is completed and the insured's address is the same as the patient's, enter SAME. If the insured's address is different, enter the mailing address and telephone number of the person listed in IN 4.
8	Select the appropriate boxes for marital status and employment status. Select Other for patients who are unmarried domestic partners or who are covered under a child's plan. If the patient is neither employed nor a student, leave the employment status box blank.
9	Secondary claim: enter patient's name in last, first, and middle initial order.
9a	Secondary claim: enter the policy or group number of that insurance.
9b	Secondary claim: enter the patient's date of birth and gender.
9c	Secondary claim: enter employer's name, if applicable.
9d	Secondary claim: enter the name of the secondary plan.
10a–10c	Choose the appropriate box to indicate whether the patient's condition is the result of a work injury, an automobile accident, or another type of accident. If any Yes is selected, the claim should be sent first to the liable party (workers' compensation, auto insurance, or other) and then a secondary claim sent to the patient's plan. The state postal code must be shown if Yes is checked in IN 10b for Auto Accident.
10d	Varies with the insurance plan; complete if instructed.
11	Enter the group number if it appears on the insurance identification card.
11a	Enter the insured's date of birth and sex if the patient is not the same person as the insured.
11b	If the policy is under a group, enter the name of the employer, school, or entity.
11c	Enter the name of the HMO, PPO, or other private plan. Note that some payers require the payer identification number of the primary insurer in this field.
11d	Select Yes if the patient is covered by additional (secondary or tertiary) insurance. If yes, IN 9a–9d must be completed.
12	Enter "Signature on File,""SOF," or a legal signature per practice policy.
13	Enter "Signature on File," "SOF," or a legal signature to indicate that there is a signature on file assigning benefits to the provider from the primary carrier. Note that many plans require assignment of benefits under their policies.
14	Enter the date documented in the medical record that symptoms first began for the current illness, injury, or pregnancy. For pregnancy, enter the first date of the last menstrual period (LMP). Previous pregnancies are not a similar illness. The date may be either before or on the current date of service. Leave blank if unknown.
15	If the patient has consulted the provider for treatment of the same or a similar condition, enter the first date.
16	Enter the dates the patient is employed but unable to work in the current occupation. (From: the first full day of disability; To: the last day of disability before returning to work.)
17	Enter the name (first name, middle initial, last name) and credentials of the professional who referred or ordered the service(s) or supply(s) on the claim.
17a	Enter the appropriate identifying number(s) (either NPI or non-NPI, a payer-assigned unique identifier) for the referring physician.
18	If the services provided are needed because of a related inpatient hospitalization, the admission and discharge dates are entered. For patients still hospitalized, the admission date is listed in the From box, and the To box is left blank.
19	Complete according to the payer's instructions.

(continued on next page)

TABLE 9.4	Private Payer CMS-1500 (08/05) Claim Completion *continued*
Item Number	**Content**
20	Complete if billing for outside lab services. Choosing No means that tests were performed by the billing physician or laboratory. Choosing Yes means that the test was done outside of the office of the physician who is billing for it. When Yes is selected, enter the purchase charge and complete IN 32. When billing for multiple purchased lab services, each service should be submitted on a separate claim.
21	Enter up to four ICD-9-CM codes in priority order. At least one code must be reported. Relate lines 1, 2, 3, 4 to the lines of service in IN 24E by line number. Do not provide narrative description in this box. The codes used should specify the highest level of detail possible, including the use of a fifth digit when appropriate.
22	Leave blank; Medicaid-specific.
23	Some procedures and diagnostic tests require preauthorization. If required, enter the preauthorization number assigned by the payer.
24	The service line information section is used to report the procedures performed for the patient. Each item of service line information has a procedure code and a charge, with additional information as detailed below.
24A	Enter the date(s) of service, from and to. If there is only one date of service, enter that date under From, and leave To blank or reenter the From date. If grouping services, the place of service, procedure code, charges, and individual provider for each line must be identical for that service line. Grouping is allowed only for services on consecutive days. The number of days must correspond to the number of units in IN 24G.
24B	Enter the place of service (POS) code that describes the location at which the service was provided. If the service was provided to a hospitalized inpatient (POS 21), enter the hospital's provider information in IN 32.
24C	Check with the payer to determine whether this element (emergency indicator) is necessary. If required, enter "Y" (Yes) or "N" (No) in the unshaded bottom portion of the field.
24D	Enter the CPT/HCPCS codes, applicable modifiers, and anesthesia time in minutes for services provided. Do not use hyphens.
24E	Using the numbers (1, 2, 3, 4) listed to the left of the diagnosis codes in IN 21, enter the diagnosis for the each service listed in IN 24D.
24F	For each service listed in IN 24D, enter charges without dollar signs or decimals. If the claim reports an encounter with no charge, such as a capitated visit, a value of zero (0) may be used.
24G	Enter the number of days or units, as applicable. This field is most commonly used for multiple visits, units of supplies, anesthesia units or minutes, or oxygen volume. If only one service is performed, the numeral 1 must be entered.
24H	Leave blank; Medicaid-specific.
24I–24J	IN 24I and IN 24J work together. These boxes are used to enter an ID number for the rendering provider of the service. If the number is an NPI, it goes in IN 24J in the unshaded area next to the 24I label *NPI*. If the number is a non-NPI (other ID number), the qualifier identifying the type of number goes in IN 24I next to the number in 24J.
25	Enter the physician's or supplier's federal tax identification number (either a Social Security number or an Employer Identification Number). Check the appropriate box for SSN or EIN.
26	Enter the patient account number used by the practice's accounting system.
27	If the physician accepts assignment, select Yes.
28	Enter the total of all charges in IN 24F. If the claim is to be submitted on paper and there are more services to be billed, put "continued" here, and put the total charge on the last claim form page.
29	Amount of the payments received for the services listed on this claim. If no payment was made, enter "None" or 0.00.
30	Enter the balance resulting from subtracting the amount in IN 29 from the amount in IN 28.
31	Enter the provider's or supplier's signature, the date of the signature, and the provider's credentials (such as MD).
32	Enter the name, address, city, state, and ZIP code of the location where the services were rendered if not the physician's office or the patient's home, or enter SAME. A supplier's NPI is entered IN 32a. Enter the payer-assigned identifying non-NPI number/qualifier of the service facility in IN 32b.
33	Enter the billing provider's or supplier's name, address, ZIP code, telephone number, NPI, non-NPI number and appropriate qualifier. The NPI is entered in IN 33a. Enter the identifying non-NPI number and qualifier of the billing provider in box 33b.

1500

HEALTH INSURANCE CLAIM FORM

PICA

1. MEDICARE / MEDICAID / TRICARE CHAMPUS / CHAMPVA / GROUP HEALTH PLAN [X] (SSN or ID) / FECA BLK LUNG / OTHER

1a. INSURED'S I.D. NUMBER: GH 331240789

2. PATIENT'S NAME (Last Name, First Name, Middle Initial): CARUTHERS ROBIN

3. PATIENT'S BIRTH DATE: 03 29 1979 — SEX: F [X]

4. INSURED'S NAME (Last Name, First Name, Middle Initial):

5. PATIENT'S ADDRESS (No., Street): 167 CHEVY LANE

6. PATIENT RELATIONSHIP TO INSURED: Self [X]

7. INSURED'S ADDRESS (No., Street):

CITY: CLEVELAND — STATE: OH

8. PATIENT STATUS: Married [X]; Employed [X]

ZIP CODE: 44101 — TELEPHONE (Include Area Code): (555) 629 0347

9. OTHER INSURED'S NAME (Last Name, First Name, Middle Initial):

10. IS PATIENT'S CONDITION RELATED TO:
a. EMPLOYMENT? (CURRENT OR PREVIOUS) NO [X]
b. AUTO ACCIDENT? NO [X]
c. OTHER ACCIDENT? NO [X]
10d. RESERVED FOR LOCAL USE

11. INSURED'S POLICY GROUP OR FECA NUMBER: OH 4071
a. INSURED'S DATE OF BIRTH / SEX
b. EMPLOYER'S NAME OR SCHOOL NAME: THE KAUFMAN GROUP
c. INSURANCE PLAN NAME OR PROGRAM NAME: ANTHEM BCBS PPO
d. IS THERE ANOTHER HEALTH BENEFIT PLAN? NO [X] *If yes,* return to and complete item 9 a-d.

READ BACK OF FORM BEFORE COMPLETING & SIGNING THIS FORM.

12. PATIENT'S OR AUTHORIZED PERSON'S SIGNATURE I authorize the release of any medical or other information necessary to process this claim. I also request payment of government benefits either to myself or to the party who accepts assignment below.

SIGNED: SOF — DATE

13. INSURED'S OR AUTHORIZED PERSON'S SIGNATURE I authorize payment of medical benefits to the undersigned physician or supplier for services described below.

SIGNED: SOF

14. DATE OF CURRENT: ILLNESS (First symptom) OR INJURY (Accident) OR PREGNANCY(LMP)
15. IF PATIENT HAS HAD SAME OR SIMILAR ILLNESS. GIVE FIRST DATE
16. DATES PATIENT UNABLE TO WORK IN CURRENT OCCUPATION FROM / TO
17. NAME OF REFERRING PHYSICIAN OR OTHER SOURCE — 17a. — 17b. NPI
18. HOSPITALIZATION DATES RELATED TO CURRENT SERVICES FROM / TO
19. RESERVED FOR LOCAL USE
20. OUTSIDE LAB? NO [X] — $ CHARGES
21. DIAGNOSIS OR NATURE OF ILLNESS OR INJURY. (Relate Items 1,2,3 or 4 to Item 24e by Line)
1. 427 31
22. MEDICAID RESUBMISSION CODE — ORIGINAL REF. NO.
23. PRIOR AUTHORIZATION NUMBER

	24. A. DATE(S) OF SERVICE From	To	B. PLACE OF SERVICE	C. EMG	D. CPT/HCPCS	MODIFIER	E. DIAGNOSIS POINTER	F. $ CHARGES	G. DAYS OR UNITS	H. EPSDT Family Plan	I. ID. QUAL.	J. RENDERING PROVIDER ID. #
1	10 01 2008		11		99213		1	62 00	1		NPI	
2	10 01 2008		11		93000		1	70 00	1		NPI	
3											NPI	
4											NPI	
5											NPI	
6											NPI	

25. FEDERAL TAX I.D. NUMBER: 16 1234567 — SSN EIN [X]
26. PATIENT'S ACCOUNT NO.: CARUTRO0
27. ACCEPT ASSIGNMENT? (For govt. claims, see back) YES / NO
28. TOTAL CHARGE: $ 132 00
29. AMOUNT PAID: $ 15 00
30. BALANCE DUE: $

31. SIGNATURE OF PHYSICIAN OR SUPPLIER INCLUDING DEGREES OR CREDENTIALS (I certify that the statements on the reverse apply to this bill and are made a part thereof.)

SIGNED: SOF — DATE

32. SERVICE FACILITY LOCATION INFORMATION: SAME
a. NPI — b.

33. BILLING PROVIDER INFO & PHONE #: (720) 554 1222
CHRISTOPHER CONNOLLY
1400 WEST CENTER ST
TOLEDO OH 43601 0213
a. 1286927799 — b.

NUCC Instruction Manual available at: www.nucc.org

CARRIER — PATIENT AND INSURED INFORMATION — PHYSICIAN OR SUPPLIER INFORMATION

FIGURE 9.13 CMS-1500 (08/05) Completion for Private Payers

Following are some claim preparation tips:

- *Taxonomy codes:* The participation contract may state that certain specialties receive higher rates for various procedures. For example, if a pediatrician is board-certified in pediatric cardiology, the correct taxonomy code—either for pediatrician or for pediatric cardiology—would be reported with the associated service.
- *Identifying numbers:* Until the NPI program is fully implemented, many private payers require the claim to contain the providers' identifying numbers. BCBS plans usually require the Blue Provider Number.
- *Contract information:* The participation contract may require a contract-type code, contract amount, contract percent, contract code, discount percent, or contract version identifier.
- *Description of services for modifiers –22 and –23*: Many plans require a complete description of the services including supporting documentation when these modifiers are used.

Billing Tip

Audits
Internal claim audits before transmission are the best way to check claims. During this review, a staff member other than the claim preparer checks the claim's coding and billing compliance for the payer.

The plan's claim submission guidelines are also followed. Contact the payer representative to clarify the procedure for claim attachments or other points.

Communications with Payers

Good communication between payers and the medical insurance staff is essential for effective contract and claim management. As claims are processed, questions and requests for information go back and forth between the practice staff and the payer's claim processing group. When claims are long overdue or there are repeated difficulties, however, these problems are the responsibility of the payer's provider representatives.

To avoid major problems, many practices routinely meet with payers to address the practice's specific problems and questions. A meeting should also be held when a new participation contract is signed to discuss the payer's major guidelines, fee schedule, and medical record documentation requirements.

Billing Tip

Secondary Claims and Coordination of Benefits
Chapters 14 and 15 discuss processing RAs/EOBs, secondary claims, coordination of benefits, and appeals for private payers.

Capitation Management

When the practice has a capitated contract, careful attention must be paid to patient eligibility, referral requirements, encounter reports, claim write-offs, and billing procedures.

Patient Eligibility

Under most capitated agreements with primary care physicians, providers receive monthly payments that cover the patients who chose them as their PCPs for that month. The **monthly enrollment list** that the plan sends with the payment should list the current members. This list, also called a "provider patient listing" or "roster," contains patients' names, identification numbers, dates of birth, type of plan or program, and effective date of registration to the PCP.

At times, however, the list is not up to date. To be sure that the patient is eligible for services, the insurance coverage is always verified.

Referral Requirements

An HMO may require a PCP to refer a patient to an in-network provider or to get authorization from the plan to refer a patient to an out-of-network provider. Patients who self-refer to nonparticipating providers may be balance-billed for those services. Both PCPs and specialists may be required to keep logs of referral activities.

Encounter Reports and Claim Write-offs

Most HMOs require capitated providers to submit encounter reports for patient encounters. Some do not require regular procedural coding and charges on the reports; the payer's form may just list "office visit" to be checked off. However, some plans do require the use of a regular claim with CPT codes.

The practice management program (PMP) is set up so that charges for service under capitated plans are written off as an adjustment to the patient's account. The billing staff knows not to expect additional payment based on a claim for a capitated-plan patient. If the service charges were not written off, the PMP would double-count the revenue for these patient encounters—once at the beginning of the month when the capitated payment was entered for a patient, and then again when a claim was created for a patient who has had an encounter during the month. Thus, the regular charges for the services that are included in the cap rate are written off by the biller. Only the monthly capitated payment remains on the patient's account—unless the patient has incurred charges beyond those items.

Billing for Excluded Services

Under a capitated contract, providers bill patients for services not covered by the cap rate. Medical insurance specialists need to organize this information for billing. For example, a special encounter form for the capitated plan might list the CPTs covered under the cap rate and then list the CPTs that can be billed. The plan's summary grid should indicate the plan's payment method for the additional services to be balance-billed, such as discounted fee-for-service.

Thinking it Through — 9.4

Audit the private-payer primary claim on page 322. What problems do you find in the preparation of the claim? List the item number and the problem or question you would raise.

1500

HEALTH INSURANCE CLAIM FORM

APPROVED BY NATIONAL UNIFORM CLAIM COMMITTEE 08/05

PICA | PICA

CARRIER

1. MEDICARE (Medicare #) / MEDICAID (Medicaid #) / TRICARE CHAMPUS (Sponsor's SSN) / CHAMPVA (Member ID#) / GROUP HEALTH PLAN (SSN or ID) / FECA BLK LUNG (SSN) / OTHER (ID)	GROUP HEALTH PLAN [X]
1a. INSURED'S I.D. NUMBER (For Program in Item 1)	
2. PATIENT'S NAME (Last Name, First Name, Middle Initial)	BELLINI JIMMY
3. PATIENT'S BIRTH DATE (MM DD YY) / SEX	03 04 2001 / M [X] F [ ]
4. INSURED'S NAME (Last Name, First Name, Middle Initial)	BELLINI GEORGE I
5. PATIENT'S ADDRESS (No., Street)	4144 BARKER AVE
6. PATIENT RELATIONSHIP TO INSURED (Self / Spouse / Child / Other)	Child [X]
7. INSURED'S ADDRESS (No., Street)	SAME
CITY	JACKSONVILLE
STATE	FL
8. PATIENT STATUS (Single / Married / Other)	Single [X]
CITY (insured)	
STATE (insured)	
ZIP CODE	35000
TELEPHONE (Include Area Code)	(941) 555 1287
Employed / Full-Time Student / Part-Time Student	Full-Time Student [X]
ZIP CODE (insured)	
TELEPHONE (INCLUDE AREA CODE) (insured)	( )
9. OTHER INSURED'S NAME (Last Name, First Name, Middle Initial)	
10. IS PATIENT'S CONDITION RELATED TO:	
11. INSURED'S POLICY GROUP OR FECA NUMBER	21 B
a. OTHER INSURED'S POLICY OR GROUP NUMBER	
a. EMPLOYMENT? (CURRENT OR PREVIOUS)	YES [ ] NO [X]
a. INSURED'S DATE OF BIRTH (MM DD YY) / SEX	M [X] F [ ]
b. OTHER INSURED'S DATE OF BIRTH (MM DD YY) / SEX	M [ ] F [ ]
b. AUTO ACCIDENT? PLACE (State)	YES [ ] NO [X]
b. EMPLOYER'S NAME OR SCHOOL NAME	SOUTHERN BANK
c. EMPLOYER'S NAME OR SCHOOL NAME	
c. OTHER ACCIDENT?	YES [ ] NO [X]
c. INSURANCE PLAN NAME OR PROGRAM NAME	AETNA WORLD PLAN
d. INSURANCE PLAN NAME OR PROGRAM NAME	
10d. RESERVED FOR LOCAL USE	
d. IS THERE ANOTHER HEALTH BENEFIT PLAN?	YES [ ] NO [X] *If yes*, return to and complete item 9 a-d.

READ BACK OF FORM BEFORE COMPLETING & SIGNING THIS FORM.

12. PATIENT'S OR AUTHORIZED PERSON'S SIGNATURE I authorize the release of any medical or other information necessary to process this claim. I also request payment of government benefits either to myself or to the party who accepts assignment below.

SIGNED George Bellini DATE 3/15/2008

13. INSURED'S OR AUTHORIZED PERSON'S SIGNATURE I authorize payment of medical benefits to the undersigned physician or supplier for services described below.

SIGNED

PATIENT AND INSURED INFORMATION

14. DATE OF CURRENT: ILLNESS (First symptom) OR INJURY (Accident) OR PREGNANCY(LMP) (MM DD YY)	
15. IF PATIENT HAS HAD SAME OR SIMILAR ILLNESS. GIVE FIRST DATE (MM DD YY)	
16. DATES PATIENT UNABLE TO WORK IN CURRENT OCCUPATION (FROM / TO)	
17. NAME OF REFERRING PHYSICIAN OR OTHER SOURCE	
17a.	
17b. NPI	
18. HOSPITALIZATION DATES RELATED TO CURRENT SERVICES (FROM / TO)	
19. RESERVED FOR LOCAL USE	
20. OUTSIDE LAB? / $ CHARGES	YES [ ] NO [X]
21. DIAGNOSIS OR NATURE OF ILLNESS OR INJURY. (Relate Items 1,2,3 or 4 to Item 24e by Line)	1. V20 . 2 / 2. V06 . 4 / 3. / 4.
22. MEDICAID RESUBMISSION CODE / ORIGINAL REF. NO.	
23. PRIOR AUTHORIZATION NUMBER	

	24. A. DATE(S) OF SERVICE From (MM DD YY)	To (MM DD YY)	B. PLACE OF SERVICE	C. EMG	D. PROCEDURES, SERVICES, OR SUPPLIES (Explain Unusual Circumstances) CPT/HCPCS	MODIFIER	E. DIAGNOSIS POINTER	F. $ CHARGES	G. DAYS OR UNITS	H. EPSDT Family Plan	I. ID. QUAL.	J. RENDERING PROVIDER ID. #
1	03 15 2008				99382		1	132 00	1		NPI	
2	03 15 2008				90707		2	82 00	1		NPI	
3	03 15 2008				90701		2	70 00	1		NPI	
4	03 15 2008				90471		2	20 00	1		NPI	
5	03 15 2008				90472		2	20 00	1		NPI	
6											NPI	

25. FEDERAL TAX I.D. NUMBER / SSN EIN	214809186 / EIN [X]
26. PATIENT'S ACCOUNT NO.	BEI20
27. ACCEPT ASSIGNMENT? (For govt. claims, see back)	YES [ ] NO [ ]
28. TOTAL CHARGE	$ 314 00
29. AMOUNT PAID	$ 15 00
30. BALANCE DUE	$ 299 00
31. SIGNATURE OF PHYSICIAN OR SUPPLIER INCLUDING DEGREES OR CREDENTIALS (I certify that the statements on the reverse apply to this bill and are made a part thereof.)	SIGNATURE ON FILE
SIGNED / DATE	
32. SERVICE FACILITY LOCATION INFORMATION	SAME
a. NPI / b.	
33. BILLING PROVIDER INFO & PHONE # ( )	FRANCES G FERRONE MD / FAMILY GROUP HEALTH / JACKSONVILLE FL
a. / b.	NPI 8876427755

PHYSICIAN OR SUPPLIER INFORMATION

NUCC Instruction Manual available at: www.nucc.org

Item No.	Problem
1.	
2.	
3.	
4.	
5.	
6.	

Review

Steps to Success

- ❒ Read this chapter and review the Key Terms and the Chapter Summary.
- ❒ Answer the Review Questions and Applying Your Knowledge in the Chapter Review.
- ❒ Access the chapter's websites and complete the Internet Activities to learn more about available professional resources.
- ❒ Complete the related chapter in the *Medical Insurance Workbook* to reinforce your understanding of private payer plans and billing procedures.

Chapter Summary

1. Employer-sponsored group health plans are organized by employers to provide heath care benefits to employees. The insurance coverage is purchased from an insurance carrier or managed care organization. Group health plans are subject to state laws for coverage and payment. Self-funded health plans are also organized by employers, but the employers insure the plan's members themselves rather than buying insurance coverage. Self-funded plans often hire third-party administrators and have administrative services only contracts for tasks such as subscriber enrollment and claims processing. These plans are controlled by federal ERISA law rather than by state law.
2. Group health plans establish and regulate health plans for employees, deciding on basic plan coverage and optional riders; eligibility requirements; and premiums and deductibles. The federal COBRA and HIPAA laws must be observed by the plans to ensure portability and coverage as required
3. Under preferred provider organizations (PPOs), providers are paid under a discounted fee-for-service structure. In health maintenance organizations (HMOs) and point-of-service (POS) plans, the payment may be a salary or capitated rate, depending on the business model. Indemnity plans basically pay from the physician's fee schedule.
4. Consumer-driven health plans are intended to shift costs and responsibilities for health care decisions to consumers. A consumer-driven health plan combines a high-deductible health plan (HDHP) that is usually a PPO for catastrophic coverage with one or more employer or employee funding options for out-of-pocket medical expenses.
5. Three types of funding options are used for out-of-pocket expenses in consumer-driven heath plans. A health reimbursement account (HRA) is set up by an employer to give tax-advantaged funds for employees' expenses. Health savings accounts (HSA) and flexible savings accounts (FSA) both can be funded by employees and employers on a tax-advantaged basis. HSA funds can be rolled over and taken by the individual to another job or into retirement, like an IRA. FSAs do not roll over.
6. Participation contracts have five main parts. The introductory section provides the names of the parties to the agreement, contract definitions, and the payer. The contract purpose and covered medical services section lists the type and purpose of the plan and the medical services it covers for its enrollees. The third section covers the physician's responsibilities as a participating provider. The fourth section covers the plan's responsibilities toward the participating provider. The fifth section lists the compensation and billing guidelines, such as fees, billing rules, filing deadlines, patients' financial responsibilities, and coordination of benefits.
7. Under participation contracts, most plans require copayments to be subtracted from the usual fees that are billed to the plans. To bill for

elective surgery requires precertification (also commonly called preauthorization) from the plan. Providers must notify plans about emergency surgery within the specified timeline after the procedure.

8. Plan summary grids list key information about each contracted plan and provide a shortcut reference for the billing and reimbursement process, including collecting payments at the time of service and completing claims.

9. The medical billing process is followed to prepare correct claims. (a) The general guidelines apply to the preregistration process for private health plan patients, when basic demographic and insurance information are collected; (b) the financial responsibility for the visit is established by verifying insurance eligibility and coverage with the payer for the plan, coordinating benefits, and meeting preauthorization requirements; (c) copayments are collected before the encounter; (d) any other payments due at the end of the encounter, such as deductible, charges for noncovered services, and balances due, are collected according to the practice's financial policy; (e) coding compliance is checked, verifying the use of correct codes as of the date of service that show medical necessity; (f) billing compliance with the plan's rules is checked; and (g) claims are completed, checked, and transmitted in accordance with the payer's billing and claims guidelines.

10. Under capitated contracts, medical insurance specialists verify patient eligibility with the plan because enrollment data are not always up to date. Encounter information, whether it contains complete coding or just diagnostic coding, must accurately reflect the necessity for the provider's services.

Review Questions

Match the key terms with their definitions.

A. monthly enrollment list
B. precertification
C. rider
D. high-deductible health plan
E. carve out
F. utilization review organization
G. Employee Retirement Income Security Act of 1974
H. home plan
I. stop-loss provision
J. elective surgery

____ 1. Payer preauthorization for elective hospital-based services and outpatient surgeries
____ 2. Insurance plan, usually a PPO, that requires a large amount to be paid before benefits begin; part of a consumer-driven health plan
____ 3. A federal law that provides incentives and protection against litigation for companies that set up employee health and pension plans
____ 4. A part of a standard health plan that is changed under a negotiated employer-sponsored plan
____ 5. Document of eligible members of a capitated plan registered with a particular PCP for a monthly period
____ 6. Document that modifies an insurance contract
____ 7. Surgical procedure that can be scheduled in advance
____ 8. In a BlueCard program, the provider's local BCBS plan
____ 9. A company hired by a payer to evaluate the appropriateness and medical necessity of hospital-based health care services
____ 10. Contractual guarantee against a participating provider's financial loss due to an unusually large demand for high-cost services

Decide whether each statement is true or false.

____ 1. Preferred provider organizations are the most popular type of managed care plan.
____ 2. A carve out may be used by an employer to omit a specific plan benefit that is usually covered by a health plan.

____ 3. Self-funded health plans are required by ERISA to use pharmacy benefit managers.

____ 4. The introductory section of a participation contract specifies the payer.

____ 5. Stop-loss provisions protect the plan from the financial impact of an unusually high number of expensive claims.

____ 6. If the participation contract states that copayments apply, the payer subtracts the patient's copayment from the provider's reimbursement.

____ 7. Elective surgery is not reimbursed because it is not medically necessary.

____ 8. Elective surgery requires preauthorization (precertification).

____ 9. Claims for private payers are sent first to patients, who then send them to the employer.

____ 10. A consumer-driven health plan involves a high-deductible health plan coupled with a funding option such as a health savings account.

Select the letter that best completes the statement or answers the question.

____ 1. The largest employer-sponsored health program in the United States is
- A. Medicare
- B. Medicaid
- C. Federal Employees Health Benefits program
- D. workers' compensation

____ 2. In employer-sponsored health plans, employees may choose their plan during the
- A. carve out
- B. open enrollment period
- C. contract period
- D. birthday rule period

____ 3. The portability of health insurance is governed by which laws?
- A. ERISA and HIPAA
- B. COBRA and HIPAA
- C. PPO and HMO
- D. FEHB and ERISA

____ 4. Self-funded health plans are regulated by
- A. PHI
- B. PPO
- C. FEHB
- D. ERISA

____ 5. Blue Cross and Blue Shield Association member plans offer
- A. all major types of health plans
- B. indemnity plans only
- C. PPOs only
- D. HMOs only

____ 6. Emergency surgery usually requires
- A. a deductible paid to the hospital or clinic
- B. precertification (preauthorization) within a specified time after the procedure
- C. a referral before the procedure
- D. none of the above

____ 7. Providers who participate in a PPO are paid
   A. a capitated rate
   B. a discounted fee-for-service
   C. an episode-of-care payment
   D. according to their usual physician fee schedule

____ 8. Under a capitated HMO plan, the physician practice receives
   A. an encounter report
   B. precertification for services
   C. a monthly enrollment list
   D. a secondary insurance identification number

____ 9. What document is researched to uncover rules for private payers' definitions of insurance-related terms?
   A. ERISA
   B. participation contract
   C. HIPAA Security Rule
   D. none of the above

____ 10. Consumer-driven health plans have what effect on a practice's cash flow?
   A. A high-deductible payment from the patient takes longer to collect than does a copayment.
   B. The health plan's payment arrives faster than under other types of plans.
   C. There is no effect on cash flow.
   D. The effect is the same as the effect of a capitated plan.

Answer the following questions.

1. List the five main parts of participation contracts.
2. List the seven steps of the medical billing process that lead to completion of correct private payer claims.

(1) ____________________
(2) ____________________
(3) ____________________
(4) ____________________
(5) ____________________
(6) ____________________
(7) ____________________

Applying Your Knowledge

Case 9.1 Abstracting Insurance Information

Based on the following notes, fill out the precertification form for Betty Sinowitcz.

Encounter Data: 5/4/2007
Patient: Elizabeth R. Sinowitcz
Date of Birth: 8/2/1937
Address: 45 Maple Hill Road, Apt. 12-B, Rangeley, MN 55555
Home Telephone: 555-123-9887
Employer: Argon Electric Company, 238 Industry Way, Rangeley, MN 55554
Work Telephone: 555-124-8754

PRECERTIFICATION FORM

Insurance carrier ______________________________

Certification for [ ] admission and/or [ ] surgery and/or [ ] ______________

Patient name ______________________________

Street address ______________________________

City/state/zip ______________________________

Telephone ______________ Date of birth ______________

Subscriber name ______________________________

Employer ______________________________

Member no. ______________ Group no. ______________

Admitting physician ______________________________

Provider no. ______________________________

Hospital/facility ______________________________

Planned admission/procedure date ______________________________

Diagnosis/symptoms ______________________________

Treatment/procedure ______________________________

Estimated length of stay ______________________________

Complicating factors ______________________________

Second opinion required [ ] Yes [ ] No If yes, [ ] Obtained

Corroborating physician ______________________________

Insurance carrier representative ______________________________

Approval [ ] Yes [ ] No If yes, certification no. ______________

If no, resason(s) for denial ______________________________

Betty is on Medicare. She also has insurance coverage through Argon Electric in the Horizon PPO. Her insurance card shows her member number as 65-PO; no group number is shown.

Betty was referred to Dr. Hank R. Ferrara, a Horizon-participating ophthalmologist (PIN 349-00-G), for evaluation of her blurred and dimmed vision. After conducting an examination and taking the necessary history, Dr. Ferrara diagnoses the patient's condition as a cataract of the left eye that is close to mature (ICD-9-CM 366.10). Dr. Ferrara decides to schedule Betty for lens extraction; the procedure is ambulatory care surgery with same-day admission and discharge. The procedure will be done at Mischogie Hospital's Outpatient Clinic on 5/10. Horizon PPO requires precertification for this procedure (CPT 66984).

Case 9.2 Applying Insurance Rules

Jan Wommelsdorf, of Fargo, North Dakota, was on vacation in Portland, Oregon, when she became ill. She has BCBS BlueCard insurance, so she telephoned the BlueCard toll-free number to find a provider near her in Portland. She was examined by Dr. Vijay Sundaram and provided with a special diet to follow until she returns home and visits her regular physician.

A. Who submits the claim, Jan Wommelsdorf or Dr. Sundaram?

B. Is the claim submitted to Jan's local BCBS plan in North Dakota or to Dr. Sundaram's local plan in Oregon?

Case 9.3 Calculating Insurance Math

A. A physician's usual fee for a routine eye examination is $80. Under the discounted fee-for-service arrangement the doctor has with Plan A, the fee is discounted 15 percent for Plan A members. This month, the doctor has seen five Plan A members for routine eye exams.

1. What is the physician's usual fee for the five patients?
2. What will the physician be paid for one Plan A member's exam?
3. What will the physician be paid for the five Plan A eye exams?

B. Using this fee schedule for three different payers for orthopedic procedures, complete the questions that follow.

Code	Description	BCBS	United	Medicare
29871	Knee arthroscopy, surgical; for infection, lavage and drain	$ 908.95	$1,179.12	$485.06
29876	Knee arthroscopy, surgical; major synovectomy	$1,097.78	$1,356.58	$584.21
29877	Knee arthroscopy, surgical; debridement	$1,031.60	$1,240.64	$549.58
29880	Knee arthroscopy, surgical; with meniscectomy, medial AND lateral	$1,167.23	$1,385.82	$621.21
29881	Knee arthroscopy, surgical; with meniscectomy, medial OR lateral	$1,080.44	$1,292.96	$575.04

1. A patient with BCBS PPO coverage had surgical knee arthroscopy with medial and lateral meniscectomy. The plan has an 80/20 coinsurance, with no copayment for surgical procedures. The annual deductible is met. What will the plan pay, and what amount does the patient owe?
2. A United patient has a high-deductible plan with a $1,200 deductible for this year that has not been met and 75/25 coinsurance. He has surgical knee arthroscopy with debridement. What will the plan pay, and what amount does the patient owe?
3. Another payer offers the practice a contract based on 115 percent of the Medicare Fee Schedule. What amounts are offered for the codes above?

Case 9.4 Completing Correct Claims

The objective of these exercises is to correctly complete private-payer claims, applying what you have learned in the chapter. Following the information about the provider for the cases are two sections. The first section contains information about the patient, the insurance coverage, and the current medical condition. The second section is an encounter form for Valley Associates, P.C.

If you are using Medisoft to complete the cases, read the *Guide to Medisoft* before beginning. Information from the first section, the patient information form, has already been entered in the program for you. You must enter information from the second section, the encounter form, to complete the claim. If you are gaining experience by completing a paper CMS-1500 claim form, use the blank claim form supplied to you (from Appendix D or printed from the Student Data Template CD ROM) and follow the instructions on pages 317–318.

The following provider information, which is also preloaded in the Medisoft database, should be used for Cases 9.4A and 9.4B.

Provider Information

Name	David Rosenberg, M.D.
Practice Name	Valley Associates, P.C.
Address	1400 West Center Street Toledo, OH 43601-0213
Telephone	555-967-0303
Employer ID Number	16-2345678
NPI	1288560027
BCBS PIN	18A09
Aetna PIN:	RZX334
Assignment	Accepts
Signature	On File (1-1-2008)

Also note the following fee schedule information, which applies to all the claim-completion exercises in this and subsequent chapters.

Price Code A: Standard fees, used for all payers except Medicare and Medicaid

Price Code B: Reduced fees, used for Medicare (Medicare Nationwide and Medicare HMO) and Medicaid payers

The amounts shown on the encounter forms in the claim-completion cases reflect the appropriate fee schedules.

Internet Activities

1. FEHB beneficiaries have an annual open enrollment season during which they can decide whether to remain in their current health plan or switch to a different plan. Access http://www.opm.gov and explore Employment and Benefits. Investigate the options under FEHB and their FSA plans.
2. Explore the website for the national Blue Cross and Blue Shield Association at http://www.bluecares.com. Enter your ZIP code, and look up information about the Blue Cross and Blue Shield affiliate for the state in which you live. What types of plans are offered?
3. Private payers have valuable information for providers on their websites, such as coverage bulletins, provider manuals, and referral/authorization requirements. Investigate the website of a major payer, and explore the Providers tab to see what transactions can be handled. Is it possible, for example, to check eligibility, benefits, claims, referrals, and precertification status online?
4. Use a search engine to access the America's Health Insurance Plans (AHIP) website and review current information on health savings accounts. For example, research whether unused funds left in HSAs at the end of a year are considered taxable income to the insured.

A. Based on the following patient and encounter information, complete a claim for the patient.

From the Patient Information Form:

Name	David Belline	*Employer*	Kinko's
Sex	M	*Health Plan*	Anthem BCBS PPO
Birth Date	01/22/1951	*Insurance ID Number*	35Z29005
Marital Status	Married	*Assignment of Benefits*	Y
SSN	439-01-3349	*Signature on File*	Y (06/01/2008)
Address	250 Milltown Rd. Alliance, OH 44601-3456	*Condition unrelated to Employment, Auto Accident, or Other Accident*	
Telephone	555-239-0226		
Employment status	Full-time		

VALLEY ASSOCIATES, PC
David Rosenberg, MD - Dermatology
555-967-0303
FED I.D. #16-2345678

PATIENT NAME	APPT. DATE/TIME
Belline, David S.	10/13/2008 10:00 am
PATIENT NO.	**DX**
BELLIDA0	1. 250.00 diabetes mellitus, type II 2. 3. 4.

DESCRIPTION	✓	CPT	FEE	DESCRIPTION	✓	CPT	FEE
OFFICE VISITS				**PROCEDURES**			
New Patient				Acne Surgery		10040	
LI Problem Focused		99201		I&D, Abscess, Smpl		10060	
LII Expanded		99202		I&D, Abscess, Mult		10061	
LIII Detailed		99203		I&D, Pilonidal Cyst, Smpl		10080	
LIV Comp./Mod.		99204		I&D, Pilonidal Cyst, Compl		10081	
LV Comp./High		99205		I&R, Foreign Body, Smpl		10120	
Established Patient				I&R, Foreign Body, Compl		10121	
LI Minimum		99211		I&D Hematoma		10140	
LII Problem Focused		99212		Puncture Aspiration		10160	
LIII Expanded		99213		Debride Skin, To 10%		11000	
LIV Detailed		99214		Each Addl 10%		11001	
LV Comp./High		99215		Pare Benign Skin Lesion		11055	
				Pare Benign Skin Lesion, 2-4		11056	
CONSULTATION: OFFICE/OP				Pare Benign Skin Lesion, 4+		11057	
Requested By:				Skin Biopsy, Single Les.		11100	
LI Problem Focused		99241		Skin Biopsy, Mult Les.		+11101	
LII Expanded		99242		Remove Skin Tags, 1-15		11200	
LIII Detailed		99243		Remove Skin Tags, Addl 10		+11201	
LIV Comp./Mod.		99244		Trim Nails		11719	
LV Comp./High		99245		Debride Nails, 1-5		11720	
				Debride Nails, 6+		11721	
CARE PLAN OVERSIGHT				Avulsion of Nail Plate,1	✓	11730	107
Supervision, 15-29 min.		99339		Avulsion of Nail Plate,Addl 1		+11732	
Supervision, 30+ min.		99340		Nail Biopsy		11755	
				Repair Nail Bed		11760	
				Excision, Ingrown Toenail		11765	
				TOTAL FEES			

B. Based on the following patient and encounter information, complete a claim for the patient.

From the Patient Information Form:

Name	Gwen Remarky	*Employment status*	Full-time
Sex	F	*Employer*	Brooklyn Day Care
Birth Date	11/05/1962	*Health Plan*	Aetna Choice
Marital Status	Married	*Insurance ID Number*	BP3333-X89
SSN	221-84-3902	*Assignment of Benefits*	Y
Address	9 Sealcrest Drive.	*Signature on File*	Y (01/01/2008)
	Brooklyn, OH 44144-6789	*Condition unrelated to Employment,*	
Telephone	555-666-4355	*Auto Accident, or Other Accident*	

VALLEY ASSOCIATES, PC
David Rosenberg, MD - Dermatology
555-967-0303
FED I.D. #16-2345678

PATIENT NAME	APPT. DATE/TIME
Remarky, Gwen	10/13/2008 11:30 am
PATIENT NO.	**DX**
REMARGWE0	1. 681.11 chronic paronychia, right big toe 2. 3. 4.

DESCRIPTION	✓	CPT	FEE	DESCRIPTION	✓	CPT	FEE
OFFICE VISITS				**PROCEDURES**			
New Patient				Acne Surgery		10040	
LI Problem Focused		99201		I&D, Abscess, Smpl		10060	
LII Expanded		99202		I&D, Abscess, Mult		10061	
LIII Detailed		99203		I&D, Pilonidal Cyst, Smpl		10080	
LIV Comp./Mod.		99204		I&D, Pilonidal Cyst, Compl		10081	
LV Comp./High		99205		I&R, Foreign Body, Smpl		10120	
Established Patient				I&R, Foreign Body, Compl		10121	
LI Minimum		99211		I&D Hematoma		10140	
LII Problem Focused	✓	99212	46	Puncture Aspiration		10160	
LIII Expanded		99213		Debride Skin, To 10%		11000	
LIV Detailed		99214		Each Addl 10%		11001	
LV Comp./High		99215		Pare Benign Skin Lesion		11055	
				Pare Benign Skin Lesion, 2-4		11056	
CONSULTATION: OFFICE/OP				Pare Benign Skin Lesion, 4+		11057	
Requested By:				Skin Biopsy, Single Les.		11100	
LI Problem Focused		99241		Skin Biopsy, Mult Les.		+11101	
LII Expanded		99242		Remove Skin Tags, 1-15		11200	
LIII Detailed		99243		Remove Skin Tags, Addl 10		+11201	
LIV Comp./Mod.		99244		Trim Nails		11719	
LV Comp./High		99245		Debride Nails, 1-5		11720	
				Debride Nails, 6+		11721	
CARE PLAN OVERSIGHT				Avulsion of Nail Plate, 1		11730	
Supervision, 15-29 min.		99339		Avulsion of Nail Plate, Addl 1		+11732	
Supervision, 30+ min.		99340		Nail Biopsy		11755	
				Repair Nail Bed		11760	
				Excision, Ingrown Toenail		11765	
				TOTAL FEES			

Chapter 10

Medicare

CHAPTER OUTLINE

The Medicare Program

Medicare Coverage and Benefits

Medicare Participating Providers

Nonparticipating Providers

Original Medicare Plan and Medicare Advantage Plans

Medigap Insurance

Medicare Billing and Compliance

Preparing Primary Medicare Claims

Learning Outcomes

After studying this chapter, you should be able to:

1. List the eligibility requirements for Medicare program coverage.
2. Describe the coverage provided by each of the four parts of the Medicare program.
3. Discuss medical and preventive services that are covered or excluded under Medicare Part B.
4. Discuss the billing rules governing Medicare participating providers.
5. Explain the calculations used to determine nonparticipating provider payments for assigned and unassigned claims under Medicare.
6. Describe the features of the Original Medicare Plan.
7. Discuss the features and coverage offered under Medicare Advantage plans.
8. Discuss Medigap insurance plans, and explain the coverage they offer.
9. Discuss the Medicare Medical Review (MR) Program.
10. Prepare correct Medicare primary claims.

Key Terms

Additional Documentation Request
advance beneficiary notice (ABN)
carrier
Clinical Laboratory Improvement Amendments (CLIA)
Common Working File (CWF)
fiscal intermediary
Health Professional Shortage Area (HPSA)
incident to
initial preventive physical examination (IPPE)
limiting charge
local coverage determination (LCD)
Medical Review (MR) Program
Medical Savings Account (MSA)
Medicare Advantage
Medicare card
Medicare health insurance claim number (HICN)
Medicare Modernization Act (MMA)
Medicare Part A (Hospital Insurance [HI])
Medicare Part B (Supplementary Medical Insurance [SMI])
Medicare Part C
Medicare Part D
Medicare Summary Notice (MSN)
Medigap
national coverage determination (NCD)
Notice of Exclusions from Medicare Benefits (NEMB)
Original Medicare Plan
Quality Improvement Organization (QIO)
roster billing
screening service
urgently needed care
waived tests

Medicare is a federal medical insurance program established in 1965 under Title XVIII of the Social Security Act. The first benefits were paid in January 1966. Medicare now provides benefits to more than 40 million people. The Medicare program is managed by the Centers for Medicare and Medicaid Services (CMS) under the Department of Health and Human Services (HHS). Although it has just four parts, it is arguably the most complex program that medical practices deal with, involving numerous rules and regulations that must be followed for claims to be paid. To complicate matters, these rules change frequently, and keeping up with the changes is a challenge for providers and medical insurance specialists alike.

The Medicare Program

Medicare is a defined benefits program, meaning that, to be covered, an item or service must be in a benefit category established by law and not otherwise excluded.

To receive benefits, individuals must be eligible under one of six beneficiary categories:

1. *Individuals age sixty-five or older:* Persons age sixty-five or older who have paid FICA taxes or railroad retirement taxes for at least forty calendar quarters.
2. *Disabled adults:* Individuals who have been receiving Social Security disability benefits or Railroad Retirement Board disability benefits for more than two years. Coverage begins five months after the two years of entitlement.
3. *Individuals disabled before age eighteen:* Individuals under age eighteen who meet the disability criteria of the Social Security Act.
4. *Spouses of entitled individuals:* Spouses of deceased, disabled, or retired individuals who are (or were) entitled to Medicare benefits.
5. *Retired federal employees enrolled in the Civil Service Retirement System (CSRS):* Retired CSRS employees and their spouses.
6. *Individuals with end-stage renal disease (ESRD):* Individuals of any age who receive dialysis or a renal transplant for ESRD. Coverage typically begins

on the first day of the month following the start of dialysis treatments. In the case of a transplant, entitlement begins the month the individual is hospitalized for the transplant (the transplant must be completed within two months). The donor is covered for services related to the donation of the organ only.

Medicare Part A

> **Billing Tip**
>
> **Part A Premium and Deductible**
> The 2007 premium is $410. The 2007 deductible is $992.

Medicare Part A, which is also called **Hospital Insurance (HI)**, pays for inpatient hospital care, skilled nursing facility care, home health care, and hospice care. Anyone who receives Social Security benefits is automatically enrolled in Part A by the Social Security Administration. Eligible beneficiaries do not pay premiums. Individuals age sixty-five or older who are not eligible for Social Security benefits may enroll in Part A, but they must pay premiums for the coverage. Details of Part A coverage are provided in Table 10.1

Medicare Part B

Medicare Part B, which is also called **Supplementary Medical Insurance (SMI)**, helps beneficiaries pay for physician services, outpatient hospital services, medical equipment, and other supplies and services. Individuals entitled to Part A benefits are automatically qualified to enroll in Part B. U.S. citizens and permanent residents over the age of sixty-five are also eligible.

Part B is a voluntary program; eligible persons choose whether to take part in it. Those desiring Part B coverage must enroll; coverage is not automatic. If enrollment takes place more than twelve months after a person's initial enrollment period, there is a permanent 10 percent increase in the premium for each year the beneficiary failed to enroll.

TABLE 10.1 Medicare Part A Coverage

Coverage
Inpatient hospital stays: semiprivate room, meals, general nursing and other hospital services and supplies, including blood.
Stays at a skilled nursing facility (SNF) following a related, covered three-day hospital stay. At a SNF, skilled nursing and rehabilitation care are provided, in contrast to a nursing home that provides custodial care. Coverage includes semiprivate room, meals, skilled nursing and rehabilitative services, other services and supplies, including blood.
Home health care: intermittent skilled nursing care, physical therapy, occupational therapy, speech-language pathology, home health aide services, durable medical equipment, but not prescription drugs.
Psychiatric inpatient care.
Hospice care: pain and symptom relief and supportive services.
Benefits Periods and Patient's Responsibility
Medicare Part A coverage is tied to a benefit period of sixty days for a spell of illness. A spell of illness benefit period commences on the first day of the patient's stay in a hospital or in a skilled nursing facility and continues until sixty consecutive days have lapsed and the patient has received no skilled care. Medicare does not cover care that is or becomes primarily custodial, such as assistance with bathing and eating.
The patient benefit period with Medicare, the spell of illness, does not end until sixty days after discharge from the hospital or the skilled nursing facility. Therefore, if the patient is readmitted within those sixty days, the patient is considered to be in the same benefit period and is not subject to another deductible. A new spell of illness begins if the patient is readmitted more than sixty days after discharge. There is no limit on the number of spells of illness Medicare will cover in a patient's lifetime.
For the first sixty days, the patient's responsibility is the annual deductible (the amount changes each year). For days 61–90, there is a per-day copayment, and another per-day copayment for days 91–150. Beyond 150 days, Medicare Part A does not make any payment.

Beneficiaries pay a monthly premium. They are also subject to an annual deductible and coinsurance, which are established by federal law. The two basic types of plans available under Medicare Part B—the Original Medicare Plan and Medicare Advantage plans—are discussed on pages 346–349.

Medicare Part C

In 1997, **Medicare Part C** (originally called Medicare + Choice) became available to individuals who are eligible for Part A and enrolled in Part B. Under Part C, private health insurance companies contract with CMS to offer Medicare beneficiaries Medicare Advantage plans that compete with the Original Medicare Plan.

In 2003, under the Medicare Prescription Drug, Improvement, and Modernization Act (commonly called the **Medicare Modernization Act**, or **MMA**), Advantage became the new name for Medicare + Choice plans, and certain rules were changed to give Part C enrollees better benefits and lower costs.

Medicare Part D

Medicare Part D, authorized under the MMA, provides voluntary Medicare prescription drug plans that are open to people who are eligible for Medicare.

All Medicare prescription drug plans are private insurance plans, and most participants pay monthly premiums to access discounted prices. There are two types of plans. The prescription drug plan covers only drugs and can be used with an Original Medicare Plan and/or a Medicare supplement plan. The other type combines a prescription drug plan with a Medicare Advantage plan that includes medical coverage for doctor visits and hospital expenses. This kind of plan is called Medicare Advantage Plus Prescription Drug. The Medicare prescription drug plan has a list of drugs it covers, often structured in payment tiers. Under an approach called "step therapy," plans may require patients to first try a generic or less expensive drug rather than the presribed medication; if it does not work as well, the physician may request coverage for the original prescription.

Billing Tip

Part B Premium and Deductible
The 2007 standard premium is $93.50 a month. Higher-income beneficiaries pay a surcharge (from $12.50 to $68.60) monthly. The 2007 deductible is $131.

Current Deductible, Coinsurance, and Premium

http://medicare.org/medicarepart_b.cfm

Medicare Coverage and Benefits

Each Medicare enrollee receives a **Medicare card** issued by the Social Security Administration (see Figure 10.1 on page 336). This card lists the beneficiary's name and sex, the effective dates for Part A and Part B coverage, and the Medicare number. The Medicare number is most often called the **Medicare health insurance claim number (HICN)**. It usually consists of nine digits followed by a numeric or alphanumeric suffix. The suffix indicates whether the benefits are drawn from the patient's work history or someone else's. Common suffixes are:

A	Primary wage earner (male or female)
B	Aged wife, first claimant (female)
B1	Husband, first claimant (male)
C1–C9	Child or grandchild, disabled/student
D	Aged widow, first claimant
T	Federal employee

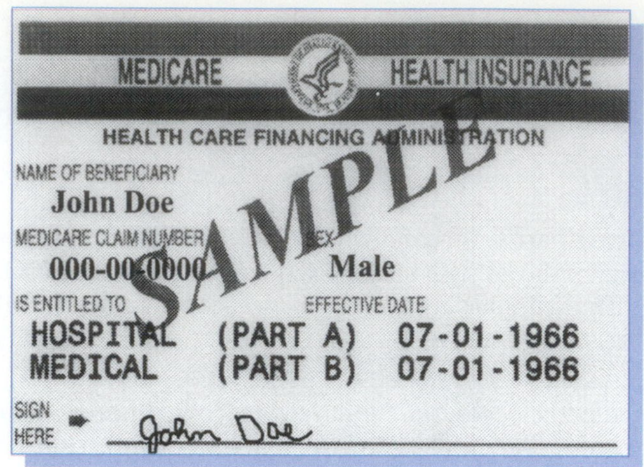

FIGURE 10.1 Medicare Card Showing Medicare Eligibility and Medicare Health Insurance Claim Number

Billing Tips

Use Exact Name and HICN
Be sure to use the patient's name and HICN exactly as they appear on the Medicare card. This information must match Medicare's Common Working File (CWF), the Medicare claim processing system.

Wrong Information on Card
Advise patients who insist that their cards are not correct to contact the local Social Security field office or to use online access to get a correct card.

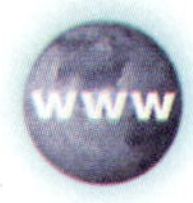

Part A Intermediaries and Part B Carriers by State
http://www.cms.hhs.gov/apps/contacts/incardir.asp#1

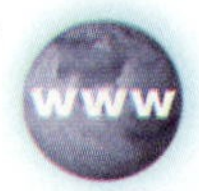

CMS Regional Offices
http://www.cms.hhs.gov/about/regions/professionals.asp

When the beneficiary's card shows a prefix (such as A, MA, WA, or WD) instead of a suffix, the patient is eligible for railroad retirement benefits, and claims must be submitted to the Railroad Medicare Part B claim office:

Palmetto GBA (Government Benefits Administrator)
Railroad Retirees Benefits Medicare Claim Office
PO Box 10066
Augusta, GA 30999-0001
1-877-288-7600

Medicare Claim Processing

The federal government does not pay Medicare claims directly; instead, it hires contractors to process its claims. Contractors are usually major national insurance companies such as Blue Cross and Blue Shield member plans. Contractors that process claims sent by hospitals, skilled nursing facilities, intermediate care facilities, long-term care facilities, and home health care agencies are known as **fiscal intermediaries**. Those that process claims sent by physicians, providers, and suppliers are referred to as **carriers**. Regional contractors handle durable medical equipment supplies and drugs billed by physicians (see Chapter 6) that may not be billed to the local carrier.

In addition to a headquarters office in Baltimore, Maryland, there are ten CMS regional offices that can answer questions when the carrier does not have sufficient information. The regions are located in:

Boston, Massachusetts	Dallas, Texas
New York, New York	Kansas City, Missouri
Philadelphia, Pennsylvania	Denver, Colorado
Atlanta, Georgia	San Francisco, California
Chicago, Illinois	Seattle, Washington

Figure 10.2 illustrates the coverage of each region.

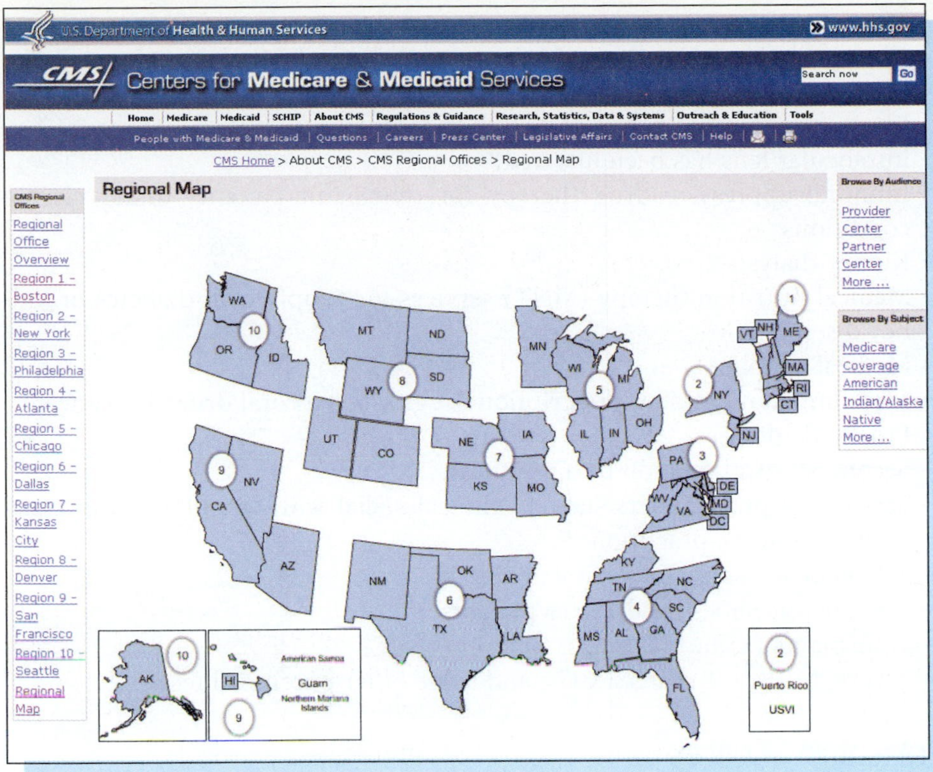

FIGURE 10.2 CMS Regional Map

Medical Services and Other Services

Regular Medicare Part B benefits are shown below.

Covered Services	Patient Payment (Par Provider)
Medical Services Physicians' services, including inpatient and outpatient medical and surgical services and supplies; physical, occupational, and speech therapy; diagnostic tests; and durable medical equipment (DME)	• Annual deductible • 20 percent coinsurance of approved amount after the deductible, except in the outpatient setting • 50 percent coinsurance for most outpatient mental health
Clinical Laboratory Services Blood tests, urinalysis, and so forth	Covered fully by Medicare
Home Health Care Intermittent skilled care, home health aide services, DME	• Services fully covered by Medicare • 20 percent coinsurance for DME
Outpatient Hospital Services Services for diagnoses or treatment of an illness or injury	Coinsurance or copayment that varies according to the service
Blood As an outpatient or as part of a Part B covered service	For the first three pints plus 20 percent of the approved amount for additional pints (after the deductible)

Part B also covers:

- Ambulance services when other transportation would endanger the patient's health
- Artificial eyes
- Artificial limbs that are prosthetic devices and their replacement parts

- Braces
- Chiropractic services (limited)
- Emergency care
- Eyeglasses—one pair of glasses or contact lenses after cataract surgery (if an intraocular lens has been inserted)
- Immunosuppressive drug therapy for transplant patients under certain conditions
- Kidney dialysis
- Medical nutrition therapy (MNT) services for people with diabetes or kidney disease
- Medical supplies
- Very limited outpatient prescription drugs (such as oral drugs for cancer)
- Prosthetic devices
- Second surgical opinion by a physician
- Services of practitioners such as clinical social workers, physician's assistants, and nurse-practitioners
- Telemedicine services in rural areas
- Therapeutic shoes for diabetes patients
- Transplants (some)
- X-rays, MRIs, CT scans, ECGs, and some other purchased tests

Billing Tip

Counseling Services
Medicare covers smoking and tobacco-use cessation counseling services.

Preventive Services

Certain preventive services for qualified individuals are also covered:

- Bone mass measurements
- Cardiovascular disease screening
- Colorectal cancer screening
- Diabetes screening tests (for certain at-risk patients), services, and supplies
- Glaucoma screening
- **Initial preventive physical examination (IPPE)**, a once-in-a-lifetime benefit that must be received in the first six months after the date of enrollment
- Mammogram screening
- Pap test and pelvic examination (includes clinical breast examination)
- Prostate cancer screening
- Vaccinations (influenza, pneumococcal polysaccharide vaccine, hepatitis B virus)

Billing Tip

Preventive Services and Deductibles
Under Medicare Part B, some preventive services are subject to a deductible, and some are not. The Medicare plan summary grid should note these requirements.

A **screening service** is performed for a patient who does not have symptoms, abnormal findings, or any past history of the disease. The purpose is to detect an undiagnosed disease so that medical treatment can begin to prevent harm. The Medicare policy may limit screening services or their frequency according to the health status of the patient. Screenings are different from diagnostic services, which are done to treat a patient who has been diagnosed with a condition or with a high probability for it.

Excluded Services and Not Medically Necessary Services

What Medicare covers is determined by federal legislation rather than by medical practice. For this reason, Medicare does not provide coverage for certain services and procedures. Claims may be denied because the service provided is excluded by Medicare or because the service was not reasonable and necessary for the specific patient.

Excluded services are not covered under any circumstances. For example, these services were excluded in 2006:

- Routine preventive physical examinations (after the initial preventive physical examination)
- Immunizations, with the exception of influenza, hepatitis B, and pneumococcal vaccines
- Routine dental examinations
- Eye refraction
- Specific foot care procedures, including most instances of treatment or surgery for subluxation of the foot, supportive shoes, treatment of flat foot, and routine foot care
- Examinations for the prescription of hearing aids or actual hearing aid devices
- Examinations for the prescription of eyeglasses or contact lenses or actual eyeglasses or contact lenses (unless an underlying disease is the cause)
- Services provided by a nonphysician in a hospital inpatient setting that were not ordered or provided by an employee under contract with the hospital
- Services provided as a result of a noncovered procedure, such as laboratory tests ordered in conjunction with a noncovered surgical procedure
- Most custodial services, including daily administration of medication, routine care of a catheter, and routine administration of oxygen therapy
- Long-term care, such as most nursing home care
- Cosmetic surgery
- Acupuncture
- Health care received while traveling outside the United States

Other services that are not covered are classified as not medically necessary under Medicare guidelines. These services are not covered by Medicare unless certain conditions are met, such as particular diagnoses. For example, a vitamin B_{12} injection is a covered service only for patients with certain diagnoses, such as pernicious anemia, but not for a diagnosis of fatigue. If the patient does not have one of the specified diagnoses, the B_{12} injection is categorized as not reasonable and necessary. The Medicare code edits under Medicare Correct Coding Initiative (CCI; see Chapter 7) will deny the claim.

To be considered medically necessary, a treatment must be

- Appropriate for the symptoms or diagnoses of the illness or injury
- Not an elective procedure
- Not an experimental or investigational procedure
- An essential treatment; not performed for the patient's convenience
- Delivered at the most appropriate level that can safely and effectively be administered to the patient

Several common categories of medical necessity denials include the following:

- *The diagnosis does not match the service:* In this case, *match* means that the diagnosis does not justify the procedures performed. In some instances, the denial is the result of a clerical error—for example, a fifth digit was dropped from an ICD-9-CM code. In these instances, the claim can be corrected, and many times it will eventually be paid. In other situations, the diagnosis is not specific enough to justify the treatment.
- *Too many services in a brief period of time:* Examples include more than one office visit in a day or too many visits for treatment of a minor problem.
- *Level of service denials:* These Evaluation and Management (E/M) claims are either denied or downcoded (coded at a lower level) because the services were in excess of those required to adequately diagnose and/or treat the problem. Rather than deny the claim, the payer downcodes the procedure—for example, changing a CPT E/M code from 99214 to 99212.

Billing Tip

Expanding Preventive Benefits Coverage
Each year, more preventive services are covered by Medicare. For example, as of 2005, preventive benefits include a one-time physical exam for new Medicare enrollees, screening blood tests for cardiovascular disease, and tests for people at risk for diabetes.

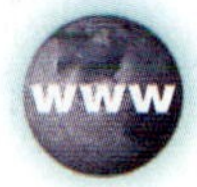

Medicare Coverage Home Page

http://www.cms.hhs.gov/coverage/default2.asp

Thinking It Through — 10.1

Vijay Sundaram sees his physician, Dr. Elliot Gold, for his annual routine checkup. He has been in the Medicare Part B program for five years. Dr. Gold examines him, orders blood work, and performs an ECG. The ECG differs from the one Dr. Gold has on file from last year, so Dr. Gold orders a cardiovascular stress test for Sundaram.

1. Is the annual examination covered under Medicare Part B?
2. Will the stress test be covered under Medicare Part B?

Medicare Participating Providers

Physicians choose whether to participate in the Medicare program. Before the start of a new year, Medicare carriers have an open enrollment period when providers who are currently enrolled can change their status and new physicians can sign participation agreements.

Medicare Physician Website
http://cms.hhs.gov/physicians/

Participating physicians agree to accept assignment for all Medicare claims and to accept Medicare's allowed charge as payment in full for services. They also agree to submit claims on behalf of the patient at no charge and to receive payment directly from Medicare on the patient's behalf. Participants are responsible for knowing the rules and regulations of the program as they affect their patients. These rules are available online at the CMS Medicare website, which contains more than twenty manuals that offer day-to-day operating instructions, policies, and procedures based on statutes and regulations, guidelines, models, and directives.

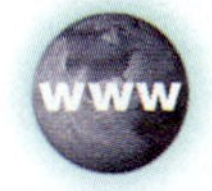

CMS Online Manual System
http://cms.hhs.gov/manuals/

To ensure that only qualified providers are enrolled in Medicare, CMS requires all providers who wish to participate or to renew contracts to complete form CMS 855, the Medicare Provider/Supplier Enrollment Application. It contains data about education and credentials as appropriate to the type of provider or supplier. Providers must attest to the accuracy of the information reported every three years.

Incentives

Medicare carriers offer incentives to physicians to encourage participation. For example:

- Medicare Physician Fee Schedule (MPFS) amounts are 5 percent higher than for nonparticipating (nonPAR) providers.
- Participating providers do not have to forward claims for beneficiaries who also have supplemental insurance coverage and who assign their supplemental insurance payments to the participating provider. The Medicare carrier automatically forwards the claim to the supplemental carrier, and payments are made directly to the provider from both the primary and secondary payers, with no extra administrative work on the provider's end.

  Participating providers are listed in the carrier's online directory of Medicare participating providers and receive referrals in some circumstances.
- Medicare has created **Health Professional Shortage Areas (HPSAs)** for primary care and mental health professionals. Providers located in such areas are eligible for 10 percent bonus payments from Medicare.

Payments

Physicians who participate agree to accept the charge amounts listed in the Medicare Physician Fee Schedule (MPFS) as payment in full for all covered services. MPFS was developed from the resource-based relative value scale (RBRVS) system (see Chapter 7).

MPFS On Line

The online Medicare Physician Fee Schedule (MPFS) lists all physician services, RVUs, and payment policies.

http://www.cms.hhs.gov/apps/pfslookup

Notice of Exclusions from Medicare Benefits

Participating providers may bill patients for services that are not covered by the Medicare program, such as routine physicals and many screening tests. Giving a patient written notification that Medicare will not pay for a service before providing it is a good policy, although it is not required. When patients are notified ahead of time, they understand their financial responsibility to pay for the service. CMS Form No. 20007, **Notice of Exclusions from Medicare Benefits (NEMB)** is available for this purpose (see Figure 10.3 on page 342). Providers use NEMBs on an entirely voluntary basis. Their purpose is to advise beneficiaries, before they receive services that are not Medicare benefits, that Medicare will not pay for them and to provide beneficiaries with an estimate of how much they may have to pay. Providers may also choose to design their own NEMBs based on the services they offer.

Notice of Exclusions from Medicare Benefits Form

http://www.cms.hhs.gov/BNI/11_.FFSNEMBGeneral.asp

Advance Beneficiary Notice

Participating physicians also agree to not bill patients for services that Medicare declares as being not reasonable and necessary unless the patients were informed ahead of time in writing and agreed to pay for the services. **Local coverage determinations (LCDs)** and **national coverage determinations (NCDs)** issued by Medicare help sort out medical necessity issues. LCDs (formerly called Local Medicare Review Policies, or LMRPs) and NCDs contain detailed and updated information about the coding and medical necessity of specific services, including:

- A description of the service
- A list of indications (instances in which the service is deemed medically necessary)
- The appropriate CPT/HCPCS code
- The appropriate ICD-9-CM code
- A bibliography containing recent clinical articles to support the Medicare policy

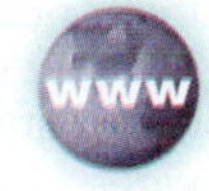

LCD/NCDs Online

http://www.cms.hhs.gov/center/coverage.asp

If a provider thinks that a procedure will not be covered by Medicare because it is not reasonable and necessary, the patient is notified of this before the treatment by means of a standard **advance beneficiary notice (ABN)** from CMS (see Figure 10.4 on page 343). A filled-in form is given to the patient for signature. The ABN form is designed to:

- Identify the service or item that Medicare is unlikely to pay for
- State the reason Medicare is unlikely to pay
- Estimate how much the service or item will cost the beneficiary if Medicare does not pay

> **Billing Tip**
>
> **NEMB or ABN?**
> NEMB = Service not covered under Medicare.
> ABN = Medicare does not consider a service reasonable and necessary in this situation.

The ABN for general use is form CMS-R-131-G. Variations of the form for laboratory use (CMS-R-131-L) and home health care (CMS-R-296) are also available.

ABNs are not for excluded services. They are used only for services that may not be reasonable and necessary under Medicare. As with a NEMB, the purpose of the ABN is to help the beneficiary make an informed decision

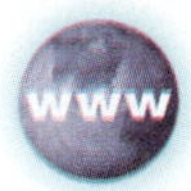

Advance Beneficiary Notice Form

http://www.cms.hhs.gov/cmsforms/downloads/cmsr-131-g.pdf

NOTICE OF EXCLUSIONS FROM MEDICARE BENEFITS (NEMB)

There are items and services for which Medicare will not pay.

- Medicare does **not** pay for all of your health care costs. Medicare only pays for covered benefits. **Some items and services are not Medicare benefits and Medicare will not pay for them.**
- When you receive an item or service that is not a Medicare benefit, **you are responsible to pay for it,** personally or through any other insurance that you may have.

The purpose of this notice is to help you make an informed choice about whether or not you want to receive these items or services, knowing that you will have to pay for them yourself. **Before you make a decision, you should read this entire notice carefully.**

Ask us to explain, if you don't understand why Medicare won't pay.

Ask us how much these items or services will cost you (**Estimated Cost: $**__________).

Medicare will not pay for: ____;

❑ **1. Because it does not meet the definition of any Medicare benefit.**

❑ **2. Because of the following exclusion * from Medicare benefits:**

❑ Personal comfort items.
❑ Most shots (vaccinations).
❑ Hearing aids and hearing examinations.
❑ Most outpatient prescription drugs.
❑ Orthopedic shoes and foot supports (orthotics).
❑ Health care received outside of the USA.
❑ Services required as a result of war.
❑ Routine physicals and most tests for screening.
❑ Routine eye care, eyeglasses and examinations.
❑ Cosmetic surgery.
❑ Dental care and dentures (in most cases).
❑ Routine foot care and flat foot care.
❑ Services by immediate relatives.
❑ Services under a physician's private contract.
❑ Services paid for by a governmental entity that is not Medicare.
❑ Services for which the patient has no legal obligation to pay.
❑ Home health services furnished under a plan of care, if the agency does not submit the claim.
❑ Items and services excluded under the Assisted Suicide Funding Restriction Act of 1997.
❑ Items or services furnished in a competitive acquisition area by any entity that does not have a contract with the Department of Health and Human Services (except in a case of urgent need).
❑ Physicians' services performed by a physician assistant, midwife, psychologist, or nurse anesthetist, when furnished to an inpatient, unless they are furnished under arrangements by the hospital.
❑ Items and services furnished to an individual who is a resident of a skilled nursing facility (a SNF) or of a part of a facility that includes a SNF, unless they are furnished under arrangements by the SNF.
❑ Services of an assistant at surgery without prior approval from the peer review organization.
❑ Outpatient occupational and physical therapy services furnished incident to a physician's services.

* **This is only a general summary of exclusions from Medicare benefits. It is not a legal document. The official Medicare program provisions are contained in relevant laws, regulations, and rulings.**

FIGURE 10.3 Notice of Exclusions from Medicare Benefits (NEMB)

about services that might have to be paid out-of-pocket. A provider who could have been expected (by Medicare) to know that a service would not be covered and who performed the service without informing the patient could be liable for the charges.

Modifiers for ABNs

Modifiers are appended to procedure codes for noncovered Medicare services on claims. There are three modifiers that indicate whether an ABN is on file or needed:

- *GZ*: An item or service is expected to be denied as not reasonable and necessary but the physician's office does *not* have a signed ABN. This might oc-

Patient's Name: Medicare # (HICN):

ADVANCE BENEFICIARY NOTICE (ABN)

NOTE: You need to make a choice about receiving these health care items or services.

We expect that Medicare will not pay for the item(s) or service(s) that are described below. Medicare does not pay for all of your health care costs. Medicare only pays for covered items and services when Medicare rules are met. The fact that Medicare may not pay for a particular item or service does not mean that you should not receive it. There may be a good reason your doctor recommended it. Right now, in your case, **Medicare probably will not pay for –**

Items or Services:
Because:

The purpose of this form is to help you make an informed choice about whether or not you want to receive these items or services, knowing that you might have to pay for them yourself. Before you make a decision about your options, you should **read this entire notice carefully.**

- Ask us to explain, if you don't understand why Medicare probably won't pay.
- Ask us how much these items or services will cost you (**Estimated Cost: $**______________), in case you have to pay for them yourself or through other insurance.

PLEASE CHOOSE **ONE** OPTION. CHECK **ONE** BOX. **SIGN & DATE** YOUR CHOICE.

☐ **Option 1. YES.** **I want to receive these items or services.**

I understand that Medicare will not decide whether to pay unless I receive these items or services. Please submit my claim to Medicare. I understand that you may bill me for items or services and that I may have to pay the bill while Medicare is making its decision. If Medicare does pay, you will refund to me any payments I made to you that are due to me. If Medicare denies payment, I agree to be personally and fully responsible for payment. That is, I will pay personally, either out of pocket or through any other insurance that I have. I understand I can appeal Medicare's decision.

☐ **Option 2. NO.** **I have decided not to receive these items or services.**

I will not receive these items or services. I understand that you will not be able to submit a claim to Medicare and that I will not be able to appeal your opinion that Medicare won't pay.

____________ ________________________

Date **Signature of patient or person acting on patient's behalf**

NOTE: Your health information will be kept confidential. Any information that we collect about you on this form will be kept confidential in our offices. If a claim is submitted to Medicare, your health information on this form may be shared with Medicare. Your health information which Medicare sees will be kept confidential by Medicare.

OMB Approval No. 0938-0566 Form No. CMS-R-131-G (June 2002)

FIGURE 10.4 Advance Beneficiary Notice (ABN)

cur in an emergency care situation, or a patient might not be available to sign the document before a specimen is tested. The –GZ modifier might be used for a noncovered screening test or a service reported with a noncovered ICD-9-CM code. The patient cannot be billed for the service if Medicare does not pay.

- *GA*: A waiver of liability statement is on file. The –GA modifier also applies when services are expected to be denied as not reasonable and necessary. However, it shows that a signed ABN is on file in the physician's office. If the claim is not paid by Medicare, the patient is responsible for payment of the charges.
- *GY*: An item or service that is statutorily excluded or does not meet the definition of a Medicare benefit. This would be used for services *never* covered by Medicare, such as routine physicals or cosmetic surgeries. It

Compliance Guidelines

Do Not Use "Blanket" or Blank ABNs

- Medicare prohibits the use of blanket ABNs given routinely to all patients just to be sure of payment.
- Never have a patient sign a blank ABN for the physician to fill in later. The form must be filled in before the patient signs it.

Billing Tips

ABNs
The ABN must be specific to the service and date, signed and dated by the patient, and filed. Best practices are to give the patient a copy of the signed document and note this on the filed copy.

–GY Modifier
Use the –GY modifier to speed Medicare denials so the amount due can be collected from the patient (or a secondary payer).

indicates that an ABN is not required. The claim will be denied by Medicare, and the patient (or a secondary payer) is responsible for payment of the charges.

Nonparticipating Providers

Nonparticipating physicians decide whether to accept assignment on a claim-by-claim basis.

Payment Under Acceptance of Assignment

Providers who elect not to participate in the Medicare program but who accept assignment on a claim are paid 5 percent less for their services than are PAR providers. For example, if the Medicare-allowed amount for a service is $100, the PAR provider receives $80 (80 percent of $100), and the nonPAR provider receives $76 ($80 minus 5 percent).

A nonparticipating provider must also provide a surgical financial disclosure—advance written notification—when performing elective surgery that has a charge of $500 or more. The form must contain specific wording and must include an estimated charge for the procedure (see Figure 10.5 for an example).

Like participating providers, nonPAR providers may bill patients for services that are excluded from coverage in the Medicare program. Therefore, it is good practice to provide patients with an NEMB notifying them that Medicare will not pay for a service before providing the service.

Dear (Patient's name):

I do not plan to accept assignment for your surgery. The law requires that where assignment is not taken and the charge is $500 or more, the following information must be provided prior to surgery. These estimates assume that you have already met the $100 annual Medicare Part B deductible.

Type of Surgery

____

Estimated charge for surgery $______

Estimated Medicare payment $______

Your estimated out-of-pocket expense $______

______________ ______

Patient signature Date

FIGURE 10.5 Advance Notice for Elective Surgery Form

Payment for Unassigned Claims: The Limiting Charge

NonPAR providers who do not accept assignment are subject to Medicare's charge limits. The Medicare Comprehensive Limiting Charge Compliance Program (CLCCP) was created to prevent nonparticipating physicians from collecting the balance from Medicare patients. (Note that more restrictive rules apply to nonPAR billing rates in some states.) A physician may not charge a Medicare patient more than 115 percent of the amount listed in the Medicare nonparticipating fee schedule. This amount—115 percent of the fee listed in the nonPAR MFS—is called the **limiting charge**. Medicare issues bulletins to physicians that list fees and limiting charges. [EX]

Nonparticipating amount	$115.26
	× 115%
Limiting charge amount	$132.55

The limiting charge does not apply to immunizations, supplies, or ambulance service. Physicians who collect amounts in excess of the limiting charge are subject to financial penalties and may be excluded from the Medicare program for a specific time period.

For a nonassigned claim, the provider can collect the full payment from the patient at the time of the visit. The claim is then submitted to Medicare. If approved, Medicare will pay 80 percent of the allowed amount on the nonPAR fee schedule rather than the limiting amount. Medicare sends this payment directly to the patient, since the physician has already been paid.

A participating provider may also be part of a clinic or group that does not participate. In this case, the beneficiary may be charged more if the visit takes place at the clinic or group location than if it takes place at the provider's private office.

The following example illustrates the different fee structures for PARs, nonPARs who accept assignment, and nonPARs who do not accept assignment.

Participating Provider	
Physician's standard fee	$120.00
Medicare fee	$60.00
Medicare pays 80% ($60.00 × 80%)	$48.00
Patient or supplemental plan pays 20% ($60.00 × 20%)	$12.00
Provider adjustment (write-off) ($120.00 - $60.00)	$60.00
Nonparticipating Provider (Accepts Assignment)	
Physician's standard fee	$120.00
Medicare nonPAR fee ($60.00 minus 5%)	$57.00
Medicare pays 80% ($57.00 × 80%)	$45.60
Patient or supplemental plan pays 20% ($57.00 × 20%)	$11.40
Provider adjustment (write-off) ($120.00 - $57.00)	$63.00
Nonparticipating Provider (Does Not Accept Assignment)	
Physician's standard fee	$120.00
Medicare nonPAR fee	$57.00
Limiting Charge (115% × $57.00)	$65.55
Patient billed	$65.55
Medicare pays patient (80% × $57.00)	$45.60
Total provider can collect	$65.55
Patient out-of-pocket expense ($65.55 - $45.60)	$19.95

Billing Tip

Limiting Charges
Limiting charges apply only to nonparticipating providers submitting nonassigned claims.

Billing Tip

Accept Assignment on Drugs and Biologics
Nonparticipating providers must accept assignment and not collect up-front payment for drugs and biologics they administer in the office, such as reimbursement for flu and pneumococcal vaccinations.

Thinking It Through — 10.2

Fill in the blanks in the following payment situations:

Participating Provider	
Physician's standard fee	$210.00
Medicare fee	$115.00
Medicare pays 80%	$_____
Patient or supplemental plan pays 20%	$_____
Provider adjustment (write-off)	$_____
Nonparticipating Provider (Accepts Assignment)	
Physician's standard fee	$210.00
Medicare nonPAR fee	$_____
Medicare pays 80%	$_____
Patient/supplemental plan pays 20%	$_____
Provider adjustment (write-off)	$_____
Nonparticipating Provider (Does Not Accept Assignment)	
Physician's standard fee	$210.00
Medicare nonPAR fee	$_____
Limiting Charge	$_____
Patient billed	$_____
Medicare pays patient	$_____
Total provider can collect	$_____
Patient out-of-pocket expense	$_____

Compliance Guideline

Avoid Waiving Patients' Payments
Under Medicare regulations, physicians should not routinely waive any payments that are due from patients, such as deductibles. Doing so may appear to be illegal inducements to patients.

Compliance Guideline

Medicare Fraud Watch
Under a special program, Medicare beneficiaries can earn rewards of up to $1,000 if they turn in providers who are proven to have committed fraud against the program. A Medicare beneficiary has the right to ask a provider for an itemized statement for any item or service for which Medicare has paid. The program instructs Medicare recipients to verify that they have received the services listed on their MSNs.

Original Medicare Plan and Medicare Advantage Plans

Medicare beneficiaries select from two main types of coverage plans: traditional fee-for-service or managed care.

Original Medicare Plan

The Medicare fee-for-service plan, referred to by Medicare as the **Original Medicare Plan**, allows the beneficiary to choose any licensed physician certified by Medicare. Each time the beneficiary receives services, a fee is billable. Part of this fee is generally paid by Medicare, and part is paid by the beneficiary or sometimes by a secondary policy.

Original Medicare Plan patients are responsible for an annual deductible. They are also responsible for the portion of the bill that Medicare does not pay (coinsurance), typically 20 percent of allowed charges. Patients receive a **Medicare Summary Notice (MSN)** that details the services they were provided over a thirty-day period, the amounts charged, and the amounts they may be billed (see Figure 10.6). This form was formerly called the Explanation of Medicare Benefits, or EOMB.

The MSN presents coverage decisions in patient-friendly language. For example, instead of the phrases *not medically necessary* and *not reasonable and necessary*, patients see message such as "the information provided does not support the need for this many services or items" and "we have approved this service at a reduced level."

355369622
Page 1 of 3

CMS CENTERS for MEDICARE & MEDICAID SERVICES

Medicare Summary Notice

October 28, 2008

CMCA30230118832T
EVE J LANE
12 GRASSY HILL RD
ROXBURY CT 06783-1812

CUSTOMER SERVICE INFORMATION

Your Medicare Number: 444-50-2225A

If you have any questions, write or call:
First Coast Service Options
321 Research Parkway
PO Box 9000
Meriden, CT 06454-9000
Toll-Free: 1-800-982-6819
TTY for Hearing Impaired: 1-866-359-3614

BE INFORMED: Do not sell your Medicare Number or Medicare Summary notice.

This is a summary of claims processed from 10/06/2008 through 10/27/2008.

PART B MEDICAL INSURANCE - ASSIGNED CLAIMS

Dates of Service	Services Provided	Amount Charged	Medicare Approved	Medicare Paid Provider	You May Be Billed	See Notes Section
Claim number 22-03266-168-770 **Deresh Ahmad M D, Suite 210,** **1305 Post Road , Fairfield, CT 06430-0000** Dr. Ahmad, Deresh						a,b
09/15/08	1 Office/outpatient visit, est (99213)	$95.00	$56.29	$45.03	$11.26	
Claim number 22-03289-263-180 **Deresh Ahmad M D, Suite 210,** **1305 Post Road , Fairfield, CT 06430-0000** Dr. Ahmad, Deresh						b
09/26/08	1 Office/outpatient visit, est (99213)	$95.00	$56.29	$45.03	$11.26	

Notes Section:

a A copy of this notice will not be forwarded to your Medigap insurer because the information was incomplete or invalid. Please submit a copy of this notice to your Medigap insurer.

b This information is being sent to your private insurer(s). Send any questions regarding your benefits to them.

Deductible Information:

You have met the Part B deductible for 2008.

Appeals Information - Part B

If you disagree with any claims decision on this notice, you can request an appeal by **February 25, 2009.** Follow the instructions below:

1) Circle the item(s) you disagree with and explain why you disagree.

2) Send this notice, or a copy, to the address in the "Customer Service Information" box on Page 1. (You may also send any additional information you may have about your appeal.)

3) Sign here______________________________ Phone number (____)____________

FIGURE 10.6 Medicare Summary Notice (MSN)

Medicare Advantage Plans

Medicare also offers a group of managed care plans called **Medicare Advantage** and also called Medicare Part C (formerly Medicare + Choice). A Medicare Advantage organization (MAO) is responsible for providing all Medicare-covered services, except hospice care, in return for a predetermined capitated payment. Medicare Advantage offers three types of plans:

1. Medicare coordinated care plans (CCPs)
2. Medicare private fee-for-service plans
3. Medical Savings Accounts (MSAs)

Medicare Coordinated Care Plans

Many Medicare beneficiaries are enrolled in Medicare Advantage coordinated care plans. A coordinated care plan includes providers who are under contract to deliver the benefit package approved by CMS. Many CCPs are run by the same major payers that offer private (commercial) coverage.

CCPs may use features to control utilization, such as requiring referrals from primary care providers (PCP), and may use methods of paying providers to encourage high-quality and cost-effective care. A plan may require the patient to receive treatment within the plan's network. If a patient goes out of the network for services, the plan will not pay; the patient must pay the entire bill. This restriction does not apply to emergency treatment (which may be provided anywhere in the United States) and **urgently needed care** (care provided while temporarily outside the plan's network area).

CCP plans include the following:

- HMOs, with or without a point-of-service option. HMOs are generally the most restrictive plans. The point-of-service option permits a patient to receive some services from outside the network, for which the plan will pay a percentage of the fee rather than the entire bill. The patient is responsible for the balance of the charges, usually at least 20 percent. Under yet another option, patients may also see health care providers within or outside the plan's network; charges for services received within the network are subject to small copayments, and those outside the network are handled like other fee-for-service Medicare claims. In other words, charges for services outside the network are not paid by the managed care plan but are instead covered under regular Medicare, subject to deductibles and coinsurance. HMOs also offer extra coverage for such services as preventive care and prescription drugs at an additional cost.
- PSOs, which are the Medicare version of independent practice associations (IPAs), groups of providers who share the financial risk of the plan (see Chapter 9).
- PPOs, which are either local or one of twenty-six regional PPOs that must be licensed or otherwise authorized as managed care organizations in the states they serve. In the Medicare PPO, patients have a financial incentive to use doctors within a network, but they may choose to go outside it and pay additional costs, which may include higher copayments or higher coinsurance. A PPO contracts with a group of providers to offer health care services to patients. Unlike HMOs, many PPOs do not require the patient to select a PCP.
- Special needs plans (SNPs), which enroll either only or a greater proportion of special needs individuals: institutionalized individuals, people entitled to

Thinking It Through — 10.3

1. Does a participating provider in a traditional fee-for-service plan always get paid more for a service than a nonparticipating provider who does not accept assignment?
2. Does a patient in a traditional fee-for-service plan always pay higher fees when services are provided by a nonparticipating provider who does not accept assignment?

medical assistance under a state Medicaid plan, and other high-risk groups of chronically ill or disabled individuals.

- Religious fraternal benefits plans (RFBs), which limit enrollment to a religious fraternal benefits society.

To maintain uniform coverage within a geographic area, CMS requires managed care plans to provide all of the Medicare benefits available in the service area. Beyond that restriction, plans are free to offer coverage for additional services not covered under fee-for-service plans, such as prescription drugs, preventive care (including physical examinations and inoculations), eyeglasses and hearing aids, dental care, and care for treatment received while traveling overseas.

Medicare Private Fee-for-Service (PFFS)

Under a Medicare private fee-for-service plan, patients receive services from Medicare-approved providers or facilities of their choosing. The plan is operated by a private insurance company that contracts with Medicare but pays on a fee-for-service basis.

Medical Savings Accounts

The Medicare Modernization Act created a new plan for Medicare called a **Medical Savings Account (MSA).** Similar to a private medical savings account, it combines a high-deductible fee-for-service plan with a tax-exempt trust to pay for qualified medical expenses. The maximum annual MSA plan deductible is set by law. CMS pays premiums for the insurance policies and makes a contribution to the MSA; the beneficiary puts in the rest of the fund. Beneficiaries use the money in their MSAs to pay for their health care before the high deductible is reached. At that point, the Medicare Advantage plan offering the MSA pays for all expenses for covered services.

Medigap Insurance

Individuals enrolled in Medicare Part B Original Medicare Plan often have additional insurance, either Medigap insurance they purchase or insurance provided by a former employer. These plans frequently pay the patient's Part B deductible and additional procedures that Medicare does not cover. If Medicare does not pay a claim because of lack of medical necessity, Medigap and supplemental carriers are not required to pay the claim either.

Compliance Guideline

Medigap

Medigap plans can legally be sold only to people covered by the Medicare fee-for-service plan (Original Medicare Plan). Patients covered by a Medicare managed care plan or by Medicaid (see Chapter 11) do not need Medigap policies.

Medigap Insurance

Medigap is private insurance that beneficiaries may purchase to fill in some of the gaps—unpaid amounts—in Medicare coverage. These gaps include the annual deductible, any coinsurance, and payment for some noncovered services. Even though private insurance carriers offer Medigap plans, coverage and standards are regulated by federal and state law.

Medigap policyholders pay monthly premiums. Ten plans are available, labeled A through J. Monthly premiums vary widely across the different plan levels, as well as within a single plan level, depending on the insurance company selected. However, a set of core benefits is common to all Medigap plans:

- Part A daily coinsurance for days 61 to 90 of hospitalization
- Part A daily coinsurance for each of Medicare's 60 lifetime inpatient hospital days
- 100 percent of covered hospital charges for 365 additional days after all Medicare hospital benefits have been used
- Part B coinsurance amount (usually 20 percent of approved charges) after the deductible
- First three pints of blood per calendar year

Billing Tip

List of Medigap Companies

Medicare carriers maintain lists of Medigap companies on their websites. Check the list for current Payer IDs for claims.

Plans B through J also pay the Part A hospital deductible for each hospitalization. See Figure 10.7 for a complete listing of Medigap plans and the coverage they provide.

After a Medicare carrier processes a claim for a patient with Medigap coverage, the carrier automatically forwards the claim to the Medigap payer, indicating the amount Medicare approved and paid for the procedures. Once the Medigap carrier adjudicates the claim, the provider is paid directly, eliminating the need for the practice to file a separate Medigap claim. The beneficiary receives copies of the Medicare Summary Notices that explain the charges paid and due.

A	B	C	D	E	F	G	H	I	J*
Basic Benefit	Basic Benefit	Basic Benefit	Basic Benefit	Basic Benefit	Basic Benefit	Basic Benefit	Basic Benefit	Basic Benefit	Basic Benefit
		Skilled Nursing Coinsurance	Skilled Nursing Coinsurance	Skilled Nursing Coinsurance	Skilled Nursing Coinsurance	Skilled Nursing Coinsurance	Skilled Nursing Coinsurance	Skilled Nursing Coinsurance	Skilled Nursing Coinsurance
	Part A Deductible	Part A Deductible	Part A Deductible	Part A Deductible	Part A Deductible	Part A Deductible	Part A Deductible	Part A Deductible	Part A Deductible
		Part B Deductible			Part B Deductible				Part B Deductible
					Part Excess (100%)	Part Excess (80%)		Part Excess (100%)	Part Excess (100%)
		Foreign Travel Emergency	Foreign Travel Emergency	Foreign Travel Emergency	Foreign Travel Emergency	Foreign Travel Emergency	Foreign Travel Emergency	Foreign Travel Emergency	Foreign Travel Emergency
			At-Home Recovery			At-Home Recovery		At-Home Recovery	At-Home Recovery
							Basic Drug Benefit (50%) ($3,000 Limit)	Basic Drug Benefit (50%) ($3,000 Limit)	Extended Drug Benefit ($3,000 Limit)
				Preventive Care ($120 Limit)					Preventive Care ($120 Limit)

*High-deductible plans available.

FIGURE 10.7 Medigap Coverage, Plans A-J

Supplemental Insurance

Supplemental insurance is a plan an individual may receive when retiring from a company. A supplemental plan is designed to provide additional coverage for an individual receiving benefits under Medicare Part B. Supplemental policies provide benefits similar to those offered in the employer's standard group health plan. CMS does not regulate the supplemental plan's coverage, in contrast to what it does with Medigap insurance. Some supplemental plans require preauthorization for surgery and diagnostic tests.

> **Billing Tip**
>
> **Medicare As The Secondary Payer**
> In certain situations, Medicare pays benefits on a claim only after another insurance carrier—the primary carrier—has processed the claim. The medical information specialist is responsible for knowing when Medicare is the secondary payer and, in those cases, for submitting claims to the primary payer first. This is explained in Chapter 14.

Medicare Billing And Compliance

Billing Medicare can be complex. The flow of claims from the provider to the carrier and back is illustrated in Figure 10.8. A medical insurance specialist must be familiar with the rules and regulations for the practice's Medicare carrier, including the common topics discussed below.

CCI Edits and Global Surgical Packages

Medicare requires the use of the Healthcare Common Procedure Coding System (CPT/HCPCS) for coding services (see Chapters 5 and 6). Medicare's Correct Coding Initiative (CCI, see Chapter 7) is a list of CPT code combinations that, if used, would cause a claim to be rejected. The list is updated every quarter and must be followed closely for compliant billing. Many practices use a software tool to check Medicare claims against the CCI before transmitting them.

The CCI edits enforce Medicare regulations under which a physician cannot bill separately for each visit or procedure that is part of a bundled surgical procedure. Instead, a charge for a global surgical package includes services provided by the physician for a specified preoperative and follow-up period. The source for the regulations on global packages is the Medicare Physician Fee Schedule (MPFS).

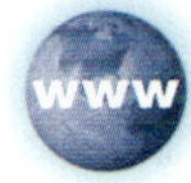

Medicare Physician Fee Schedule
http://www.cms.hhs.gov/PhysicianFeeSched/

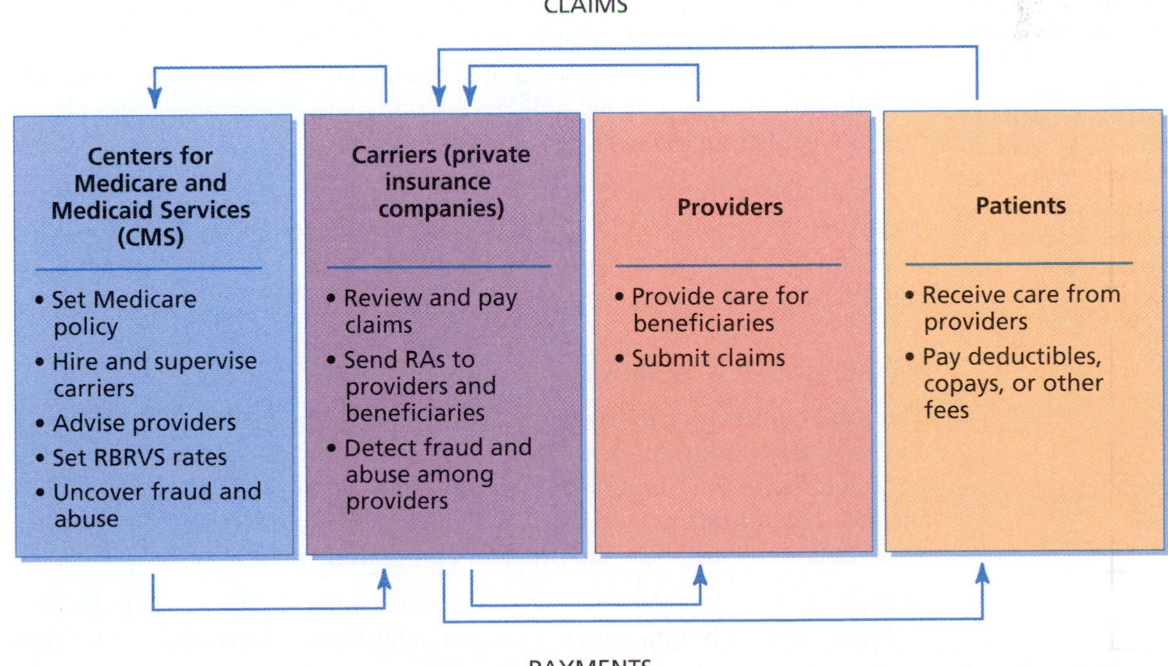

FIGURE 10.8 The Medicare Claims Process

Billing Tip

Bill Unrelated Services During the Global Period
Services during a global period that are unrelated to the procedure can be billed. For example, a patient's skin biopsy that occurs during a global follow-up period for ankle reconstruction is billable.

The MPFS lists all the CPT/HCPCS codes and includes a column labeled *Global Period* containing one of these indicators:

- 000 No global days are assigned to the code.
- 010 Minor surgery; a ten-day postoperative care period.
- 090 Major surgery; one day of preoperative and ninety days of postoperative care.
- MMM Maternity code; global period does not apply.
- XXX The global concept does not apply to the code.
- YYY Carrier decides what the global period will be.
- ZZZ The code is related to another service and is always included in that service's global period.

Following these guidelines for correct billing:

- Keep track of Medicare patients' visits after surgery and determine what the follow-up period is. All visits within that period that are *unrelated* to the surgery must be billed with a modifier –24.
- Note that all procedures in the surgical section of CPT are subject to the global period, even minor procedures like joint injections. Some procedures in the medicine section of CPT, such as cardiac catheterization, are also subject to global surgery rules.

Timely Filing

Medicare law sets specific time limits for submission of claims for physician and other Part B services payable on a reasonable-charge or fee-schedule basis. For these services, the law requires the claim to be filed no later than the end of the calendar year following the year in which the service was furnished, except as follows:

Billing Tip

Filing Late Claims
When filing a late claim, be sure to include an explanation of the reason and have evidence to support it. Claims may be paid if the filing is late for a good reason, such as because of a Medicare administrative error, unavoidable delay, or accidental record damage.

- The time limit on filing claims for services furnished in the last three months of a year is the same as if the services had been furnished in the subsequent year. In other words, the time limit on filing claims for services furnished in the last three months of the year is December 31 of the second year following the year in which the services were rendered.
- When the last day for timely filing of a claim falls on a Saturday, Sunday, federal non-workday, or legal holiday, the filing will be considered timely if the claim is filed on the next workday.

For example, for surgery in August 2007, a claim for payment must be filed on or before December 31, 2008. A claim for a service provided in October 2007 must be filed on or before December 31, 2009. A claim received by a carrier after the time limit is subject to a 10 percent reduction.

Medical Review Program

Medicare contractors audit claim data on an ongoing basis under the **Medical Review (MR) Program**, in which they check for inappropriate billing. These contractors use the Comprehensive Error Rate Testing (CERT) program information to determine which services are being billed incorrectly. They then analyze data to identify specific providers for a probe review:

- *Probe review*: Providers may be selected for medical review when the carrier finds atypical billing patterns or particular errors. First, the carrier does a probe review, checking twenty to forty claims for provider-specific problems. Providers are notified that a probe review is being conducted and are asked to provide more documentation. If the probe review verifies that an error exists, the carrier classifies it as minor, moderate, or severe. Providers are then educated on correct billing procedures.

- *Prepayment review*: The provider may be placed on prepayment review, in which a percentage of claims are subject to MR before being paid. Once providers have shown they know how to bill correctly, they are removed from prepayment review.
- *Postpayment review*: The provider may instead be placed on postpayment review, which uses a sampling of submitted claims to estimate overpayments instead of pulling all the records.

At any time during the medical review process, the carrier may ask for additional documentation by issuing an **Additional Documentation Request (ADR).** ADRs require the provider to respond within thirty days.

When a series of requests leads to a comprehensive medical review, the matter is especially serious. When this level of audit is requested by Medicare, medical insurance specialists should:

- Notify the compliance officer
- Send the complete documentation available for each medical record, including all notes, correspondence, and test results (this does not violate HIPAA)
- Keep copies of everything that has been sent

The Medicare carrier notifies the practice of the audit's results, listing whether each charge on the audited claims was accepted, denied, or downcoded. If payments were previously received from Medicare for charges that are now denied or reduced, the resulting overpayments must be reimbursed to the Medicare program. Providers may also wish to appeal decisions (see Chapter 14).

If warranted by possible fraudulent patterns, Medicare may refer the case to the Office of the Inspector General (OIG) for fraud and abuse investigation. OIG attorneys must follow certain procedures before they allege that a physician has violated the False Claims Act.

Compliance Guideline

Checking Medicare Payments
To safeguard against fraud by outside billing services, all payments from carriers are made in the name of the provider and transmitted to the pay-to provider. Providers are also required to review monthly RAs when a billing service is used and to notify CMS if they believe false claims have been generated. CMS's PECOS (Provider Enrollment, Chain, and Ownership System) records data about the billing service or clearinghouse providers use.

Duplicate Claims

Medicare defines duplicate claims as those sent to one or more Medicare contractors from the same provider for the same beneficiary, the same service, and the same date of service. A practice should not

- Send a second claim if the first one has not been paid. Instead, contact the payer after thirty days if a claim is unpaid, using the telephone or electronic claim status inquiries.
- Bill both a Part B carrier and a Durable Medical Equipment Regional Carrier for the same beneficiary, service, and date of service.

Split Billing

If covered and noncovered services are both performed for a patient on the same date, practices split the bill when preparing the claim by subtracting the cost of the covered service from the exam cost and reporting it with an appropriate ICD-9-CM code.

This issue is complicated when billing an office visit on the same day as a preventive medicine visit. In general, Medicare considers a covered physician service provided at the same place on the same date as a preventive service to be separate and billable (with a –25 modifier to show that a significant, separately identifiable evaluation and management service has been provided).

Preauthorization

Some surgical procedures require preauthorization from qualified independent organizations, formerly known as peer review organizations (PROs). A **Quality Improvement Organization (QIO)** is a state-based group of physicians who are paid by the government to review aspects of the Medicare program, including the quality and appropriateness of services provided and fees charged.

Clinical Laboratory Improvement Amendments

Lab work may be done either in physicians' offices or in off-site labs. All lab work is regulated by **Clinical Laboratory Improvement Amendments (CLIA)** rules. Most offices do easy-to-administer, low-risk tests (ovulation, blood glucose, dipstick or tablet reagent urinalyses, and rapid strep test), which are "waived" under CLIA and are subject to minimal requirements. Medicare providers who want to perform these **waived tests** file an application and pay a small fee. Offices that handle more complex testing (like CBCs, PSAs, routine chemistry panels, and antibiotic susceptibility tests) must apply and be certified and inspected for accreditation.

To bill Medicare for waived tests, the office must have a CLIA certificate of waiver; follow the manufacturers' test instructions; include the CLIA number on the claims; and add modifier -QW (for CLIA waived test) to the codes. (Note that this modifier does not apply to private payers.) Examples are:

CPT Code/Modifier	Description
81025–QW	Urine pregnancy test (various manufacturers)
86318–QW	Acon® *H. pylori* Test Device
85018–QW	HemoCue Hemoglobin 201
83001–QW	Synova Healthcare Menocheck Pro

Incident-to Billing

CLJA Categorization of Tests
http://cms.hss.gov/CLIA

Medicare pays for services and supplies that are furnished **incident to** a physician's services, that are commonly included in bills, and for which payment is not made under a separate benefit category. Incident-to services and supplies are performed or provided by medical staff members other than the physician—such as physician assistants (PAs) and nurse practitioners (NPs) and are supervised by the physician. The deciding factor for billing is the direct supervision by the physician. Specific rules concerning which Medicare identifier numbers and fees to use must be researched before incident-to claims are submitted.

Billing Tip

Check Diagnosis Code Requirements
Check the ICD-9-CM code requirements given in local coverage determinations after the new diagnosis codes are announced each year, paying special attention to screening services. Different codes may be needed for low- versus high-risk patients.

Roster Billing

Roster billing is a simplified process that allows a provider to submit a single paper claim with the names, health insurance claim numbers, dates of birth, sex, dates of service, and signatures for Medicare patients who received vaccinations for influenza and pneumococcal vaccines covered by Medicare. These claims do not have to be sent electronically. Annual Part B deductible and coinsurance amounts do not apply to these vaccines. Assuming that the patient received no services other than the shot, administering seasonal shots is coded

- G0008 for influenza virus vaccine administration
- G0009 for pneumococcal vaccine administration
- G0010 for hepatitis B vaccine

Also report the appropriate vaccine product code and a V code (from the ICD-9-CM) to show the need for the shot.

Preparing Primary Medicare Claims

Under HIPAA, electronic billing complying with HIPAA standards is mandatory for physician practices except offices with fewer than ten full-time (or equivalent) employees. Some practices mistakenly submit claims on paper rather than electronically when attachments such as an operative report, nurse's notes, doctor's orders, RA/EOB, or other documents are needed. However, carriers do not require submitting a claim on paper in order to send accompanying documentation on paper.

Sending any claims on paper slows cash flow, because by law paper claims must be held longer than HIPAA-compliant electronic claims before payment can be released. Paper claims cannot be paid before the 29th day after receipt of the claim, according to CMS guidelines. Most carriers prefer electronic claims, and in the rare instances when they need additional information to complete processing of an electronic claim, they will ask for it.

Billing Tip

Which Carrier?
Claims should be sent to the carrier for the state where the service was provided, not the carrier for the state where the patient resides. Payment is based on the ZIP code for the place of service except when service was provided in the patient's home. In that case Medicare uses the beneficiary address on file to determine the geographical payment.

Medicare Required Data Elements on the HIPAA 837 Claim

In addition to the standard data elements that are required on HIPAA claims (see Chapter 8), medical insurance specialists should be alert for the data discussed below.

Information in the Notes Segment

A section of the HIPAA 837 claim called NTE (meaning "notes") should be used to report any information Medicare needs to process an electronic claim that is not appropriately reported elsewhere. The NTE segment is used for the following types of information:

- Descriptions of unlisted surgery codes (codes that end in –99)
- Dosages and drug names for unlisted drug and injection codes
- Description of why a service is unusual (modifier –22)
- Details on the reason for an ambulance trip
- Periods (dates) of care when billing postoperative care
- Reason for a reduced service (modifier –52)
- Information on discontinued procedures (modifier –53)

Billing Tip

NTE Segment
Each claim line allows for eighty characters of data to be reported in the NTE segment. The practice management program (PMP) should be set up to create the NTE segment when billing claims electronically.

Diagnosis Codes

The HIPAA 837 claim allows a maximum of eight ICD-9-CM codes to be reported for each claim. All are automatically considered when the claim is processed.

Billing Tip

Rejections Because of Invalid or Missing ICD-9-CM Codes
Claims that have invalid or missing diagnosis codes will be returned as unprocessable. A fine may also be charged for each violation of the HIPAA standard.

Medicare Assignment Code

The Medicare assignment code indicates whether the provider accepts Medicare assignment. The choices are as follows:

Code	*Definition*
A	Assigned
B	Assignment accepted on clinical lab services only
C	Not assigned
P	Patient refuses to assign benefits

Insurance Type Code

An insurance type code is required for a claim being sent to Medicare when Medicare is not the primary payer. Choices include:

Code	*Definition*
AP	Auto insurance policy
C1	Commercial
CP	Medicare conditionally primary
GP	Group policy
HM	Health maintenance organization (HMO)
IP	Individual policy
LD	Long-term policy
LT	Litigation
MB	Medicare Part B
MC	Medicaid
MI	Medigap Part B
MP	Medicare primary
OT	Other
PP	Personal payment (cash—no insurance)
SP	Supplemental policy

Assumed Care Date/Relinquished Care Date

This information is required when providers share postoperative care; the date a provider assumed or gave up care is reported.

Billing Tip

Medicare Instructions May Vary
The NUCC instructions do not address any particular payer. Best practice for paper claims is to check with the Medicare carrier for specific information required on the form.

CMS-1500 Claim Completion

When the CMS-1500 paper claim is required for a primary Medicare claim, follow the general guidelines described in Table 10.2 and illustrated in Figure 10.9 on page 359.

If a patient is covered by both Medicare and a Medigap plan, a single claim is sent to Medicare; Medicare will automatically send it to the Medigap plan for secondary payment. In this case, if a paper claim is completed, the Item Numbers are as indicated in Table 10.3 on page 360 and shown in Figure 10.10 on page 362.

Billing Tip

Secondary Claims/COB
Chapters 14 and 15 discuss processing RAs/EOBs, secondary claims, coordination of benefits, and appeals for Medicare.

Item Number 19

Many claim details can be entered in IN 19 under CMS guidelines, such as:

- Enter the date a patient was last seen and the NPI of the attending physician when an independent physical or occupational therapist submits claims or a physician providing routine foot care submits claims. For physical and occupational therapists, entering this information certifies that the necessary physician certification (or recertification) is being kept on file, per Medicare requirements.
- Enter the x-ray date for chiropractor services (if an x-ray, rather than a physical examination was the method used to demonstrate the subluxation). By entering an x-ray date and the initiation date for course of chiropractic treatment in Item Number 14, the chiropractor is certifying that all the relevant information requirements (including level of subluxation) are on file, along with the appropriate x-ray and all are available for carrier review.

Table 10.2 Medicare CMS-1500 (08/05) Claim Completion

Item Number	*Content*
1	Indicate Medicare.
1a	Enter the Medicare health insurance claim number that appears on the patient's Medicare card.
2	Record the patient's name *exactly* as it appears on the Medicare card, entering it in last name, first name, middle initial order.
3	Enter the patient's date of birth in eight-digit format; make the appropriate selection for male or female.
4	Enter the name of the insured person, if not the patient.
5	Enter the patient's mailing address, including the number and street, city, state, ZIP code, and the home telephone number.
6	Select the appropriate box for the relationship: Self, spouse, child, or other.
7	Address and telephone number of the insured person listed in IN 4 if not the same as the patient's address.
8	Select the appropriate boxes for marital status and employment status.
9	Leave blank.
9a-c	Leave blank.
10a-10c	Choose the appropriate box to indicate whether the patient's condition is the result of a work injury, an automobile accident, or another type of accident. If any Yes is selected, the claim should be sent first to the liable party (workers' compensation, auto insurance, or other) and then a secondary claim sent to the Medicare. The state postal code must be shown if Yes is checked in IN 10b for Auto Accident.
10d	Varies with the insurance plan; complete if instructed.
11	Enter NONE.
11a-d	Leave blank.
12	Enter "Signature on File," "SOF," or a legal signature, per practice policy.
13	Leave blank.
14	Enter the date that symptoms first began for the current illness, injury, or pregnancy, as documented in the medical record. For pregnancy, enter the first date of the last menstrual period (LMP). Previous pregnancies are not a similar illness. If a Medicare patient is receiving chiropractic services, enter the date that this course of treatment began.
15	Leave blank.
16	Enter the dates the patient is employed but unable to work in the current occupation. (From: the first full day of disability/To: the last day of disability before returning to work.)
17	Enter the name (first name, middle initial, last name) and credentials of the professional who referred or ordered the services or supplies on the claim.
17a	Enter the appropriate identifying number (either NPI or non-NPI/qualifier) for the referring physician.
18	If the services provided are needed because of a related inpatient hospitalization, the admission and discharge dates are entered. For patients still hospitalized, the admission date is listed in the From box, and the To box is left blank.
19	Complete according to the carrier's instructions.
20	Complete if billing for outside lab services. Choosing No means that tests were performed by the billing physician or laboratory. Choosing Yes means that the test was done outside of the office of the physician who is billing for it. When Yes is selected, enter the purchase charge and complete IN 32. When billing for multiple purchased lab services, each service should be submitted on a separate claim.
21	Enter up to four ICD-9-CM codes in priority order. At least one code must be reported. Relate lines 1, 2, 3, 4 to the lines of service in IN 24E by line number. Do not provide narrative description in this box. The codes used should specify the highest level of detail possible, including the use of a fifth digit when appropriate.
22	Leave blank; Medicaid-specific.
23	Enter the preauthorization number assigned by the payer or a CLIA number.
24	The service line information section is used to report the procedures performed for the patient. Each item of service line information has a procedure code and a charge, with additional information as detailed below.
24A	Enter the date(s) of service, from and to. If there is only one date of service, enter that date under From and leave To blank or reenter the From date. If grouping services, the place of service, procedure code, charges, and individual provider for each line must be identical for that service line. Grouping is allowed only for services on consecutive days. The number of days must correspond to the number of units in IN 24G.
24B	Enter the place of service (POS) code that describes the location at which the service was provided. If the service was provided to a hospitalized inpatient (POS 21), enter the hospital's provider information in IN 32.
24C	Check with the payer to determine whether this element (emergency indicator) is necessary. If required, enter Y (yes) or N (no) in the unshaded bottom portion of the field.
24D	Enter the CPT/HCPCS codes and applicable modifiers for services provided. Do not use hyphens.

TABLE 10.2	Medicare CMS-1500 (08/05) Claim Completion—*continued*
Item Number	***Content***
24E	Using the numbers (1, 2, 3, 4) listed to the left of the diagnosis codes in IN 21, enter the diagnosis for the each service listed in IN 24D.
24F	For each service listed in IN 24D, enter charges without dollar signs or decimals. If the claim reports an encounter with no charge, such as a capitated visit, a value of zero (0) may be used.
24G	Enter the number of days or units, as applicable. This field is most commonly used for multiple visits, units of supplies, anesthesia units or minutes, or oxygen volume. If only one service is performed, the numeral 1 must be entered.
24H	Leave blank; Medicaid-specific.
24I–24J	IN 24I and IN 24J work together. These boxes are used to enter an ID number for the rendering provider of the service. If the number is an NPI, it goes in IN 24J in the unshaded area next to the 24I label *NPI.* If the number is a non-NPI (other ID number), the qualifier identifying the type of number goes in IN 24I next to the number in 24J.
25	Enter the physician's or supplier's federal tax identification number (either a Social Security number or an Employer Identification Number). Check the appropriate box for SSN or EIN.
26	Enter the patient account number used by the practice's accounting system.
27	If the physician accepts assignment, select Yes. If the patient is also covered by a Medigap plan and the patient has authorized payment directly to the provider, the provider must also be a Medicare participating physician and must accept assignment.
28	Enter the total of all charges in IN 24F. If the claim is to be submitted on paper and there are more services to be billed, put "continued" here and put the total charge on the last claim form page.
29	Amount of the payments received for the services listed on this claim. If no payment was made, enter "none" or "0.00."
30	Enter the balance resulting from subtracting the amount in IN 29 from the amount in IN 28.
31	Enter the provider's or supplier's signature, the date of the signature, and the provider's credentials (such as MD).
32	Enter the name, address, city, state, and ZIP code of the location where the services were rendered if not the physician's office or the patient's home. Physicians billing for purchased diagnostic tests must identify the supplier's name, address, ZIP code, and NPI in IN 32a. Enter the payer-assigned identifying non-NPI number and qualifier of the service facility in IN 32b.
33	Enter the billing provider's or supplier's name, address, ZIP code, telephone number, NPI, non-NPI number, and appropriate qualifier. The NPI should be placed in IN 33a. Enter the identifying non-NPI number and qualifier of the billing provider in IN 33b.

- Enter the drug's name and dosage when submitting a claim for Not Otherwise Classified (NOC) drugs.
- Enter a concise description of an "unlisted procedure code" or a "*not otherwise classified*" (NOC) code if one can be given within the confines of this box. Otherwise an attachment *must* be submitted with the claim.
- Enter all applicable modifiers when modifier -99 (multiple modifiers) is entered in Item Number 24D. If modifier -99 is entered on multiple line items of a single claim form, all applicable modifiers for each line item containing a –99 modifier should be listed as follows: 1=(mod), where the number 1 represents the line item and "mod" represents all modifiers applicable to the referenced line item. Modifier 99 is only appropriate when more than four modifiers are necessary per claim line. When four or less modifiers apply, each modifier can be entered in the existing space in Item 24D on the CMS-1500 claim form.
- When billing for radiation oncology services, the date span and the number of fractions must be reported in IN 24A or 19.
- Enter the statement "Homebound" when an independent laboratory renders an EKG tracing or obtains a specimen from a homebound or institutionalized patient.
- Enter the statement, "Patient refuses to assign benefits" when the beneficiary absolutely refuses to assign benefits to a participating provider. In this case, no payment may be made on the claim.

1500

HEALTH INSURANCE CLAIM FORM

APPROVED BY NATIONAL UNIFORM CLAIM COMMITTEE 08/05

PICA | PICA

CARRIER

1. MEDICARE [X] (Medicare #) | MEDICAID (Medicaid #) | TRICARE CHAMPUS (Sponsor's SSN) | CHAMPVA (Member ID#) | GROUP HEALTH PLAN (SSN or ID) | FECA BLK LUNG (SSN) | OTHER (ID)

1a. INSURED'S I.D. NUMBER (For Program in Item 1): 456 22 1234A

2. PATIENT'S NAME (Last Name, First Name, Middle Initial): NAPJER JOHN D

3. PATIENT'S BIRTH DATE MM DD YY: 05 05 1938 SEX M [X] F

4. INSURED'S NAME (Last Name, First Name, Middle Initial)

5. PATIENT'S ADDRESS (No., Street): 47 CARRIAGE DR

6. PATIENT RELATIONSHIP TO INSURED: Self [X] Spouse Child Other

7. INSURED'S ADDRESS (No., Street)

CITY: CHESHIRE STATE: CO

8. PATIENT STATUS: Single Married [X] Other

CITY STATE

ZIP CODE: 80034 TELEPHONE (Include Area Code): (720) 123 5555

Employed Full-Time Student Part-Time Student

ZIP CODE TELEPHONE (INCLUDE AREA CODE) ( )

9. OTHER INSURED'S NAME (Last Name, First Name, Middle Initial)

10. IS PATIENT'S CONDITION RELATED TO:

11. INSURED'S POLICY GROUP OR FECA NUMBER

a. OTHER INSURED'S POLICY OR GROUP NUMBER

a. EMPLOYMENT? (CURRENT OR PREVIOUS) YES NO [X]

a. INSURED'S DATE OF BIRTH MM DD YY SEX M F

b. OTHER INSURED'S DATE OF BIRTH MM DD YY SEX M F

b. AUTO ACCIDENT? YES NO [X] PLACE (State)

b. EMPLOYER'S NAME OR SCHOOL NAME

c. EMPLOYER'S NAME OR SCHOOL NAME

c. OTHER ACCIDENT? YES NO [X]

c. INSURANCE PLAN NAME OR PROGRAM NAME

d. INSURANCE PLAN NAME OR PROGRAM NAME

10d. RESERVED FOR LOCAL USE

d. IS THERE ANOTHER HEALTH BENEFIT PLAN? YES NO *If yes*, return to and complete item 9 a-d.

READ BACK OF FORM BEFORE COMPLETING & SIGNING THIS FORM.

12. PATIENT'S OR AUTHORIZED PERSON'S SIGNATURE I authorize the release of any medical or other information necessary to process this claim. I also request payment of government benefits either to myself or to the party who accepts assignment below.

SIGNED SOF DATE

13. INSURED'S OR AUTHORIZED PERSON'S SIGNATURE I authorize payment of medical benefits to the undersigned physician or supplier for services described below.

SIGNED

PATIENT AND INSURED INFORMATION

14. DATE OF CURRENT: ILLNESS (First symptom) OR INJURY (Accident) OR PREGNANCY(LMP) MM DD YY: 10 01 2008

15. IF PATIENT HAS HAD SAME OR SIMILAR ILLNESS. GIVE FIRST DATE MM DD YY

16. DATES PATIENT UNABLE TO WORK IN CURRENT OCCUPATION FROM MM DD YY TO MM DD YY

17. NAME OF REFERRING PHYSICIAN OR OTHER SOURCE

17a.

17b. NPI

18. HOSPITALIZATION DATES RELATED TO CURRENT SERVICES FROM MM DD YY TO MM DD YY

19. RESERVED FOR LOCAL USE

20. OUTSIDE LAB? YES NO [X] $ CHARGES

21. DIAGNOSIS OR NATURE OF ILLNESS OR INJURY. (Relate Items 1,2,3 or 4 to Item 24e by Line)

1. 78 06

2. 78 56

3.

4.

22. MEDICAID RESUBMISSION CODE ORIGINAL REF. NO.

23. PRIOR AUTHORIZATION NUMBER

	24. A. DATE(S) OF SERVICE From MM DD YY	To MM DD YY	B. PLACE OF SERVICE	C. EMG	D. PROCEDURES, SERVICES, OR SUPPLIES (Explain Unusual Circumstances) CPT/HCPCS	MODIFIER	E. DIAGNOSIS POINTER	F. $ CHARGES	G. DAYS OR UNITS	H. EPSDT Family Plan	I. ID. QUAL.	J. RENDERING PROVIDER ID. #
1	10 02 2008		11		99203		1,2	95 00	1		NPI	8221238999
2											NPI	
3											NPI	
4											NPI	
5											NPI	
6											NPI	

25. FEDERAL TAX I.D. NUMBER: 123 45 9666 SSN [X] EIN

26. PATIENT'S ACCOUNT NO.: NAP0123

27. ACCEPT ASSIGNMENT? (For govt. claims, see back) YES [X] NO

28. TOTAL CHARGE $ 95 00

29. AMOUNT PAID $ 0 00

30. BALANCE DUE $ 95 00

31. SIGNATURE OF PHYSICIAN OR SUPPLIER INCLUDING DEGREES OR CREDENTIALS (I certify that the statements on the reverse apply to this bill and are made a part thereof.)

SIGNED SOF DATE

32. SERVICE FACILITY LOCATION INFORMATION: SAME

a. NPI b.

33. BILLING PROVIDER INFO & PHONE # (720) 554 1222

CENTER CLINIC

3810 EXECUTIVE BLVD

RAYTOWN CO 80033

a. 4455667788 b.

PHYSICIAN OR SUPPLIER INFORMATION

NUCC Instruction Manual available at: www.nucc.org

FIGURE 10.9 CMS-1500 (08/05) Completion for Medicare Primary Claims

Table 10.3 Medicare/Medigap CMS-1500 (08/05) Claim Completion

Item Number	*Content*
1	Indicate Medicare and check Group or Other for the patient's Medigap plan.
1a	Enter the Medicare health insurance claim number that appears on the patient's Medicare card.
2	Record the patient's name *exactly* as it appears on the Medicare card, entering it in last name, first name, middle initial order.
3	Enter the patient's date of birth in eight-digit format; select male or female.
4	Enter the name of the insured if not the patient.
5	Enter the patient's mailing address.
6	Select the appropriate box for the relationship.
7	If the insured's address is different, enter it.
8	Select the appropriate boxes for marital status and employment status.
9	INs 9–9D refer to Medigap policies. IN 9 is completed when a Medicare patient agrees to assign benefits of a Medigap policy to a Medicare participating provider. Enter SAME or the insured's name.
9a	"Medigap," "Mgap," or "MG" followed by the policy number.
9b	If other than patient, the Medigap policyholder's date of birth.
9c	Claims processing address for the Medigap insurer, which is usually found on the enrollee's Medigap identification card.
9d	Medigap insurance plan name or the Medigap insurer's identifier.
10a–10c	Choose the appropriate box to indicate whether the patient's condition is the result of a work injury, an automobile accident, or another type of accident.
10d	Varies with the insurance plan; complete if instructed.
11	IN 11 indicates whether the patient has any insurance primary to Medicare. If there is no plan primary to Medicare, enter NONE. If there is coverage primary to Medicare, the insured's policy identification number is entered, and INs 11a–11c must also be completed.
11d	Leave blank.
12	Enter "Signature on File," "SOF," or a legal signature, per practice policy.
13	Enter "Signature on File," "SOF," or a legal signature if authorizing payment of medical benefits to the provider for Medigap.
14	Enter the date that symptoms first began for the current illness, injury, or pregnancy.
15	Leave blank.
16	Enter the dates the patient is employed but unable to work in the current occupation. (From: the first full day of disability/To*:* the last day of disability before returning to work.)
17	Enter the name (first name, middle initial, last name) and credentials of the professional who referred or ordered the services or supplies on the claim.
17a	Enter the appropriate identifying number (either NPI or non-NPI/qualifier) for the referring physician.
18	If the services provided are needed because of a related inpatient hospitalization, the admission and discharge dates are entered. For patients still hospitalized, the admission date is listed in the From box, and the To box is left blank.
19	Complete according to the carrier's instructions.
20	Complete if billing for outside lab services.
21	Enter up to four ICD-9-CM codes in priority order. At least one code must be reported.
22	Leave blank; Medicaid-specific.
23	Enter the preauthorization number assigned by the payer or a CLIA number.
24A	Enter the date(s) of service, from and to.
24B	Enter the place of service (POS) code that describes the location at which the service was provided.
24C	Check with the payer to determine whether this element (emergency indicator) is necessary. If required, enter Y (yes) or N (no) in the unshaded bottom portion of the field.
24D	Enter the CPT/HCPCS codes and applicable modifiers for services provided. Do not use hyphens.
24E	Using the numbers (1, 2, 3, 4) listed to the left of the diagnosis codes in IN 21, enter the diagnosis for the each service listed in IN 24D.
24F	For each service listed in IN 24D, enter charges without dollar signs or decimals. If the claim reports an encounter with no charge, such as a capitated visit, a value of zero (0) may be used.
24G	Enter the number of days or units, as applicable. If only one service is performed, the numeral 1 must be entered.
24H	Leave blank; Medicaid-specific.

Table 10.3 Medicare/Medigap CMS-1500 (08/05) Claim Completion

Item Number	Content
24I–24J	Enter the NPI or non-NPI/qualifier.
25	Enter the physician's or supplier's federal tax identification number and check the appropriate box for SSN or EIN.
26	Enter the patient account number used by the practice's accounting system.
27	If the physician accepts assignment, select Yes. If the patient is also covered by a Medigap plan and the patient has authorized payment directly to the provider, the provider must also be a Medicare participating physician and must accept assignment.
28	Enter the total of all charges in IN 24F.
29	Amount of the payments received for the services listed on this claim. If no payment was made, enter "none" or "0.00."
30	Leave blank.
31	Enter the provider's or supplier's signature, the date of the signature, and the provider's credentials (such as MD).
32	Enter the name, address, city, state, and ZIP code of the location where the services were rendered if not the physician's office or the patient's home, or enter SAME. The supplier's NPI is entered in IN 32a. Enter the payer-assigned identifying non-NPI number and qualifier of the service facility in IN 32b.
33	Enter the billing provider's or supplier's name, address, ZIP code, telephone number, NPI, non-NPI number, and appropriate qualifier. The NPI should be placed in IN 33a. Enter the identifying non-NPI number and qualifier of the billing provider in IN 33b.

- Enter the statement, "Testing for hearing aid" when the beneficiary absolutely refuses to assign benefits to a participating provider. In this case, no payment may be made on the claim. When billing services involving the testing of a hearing aid(s), use a claim to obtain intentional denials when other payers may provide coverage.
- When dental examinations are billed, enter the specific surgery for which the exam is being performed.
- Enter the specific name and dosage amount when low osmolar contrast material is billed, but only if HCPCS codes do not cover them.
- Enter the date assumed and/or relinquished date for a global surgery claim when providers share postoperative care.
- Enter demonstration ID number "30" for all national emphysema treatment trial claims.
- Enter the NPI/PIN of the physician who is performing a purchased interpretation of a diagnostic test.

1500

HEALTH INSURANCE CLAIM FORM

APPROVED BY NATIONAL UNIFORM CLAIM COMMITTEE 08/05

PICA | PICA

CARRIER

1. MEDICARE [X] (Medicare #) MEDICAID (Medicaid #) TRICARE CHAMPUS (Sponsor's SSN) CHAMPVA (Member ID#) GROUP HEALTH PLAN (SSN or ID) FECA BLK LUNG (SSN) OTHER [X] (ID)

1a. INSURED'S I.D. NUMBER (For Program in Item 1): 581126612AA

2. PATIENT'S NAME (Last Name, First Name, Middle Initial): CARVELL JANICE G

3. PATIENT'S BIRTH DATE MM DD YY: 08 03 1933 SEX M [ ] F [X]

4. INSURED'S NAME (Last Name, First Name, Middle Initial)

5. PATIENT'S ADDRESS (No., Street): GATEWAY ROAD, UNIT 11 G

6. PATIENT RELATIONSHIP TO INSURED: Self [X] Spouse [ ] Child [ ] Other [ ]

7. INSURED'S ADDRESS (No., Street)

CITY: FREDERICK STATE: MD

8. PATIENT STATUS: Single [X] Married [ ] Other [ ]; Employed [ ] Full-Time Student [ ] Part-Time Student [ ]

CITY STATE

ZIP CODE: 21701 1004 TELEPHONE (Include Area Code): (555) 682 0311

ZIP CODE TELEPHONE (INCLUDE AREA CODE) ( )

9. OTHER INSURED'S NAME (Last Name, First Name, Middle Initial): SAME

10. IS PATIENT'S CONDITION RELATED TO:

11. INSURED'S POLICY GROUP OR FECA NUMBER: NONE

a. OTHER INSURED'S POLICY OR GROUP NUMBER: MEDIGAP G214120

a. EMPLOYMENT? (CURRENT OR PREVIOUS) [ ] YES [X] NO

a. INSURED'S DATE OF BIRTH MM DD YY SEX M [ ] F [ ]

b. OTHER INSURED'S DATE OF BIRTH MM DD YY SEX M [ ] F [ ]

b. AUTO ACCIDENT? [ ] YES [X] NO PLACE (State)

b. EMPLOYER'S NAME OR SCHOOL NAME

c. EMPLOYER'S NAME OR SCHOOL NAME: AARP/BALTIMORE MD

c. OTHER ACCIDENT? [ ] YES [X] NO

c. INSURANCE PLAN NAME OR PROGRAM NAME

d. INSURANCE PLAN NAME OR PROGRAM NAME: AARP LEVEL1 PLAN

10d. RESERVED FOR LOCAL USE

d. IS THERE ANOTHER HEALTH BENEFIT PLAN? [ ] YES [ ] NO *If yes*, return to and complete item 9 a-d.

READ BACK OF FORM BEFORE COMPLETING & SIGNING THIS FORM.

12. PATIENT'S OR AUTHORIZED PERSON'S SIGNATURE I authorize the release of any medical or other information necessary to process this claim. I also request payment of government benefits either to myself or to the party who accepts assignment below.

SIGNED SIGNATURE ON FILE DATE

13. INSURED'S OR AUTHORIZED PERSON'S SIGNATURE I authorize payment of medical benefits to the undersigned physician or supplier for services described below.

SIGNED SIGNATURE ON FILE

PATIENT AND INSURED INFORMATION

14. DATE OF CURRENT: ILLNESS (First symptom) OR INJURY (Accident) OR PREGNANCY(LMP) MM DD YY: 10 09 2008

15. IF PATIENT HAS HAD SAME OR SIMILAR ILLNESS. GIVE FIRST DATE MM DD YY

16. DATES PATIENT UNABLE TO WORK IN CURRENT OCCUPATION MM DD YY FROM TO

17. NAME OF REFERRING PHYSICIAN OR OTHER SOURCE

17a.

17b. NPI

18. HOSPITALIZATION DATES RELATED TO CURRENT SERVICES MM DD YY FROM TO

19. RESERVED FOR LOCAL USE

20. OUTSIDE LAB? [ ] YES [ ] NO $ CHARGES

21. DIAGNOSIS OR NATURE OF ILLNESS OR INJURY. (Relate Items 1,2,3 or 4 to Item 24e by Line)

1. 465 . 9

2. ___ . ___

3. ___ . ___

4. ___ . ___

22. MEDICAID RESUBMISSION CODE ORIGINAL REF. NO.

23. PRIOR AUTHORIZATION NUMBER

	24. A. DATE(S) OF SERVICE From MM DD YY	To MM DD YY	B. PLACE OF SERVICE	C. EMG	D. PROCEDURES, SERVICES, OR SUPPLIES (Explain Unusual Circumstances) CPT/HCPCS	MODIFIER	E. DIAGNOSIS POINTER	F. $ CHARGES	G. DAYS OR UNITS	H. EPSDT Family Plan	I. ID. QUAL.	J. RENDERING PROVIDER ID.#
1	10 11 2008	10 11 2008	11		99202		1	89 00	1		NPI	
2	10 11 2008	10 11 2008	11		93000		1	29 00	1		NPI	
3											NPI	
4											NPI	
5											NPI	
6											NPI	

25. FEDERAL TAX I.D. NUMBER: 758126007 SSN [ ] EIN [X]

26. PATIENT'S ACCOUNT NO.: C15889X4

27. ACCEPT ASSIGNMENT? (For govt. claims, see back) [X] YES [ ] NO

28. TOTAL CHARGE $

29. AMOUNT PAID $

30. BALANCE DUE $

31. SIGNATURE OF PHYSICIAN OR SUPPLIER INCLUDING DEGREES OR CREDENTIALS (I certify that the statements on the reverse apply to this bill and are made a part thereof.)

SIGNATURE ON FILE

SIGNED DATE

32. SERVICE FACILITY LOCATION INFORMATION

SAME

a. NPI b.

33. BILLING PROVIDER INFO & PHONE # (301) 662 5555

MARTHA R BENG MD
43 CENTRAL AVE
FREDERICK MD 21701 1214

a. NPI 6677541234 b.

PHYSICIAN OR SUPPLIER INFORMATION

NUCC Instruction Manual available at: www.nucc.org

FIGURE 10.10 CMS-1500 (08/05) Completion for Medicare/Medigap Claims

Review

Steps to Success

- ❒ Read this chapter and review the Key Terms and the Chapter Summary.
- ❒ Answer the Review Questions and Applying Your Knowledge in the Chapter Review.
- ❒ Access the chapter's websites and complete the Internet Activities to learn more about available professional resources.
- ❒ Complete the related chapter in the *Medical Insurance Workbook* to reinforce your understanding of Medicare coverage and billing procedures.

Chapter Summary

1. Individuals eligible for Medicare are in one of six categories: (a) age sixty-five or older; (b) disabled adults; (c) disabled before age eighteen; (d) spouses of deceased, disabled, or retired employees; (e) retired federal employees enrolled in the Civil Service Retirement System (CSRS); or (f) individuals of any age diagnosed with end-stage renal disease (ESRD).
2. Medicare Part A provides coverage for care in hospitals and skilled nursing facilities, for home health care, and for hospice care. Part B provides outpatient medical coverage. Part C offers managed care plans called Medicare Advantage as an option to the traditional fee-for-service coverage under the Original Medicare Plan. Part D is a prescription drug benefit.
3. Medicare Part B covers physician services, diagnostic X-rays and laboratory tests, some preventive care examinations and tests, outpatient hospital visits, durable medical equipment, and other nonhospital services. It does not cover most routine and custodial care, examinations for eyeglasses or hearing aids, some foot care procedures, services not ordered by a physician, cosmetic surgery, health care received while traveling outside the United States, and procedures deemed not reasonable and medically necessary.
4. Participating providers agree to accept assignment for all Medicare claims and to accept Medicare's fee as payment in full for services. They are responsible for informing patients when services will not, or are not likely to be, paid by the program. They must also comply with numerous billing rules such as global periods.
5. Nonparticipating providers choose whether to accept assignment on a claim-by-claim basis. NonPAR providers are allowed 5 percent less than PAR providers on assigned claims; on unassigned claims, nonPAR providers are subject to Medicare's limiting charges.
6. The Original Medicare Plan is a fee-for-service plan that provides maximum freedom of choice when selecting a provider or specialist.
7. Medicare Advantage plans offer additional services but restrict beneficiaries to a network of providers, a preferred provider organization (PPO) plan, private fee-for-service, or Medical Savings Account.
8. Medigap insurance pays for services that are not covered by Medicare. Coverage varies with specific Medigap plans, but all provide coverage for patient deductibles and coinsurance. Some also cover excluded services such as prescription drugs and limited preventive care.
9. The Medicare Medical Review (MR) Program is implemented by contractors to ensure correct billing. Under this program, a carrier may audit claims by sampling codes to see if they match national averages, and may request documentation (medical records) to check on certain claims.

Review Questions

Match the key terms with their definitions.

A. advance beneficiary notice (ABN)

B. carrier

C. Medicare Advantage

D. Medigap

E. limiting charge

F. fiscal intermediary

G. Notice of Exclusions from Medicare Benefits (NEMB)

H. quality improvement organization (QIO)

I. urgently needed care

J. Medicare Summary Notice (MSN)

____ 1. An organization that has a contract with Medicare to process insurance claims from physicians, providers, and suppliers

____ 2. A group of insurance plans offered under Medicare Part B that are intended to provide beneficiaries with a wider selection of plans

____ 3. Nonparticipating physicians cannot charge more than 115 percent of the Medicare Fee Schedule on unassigned claims

____ 4. A form given to patients when the practice thinks that a service to be provided will not be considered medically necessary or reasonable by Medicare

____ 5. Emergency treatment needed by a managed care patient while traveling outside the plan's network area

____ 6. A form that advises beneficiaries, before services that are not Medicare benefits are furnished, that Medicare will not pay for them and that provides an estimate of how much the beneficiaries may have to pay

____ 7. A document furnished to Medicare beneficiaries by the Medicare program that lists the services they received and the payments the program made for them

____ 8. A Medicare Part B contractor

____ 9. A type of federally regulated insurance plan that provides coverage in addition to Medicare Part B

____ 10. A group of physicians paid by the government to review aspects of the Medicare program, including the quality and appropriateness of services provided and fees charged

Decide whether each statement is true or false.

____ 1. Fiscal intermediaries are the claims processors for Medicare Part B.

____ 2. Screening mammograms are excluded services for Medicare Part B.

____ 3. A procedure is classified as not medically necessary if it is an elective procedure.

____ 4. Physicians who agree to participate can choose to accept assignment on a claim-by-claim basis.

____ 5. Participating and nonparticipating providers may bill patients at their standard rates for services excluded from Medicare coverage.

____ 6. Medicare Advantage plans usually offer coverage for some services that are not covered by the Original Medicare Plan.

____ 7. All Medigap policies provide coverage for Part B coinsurance.

____ 8. Medicare is the secondary payer for all beneficiaries over age sixty-five and working.

____ 9. Local coverage determinations (LCDs) are notices sent to physicians about the coding and medical necessity of specific services.

____ 10. An ABN should be signed by the patient when the provider has reason to think that services will not be covered by Medicare due to lack of medical necessity.

Select the letter that best completes the statement or answers the question.

____ 1. Medicare Part A covers
- A. physician services
- B. prescription drugs
- C. hospital services
- D. carriers

____ 2. The Original Medicare Plan requires a premium, a deductible, and
- A. Medigap
- B. supplemental insurance
- C. coinsurance
- D. HIPAA TCS

____ 3. Which ABN modifier indicates that a service that was done is not covered when no ABN was signed?
- A. AB
- B. GA
- C. GY
- D. GZ

____ 4. Which modifier indicates that a signed ABN is on file?
- A. AB
- B. GA
- C. GZ
- D. GY

____ 5. Under Medicare's global surgical package regulations, a physician may bill a patient separately for
- A. supplies used during the surgical procedure
- B. procedures performed after the surgery to minimize pain
- C. diagnostic tests required to determine the need for surgery
- D. the removal of tubes, sutures, or catheters

____ 6. HIPAA regulations require the Medicare program to comply with
- A. the Privacy Rule
- B. the Security Rule
- C. the Transactions and Code Sets standards
- D. all of the above

____ 7. Under Medicare Advantage, a PPO __________________ an HMO.
- A. is more restrictive than
- B. is less restrictive than
- C. has the same network as
- D. has the same deductible as

____ 8. Under the Medicare Part B traditional fee-for-service plan, Medicare pays ______ percent of the allowed charges.
- A. 75
- B. 80
- C. 90
- D. 100

____ 9. Medicare Part D covers
- A. prescription drugs
- B. mammography
- C. screening for cancer
- D. none of the above

____10. Medicare medical review is conducted by
A. the physician
B. the Medicare carrier
C. the primary payer
D. the Medigap payer

Answer the following questions

1. What is the difference between excluded services and services that are not reasonable and necessary?

___

___

2. If a patient who lives in Texarkana, Arkansas, sees a physician for Medicare Part B services in Newark, New Jersey, to which location's carrier should the claim be sent?

___

Applying Your Knowledge

The objective of these exercises is to correctly complete Medicare claims, applying what you have learned in the chapter. Following the information about the provider for the cases are two sections. The first section contains information about the patient, the insurance coverage, and the current medical condition. The second section is an encounter form for Valley Associates, P.C.

If you are using Medisoft to complete the cases, read the *Guide to Medisoft* before beginning. Information from the first section, the patient information form, has already been entered in the program for you. You must enter information from the second section, the encounter form, to complete the claim. If you are gaining experience by completing a paper CMS-1500 claim form, use the blank claim form supplied to you (from the back of the book or printed from the Student Data Template CD ROM) and follow the instructions on pages 357–358.

The following provider information, which is also preloaded in the Medisoft database, should be used for Cases 10.1, 10.2, and 10.3.

Provider Information

Name	Christopher M. Connolly, M.D.
Practice Name	Valley Associates, P.C.
Address	1400 West Center Street Toledo, OH 43601-0213
Phone	555-967-0303
Employer ID Number	16-1234567
NPI	8877365552
Assignment	Accepts
Signature	On File 01/01/08

Case 10.1

From the Patient Information Form

Name	Donald Martone	*Health Plan*	Medicare Nationwide
Sex	M	*Health Insurance No.*	312460239A
Birth Date	06/24/1934	*Signature*	On File *01/01/2008*
Marital Status	S	*Condition Related to:*	
Employer	Retired	*Employment*	No
		Auto Accident	*No*
		Other Accident	*No*
SSN	312-46-0239	*Accept Assignment*	Yes
Telephone	555-333-0412		

VALLEY ASSOCIATES, PC
Christopher M. Connolly, MD - Internal Medicine
555-967-0303
FED I.D. #16-1234567

PATIENT NAME	APPT. DATE/TIME
Martone, Donald	10/6/2008 9:30 am
PATIENT NO.	**DX**
MARTODO0	1. 465.9 upper respiratory infection 2. 786.2 cough 3. 780.6 fever 4.

DESCRIPTION	✓	CPT	FEE	DESCRIPTION	✓	CPT	FEE
OFFICE VISITS				**PROCEDURES**			
New Patient				Diagnostic Anoscopy		46600	
LI Problem Focused		99201		ECG Complete		93000	
LII Expanded		99202		I&D, Abscess		10060	
LIII Detailed		99203		Pap Smear		88150	
LIV Comp./Mod.		99204		Removal of Cerumen		69210	
LV Comp./High		99205		Removal 1 Lesion		17000	
Established Patient				Removal 2-14 Lesions		17003	
LI Minimum		99211		Removal 15+ Lesions		17004	
LII Problem Focused	✓	99212	28	Rhythm ECG w/Report		93040	
LIII Expanded		99213		Rhythm ECG w/Tracing		93041	
LIV Detailed		99214		Sigmoidoscopy, diag.		45330	
LV Comp./High		99215					
				LABORATORY			
PREVENTIVE VISIT				Bacteria Culture		87081	
New Patient				Fungal Culture		87101	
Age 12-17		99384		Glucose Finger Stick		82948	
Age 18-39		99385		Lipid Panel		80061	
Age 40-64		99386		Specimen Handling		99000	
Age 65+		99387		Stool/Occult Blood		82270	
Established Patient				Tine Test		85008	
Age 12-17		99394		Tuberculin PPD		85590	
Age 18-39		99395		Urinalysis		81000	
Age 40-64		99396		Venipuncture		36415	
Age 65+		99397					
				INJECTION/IMMUN.			
CONSULTATION: OFFICE/OP				Immun. Admin.		90471	
Requested By:				Ea. Addl.		90472	
LI Problem Focused		99241		Hepatitis A Immun		90632	
LII Expanded		99242		Hepatitis B Immun		90746	
LIII Detailed		99243		Influenza Immun		90659	
LIV Comp./Mod.		99244		Pneumovax		90732	
LV Comp./High		99245					
				TOTAL FEES			

Case 10.2

From the Patient Information Form

Name	Carmen Perez
Sex	M
Birth Date	05/15/1929
Marital Status	M
Employer	Retired
Address	225 Potomac Dr Shaker Heights, OH 44118-2345
Telephone	555-692-3314
SSN	140-24-6113
Signature	On File (1-1-2008)

Condition unrelated to Employment, Auto Accident, or Other Accident

Accept Assignment	Yes

Primary Insurance Information

Insured	Monica Perez
Pt Relationship to Insured	Spouse
Insured's Date of Birth	03/14/1931
Insured's Employer	Kinko's
SSN	140-60-3312
Insurance Plan	Cigna HMOPlus
Insurance ID No.	140603312X

Secondary Insurance Information

Health Plan	Medicare Nationwide
Health Insurance No.	140246113A

VALLEY ASSOCIATES, PC

Christopher M. Connolly, MD - Internal Medicine
555-967-0303
FED I.D. #16-1234567

PATIENT NAME	APPT. DATE/TIME
Perez, Carmen	10/8/2008 2:00 pm
PATIENT NO.	**DX**
PEREZCA0	1. 493.00 extrinsic asthma 2. 3. 4.

DESCRIPTION	✓	CPT	FEE	DESCRIPTION	✓	CPT	FEE
OFFICE VISITS				**PROCEDURES**			
New Patient				Diagnostic Anoscopy		46600	
LI Problem Focused		99201		ECG Complete		93000	
LII Expanded		99202		I&D, Abscess		10060	
LIII Detailed		99203		Pap Smear		88150	
LIV Comp./Mod.		99204		Removal of Cerumen		69210	
LV Comp./High		99205		Removal 1 Lesion		17000	
Established Patient				Removal 2-14 Lesions		17003	
LI Minimum	✓	99211	30	Removal 15+ Lesions		17004	
LII Problem Focused		99212		Rhythm ECG w/Report		93040	
LIII Expanded		99213		Rhythm ECG w/Tracing		93041	
LIV Detailed		99214		Sigmoidoscopy, diag.		45330	
LV Comp./High		99215					
				LABORATORY			
PREVENTIVE VISIT				Bacteria Culture		87081	
New Patient				Fungal Culture		87101	
Age 12-17		99384		Glucose Finger Stick		82948	
Age 18-39		99385		Lipid Panel		80061	
Age 40-64		99386		Specimen Handling		99000	
Age 65+		99387		Stool/Occult Blood		82270	
Established Patient				Tine Test		85008	
Age 12-17		99394		Tuberculin PPD		85590	
Age 18-39		99395		Urinalysis		81000	
Age 40-64		99396		Venipuncture		36415	
Age 65+		99397					
				INJECTION/IMMUN.			
CONSULTATION: OFFICE/OP				Immun. Admin.		90471	
Requested By:				Ea. Add'l.		90472	
LI Problem Focused		99241		Hepatitis A Immun		90632	
LII Expanded		99242		Hepatitis B Immun		90746	
LIII Detailed		99243		Influenza Immun		90659	
LIV Comp./Mod.		99244		Pneumovax		90732	
LV Comp./High		99245					
				TOTAL FEES			

Case 10.3

From the Patient Information Form

Name	Hector Munoz
Sex	M
Birth Date	10/19/1926
Marital Status	M
Employer	Retired
Telephone	555-326-1742
SSN	301-46-2901
Health Plan	Medicare Nationwide
Health Insurance No.	301462901A
Signature	On File 01/01/08

Secondary Insurance Information

Insured	Same
Pt Relationship to Insured	
Insured's Date of Birth	
Insured's Employer	
SSN	
Insurance Plan	AARP Medigap
Insurance ID No.	301462901B
Insurance Group No.	
Condition Related to:	
Employment	No
Auto Accident	No
Other Accident	No
Accept Assignment	Yes

VALLEY ASSOCIATES, PC
Christopher M. Connolly, MD - Internal Medicine
555-967-0303
FED I.D. #16-1234567

PATIENT NAME	APPT. DATE/TIME
Munoz, Hector	10/10/2008 9:30 am
PATIENT NO.	**DX**
MUNOZHE0	1. 682.0 abscess on chin 2. 3. 4.

DESCRIPTION	✓	CPT	FEE	DESCRIPTION	✓	CPT	FEE
OFFICE VISITS				**PROCEDURES**			
New Patient				Diagnostic Anoscopy		46600	
LI Problem Focused		99201		ECG Complete		93000	
LII Expanded	✓	99202	50	I&D, Abscess	✓	10060	57
LIII Detailed		99203		Pap Smear		88150	
LIV Comp./Mod.		99204		Removal of Cerumen		69210	
LV Comp./High		99205		Removal 1 Lesion		17000	
Established Patient				Removal 2-14 Lesions		17003	
LI Minimum		99211		Removal 15+ Lesions		17004	
LII Problem Focused		99212		Rhythm ECG w/Report		93040	
LIII Expanded		99213		Rhythm ECG w/Tracing		93041	
LIV Detailed		99214		Sigmoidoscopy, diag.		45330	
LV Comp./High		99215					
				LABORATORY			
PREVENTIVE VISIT				Bacteria Culture		87081	
New Patient				Fungal Culture		87101	
Age 12-17		99384		Glucose Finger Stick		82948	
Age 18-39		99385		Lipid Panel		80061	
Age 40-64		99386		Specimen Handling		99000	
Age 65+		99387		Stool/Occult Blood		82270	
Established Patient				Tine Test		85008	
Age 12-17		99394		Tuberculin PPD		85590	
Age 18-39		99395		Urinalysis		81000	
Age 40-64		99396		Venipuncture		36415	
Age 65+		99397					
				INJECTION/IMMUN.			
CONSULTATION: OFFICE/OP				Immun. Admin.		90471	
Requested By:				Ea. Add'l.		90472	
LI Problem Focused		99241		Hepatitis A Immun		90632	
LII Expanded		99242		Hepatitis B Immun		90746	
LIII Detailed		99243		Influenza Immun		90659	
LIV Comp./Mod.		99244		Pneumovax		90732	
LV Comp./High		99245					
				TOTAL FEES			

Internet Activities

1. Visit the official U.S. government website for Medicare beneficiaries at http://www.medicare.gov. Use the Medicare Personal Plan Finder to help you decide on the right Medicare health plan for a senior family member or friend. Compare benefits, costs, options, and provider quality information.
2. Go to the Centers for Medicare and Medicaid Services (CMS) website at http://www.cms.hhs.gov. Select the link for the Quarterly Provider Update, which contains quarterly updates on all changes to Medicare's regulations and instructions that affect providers. Click the link for the latest issue's table of contents, and then select the link for Physicians in the list of specific Medicare providers. Read about one Medicare regulation that physicians should know about that is currently undergoing change.
3. Go to the CMS website for Medicare physicians at http://www.cms.hhs.gov/physicians/. Look up information on a topic under billing and payment.
4. CMS has a series of online educational articles called *MLN Matters* that inform physicians about the latest changes to the Medicare program. Visit http://www.cms.hhs.gov/MLNMattersArticles/. Report on an article posted to this website in the last year.

Chapter 11

Medicaid

CHAPTER OUTLINE

The Medicaid Program

Federal Eligibility

State Programs

Medicaid Enrollment Verification

Covered and Excluded Services

Types of Plans

Payment for Services

Third-Party Liability

Claim Filing Guidelines

Medicaid Claim Completion

Learning Outcomes

After studying this chapter, you should be able to:

1. Describe the federal Medicaid eligibility requirements.
2. Discuss the effects of the Welfare Reform Act on Medicaid eligibility.
3. Explain the difference between categorically needy and medically needy.
4. Describe the income and asset guidelines used by most states to determine eligibility.
5. List the services that Medicaid usually does not cover.
6. List the types of plans that states offer to Medicaid recipients.
7. Discuss the claim filing procedures when a Medicaid recipient has other insurance coverage.
8. Prepare correct Medicaid claims.

Key Terms

categorically needy
crossover claim
dual-eligible
Early and Periodic Screening, Diagnosis, and Treatment (EPSDT)
Federal Medicaid Assistance Percentage (FMAP)
MediCal
medically needy
Medi-Medi beneficiary
payer of last resort
restricted status
spend-down
State Children's Health Insurance Program (SCHIP)
Temporary Assistance for Needy Families (TANF)
Welfare Reform Act

The Medicaid program covers more than 50 million low-income people, pays for more than one-third of births, and finances care for two-thirds of nursing home residents. The cost of the program, financed jointly by the federal government and the states, exceeds $300 billion a year.

Medicaid is the nation's largest non-employer-sponsored health insurance program. Because Medicaid is run by states, rather than by the federal government, medical insurance specialists refer to the laws and regulations of their state Medicaid programs to correctly process claims for these patients.

The Medicaid Program

The Medicaid program was established under Title XIX of the Social Security Act of 1965 to pay for the health care needs of individuals and families with low incomes and few resources. The federal government makes payments to states under the **Federal Medicaid Assistance Percentage (FMAP)**. The amount is based on the state's average per capita income in relation to the national income average.

People applying for Medicaid benefits must meet minimum federal requirements and any additional requirements of the state in which they live. A person eligible in one state may be denied coverage in another state. Coverage also varies, with some states providing coverage for fewer than 40 percent of residents below the poverty level and other states covering as much as 60 percent of the same population. Because of this variation and because Medicaid rules change frequently, this chapter presents a general overview of the program.

To apply for Medicaid benefits, individuals must call or write their local Income Maintenance office or Department of Social Services and request an application. Once completed, the application is returned to the office, along with proof of income, assets, and any other relevant proof of eligibility. Medicaid coverage may begin as early as the third month prior to application—if the person would have been eligible for Medicaid had he or she applied during that time. Medicaid coverage generally stops at the end of the month in which a person no longer meets the eligibility criteria. (States may provide twelve months of continuous Medicaid coverage for eligible children under the age of nineteen.) Denied coverage may be appealed through a Fair Hearing. Beneficiaries must notify the agency immediately if their income, assets, or living situations change.

Federal Eligibility

Federal guidelines mandate coverage for individuals referred to as **categorically needy**—people with low incomes and few resources, including certain Medicare beneficiaries with low incomes. The categorically needy typically include families with dependent children who receive some form of cash assistance, individuals eligible to receive Supplemental Security Income (SSI), pregnant women with low incomes, and infants and children who meet low-income requirements.

The federal government requires states to offer benefits to the following groups:

- People with low incomes and few resources who receive financial assistance under **Temporary Assistance for Needy Families (TANF)**
- People who are eligible for TANF but who do not receive financial assistance
- People who receive foster care or adoption assistance under Title IV-E of the Social Security Act
- Children under six years of age who meet TANF requirements or whose family income is below 133 percent of the poverty level
- People in some groups who lose cash assistance when their work income or Social Security benefits exceed allowable limits (temporary Medicaid eligibility)
- Pregnant women whose family income is below 133 percent of the poverty level (coverage limited to pregnancy-related medical care)
- Infants born to Medicaid-eligible pregnant women
- People who are age sixty-five and over, legally blind, or totally disabled and who receive Supplemental Security Income (SSI)
- Certain low-income Medicare recipients

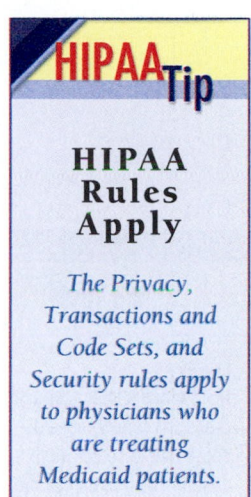

HIPAA Tip
HIPAA Rules Apply
The Privacy, Transactions and Code Sets, and Security rules apply to physicians who are treating Medicaid patients.

State Children's Health Insurance Program

From time to time, the federal government enacts legislation that affects the Medicaid program. The **State Children's Health Insurance Program (SCHIP)**, part of the Balanced Budget Act of 1997, offers states the opportunity to develop and implement plans for health insurance coverage for uninsured children. Children served by SCHIP come from low-income families whose incomes are not low enough to qualify for Medicaid. The program covers children up to age nineteen.

The SCHIP program is funded jointly by the federal government and the states. It provides coverage for many preventive services, physician services, and inpatient and outpatient services. A state may meet SCHIP requirements by expanding its current Medicaid program to include uninsured children, by establishing a new program, or by some combination of the two methods. Once a state's plan is approved, the federal government provides matching funds. In recent years, through state waivers, states have been given greater flexibility to expand their insurance coverage to the uninsured. This has resulted in increased enrollment in Medicaid and SCHIP. In 2003, 5 million children were estimated to be covered under SCHIP. Unlike in previous years, legislation introduced in 2003 allowed states to start carrying over a certain amount of unspent SCHIP money from previous years, making more money available to the expanding program.

Early and Periodic Screening, Diagnosis, and Treatment

Early and Periodic Screening, Diagnosis, and Treatment (EPSDT) provides health care benefits to children under age twenty-one who are enrolled in Medicaid. States are required by federal law to inform all Medicaid-eligible people who are under age twenty-one of the availability of EPSDT and immunizations. Patients are not charged fees for EPSDT services, but some families do pay monthly premiums.

The EPSDT program emphasizes preventive care. Medical, vision, hearing, and dental health screenings (known as well-child checkups) are performed at regular intervals. These examinations must include at least the following nine components:

1. A comprehensive health and developmental history, including assessment of both physical and mental health
2. A comprehensive, unclothed physical examination
3. Appropriate immunizations
4. Laboratory tests (including lead blood testing at twelve and twenty-four months and otherwise, according to age and risk factors)
5. Health education, including anticipatory guidance
6. Vision services
7. Dental services
8. Hearing services
9. Other necessary health care (diagnosis services, treatment, and other measures necessary to correct or ameliorate problems discovered by the screening services)

Billing Tip

EPSDT
Most practice management programs (PMPs) have a check box to select when a patient's visit is part of the Medicaid EPSDT program.

EPSDT also covers health care services other than periodic screenings. All mandatory and optional services covered under Medicaid—even if such services are not covered for adults—are covered by the EPSDT program. A child may be referred for an additional screening by a parent, a guardian, a teacher, or another party.

The Ticket to Work and Work Incentives Improvement Act

The Ticket to Work and Work Incentive's Improvement Act of 1999 (TWWIIA) expands the availability of health care services for workers with disabilities. Previously, people with disabilities often had to choose between health care and work. TWWIIA gives states the option of allowing individuals with disabilities to purchase Medicaid coverage that is necessary to enable them to maintain employment.

New Freedom Initiative

The New Freedom Initiative was launched in 2001 as the president's comprehensive plan to reduce barriers to full community integration for people with disabilities and long-term illnesses. Under the initiative, various departments throughout the government, including the Department of Health and Human Services, were directed to partner with states to provide necessary supports to allow elders and people with disabilities to fully participate in community life. For example, through the use of Medicaid grants for community living, the initiative aims at promoting the use of at-home and community-based care as an alternative to nursing homes. Medicaid grants for aging and disability resource centers are another part of the initiative.

Spousal Impoverishment Protection

Federal Spousal Impoverishment legislation limits the amount of a married couples' income and assets that must be used before one of them can become eligible for Medicaid coverage in a long-term care facility. Before this legislation, a couples' income and assets were so depleted by the time one partner qualified for Medicaid that the other spouse was left with few resources.

The legislation applies to situations in which one member of the couple is in a nursing facility or medical institution and is expected to remain there for at least thirty days. When the couple applies for Medicaid coverage, their joint resources are evaluated. All resources held by both spouses are considered to be available to the spouse in the medical facility except for certain assets, such as a home, household goods, an automobile, and burial funds.

Welfare Reform Act

Traditionally, people eligible for cash assistance through another government program, such as the Aid to Families with Dependent Children (AFDC) and Supplemental Security Income (SSI), were considered eligible for Medicaid benefits. The Personal Responsibility and Work Opportunity Reconciliation Act of 1996 (P.L. 104-193), commonly known as the **Welfare Reform Act**, replaced the AFDC program with TANF. Under this more stringent legislation, some individuals receiving TANF payments are limited to a five-year benefit period. At the end of five years, cash assistance ceases.

Eligibility for TANF assistance is determined at the county level. Answers to the following questions are taken into account:

- Is the income below set limits?
- Are the resources (including property) equal to or less than set limits?
- Does the household include at least one child under eighteen?
- Is at least one parent unemployed, incapacitated, or absent from the home?
- Does the individual have a Social Security number and a birth certificate?
- Does the individual receive adoptive or foster care assistance?

Many states have employability assessment or job search requirements for applicants or require child immunization or school attendance, making eligibility standards more stringent. The Welfare Reform Act also affected eligibility rules for several other groups, including disabled children and immigrants. While the Welfare Reform Act made it more difficult for some groups to gain access to Medicaid benefits, individual states still have a great deal of latitude when implementing the program.

State Programs

Although the federal government sets broad standards for Medicaid coverage, there is variation among the states. States establish their own eligibility standards; their own type, amount, duration, and scope of services; and their own payments to providers. Table 11.1 on page 379 provides a list of state websites to research the state's standards.

A state's income limits usually consider the applicant's income relative to the federal poverty level (FPL), taking household size into account.

Most states also provide Medicaid coverage to **medically needy** individuals—people with high medical expenses and low financial resources (but not low enough to receive cash assistance). States may choose their own names for these programs. For example, California's program is called **MediCal**.

Examples of groups covered by state rules but not federal guidelines are:

- Aged, blind, or disabled people with incomes below the federal poverty level who do not qualify under federal mandatory coverage rules
- People who are institutionalized who do not qualify under federal rules, but who meet special state income requirements
- People who would be eligible if institutionalized, but who are receiving home or community care
- Children under age twenty-one who meet the TANF income and resources limits
- Infants up to one year old who do not qualify under federal rules, but who meet state income limit rules
- Pregnant women who do not qualify under federal rules, but who meet state income limit rules
- Optional targeted low-income children
- Recipients of state supplementary payments
- TB-infected people who would be financially eligible for Medicaid at the SSI level (only for TB-related ambulatory services and TB drugs)
- Uninsured low-income women identified through the Centers for Disease Control and Prevention (CDC) National Breast and Cervical Cancer Early Detection Program (NBCCEDP) as needing breast or cervical cancer treatment

Income and Asset Guidelines

In most states, general income and asset guidelines are as follows:

- People who receive income from employment may qualify for Medicaid depending on their income, since a portion of their earned income is not counted toward the Medicaid income limit (income required for necessary expenditures).
- Only a portion of unearned income from Social Security benefits, Supplemental Security Income (SSI), and veterans' benefits and pensions is counted toward income limits.
- Assets are taken into account when determining eligibility. Assets include cash, bank accounts, certificates of deposit, stocks and bonds, cash surrender value of life insurance policies, and property other than homes. The applicant's residence is not counted in arriving at the total asset calculation. Assets may be owned solely by the applicant or jointly by the applicant and another party.
- Some other possessions are not counted as assets, including essential personal property such as clothing, furniture, and personal effects, and a burial plot and money put aside for burial.
- Applicants who enter a long-term care facility have their homes counted as an asset unless they are in for a short-term stay and are expected to return home shortly, or if certain relatives will continue to live in the home. These relatives include a spouse, a disabled or blind child, a child who is less than twenty-one years of age, or a child or sibling under certain other circumstances.
- Assets that have been transferred into another person's name are closely examined. The asset may be included in the applicant's asset total depending on when the asset was transferred, to whom it was transferred, the amount paid in return for the asset, and the state in which the applicant resides.
- Information provided on the application is checked and verified using other sources of information, including the Social Security Administration, the Internal Revenue Service, the state Motor Vehicle Agency, and the state Department of Labor, among others.

Table 11.1 Medicaid State Websites

ALABAMA	AL	http://www.medicaid.state.al.us/
ALASKA	AK	http://www.hss.state.ak.us/dhcs/Medicaid/
ARIZONA	AZ	http://www.ahcccs.state.az.us/site/
ARKANSAS	AR	http://www.medicaid.state.ar.us/
CALIFORNIA	CA	http://www.dhs.ca.gov/mcs/
COLORADO	CO	http://www.chcpf.state.co.us/default.asp
CONNECTICUT	CT	http://www.ct.gov/dss/
DELAWARE	DE	http://www.dhss.delaware.gov/
DISTRICT OF COLUMBIA	DC	http://doh.dc.gov/doh/site/default.asp
FLORIDA	FL	http://www.fdhc.state.fl.us/Medicaid/
GEORGIA	GA	http://dch.georgia.gov
HAWAII	HI	http://med-quest.us/
IDAHO	ID	http://www.healthandwelfare.idaho.gov/
ILLINOIS	IL	http://www.hfs.illinois.gov/medical/
INDIANA	IN	http://www.state.in.us/
IOWA	IA	http://www.dhs.state.ia.us/
KANSAS	KS	http://da.state.ks.us/hpf/
KENTUCKY	KY	http://chfs.ky.gov
LOUISIANA	LA	http://www.dhh.state.la.us/
MAINE	ME	http://www.maine.gov/
MARYLAND	MD	http://www.dhmh.state.md.us/
MASSACHUSETTS	MA	http://www.mass.gov/
MICHIGAN	MI	http://www.Michigan.gov/mdch
MINNESOTA	MN	http://www.dhs.state.mn.us/
MISSISSIPPI	MS	http://www.medicaid.state.ms.us/
MISSOURI	MO	http://www.dss.mo.gov/
MONTANA	MT	http://www.dphhs.mt.gov
NEBRASKA	NE	http://hhs.state.ne.us/
NEVADA	NV	http://dhcfp.state.nv.us/
NEW HAMPSHIRE	NH	http://www.dhhs.state.nh.us/
NEW JERSEY	NJ	http://www.state.nj.us/
NEW MEXICO	NM	http://www.state.nm.us/
NEW YORK	NY	http://www.health.state.ny.us/
NORTH CAROLINA	NC	http://www.dhhs.state.nc.us/
NORTH DAKOTA	ND	http://www.nd.gov/humanservices/
OHIO	OH	http://jfs.ohio.gov/ohp/
OKLAHOMA	OK	http://www.ohca.state.ok.us/
OREGON	OR	http://www.oregon.gov/DHS/
PENNSYLVANIA	PA	http://www.dpw.state.pa.us/
RHODE ISLAND	RI	http://www.dhs.state.ri.us/
SOUTH CAROLINA	SC	http://www.dhhs.state.sc.us/
SOUTH DAKOTA	SD	http://www.state.sd.us/
TENNESSEE	TN	http://www.state.tn.us/tenncare/
TEXAS	TX	http://www.hhsc.state.tx.us/Medicaid/
UTAH	UT	http://health.utah.gov/medicaid/
VERMONT	VT	http://www.ovha.state.vt.us/medicaid.cfm
VIRGINIA	VA	http://www.dmas.virginia.gov/
WASHINGTON	WA	http://fortress.wa.gov/dshs/maa/
WEST VIRGINIA	WV	http://www.wvdhhr.org/bms/
WISCONSIN	WI	http://www.dhfs.state.wi.us/medicaid/
WYOMING	WY	http://wyequalitycare.acs-inc.com/

Thinking it Through — 11.1

Unlike Medicare, Medicaid eligibility coverage varies from state to state. An individual ruled ineligible in one state may qualify for coverage in another state.

1. Why do Medicaid eligibility rules and coverage vary while Medicare's do not?
2. What are the advantages and disadvantages of the current state-oriented system?

Spend-Down Programs

Some states have what are known as **spend-down** programs. In a spend-down program, individuals are required to spend a portion of their income or resources on health care until they reach or drop below the income level specified by the state. The concept is similar to an annual deductible, except that it resets at the beginning of every month. Each month, the enrollee pays a portion of incurred medical bills, up to a certain amount, before the Medicaid fee schedule takes effect and Medicaid takes over payments.

For example, a patient who has a $100 spend-down visits the physician on March 3 and is billed $75. The patient is responsible for paying the entire $75. Later in the month, she visits the physician again and is charged $60. She must pay $25, and Medicaid will pay the remaining $35. At the beginning of the next month, she is once again responsible for the first $100 of charges. The spend-down amount varies depending on the patient's financial resources.

Many states also extend benefits to other groups of individuals. For example, most states offer coverage to people described as medically needy.

Medicaid Enrollment Verification

Medicaid cards or coupons may be issued to qualified individuals. Some states issue cards twice a month, some once a month, and others every two months or every six months. Figure 11.1 shows sample ID cards. Figure 11.2 on page 382 displays a sample ID coupon.

Compliance Guideline

Fraud and Abuse
The Medicaid Alliance for Program Safeguards has members from CMS regional offices and a technical advisory group called the Medicaid Fraud and Abuse Control Technical Advisory Group, or TAG. This alliance works together to exchange experiences, resources, and solutions to prevent as well as detect Medicaid fraud and abuse.

Insurance Procedures

Patients' eligibility should be checked each time they make an appointment and before they see the physician. Most states are moving to electronic verification of eligibility under the Electronic Medicaid Eligibility Verification System (EMEVS). Many states have both online and telephone verification systems. In addition to eligibility dates, the system also specifies whether the patient is required to pay a copayment or coinsurance.

Some patients may require treatment before their eligibility can be checked. Figure 11.3 on page 383 is an example of an eligibility verification log for patients who have not yet been assigned ID numbers or who have misplaced their cards.

Some individuals enrolled in Medicaid are assigned **restricted status**. In restricted status, the patient is required to see a specific physician and/or use a

COMMUNITY HEALTH NETWORK
OF CONNECTICUT

4808 PAID Prescription, Inc.

GROUP # MEMBER #

Name:
Birth Date:
Primary Care Provider's Phone #:
Provider:

Members

- For questions about your Prescription Drug plan, call 1-800-903-8638.
- To obtain Mental Health/Substance Information or Services, call 1-800-666-9578.
- In case of Medical Emergency, call your Primary Care Provider. In life-threatening cases, go to the nearest hospital and present your I.D. card. For more information, call 1-800-859-9889.

Providers

- Except for primary care/family planning, all services MUST receive prior authorization from the Primary Care Provider. Any questions, please call 1-800-440-5071.

Only the person named on this card can use this card to receive services.

COMMUNITY HEALTH NETWORK
OF CONNECTICUT
290 Pratt St., Meriden, CT. 06450 (203) 237-4000

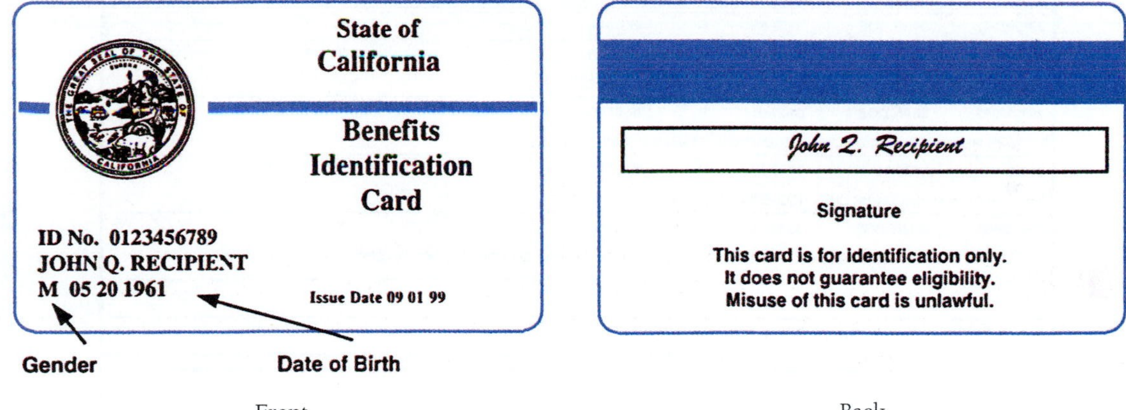

Front Back

FIGURE 11.1 Sample Medicaid Identification Cards

specific pharmacy. This physician's name is listed on the patient's ID card. If the patient sees a provider other than the one listed on the card, Medicaid benefits will be denied. Likewise, a restricted status patient is limited to a certain pharmacy for filling prescriptions. People are assigned restricted status because of past abuse of Medicaid benefits.

After a patient's Medicaid enrollment status has been verified, most practices also require a second form of identification. A driver's license or other cards may be requested to confirm the patient's identity.

Medicaid Identification (Form 3087) Sample

P.O. BOX 179030 952-X EROX 01-00001
AUSTIN, TEXAS 78714-9030

TEXAS DEPARTMENT OF HUMAN SERVICES
MEDICAID IDENTIFICATION
IDENTIFICATION PARA MEDICAID

Date Run	BIN	BP	TP	Cat	Case No.	GOOD THROUGH: VALIDA HASTA:	
10/25/99	610098		01	02	123456789		NOVEMBER 30, 1999

952-X 123456789 01 02 990930
JANE DOE
338 WEST BOONE STREET
BELVIDERE TX 78069

ANYONE LISTED BELOW
CAN GET MEDICAID SERVICES

Under 21 years old? Please call your doctor, nurse, or dentist to schedule a checkup if you see a reminder under your name. If there is no reminder, you can still use Medicaid to get health care that you need.

A ✓ on the line to the right of your name means that you can get that service too.

Questions about Medicaid? Please call **1-800-252-8263** for help.

CADA PERSONA NOMBRADA ABAJO
PUEDE RECIBIR SERVICIOS DE MEDICAID

¿Tiene menos de 21 años? Por favor, llame a su doctor, enfermera, o dentista para hacer una cita si hay una nota debajo de su nombre. Aunque no haya ninguna nota, puede usar Medicaid para recibir la atención médica que necesite.

Las marcas ✓ a la derecha en el mismo renglón donde está su nombre significan que usted puede recibir esos servicios también.

¿Tiene preguntas sobre Medicaid? Por favor, llame al **1-800-252-8263**.

ID NO.	NAME	DATE OF BIRTH	SEX	ELIGIBILITY DATE	TPR	MEDICARE NO.	EYE EXAM	EYE GLASSES	HEARING AID	ICF-MR DENTAL	PRESCRIPTIONS Up to 3	PRESCRIPTIONS More than 3	MEDICAL SERVICES
999999991	JANE DOE	03-02-63	F	07-01-99			✓	✓	✓		✓		✓
999999992	JOHN DOE	08-06-90	M	07-01-99			✓	✓	✓			✓	✓
THSTEPS MEDICAL CHECK-UP DUE / NECESITA SU EXAMEN MEDICO DE THSTEPS													
999999993	JEAN DOE	08-27-91	F	07-01-99			✓	✓	✓			✓	✓
THSTEPS MEDICAL CHECK-UP DUE / NECESITA SU EXAMEN MEDICO DE THSTEPS													
999999994	JAMES DOE	09-14-93	M	07-01-99			✓	✓	✓			✓	✓
THSTEPS DENTAL CHECK-UP DUE / NECESITA SU EXAMEN DENTAL DE THSTEPS													
999999995	JAMIE DOE	03-11-95	F	07-01-99			✓	✓	✓			✓	✓
THSTEPS MEDICAL AND DENTAL CHECK-UP DUE / NECESITA SU EXAMEN MEDICO Y DENTAL DE THSTEPS													

Form 3087/10-96

FIGURE 11.2 Sample Medicaid Identification Coupon

Medicaid Fraud and Abuse

Under the Deficit Reduction Act of 2005 the federal False Claims Act was expanded to allow states to enact their own False Claims Acts, which can bring increased recovery amounts if their act is as strong as the one enacted by the federal government. For example, if a state's federal matching rate was 57 percent, it would only receive 43 percent of the amount recovered. However, if the

Medicaid Verification Letter (Form 1027-A) Sample

Texas Department of Human Services

Form 1027-A/10-93

MEDICAL ELIGIBILITY VERIFICATION
CONFIRMACIÓN DE ELEGIBILIDAD MÉDICA

Name of Doctor/Nombre del Doctor	Name of Pharmacy/Nombre de la Farmacia

Each person listed below has applied and is eligible for MEDICAID BENEFITS, but has not yet received a recipient number. Do not submit a claim until you are given a recipient number. Pharmacists have 60 days from the date the number is issued to file claims. However, check your provider manual because other providers may have up to 90 days to file claims. Call the eligibility worker named below if you have not been given the recipient number(s) within 15 days.

Each person listed below is eligible for MEDICAID BENEFITS during the current calendar month. His Medical Care Identification form is lost or late. The recipient number must appear on all claims for health services.

Date Eligibility Verified	Verification Method	BIN
	☐ Local DCU ☐ SAVERR Direct Inquiry ☐ Regional Procedure ☐ S.O. DCU (A & d Staff only)	610098

RECIPIENT NAME / NOMBRE DEL BENEFICIARIO	DATE OF BIRTH / FECHA DE NACIMIENTO	RECIPIENT NO. / BENEFICIARIO NUM.	COVERAGE DATES / PERIODO CUBIERTO FROM/DESDE THROUGH/HASTA	MEDICARE CLAIM NO. / NUM. DE RECLAMO DE MEDICARE	DRUG RECORD: SERVICE DATE	VENDOR NO.	Rx NO.	SERVICE DATE	VENDOR NO.	Rx NO.	SERVICE DATE	VENDOR NO.	Rx NO.
					DESCRIPTION OF DRUG			DESCRIPTION OF DRUG			DESCRIPTION OF DRUG		

This form (for Medicaid eligibility) covers only the dates shown above. It is not valid for any days before or after these dates.

Esta confirmación de elegibilidad para Medicaid cubre sólo el periodo especificado arriba. No es válida ni un día antes ni un día después de la fechas especificadas.

I hereby certify, under penalty of perjury and/or fraud, that the above recipient(s) have lost, have not received, or have no access to the Medical Care Identification (Form 3087) for the current month. I have requested and received Form 1027-A, Medical Eligibility Verification, to use as proof of eligibility for the coverage dates shown above. I understand that unlimited prescriptions include prescribed family planning drugs/supplies, prescriptions for people under age 21, for nursing facility residents, and for LONESTAR recipients. For all other prescriptions, the Texas Medicaid program will pay for only three prescription drugs per recipient each month. The recipient must pay for any additional drugs. I also understand that using this form to obtain more than the allowed number of drugs per recipient each month, or to obtain drugs for people not listed above is fraud. It is punishable by fine and/or imprisonment.

Por este medio certifico bajo pena de perjurio o fraude que nosotros, los beneficiarios nombrados arriba, no hemos recibido, hemos perdido, o por otra razón no tenemos en nuestro poder la identificación para Servicios Médicos (Form 3087) del corriente mes. Solicité y recibí esta Confirmación de Elegibilidad Médica (Form 1027-A), para comprobar nuestra elegibilidad durante el periodo cubierto especificado arriba. Sé que Medicadi no limita medinas y provisiones recetadas para la planificación familiar, recetas para personas menores de 21 años de edad, para residentes de una casa para convalecientes, ni para los clientes de LONESTAR. Para todos los demás casos, Medicaid de Texas pagará sólo tres medicinas de receta al mes para cada cliente. El cliente tiene que pagar cualquier medicina adicional. Comprendo, además, que usar esta confirmación para obtener más medicinas que las permitidas para algún beneficiario o para obtener medicinas para alguna persona no nonmbrada arriba como beneficiario constituye fraude y es castigable con una multa y/o la cárcel.

Signature-Recipient or Representative/Firma-Beneficiario o Representante Date/Fecha

Office Address and Telephone No. / Oficina y Teléfono

* or Authorized Lead Worker/*or Trabajador Encargado

Name of Worker (type)/Nombre del Trabajador	Worker BJN	Worder Signature	Date
Name of Supervisor (type)*/Nombre del Supervisor*	Supervisor* BJN	Supervisor Signature	Date

FIGURE 11.3 Sample Medicaid Eligibility Verification Log

state enacts a False Claims Act meeting the government's standard it would receive 53 percent of the recovered amount.

In addition, the federal government has a provision that requires large facilities that receive Medicaid payments of or exceeding $5 million, such as hospitals, to include the provisions of the False Claims Act and the rights of whistleblowers in their employee handbook.

Covered and Excluded Services

Since plans are administered at a state level, each state determines coverage and coverage limits and sets payment rates, subject to federal guidelines established under Title XIX of the Social Security Act.

Covered Services

To receive federal matching funds, states must cover certain services, including:

- Inpatient hospital services
- Outpatient hospital services
- Physician services
- Emergency services
- Laboratory and X-ray services
- Prenatal care
- EPSDT services for people under age twenty-one, including physical examinations, immunizations, and certain age-relevant services
- Skilled nursing facility services for people age twenty-one and older
- Home health care services for people eligible for skilled nursing services
- Vaccines for children
- Family planning services and supplies
- Nurse midwife services
- Pediatric and family nurse-practitioner services
- Rural health clinic services
- Federally qualified health-center (FQHC) services

Some states also provide coverage for prescription drugs, for dental or vision care, and for such miscellaneous services as chiropractic care, psychiatric care, and physical therapy. The federal government provides matching funds for some of these optional services, the most common of which include:

- Diagnostic services
- Clinic services
- Prescription drugs
- Vision care
- Prosthetic devices
- Transportation services
- Rehabilitation and physical therapy services
- Home and community-based care to certain people with chronic impairments

Billing Tip

Preauthorization
Some services covered under Medicaid require prior authorization before they are performed. If the provider does not obtain preauthorization, the plan may refuse to pay the claim.

In recent years, however, because of large state budget deficits, state laws have cut back on some of these benefits, such as prescription drug benefits and hearing, vision, and dental benefits for adults. Many states have also had to restrict eligibility for Medicaid and to reduce Medicaid payments to doctors, hospitals, nursing homes, or other providers.

Excluded Services

Rules regarding services not covered under Medicaid vary from state to state. For example, the following services may not be covered:

- Services that are not medically necessary
- Experimental or investigational procedures
- Cosmetic procedures

Types Of Plans

In most states, Medicaid offers both fee-for-service and managed care plans.

Fee-for-Service

Medicaid clients enrolled in a fee-for-service plan may be treated by the provider of their choice, as long as that provider accepts Medicaid. The provider submits the claim to Medicaid and is paid directly by Medicaid.

Managed Care

Many states have shifted the Medicaid population from fee-for-service programs to managed care plans. Client enrollment in a managed care plan is either mandatory or voluntary, depending on state regulations. Some states, such as New York, California, and Florida, are shifting increasing numbers of Medicaid beneficiaries to managed care programs.

Medicaid managed care plans restrict patients to a network of physicians, hospitals, and clinics. Individuals enrolled in managed care plans must obtain all services and referrals through their primary care provider (PCP). The PCP is responsible for coordinating and monitoring the patient's care. If the patient needs to see a specialist, the PCP must provide a referral; otherwise, Medicaid will not pay for the service. In many states, a PCP may be an internist, a general practitioner, a family physician, a pediatrician, a nurse-practitioner, or a physician's assistant.

Managed care plans offer Medicaid recipients several advantages. Some Medicaid patients experience difficulty finding a physician who will treat them, in part due to the lower fee structure. Under a managed care plan, individuals choose a primary care physician who provides treatment and manages their medical care. The patient also has access to specialists should the need arise. In addition, managed care programs offer greater access to preventive care such as immunizations and health screenings.

Medicaid managed care claims are filed differently than other Medicaid claims. Claims are sent to the managed care organization instead of to the state Medicaid department. Participating providers agree to the guidelines of the managed care organization, provided that they are in compliance with federal requirements.

Compliance Guideline

When Medicaid conducts a post-payment review, the following information about a referral is expected to be shown in the patient record:

- PCP's name
- PCP's Medicaid PIN
- Date the PCP contacted the referring provider
- Reason for the referral (clinical data)
- Patient's name
- Patient's Medicaid ID number
- Patient's date of birth

Payment for Services

A physician who wishes to provide services to Medicaid recipients must sign a contract with the Department of Health and Human Services (HHS). Managed care plans may also contract with HHS to provide services under Medicaid. Medicaid participating providers agree to certain provisions.

Providers must agree to accept payment from Medicaid as payment in full for services; they may not bill patients for additional amounts. The difference must be entered into the billing system as a write-off. The amount of payment is determined by several factors, including Title XIX of the Social Security Act, HHS regulations, and state rules.

States may require Medicaid recipients to make small payments in the form of deductibles, coinsurance, or copayments (copays are usually in the \$2 to \$5 range). These patient payments are referred to as cost-share payments. Federal

Compliance Guideline

Discrimination Is Not Permitted
Participating providers may not discriminate on the basis of race, age, color, sex, creed, national origin, or disability and must agree to treat all eligible patients.

law mandates exempting emergency services and family planning services from copayments. In addition, federal law excludes certain categories of recipients from making copayments, including children under age eighteen, pregnant women, hospital or nursing home patients who contribute the majority of their income to that institution for care, and categorically needy recipients who are enrolled in HMOs.

If Medicaid does not cover a service, the patient may be billed if the following conditions are met:

- The physician informed the patient before the service was performed that the procedure would not be covered by Medicaid.
- The physician has an established written policy for billing noncovered services that applies to all patients, not just Medicaid patients.
- The patient is informed in advance of the estimated charge for the procedure and agrees in writing to pay the charge.

If the physician has reason to believe that a service will not be covered, the patient must be informed in advance and given a form to sign. An sample form is shown in Figure 11.4.

If a claim is denied for the following reasons, the physician may not bill the patient for the amount:

- Necessary preauthorization was not obtained prior to the procedure.
- The service was not medically necessary.
- The claim was not filed within the time period for filing (typically one year after the date of service).

Providers in capitated managed care plans who are paid flat monthly fees must still file claims with the Medicaid payer, since the payer uses the claim data to assess utilization. Utilization reviews examine the necessity, appropriateness, and efficiency of services delivered.

Third-Party Liability

Before filing a claim with Medicaid, it is important to determine whether the patient has other insurance coverage.

Private Pay Agreement

I understand ______(Provider name)______ is accepting me as a private pay patient for the period of ____________________, and I will be responsible for paying for any services I receive. The Provider will not file a claim to Medicaid for services provided to me.

Signed: ______________________________

Date: ______________________________

FIGURE 11.4 Sample Private Pay Agreement

Payer of Last Resort

If the patient has coverage through any other insurance plan or if the claim is covered by another program, such as workers' compensation, the other plan is billed first, and the remittance advice from that primary payer is forwarded to Medicaid. For this reason, Medicaid is known as the **payer of last resort**, since it is always billed after another plan has been billed, if other coverage exists.

Medicare-Medicaid Crossover Claims

Some individuals, called **Medi-Medi beneficiaries** or **dual-eligibles**, are eligible for both Medicaid and Medicare benefits. Claims for these patients are first submitted to Medicare, which makes payments to the provider and then sends the claims to Medicaid with a Medicare remittance notice. Claims billed to Medicare which are automatically sent to Medicaid are called **crossover claims**.

In many instances, Medicare requires a deductible or coinsurance payment. When an individual has Medi-Medi coverage, these payments are sometimes made by Medicaid. The total amount paid by Medicare and Medicaid is subject to a maximum allowed limit. In most states, Medicaid plans do not pay for a particular service if Medicare does not.

Medicaid programs in some states pay Medicare Part B premiums for Medi-Medi patients. For example, in California, MediCal pays the Medicare Part B premiums, and physicians may not bill patients for Medicare deductible and coinsurance amounts. However, MediCal does not reimburse Medicare HMO patients for required copayments. Depending on the specific procedures and diagnoses, MediCal sometimes reimburses providers for charges denied by Medicare, including charges for services normally not covered by Medicare.

> **HIPAA Tip**
>
> **Claims and RAs**
>
> *The HIPAA 837 is used for electronic claims and for coordination of benefits. The HIPAA 835 remittance advice is the standard transaction sent by payers to Medicaid providers.*

> **HIPAA Tip**
>
> **PHI and Dual-Eligibles**
>
> *The HIPAA Privacy Rule, since it permits sharing PHI for payment purposes, allows Medicare plans and state Medicaid agencies to exchange enrollee information.*

Claim Filing Guidelines

Because Medicaid is a state-based program, coordination of the requirements for completion of the HIPAA 837 are handled by a national committee called the National Medicaid EDI HIPAA Workgroup (NMEH). This organization advises CMS about HIPAA compliance issues related to Medicaid.

Where to File

Claims are submitted to different agencies, depending on the particular state. Some states use fiscal intermediaries. These are private insurance companies that contract with Medicaid to process and pay claims. In other states, the state's Department of Health and Human Services or the county welfare agency may handle claims. Medical offices obtain specific claim filing and completion requirements from the agency responsible for processing Medicaid claims in their state.

Medicaid Coding

For the most part, Medicaid procedures and services are reported using the CPT/HCPCS coding system that is mandated by HIPAA; the ICD-9-CM is used to code diagnoses. However, since Medicaid is state-based, some payers may not recognize all standard codes. CPT modifiers are often not honored by Medicaid; and most states do not use the Medicare CCI edits.

Unacceptable Billing Practices

Physicians who contract with Medicaid to provide services may not engage in any of the following unacceptable billing practices:

- Billing for services that are not medically necessary
- Billing for services not provided, or billing more than once for the same procedure
- Submitting claims for individual procedures that are part of a global procedure
- Submitting claims using an individual provider NPI when a physician working for or on behalf of a group practice or clinic performs services

After Filing

Once a claim has been filed and approved for payment, the provider receives payment and an RA/EOB. Claims that are denied may be appealed within a certain time period, usually thirty to sixty days. Appeals should include relevant supporting documentation and a note explaining why the claim should be reconsidered. The first level of appeal is the regional agent for Medicaid. If the appeal is denied, it goes to the state's welfare department for consideration. The highest level for a Medicaid appeal is the appellate court.

Medicaid Claim Completion

Because Medicaid is a health plan that is categorized as a covered entity under HIPAA, Medicaid claims are usually submitted using the HIAA 837 claim. In some situations, however, a paper claim using the CMS-1500 format may be used, or a state-specific form may be requested.

HIPAA Claims

A number of special data elements may be required for completion of HIPAA-compliant Medicaid claims. The requirements are controlled by state guidelines. These are:

Data Element	*Meaning*
Family Planning Indicator	Y = Family planning services involvement N = No family planning services involvement
EPSDT Indicator	Y = The services are the result of a screening referral N = The services are not the result of a screening referral
Special Program Code	Codes reported for Medicaid beneficiaries such as 03 for Special Federal Funding program and 09 for Second Opinion or Surgery
Service Authorization Exception Code	Required when providers are required by state law to obtain authorization for specific services and authorization was not obtained for reasons such as emergency care

The physician's Medicaid number is reported as a secondary identifier.

CMS-1500 Paper Claims

If a CMS-1500 paper claim is required, follow the general guidelines shown in Table 11.2 and illustrated in Figure 11.5 on page 390.

Table 11.2 Medicaid CMS-1500 (08/05) Claim Completion

ITEM NUMBER	DATA
1	Choose Medicaid
1a	Medicaid ID number
2	Patient's name
3	Patient's eight-digit date of birth and gender
4	Blank
5	Patient's address
6	Blank
7	Blank
8	Blank
9	Blank
9a	Blank
9b	Blank
9c	Blank
9d	Blank
10a–10c	Choose appropriate box
10d	Blank
11	Blank
11a	Blank
11b	Blank
11c	Blank
11d	Blank
12	Blank; signature not required
13	Blank; signature not required
14	Blank
15	Blank
16	Blank
17	Name and credentials of referring or ordering physician
17a	Provider's NPI or Medicaid ID number
18	Complete as appropriate according to state guidelines
19	Complete as appropriate according to state guidelines
20	No
21	Appropriate ICD codes
22	Complete for resubmission
23	Preauthorization/precertification number
24A	Dates of service (eight-digit format); no consecutive dates permitted
24B	Appropriate POS code
24C	Emergency indicator, if required
24D	Appropriate CPT/HCPCS codes with up to three modifiers
24E	Diagnosis key number for CPT/HCPCS codes
24F	Amount charged
24G	Appropriate days or units reported (use "1" if a single service)
24H	Enter appropriate codes if services provided under EPSDT (varies by state)
24I–24J	NPI or other ID number for rendering provider
25	Follow state guidelines
26	Blank
27	Choose Yes
28	Total of charges in FL 24F
29	Blank or $0.00
30	Follow state guidelines
31	Enter the legal signature and credentials of the provider or supplier (or representative), "Signature on File," or "SOF." Enter the date the form was signed.
32	Name and address of facility where services were rendered if other than provider's office or patient's home, or enter SAME
33	Billing provider's name, address, and NPI or Medicaid ID number

Billing Tip

Medicaid Instructions May Vary
The NUCC instructions do not address any particular payer. Best practice for paper claims is to check with the payer for specific information required on the form.

Billing Tip

Secondary Claims/COB
Chapters 14 and 15 discuss processing secondary claims, coordination of benefits, and appeals for Medicaid.

1500

HEALTH INSURANCE CLAIM FORM

APPROVED BY NATIONAL UNIFORM CLAIM COMMITTEE 08/05

PICA | PICA

CARRIER

1. MEDICARE (Medicare #) ☐ MEDICAID (Medicaid #) ☒ TRICARE CHAMPUS (Sponsor's SSN) ☐ CHAMPVA (Member ID#) ☐ GROUP HEALTH PLAN (SSN or ID) ☐ FECA BLK LUNG (SSN) ☐ OTHER (ID) ☐

1a. INSURED'S I.D. NUMBER (For Program in Item 1): 80512 D

2. PATIENT'S NAME (Last Name, First Name, Middle Initial): JONES SAMANTHA

3. PATIENT'S BIRTH DATE MM DD YY: 11 20 1950 SEX M ☐ F ☒

4. INSURED'S NAME (Last Name, First Name, Middle Initial)

5. PATIENT'S ADDRESS (No., Street): 1124 BEST ST

6. PATIENT RELATIONSHIP TO INSURED: Self ☐ Spouse ☐ Child ☐ Other ☐

7. INSURED'S ADDRESS (No., Street)

CITY: RAYTOWN STATE: CO

8. PATIENT STATUS: Single ☐ Married ☐ Other ☐ Employed ☐ Full-Time Student ☐ Part-Time Student ☐

CITY STATE

ZIP CODE: 80034 TELEPHONE (Include Area Code): (720) 104 5555

ZIP CODE TELEPHONE (INCLUDE AREA CODE) ( )

9. OTHER INSURED'S NAME (Last Name, First Name, Middle Initial)

10. IS PATIENT'S CONDITION RELATED TO:

11. INSURED'S POLICY GROUP OR FECA NUMBER

a. OTHER INSURED'S POLICY OR GROUP NUMBER

a. EMPLOYMENT? (CURRENT OR PREVIOUS) ☐ YES ☒ NO

a. INSURED'S DATE OF BIRTH MM DD YY SEX M ☐ F ☐

b. OTHER INSURED'S DATE OF BIRTH MM DD YY SEX M ☐ F ☐

b. AUTO ACCIDENT? ☐ YES ☒ NO PLACE (State)

b. EMPLOYER'S NAME OR SCHOOL NAME

c. EMPLOYER'S NAME OR SCHOOL NAME

c. OTHER ACCIDENT? ☐ YES ☒ NO

c. INSURANCE PLAN NAME OR PROGRAM NAME

d. INSURANCE PLAN NAME OR PROGRAM NAME

10d. RESERVED FOR LOCAL USE

d. IS THERE ANOTHER HEALTH BENEFIT PLAN? ☐ YES ☐ NO *If yes*, return to and complete item 9 a-d.

READ BACK OF FORM BEFORE COMPLETING & SIGNING THIS FORM.

12. PATIENT'S OR AUTHORIZED PERSON'S SIGNATURE I authorize the release of any medical or other information necessary to process this claim. I also request payment of government benefits either to myself or to the party who accepts assignment below.

SIGNED ________ DATE ________

13. INSURED'S OR AUTHORIZED PERSON'S SIGNATURE I authorize payment of medical benefits to the undersigned physician or supplier for services described below.

SIGNED ________

PATIENT AND INSURED INFORMATION

14. DATE OF CURRENT: MM DD YY ILLNESS (First symptom) OR INJURY (Accident) OR PREGNANCY(LMP)

15. IF PATIENT HAS HAD SAME OR SIMILAR ILLNESS. GIVE FIRST DATE MM DD YY

16. DATES PATIENT UNABLE TO WORK IN CURRENT OCCUPATION FROM MM DD YY TO MM DD YY

17. NAME OF REFERRING PHYSICIAN OR OTHER SOURCE

17a.

17b. NPI

18. HOSPITALIZATION DATES RELATED TO CURRENT SERVICES FROM MM DD YY TO MM DD YY

19. RESERVED FOR LOCAL USE

20. OUTSIDE LAB? ☐ YES ☒ NO $ CHARGES

21. DIAGNOSIS OR NATURE OF ILLNESS OR INJURY. (Relate Items 1,2,3 or 4 to Item 24e by Line)

1. 84 31
2. ___ . ___
3. ___ . ___
4. ___ . ___

22. MEDICAID RESUBMISSION CODE ORIGINAL REF. NO.

23. PRIOR AUTHORIZATION NUMBER

	24. A. DATE(S) OF SERVICE From MM DD YY To MM DD YY	B. PLACE OF SERVICE	C. EMG	D. PROCEDURES, SERVICES, OR SUPPLIES (Explain Unusual Circumstances) CPT/HCPCS MODIFIER	E. DIAGNOSIS POINTER	F. $ CHARGES	G. DAYS OR UNITS	H. EPSDT Family Plan	I. ID. QUAL.	J. RENDERING PROVIDER ID.#
1	12 10 2008	11		99213	1	90 00	1		NPI	2121000899
2									NPI	
3									NPI	
4									NPI	
5									NPI	
6									NPI	

25. FEDERAL TAX I.D. NUMBER SSN ☐ EIN ☐

26. PATIENT'S ACCOUNT NO.: JON0010

27. ACCEPT ASSIGNMENT? (For govt. claims, see back) ☒ YES ☐ NO

28. TOTAL CHARGE $ 90 00

29. AMOUNT PAID $

30. BALANCE DUE $

31. SIGNATURE OF PHYSICIAN OR SUPPLIER INCLUDING DEGREES OR CREDENTIALS (I certify that the statements on the reverse apply to this bill and are made a part thereof.)

Julie Groat MD

SIGNED 12/12/2008 DATE

32. SERVICE FACILITY LOCATION INFORMATION: SAME

a. NPI b.

33. BILLING PROVIDER INFO & PHONE # (720) 554 1222

CENTER CLINIC
3810 EXECUTIVE BLVD
RAYTOWN CO 80033

a. NPI b.

PHYSICIAN OR SUPPLIER INFORMATION

NUCC Instruction Manual available at: www.nucc.org

FIGURE 11.5 CMS-1500 (08/05) Claim Completion for Medicaid

Review

Steps to Success

- ❒ Read this chapter and review the Key Terms and the Chapter Summary.
- ❒ Answer the Review Questions and Applying Your Knowledge in the Chapter Review.
- ❒ Access the chapter's websites and complete the Internet Activities to learn more about available professional resources.
- ❒ Complete the related chapter in the *Medical Insurance Workbook* to reinforce your understanding of Medicaid coverage and billing procedures.

Chapter Summary

1. The federal government requires the states to provide individuals in certain low-income or low-resource categories with Medicaid coverage. Coverage is available to people receiving TANF assistance; people eligible for TANF but not receiving assistance; people receiving foster care or adoption assistance under the Social Security Act; children under six years of age from low-income families; some people who lose cash assistance when their work income or Social Security benefits exceed allowable limits; pregnant women with low incomes; infants born to Medicaid-eligible pregnant women; people age sixty-five and over or legally blind or totally disabled people who receive Supplemental Security Income (SSI); and certain low-income Medicare recipients.

   At times, federal programs and initiatives are enacted that give states the opportunity to expand Medicaid coverage in particular ways to targeted groups. Recent examples include the State Children's Health Insurance Program (SCHIP), Early and Periodic Screening, Diagnosis, and Treatment (EPSDT) services for children under age twenty-one who are enrolled in Medicaid, the Ticket to Work and Work Incentives Improvement Act (TWWIIA) of 1999 for people with disabilities who want to work, and the New Freedom Initiative aimed at reducing barriers to full community integration for people with disabilities and long-term illnesses.
2. The Welfare Reform Act made it more difficult for certain groups to obtain coverage, including disabled children and immigrants.
3. Categorically needy individuals qualify for Medicaid based on their low income and lack of resources; medically needy people receive assistance from some states because they encounter high medical bills and have limited income and resources. Medically needy individuals may have incomes that exceed Medicaid limits.
4. When determining eligibility, states examine a person's income, current assets (some assets are not counted), and assets that have recently been transferred into another person's name.
5. Medicaid usually does not pay for services that are not medically necessary, procedures that are experimental or investigational, and cosmetic procedures.
6. States offer a variety of plans, including fee-for-service and managed care plans. The trend is to shift recipients from fee-for-service plans to managed care plans.
7. When a Medicaid recipient has coverage under another insurance plan, that plan is billed first. Once the remittance advice from the primary carrier has been received, Medicaid may be billed.

Review Questions

Match the key terms with their definitions.

A. medically needy
B. Temporary Assistance for Needy Families (TANF)
C. payer of last resort
D. Welfare Reform Act
E. restricted status
F. categorically needy
G. State Children's Health Insurance Program (SCHIP)
H. Federal Medicaid Assistance Percentage (FMAP) program
I. Medi-Medi beneficiaries
J. spend-down

____ 1. The program through which the federal government makes Medicaid payments to states

____ 2. A program that requires a patient to see a specific physician and/or use a specific pharmacy

____ 3. Patients who receive benefits from both Medicare and Medicaid

____ 4. A description that applies to Medicaid, since it is always billed after another plan has been billed, if other coverage exists

____ 5. Applicants who qualify based on low income and resources

____ 6. Another name for the Personal Responsibility and Work Opportunity Reconciliation Act of 1996

____ 7. A program that requires states to develop and implement plans for health insurance coverage for uninsured children

____ 8. The government financial program that provides financial assistance for people with low incomes and few resources

____ 9. A program that requires individuals to use their own financial resources to pay a portion of incurred medical bills before Medicaid makes payments

____ 10. Individuals with high medical expenses and low financial resources

Decide whether each statement is true or false.

____ 1. A person who sees a provider for family planning services may not be charged a copayment.

____ 2. Medicaid is known as the payer of last resort because an individual must exhaust all other resources before Medicaid pays for health care.

____ 3. Individuals who are employed are ineligible for Medicaid.

____ 4. After receiving payment from Medicaid, participating physicians may bill patients for the remaining amount of the charges.

____ 5. Providers in capitated managed care plans must still submit claims to Medicaid.

____ 6. Crossover claims are submitted to Medicare first, and then to Medicaid.

____ 7. Individuals must receive financial assistance from the federal government to qualify for Medicaid.

____ 8. Medicaid benefits differ from state to state.

____ 9. The SCHIP is fully funded by individual states, without funds from the federal government.

____ 10. States may extend health insurance coverage to groups excluded by Welfare Reform Act legislation.

Select the letter that best completes the statement or answers the question.

____ 1. Applicants who have high medical bills and whose incomes exceed state limits may be eligible for health care coverage under a state ______ program.
   A. TANF
   B. categorically needy
   C. restricted status
   D. medically needy

_____ 2. Under the Federal Medicaid Assistance Program, the federal government makes payment directly to
   A. states
   B. individuals eligible to receive TANF
   C. individuals who are blind or disabled
   D. categorically needy individuals

_____ 3. Most individuals receiving TANF payments are limited to a _____ -year benefit period.
   A. two
   B. five
   C. seven
   D. ten

_____ 4. Medicaid identification cards must be checked for eligibility
   A. once a year
   B. every six months
   C. only when there is a change in the patient's address
   D. every time the patient receives services

_____ 5. People classified as restricted status
   A. must select a provider within the network
   B. receive a limited set of benefits
   C. receive emergency care only
   D. must see a specific provider for treatment

_____ 6. If family planning services are provided to a patient, what data element is affected?
   A. family planning indicator
   B. the dollar amount of the charge
   C. HCPCS codes
   D. ICD-9 codes

_____ 7. If services were provided in an emergency room, what place of service code is reported?
   A. 24C
   B. 18
   C. 24I
   D. 23

_____ 8. The Medicaid Alliance for Program Safeguards
   A. specifies civil and criminal penalties for fraudulent activities
   B. audits state Medicaid payers on a regular basis
   C. is a CMS program that came about as a result of the Welfare Reform Act
   D. oversees states' fraud and abuse efforts

_____ 9. The national committee to coordinate Medicaid data elements on health care claims is called
   A. NMEH
   B. NUBC
   C. EDI
   D. HIPAA

_____ 10. Individuals apply for Medicaid benefits by contacting
   A. the Department of Health and Human Services
   B. the local Income Maintenance office
   C. the Federal Medicaid Assistance Program
   D. the insurance carrier that processes Medicaid claims in their state

Answer the following question.

What steps should be taken to verify a patient's Medicaid eligibility?

Applying Your Knowledge

The objective of these exercises is to correctly complete Medicaid claims, applying what you have learned in the chapter. Following the information about the provider for the cases are two sections. The first section contains information about the patient, the insurance coverage, and the current medical condition. The second section is an encounter form for Valley Associates, P.C.

If you are using Medisoft to complete the cases, read the *Guide to Medisoft* before beginning. Information from the first section, the patient information form, has already been entered in the program for you. You must enter information from the second section, the encounter form, to complete the claim. If you are gaining experience by completing a paper CMS-1500 claim form, use the blank claim form supplied to you (from the back of the book or printed from the Student Data Template CD ROM) and follow the instructions on page 390.

The following provider information, which is also preloaded in the Medisoft database, should be used for Cases 11.1 and 11.2

Provider Information

Name	David Rosenberg, M.D.
Practice Name	Valley Associates, P.C.
Address	1400 West Center Street Toledo, OH 43601-0213
Telephone	555-967-0303
Medicaid ID	MCD00123
NPI	1288560027
BCBS PIN	18A09
Aetna PIN	RZX334
Assignment	Accepts
Signature	On File 01/01/08

Case 11.1

From the Patient Information Form:

Name	Mary Pascale
Sex	F
Birth Date	03/22/1979
SSN	246-71-0348
Address	412 Main St., Apt. 2A Shaker Heights, OH 44118-2345
Telephone	555-324-6669
Employer	Unemployed
Insurance Plan	Medicaid
Member ID	246710348MC
Assignment of Benefits	Y
Signature on File	On File 10/01/2008

Condition unrelated to Employment, Auto Accident, or Other Accident

VALLEY ASSOCIATES, PC
David Rosenberg, MD - Dermatology
555-967-0303
FED I.D. #16-2345678

PATIENT NAME	APPT. DATE/TIME
Pascale, Mary	10/14/2008 10:30 am
PATIENT NO.	**DX**
PASCAM0	1. 693.1 contact dermatitis due to food 2. 3. 4.

DESCRIPTION	✓	CPT	FEE	DESCRIPTION	✓	CPT	FEE
OFFICE VISITS				**PROCEDURES**			
New Patient				Acne Surgery		10040	
LI Problem Focused		99201		I&D, Abscess, Smpl		10060	
LII Expanded		99202		I&D, Abscess, Mult		10061	
LIII Detailed		99203		I&D, Pilonidal Cyst, Smpl		10080	
LIV Comp./Mod.		99204		I&D, Pilonidal Cyst, Compl		10081	
LV Comp./High		99205		I&R, Foreign Body, Smpl		10120	
Established Patient				I&R, Foreign Body, Compl		10121	
LI Minimum		99211		I&D Hematoma		10140	
LII Problem Focused	✓	99212	28	Puncture Aspiration		10160	
LIII Expanded		99213		Debride Skin, To 10%		11000	
LIV Detailed		99214		Each Addl 10%		11001	
LV Comp./High		99215		Pare Benign Skin Lesion		11055	
				Pare Benign Skin Lesion, 2-4		11056	
CONSULTATION: OFFICE/OP				Pare Benign Skin Lesion, 4+		11057	
Requested By:				Skin Biopsy, Single Les.		11100	
LI Problem Focused		99241		Skin Biopsy, Mult Les.		+11101	
LII Expanded		99242		Remove Skin Tags, 1-15		11200	
LIII Detailed		99243		Remove Skin Tags, Addl 10		+11201	
LIV Comp./Mod.		99244		Trim Nails		11719	
LV Comp./High		99245		Debride Nails, 1-5		11720	
				Debride Nails, 6+		11721	
CARE PLAN OVERSIGHT				Avulsion of Nail Plate,1		11730	
Supervision, 15-29 min.		99339		Avulsion of Nail Plate,Addl 1		+11732	
Supervision, 30+ min.		99340		Nail Biopsy		11755	
				Repair Nail Bed		11760	
				Excision, Ingrown Toenail		11765	
				TOTAL FEES			

Case 11.2

From the Patient Information Form:

Name	Scott Yeager	*Telephone*	555-619-7341
Sex	M	*Employer*	Unemployed
Birth Date	11/17/1957	*Insurance Plan*	Medicaid
SSN	139-62-9748	*Member ID*	139629748MC
Address	301 Maple Ave. Sandusky, OH 44870-4567	*Assignment of Benefits*	Y
		Signature on File	On File 10/01/2008

Condition unrelated to Employment, Auto Accident, or Other Accident

VALLEY ASSOCIATES, PC
David Rosenberg, MD - Dermatology
555-967-0303
FED I.D. #16-2345678

PATIENT NAME	APPT. DATE/TIME
Yeager, Scott	10/14/2008 11:00 am
PATIENT NO.	**DX**
YEAGESCØ	1. 919.7 superficial foreign body without 2. open wound, superficial 3. 4.

DESCRIPTION	✓	CPT	FEE	DESCRIPTION	✓	CPT	FEE
OFFICE VISITS				**PROCEDURES**			
New Patient				Acne Surgery		10040	
LI Problem Focused		99201		I&D, Abscess, Smpl		10060	
LII Expanded	✓	99202	50	I&D, Abscess, Mult		10061	
LIII Detailed		99203		I&D, Pilonidal Cyst, Smpl		10080	
LIV Comp./Mod.		99204		I&D, Pilonidal Cyst, Compl		10081	
LV Comp./High		99205		I&R, Foreign Body, Smpl	✓	10120	60
Established Patient				I&R, Foreign Body, Compl		10121	
LI Minimum		99211		I&D Hematoma		10140	
LII Problem Focused		99212		Puncture Aspiration		10160	
LIII Expanded		99213		Debride Skin, To 10%		11000	
LIV Detailed		99214		Each Addl 10%		11001	
LV Comp./High		99215		Pare Benign Skin Lesion		11055	
				Pare Benign Skin Lesion, 2-4		11056	
CONSULTATION: OFFICE/OP				Pare Benign Skin Lesion, 4+		11057	
Requested By:				Skin Biopsy, Single Les.		11100	
LI Problem Focused		99241		Skin Biopsy, Mult Les.		+11101	
LII Expanded		99242		Remove Skin Tags, 1-15		11200	
LIII Detailed		99243		Remove Skin Tags, Addl 10		+11201	
LIV Comp./Mod.		99244		Trim Nails		11719	
LV Comp./High		99245		Debride Nails, 1-5		11720	
				Debride Nails, 6+		11721	
CARE PLAN OVERSIGHT				Avulsion of Nail Plate, 1		11730	
Supervision, 15-29 min.		99339		Avulsion of Nail Plate, Addl 1		+11732	
Supervision, 30+ min.		99340		Nail Biopsy		11755	
				Repair Nail Bed		11760	
				Excision, Ingrown Toenail		11765	
				TOTAL FEES			

Internet Activities

1. Access the official website for California's MediCal program at http://www.medi-cal.ca.gov. Look for publications that describe eligibility requirements. Also look up current information on HIPAA updates. What are some of the challenges unique to Medicaid HIPAA compliance?

2. Go to the Centers for Medicare and Medicaid Services website for Medicaid at http://www.cms.gov/medicaid/. Select the Gov't Info link. Read the overview of the Medicaid program. Also look up information on the Medicaid program in your state. Has the SCHIP program in your state expanded in recent years?

3. Go to the Medicaid Alliance for Program Safeguards home page at the Centers for Medicare and Medicaid Services website at http://www.cms.gov/states/fraud/. Select the underlined link at the bottom of the page for Medicaid Alliance for Program Safeguards Background. How has CMS's role evolved in overseeing states' fraud and abuse efforts? Select the underlined link for guidance and reports. Locate information about preventing Medicaid fraud and abuse in a managed care environment.

Chapter 12

TRICARE and CHAMPVA

CHAPTER OUTLINE

The TRICARE Program

TRICARE Standard

TRICARE Prime

TRICARE Extra

TRICARE Reserve Select

TRICARE and Other Insurance Plans

Filing Claims

Fraud and Abuse

CHAMPVA

Learning Outcomes

After studying this chapter, you should be able to:

1. **Discuss the eligibility requirements for TRICARE.**
2. **Compare TRICARE participating and nonparticipating providers.**
3. **Describe the purpose of a nonavailability statement.**
4. **Explain how the TRICARE Standard, TRICARE Prime, and TRICARE Extra programs differ.**
5. **Discuss the TRICARE for Life program.**
6. **Discuss the eligibility requirements for CHAMPVA.**
7. **Prepare correct TRICARE and CHAMPVA claims.**

Key Terms

catchment area
catastrophic cap
CHAMPUS
Civilian Health and Medical Program of the Department of Veterans Affairs (CHAMPVA) cost-share
Defense Enrollment Eligibility Reporting System (DEERS)
Military Treatment Facility (MTF)
nonavailability statement (NAS)
Primary Care Manager (PCM)
sponsor
TRICARE
TRICARE Extra
TRICARE for Life
TRICARE Prime
TRICARE Reserve Select (TRS)
TRICARE Standard

The government's medical insurance programs for active-duty members, their families, and disabled veterans are served by participating providers in many parts of the country. Medical insurance specialists become familiar with the benefits, coverage, and billing rules for these programs in order to correctly verify eligibility, collect payments, and prepare claims.

The TRICARE Program

TRICARE is the Department of Defense's health insurance plan for military personnel and their families. TRICARE, which includes managed care options, replaced the program known as **CHAMPUS**, the Civilian Health and Medical Program of the Uniformed Services. TRICARE is a regionally managed health care program.

The TRICARE program brings the resources of military hospitals together with a network of civilian facilities and providers to offer increased access to health care services. All military treatment facilities, including hospitals and clinics, are part of the TRICARE system. TRICARE also contracts with civilian facilities and physicians to provide more extensive services to beneficiaries.

Eligibility

Members of the following uniformed services and their families are eligible for TRICARE: the Army, Navy, Air Force, Marine Corps, Coast Guard, Public Health Service (PHS), and National Oceanic and Atmospheric Administration (NOAA). Reserve and National Guard personnel become eligible when on active duty for more than thirty consecutive days or when they retire from reserve status at age sixty. The uniformed services member is referred to as a **sponsor**, since the member's status makes other family members eligible for TRICARE coverage.

When a TRICARE patient arrives for treatment, the medical information specialist photocopies both sides of the individual's military ID card and checks the expiration date to confirm that coverage is still valid (see Figure 12.1 on page 400). Decisions about eligibility are not made by TRICARE; the various branches of military service make them. Information about patient eligibility is stored in the **Defense Enrollment Eligibility Reporting System (DEERS)**. Sponsors may contact DEERS to verify eligibility; providers may not contact DEERS directly because the information is protected by the Privacy Act.

Billing Tip

Sponsor Information
Enter the sponsor's branch of service, status, and grade in the practice management program (PMP) when creating TRICARE patient cases.

Provider Participation and Nonparticipation

TRICARE pays only for services rendered by authorized providers. Authorized providers are certified by TRICARE regional contractors to have met specific

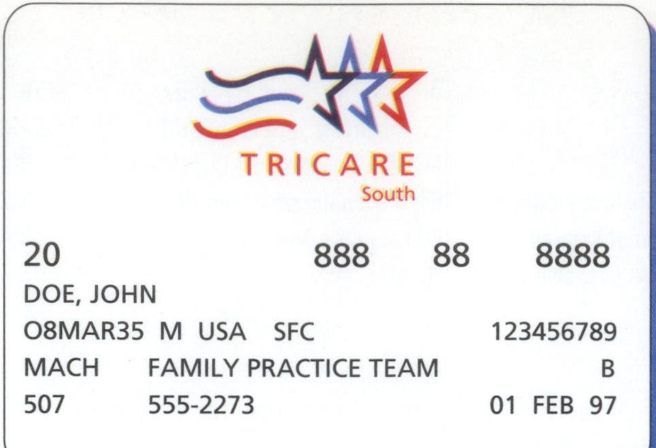

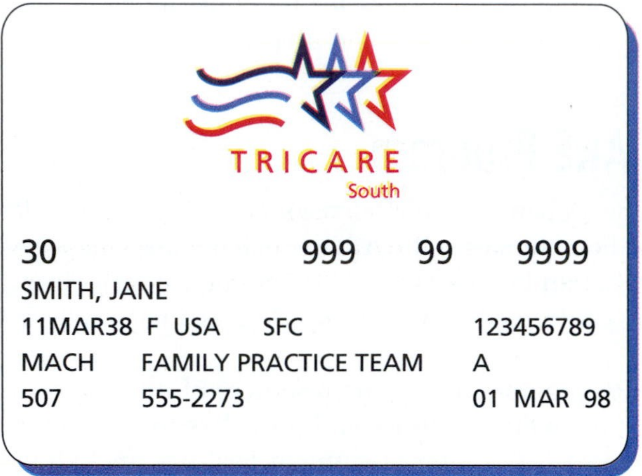

FIGURE 12.1 Sample Military (TRICARE) Identification Cards

educational, licensing, and other requirements. Once authorized, a provider is assigned a PIN and must decide whether to participate.

Participating Providers

Providers who participate agree to accept the TRICARE allowable charge as payment in full for services. Individual providers may decide whether to participate on a case-by-case basis. Participating providers are required to file claims on behalf of patients. The regional TRICARE contractor sends payment directly to the provider, and the provider collects the patient's share of the charges. Only participating providers may appeal claim decisions.

Nonparticipating Providers

A provider who chooses not to participate may not charge more than 115 percent of the allowable charge. If a provider bills more than 115 percent, the patient may refuse to pay the excess amount. For example, if the allowed charge for a procedure is $50.00, a nonparticipating provider may not charge more than $57.50 (115 percent of $50.00). If a nonparticipating provider were to charge $75.00 for the same procedure, the patient could refuse to pay the amount that exceeded 115 percent of the allowed amount. The difference of $17.50 would have to be written off by the provider. The patient would pay the cost-share (either 20 or 25 percent)—a TRICARE term for the coinsurance, the amount that is the responsibility of the patient.

Once the provider submits the claim, TRICARE pays its portion of the allowable charges, but instead of going directly to the provider, the payment is mailed to the patient. The patient is responsible for paying the provider. Payment should be collected at the time of the visit.

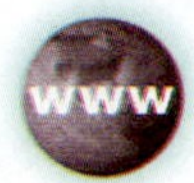

TRICARE Maxiumum Allowable Charge table

http://www.tricare.osd.mil/allowablecharges

Reimbursement

Providers who participate in the basic TRICARE plan are paid the amount specified in the Medicare Fee Schedule for most procedures. Medical supplies, durable medical equipment, and ambulance services are not subject to Medicare limits. The maximum amount TRICARE will pay for a procedure is known as the TRICARE Maximum Allowable Charge (TMAC). Providers are responsible for collecting the patients' deductibles and their cost-share portions of the charges.

Billing Tip

TRICARE Fiscal Year Different
Check the date when collecting TRICARE deductibles; TRICARE's fiscal year is from October 1 through September 30, so annual deductibles renew based on this cycle.

Network and Nonnetwork Providers

Providers who are authorized to treat TRICARE patients may also contract to become part of the TRICARE network. These providers serve patients in one of TRICARE's managed care plans. They agree to provide care to beneficiaries at contracted rates and to act as participating providers on all claims in TRICARE's managed care programs.

Providers who choose not to join the network may still provide care to managed care patients, but TRICARE will not pay for the services. The patient is 100 percent responsible for the charges.

Compliance Guideline

Covered Services
For a service to be eligible for payment, it must be:

- Medically necessary
- Delivered at the appropriate level for the condition
- At a quality that meets professional medical standards

TRICARE Standard

TRICARE offers beneficiaries access to three different health care plans. **TRICARE Standard** is a fee-for-service program that replaces the CHAMPUS program, which was also fee-for-service. The program covers medical services provided by a civilian physician or by a **Military Treatment Facility (MTF)**. Military families may receive services at an MTF, but available services vary by facility, and first priority is given to service members on active duty. When service is not available, the individual seeks treatment from a civilian provider, and TRICARE Standard benefits go into effect.

Costs

Under TRICARE Standard, medical expenses are shared between TRICARE and the beneficiary. Most enrollees pay annual deductibles. In addition, families of active-duty members pay 20 percent of outpatient charges. Retirees and their families, former spouses, and families of deceased personnel pay a 25 percent cost-share for outpatient services. If a beneficiary is treated by a provider who does not accept assignment, he or she is also responsible for the provider's additional charges, up to 115 percent of the allowable charge. See Figure 12.2 on page 402 for cost-share details.

Patient cost-share payments are subject to an annual **catastrophic cap**, a limit on the total medical expenses that beneficiaries are required to pay in one year. For active-duty families, the annual cap is $1,000, while for all other beneficiaries the limit is $3,000. Once these caps have been met, TRICARE pays 100 percent of additional charges for covered services for that coverage year.

ACTIVE-DUTY FAMILY MEMBERS			
	TRICARE Prime	TRICARE Extra	TRICARE Standard
Annual Deductible	None	$150/individual or $300/family for E-5 & above; $50/$100 for E-4 & below	$150/individual or $300/family for E-5 & above; $50/$100 for E-4 & below
Annual Enrollment Fee	None	None	None
Civilian Outpatient Visit	No cost	15% of negotiated fee	20% of allowed charges for covered service
Civilian Inpatient Admission	No cost	Greater of $25 or $14.35 per day	Greater of $25 or $14.35 per day
RETIREES, THEIR FAMILY MEMBERS, AND OTHERS			
	TRICARE Prime	TRICARE Extra	TRICARE Standard
Annual Deductible	None	$150/individual or $300/family	$150/individual or $300 family
Annual Enrollment Fee	$230/individual $460/family	None	None
Civilian Provider Copays:		20% of negotiated fee	25% of allowed charges for covered services
—Outpatient Visit	$12		
—Emergency Care	$30		
—Mental Health Visit	$25; $17 for group visit		
Civilian Inpatient Cost-Share	Greater of $11 per day or $25 per admission; no separate copayment for separately billed professional charges	Lesser of $250/day or 25% of negotiated charges plus 20% of negotiated professional fees	Lesser of $535 per day or 25% of billed charges plus 25% of allowed professional fees

FIGURE 12.2 Cost-Shares for TRICARE Standard Enrollees

Covered Services

The following services are examples of services covered under TRICARE Standard:

- Ambulatory surgery
- Diagnostic testing
- Durable medical equipment
- Family planning
- Hospice care
- Inpatient care
- Laboratory and pathology services
- Maternity care
- Outpatient care
- Prescription drugs and medicines
- Surgery
- Well-child care (birth to seventeen years)
- X-ray services

TRICARE Standard also provides many preventive benefits for enrollees, including immunizations, Pap smears, mammograms, and screening examinations for colon and prostate cancer.

Noncovered Services

TRICARE Standard generally does not cover the following services:

- Cosmetic drugs and cosmetic surgery
- Custodial care
- Unproven (experimental) procedures or treatments
- Routine physical examinations or foot care

Hospital Care and Nonavailability Statements

An individual is encouraged by TRICARE to first seek care at a military treatment facility (MTF) if living in a **catchment area**, defined as a geographic area served by a hospital, clinic, or dental clinic and usually based on Zip codes to set an approximate 40-mile radius of military inpatient treatment facilities. Formerly, a person living in a catchment area had to get a nonavailability statement before being treated for inpatient nonemergency care at a civilian hospital. A **nonavailability statement** (NAS) is an electronic document stating that the required service is not available at the nearby military treatment facility. The form is electronically transmitted to the DEERS database. Currently, under the 2002 National Defense Authorization Act, the requirement to obtain a NAS is eliminated, except for nonemergency impatient mental health care services. However, some MTFs have been given an exemption and may still require a NAS. Best practice is to advise TRICARE standard beneficiaries to check with the Beneficiary Counseling and Assistance Coordinator at the nearest MTF.

Preauthorization Requirements

TRICARE Standard does not require outpatient nonavailability statements for services other than outpatient prenatal and postpartum maternity care. A number of procedures do require preauthorization, including:

- Arthroscopy
- Cardiac catheterization
- Upper gastrointestinal endoscopy
- MRI
- Tonsillectomy or adenoidectomy
- Cataract removal
- Hernia repair

Compliance Guideline

Preauthorization
Most high-cost procedures need preauthorization. Medical information specialists should contact the TRICARE contractor for specific information.

TRICARE Prime

TRICARE Prime is a managed care plan similar to an HMO. Note that all active duty service members are automatically enrolled in TRICARE Prime, and do not have the option of choosing from among the additional TRICARE options.

After enrolling in the plan, individuals are assigned a **Primary Care Manager (PCM)** who coordinates and manages their medical care. The PCM may be a single military or civilian provider or a group of providers. In addition to most of the benefits offered by TRICARE Standard, TRICARE Prime offers preventive care, including routine physical examinations. Active-duty service members are automatically enrolled in TRICARE Prime. TRICARE Prime enrollees receive the majority of their health care services from military treatment facilities and receive priority at these facilities.

To join the TRICARE Prime program, individuals who are not active-duty family members must pay annual enrollment fees of $230 for an individual or $460 for a family. Under TRICARE Prime, there is no deductible, and no payment is required for outpatient treatment at a military facility. For active-duty family members, no payment is required for visits to civilian network providers, but different copayments apply for other beneficiaries, depending on the type of visit. For example, for retirees and their family members, outpatient visits with civilian providers require $12 copayments.

Note that TRICARE Prime also has a point-of-service (POS) option that patients may select. The POS option has a deductible and coinsurance requirements.

TRICARE Extra

TRICARE Extra is an alternative managed care plan for individuals who want to receive services primarily from civilian facilities and physicians rather than from military facilities. Since it is a managed care plan, individuals must receive health care services from a network of health care professionals. They may also seek treatment at military facilities, but active-duty personnel and other TRICARE Prime enrollees receive priority at those facilities, so care may not always be available.

TRICARE Extra is more expensive than TRICARE Prime, but less costly than TRICARE Standard. There is no enrollment fee, but there is an annual deductible of $150 for an individual and $300 for a family. TRICARE Extra beneficiaries pay 15 percent (5 percent less than TRICARE Standard enrollees) for civilian outpatient charges. Beneficiaries are not subject to additional charges of up to 115 percent of the allowable charge, since participating physicians agree to accept TRICARE's fee schedule.

TRICARE Reserve Select

Due to the large number of military reservists who have been called up for active duty, the Department of Defense implemented **TRICARE Reserve Select (TRS).** This program is a premium-based health plan available for purchase by certain members of the National Guard and Reserve activated on or after September 11, 2001. TRS provides comprehensive health care coverage similar to TRICARE Standard and Extra for TRS members and their covered family members.

TRICARE and Other Insurance Plans

If the individual has other health insurance coverage that is primary to TRICARE, that insurance carrier must be billed first. TRICARE is a secondary payer in almost all circumstances; among the few exceptions is Medicaid.

Many TRICARE beneficiaries purchase supplemental insurance policies to help pay deductible and cost-share or copayment fees. Most military associations offer supplementary plans, and so do private insurers. Supplemental plans are not regulated by TRICARE, so coverage varies. TRICARE is the primary payer; the purpose of a supplemental policy is simply to pick up the costs not paid by TRICARE.

TRICARE for Life

The Department of Defense offers a program for Medicare-eligible military retirees and Medicare-eligible family members called **TRICARE for Life.** Originally introduced in a trial program as TRICARE Senior Prime, TRICARE for Life offers the opportunity to receive health care at a military treatment facility to individuals age sixty-five and over who are eligible for both Medicare and TRICARE.

Thinking it Through — 12.1

For a Medicare-eligible retiree over age sixty-five, what are two advantages of enrolling in the TRICARE for Life program rather than in a comparable Medicare HMO?

In the past, individuals became ineligible for TRICARE once they reached sixty-five, and they were required to enroll in Medicare to obtain any health care coverage. Beneficiaries could still seek treatment at military treatment facilities, but only if space was available. Under TRICARE for Life, enrollees in TRICARE who are sixty-five and over can continue to obtain medical services at military hospitals and clinics as they did before they turned sixty-five. (Note, however, that TRICARE beneficiaries entitled to Medicare Part A based on age, disability, or end stage renal disease are required by law to enroll in Medicare Part B to retain their TRICARE benefits.) TRICARE for Life acts as a secondary payer to Medicare; Medicare pays first, and TRICARE pays the remaining out-of-pocket expenses. These claims are filed automatically. Enrollees do not need to submit a paper claim. Medicare pays its portion for Medicare covered services and automatically forwards the claim to WPS/TFL for processing. However, if the patient has other health insurance (OHI), the claim does not automatically cross over to TRICARE. Instead, the patient must submit a claim to WPS/TFL. The patient's Medicare Summary Notice along with a TRICARE paper claim (DD Form 2642) and the OHI's Explanation of Benefits (EOB) statement should be mailed by the patient to:

WPS/TFL
P.O. Box 7890
Madison, WI 53707-7890

Benefits are similar to those of a Medicare HMO, with an emphasis on preventive and wellness services. Prescription drug benefits are also included in TRICARE for Life. All enrollees in TRICARE for Life must be enrolled in Medicare Parts A and B and must have Part B premiums deducted from their Social Security check. (Individuals already enrolled in a Medicare HMO may not participate in TRICARE for Life.). Other than Medicare costs, TRICARE for Life beneficiaries pay no enrollment fees and no cost-share fees for inpatient or outpatient care at a military facility. Treatment at a civilian network facility requires a copay.

Billing Tip

Payers of Last Resort
TRICARE and TRICARE for Life are payers of the last resort.

Filing Claims

Participating providers file claims on behalf of patients. Claims are filed with the contractor for their region. Claims are submitted to the regional contractor based on the patient's home address, not the location of the facility. Contact information for regional contractors is available on the TRICARE website.

Individuals file their own claims when services are received from nonparticipating providers, using DD Form 2642, Patient's Request for Medical Payment. A copy of the itemized bill from the provider must be attached to the form.

The three administration regions (see Figure 12.3 on page 406) for TRICARE are TRICARE North, TRICARE South, and TRICARE West.

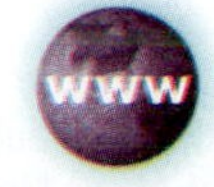

TRICARE Web Site
http://www.tricare.osd.mil

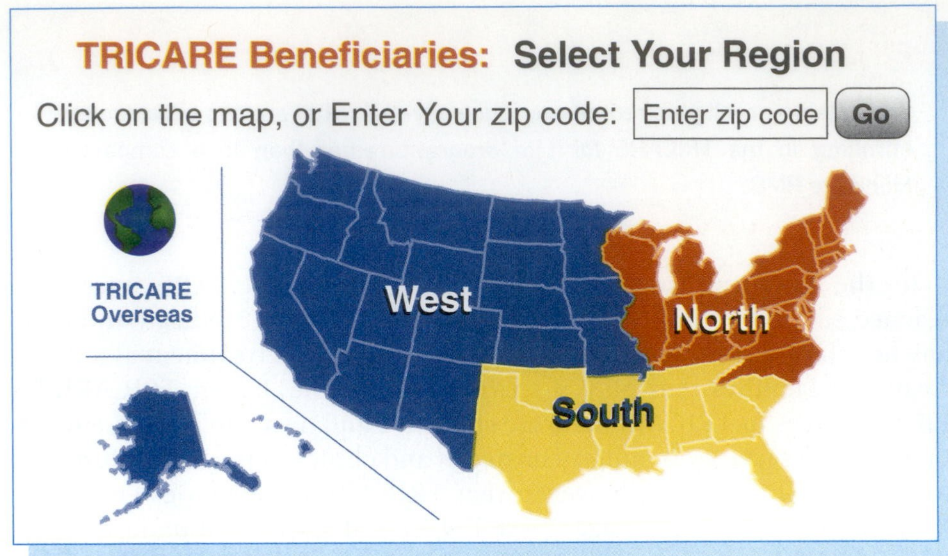

FIGURE 12.3 TRICARE Regions Map

Billing Tip

Claim Filing Deadline
TRICARE outpatient claims must be filed within one year of the date that the service was provided. For inpatient claims, the timely filing deadline is one year from the date of discharge.

HIPAA and TRICARE

The Military Health System (MHS) and the TRICARE health plan are required to comply with the HIPAA Privacy Policy and procedures for the use and disclosure of PHI. The MHS's Notice of Privacy Practices, which describes how a patient's medical information may be used and disclosed and how a patient can access the information, is posted at the TRICARE website at http://www.tricare.osd.mil.hipaa/. The HIPAA Electronic Health Care Transactions and Code Sets requirements, as well as the Security Rule, must also be followed.

Guidelines for Completing the CMS-1500

If a CMS-1500 paper claim is needed, follow the general guidelines shown in Table 12.1 and Figure 12.4 (on page 408).

Billing Tip

Payer Instructions May Vary
The NUCC instructions do not address any particular payer. Best practice for paper claims is to check with each payer for specific information required on the form.

Fraud and Abuse

The Program Integrity Office oversees the fraud and abuse program for TRICARE, working with the Office of the Inspector General Defense Criminal Investigative Service (DCIS) to identify and prosecute cases of TRICARE fraud and abuse.

TRICARE providers are also subject to a quality and utilization review similar to the process used by Medicare. A qualified independent contractor (QIC) reviews claims, documentation, and records to ensure that services were medically necessary and appropriate, that procedures were coded appropriately, and that care was up to professional medical standards.

Some examples of activities considered fraudulent include:

- Billing for services, supplies, or equipment not furnished or used by the beneficiary
- Billing for costs of noncovered services, supplies, or equipment disguised as covered items
- Billing more than once for the same service
- Billing TRICARE and the enrollee for the same services

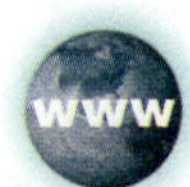

TRICARE Fraud and Abuse Link
http://www.tricare.osd.mil/fraud/

Table 12.1 TRICARE CMS-1500 (08/05) Claim Completionn

TRICARE	
Item Number	**Content**
1	Select TRICARE/CHAMPUS
1a	Sponsor's Social Security number
2	Patient's name
3	Patient's eight-digit date of birth and gender
4	Sponsor's full name, unless the sponsor is also the patient, in which case enter SAME
5	Patient's address and phone number
6	Patient's relationship to the sponsor
7	If the sponsor is on active duty, enter the duty address; if retired, the home address
8	Patient's marital and employment status
9	Enter "None"
10a–10c	If any box in 10a–10c is selected, it may be necessary to file DD Form 2527, Statement of Personal Injury—Possible Third Party Liability. If the patient was treated at a hospital for an injury possibly due to a third party, or if the patient was treated in a physician's office for a possible third-party liability injury and the charges are $500 or more, the form must be filed.
11	Enter "None"
11a–11c	Blank
11d	Choose Yes or No
12	Yes, unless there is no patient contact at the time of service—for example, if laboratory tests are conducted by an outside laboratory. In these cases, enter "Patient not present"
13–16	Blank
17–17a	Name and identification number of the referring provider or institution
18	Hospital admission and discharge dates in eight-digit format (MMDDCCYY). If the patient has been admitted but not yet discharged, enter the admission date in From, and leave To blank
19	Blank
20	Yes or No
21	Appropriate ICD codes
22	Not required
23	If a preauthorization other than a nonavailability indicator is required, attach a copy of the form
24A	Date of service (eight-digit format)
24B	Place of service code
24C	EMG: Check TRICARE contractor for information.
24D	Appropriate CPT/HCPCS codes and any modifiers
24E	Diagnosis key number for CPT/HCPCS codes
24F	Amount charged
24G	Appropriate days or units reported
24H	Blank
24I–24J	ID Qualifier/ID numbers
25	Make the appropriate selection, and enter the tax ID
26	Optional; patient account number
27	Choose Yes or No
28	Total charges
29–30	Blank
31	Check with the carrier to see if an actual signature is required
32	If the services on this claim were performed at a location other than the provider's office or the patient's home, enter the name and address of the facility; otherwise enter SAME
33	Billing provider's name, address, phone number, provider identification number, and group number

1500

HEALTH INSURANCE CLAIM FORM

APPROVED BY NATIONAL UNIFORM CLAIM COMMITTEE 08/05

PICA | PICA | CARRIER

1. MEDICARE (Medicare #) | MEDICAID (Medicaid #) | TRICARE CHAMPUS (Sponsor's SSN) [X] | CHAMPVA (Member ID#) | GROUP HEALTH PLAN (SSN or ID) | FECA BLK LUNG (SSN) | OTHER (ID)

1a. INSURED'S I.D. NUMBER (For Program in Item 1): 301694218

2. PATIENT'S NAME (Last Name, First Name, Middle Initial): RODRIGUEZ MARIE P

3. PATIENT'S BIRTH DATE MM DD YY: 01 14 1969 SEX M [ ] F [X]

4. INSURED'S NAME (Last Name, First Name, Middle Initial): RODRIGUEZ JESUS I

5. PATIENT'S ADDRESS (No., Street): 316 WASHINGTON AVE

6. PATIENT RELATIONSHIP TO INSURED: Self [ ] Spouse [X] Child [ ] Other [ ]

7. INSURED'S ADDRESS (No., Street): SAME

CITY: CLEVELAND STATE: OH

8. PATIENT STATUS: Single [ ] Married [X] Other [ ]; Employed [ ] Full-Time Student [ ] Part-Time Student [ ]

CITY | STATE

ZIP CODE: 44101-3164 TELEPHONE (Include Area Code): (555) 321 6179

ZIP CODE | TELEPHONE (INCLUDE AREA CODE) ( )

9. OTHER INSURED'S NAME (Last Name, First Name, Middle Initial)

10. IS PATIENT'S CONDITION RELATED TO:

11. INSURED'S POLICY GROUP OR FECA NUMBER: NONE

a. OTHER INSURED'S POLICY OR GROUP NUMBER

a. EMPLOYMENT? (CURRENT OR PREVIOUS) [ ] YES [X] NO

a. INSURED'S DATE OF BIRTH MM DD YY SEX M [ ] F [ ]

b. OTHER INSURED'S DATE OF BIRTH MM DD YY SEX M [ ] F [ ]

b. AUTO ACCIDENT? [ ] YES [X] NO PLACE (State)

b. EMPLOYER'S NAME OR SCHOOL NAME

c. EMPLOYER'S NAME OR SCHOOL NAME

c. OTHER ACCIDENT? [ ] YES [X] NO

c. INSURANCE PLAN NAME OR PROGRAM NAME

d. INSURANCE PLAN NAME OR PROGRAM NAME

10d. RESERVED FOR LOCAL USE

d. IS THERE ANOTHER HEALTH BENEFIT PLAN? [ ] YES [X] NO *If yes, return to and complete item 9 a-d.*

READ BACK OF FORM BEFORE COMPLETING & SIGNING THIS FORM.

12. PATIENT'S OR AUTHORIZED PERSON'S SIGNATURE I authorize the release of any medical or other information necessary to process this claim. I also request payment of government benefits either to myself or to the party who accepts assignment below.

SIGNED SIGNATURE ON FILE DATE

13. INSURED'S OR AUTHORIZED PERSON'S SIGNATURE I authorize payment of medical benefits to the undersigned physician or supplier for services described below.

SIGNED

PATIENT AND INSURED INFORMATION

14. DATE OF CURRENT: MM DD YY ILLNESS (First symptom) OR INJURY (Accident) OR PREGNANCY(LMP)

15. IF PATIENT HAS HAD SAME OR SIMILAR ILLNESS. GIVE FIRST DATE MM DD YY

16. DATES PATIENT UNABLE TO WORK IN CURRENT OCCUPATION FROM MM DD YY TO MM DD YY

17. NAME OF REFERRING PHYSICIAN OR OTHER SOURCE | 17a. | 17b. NPI

18. HOSPITALIZATION DATES RELATED TO CURRENT SERVICES FROM MM DD YY TO MM DD YY

19. RESERVED FOR LOCAL USE

20. OUTSIDE LAB? [ ] YES [X] NO $ CHARGES

21. DIAGNOSIS OR NATURE OF ILLNESS OR INJURY. (Relate Items 1,2,3 or 4 to Item 24e by Line)

1. 401.1 3. ___ . ___

2. 427.41 4. ___ . ___

22. MEDICAID RESUBMISSION CODE ORIGINAL REF. NO.

23. PRIOR AUTHORIZATION NUMBER

	24. A. DATE(S) OF SERVICE From MM DD YY	To MM DD YY	B. PLACE OF SERVICE	C. EMG	D. PROCEDURES, SERVICES, OR SUPPLIES (Explain Unusual Circumstances) CPT/HCPCS	MODIFIER	E. DIAGNOSIS POINTER	F. $ CHARGES	G. DAYS OR UNITS	H. EPSDT Family Plan	I. ID. QUAL.	J. RENDERING PROVIDER ID. #
1	10 06 2008		11		99212		1	46 00	1		NPI	
2	10 06 2008		11		93000		1, 2	70 00	1		NPI	
3											NPI	
4											NPI	
5											NPI	
6											NPI	

25. FEDERAL TAX I.D. NUMBER: 16-1246791 SSN [ ] EIN [X]

26. PATIENT'S ACCOUNT NO.: RUD210

27. ACCEPT ASSIGNMENT? (For govt. claims, see back) [X] YES [ ] NO

28. TOTAL CHARGE $ 116 00

29. AMOUNT PAID $

30. BALANCE DUE $ 80 10

31. SIGNATURE OF PHYSICIAN OR SUPPLIER INCLUDING DEGREES OR CREDENTIALS (I certify that the statements on the reverse apply to this bill and are made a part thereof.)

David Rosenberg MD

SIGNED 10/06/2008 DATE

32. SERVICE FACILITY LOCATION INFORMATION

a. NPI b.

33. BILLING PROVIDER INFO & PHONE # ( )

DAVID ROSENBERG MD

1400 WEST CENTER ST

TOLEDO OH 43601

a. NPI 12809 90812 b.

PHYSICIAN OR SUPPLIER INFORMATION

NUCC Instruction Manual available at: www.nucc.org

FIGURE 12.4 CMS-1500 (08/05) Claim Completion for TRICARE

- Submitting claims to TRICARE and other third-party payers without reporting payments already made
- Changing dates of service, frequency of service, or names of recipients
- Altering CPT codes to increase the amount of payment to the provider

Some examples of abusive activities include:

- Failure to maintain adequate clinical documentation or financial records
- Recurrent instances of waiving beneficiary cost-share payments

- Charging TRICARE beneficiaries fees that exceed those commonly charged the general public
- Recurrent instances of submitting claims for services that are not medically necessary or that are not necessary to the extent provided
- Care that is of inferior quality

Fraudulent and abusive activities can result in sanctions, exclusion from the TRICARE program, or civil or criminal penalties.

CHAMPVA

The **Civilian Health and Medical Program of the Department of Veterans Affairs (CHAMPVA)** is the government's health insurance program for veterans with 100 percent service-related disabilities and their families. Under the program, health care expenses are shared between the Department of Veterans Affairs (VA) and the beneficiary.

The Veterans Health Care Eligibility Reform Act of 1996 requires a veteran with a 100 percent disability to be enrolled in the program in order to receive benefits. Prior to this legislation, enrollment was not required.

Eligibility

The VA is responsible for determining eligibility for the CHAMPVA program. Eligible beneficiaries include:

- Dependents of a veteran who is totally and permanently disabled due to a service-connected injury
- Dependents of a veteran who was totally and permanently disabled due to a service-connected condition at the time of death
- Survivors of a veteran who died as a result of a service-related disability
- Survivors of a veteran who died in the line of duty

CHAMPVA Authorization Card

Each eligible beneficiary possesses a CHAMPVA Authorization Card, known as an A-Card. The provider's office checks this card to determine eligibility and photocopies the front and back for inclusion in the patient record.

Covered Services

CHAMPVA provides coverage for most medically necessary services. The following is a partial list of covered services:

- Inpatient services
    - Room and board
    - Hospital services
    - Surgical procedures
    - Physician services
    - Anesthesia
    - Blood and blood products
    - Diagnostic tests and procedures
    - Cardiac rehabilitation programs
    - Chemotherapy
    - Occupational therapy

Physical therapy
Prescription medications
Speech therapy
Mental health care

- Outpatient services

Maternity care
Family planning
Cancer screenings
Cholesterol screenings
HIV testing
Immunizations
Well-child care up to age six
Prescription medications
Durable medical equipment
Mental health care
Ambulance services
Diagnostic tests
Hospice services

Excluded Services

The following services are generally not covered by CHAMPVA:

- Medically unnecessary services and supplies
- Experimental or investigational procedures
- Custodial care
- Dental care (with some exceptions)

Preauthorization

Some procedures must be approved in advance; if they are not, CHAMPVA will not pay for them. It is the patient's responsibility, not the provider's, to obtain preauthorization.

Some procedures that require preauthorization are:

- Mental health and substance abuse services
- Organ and bone marrow transplants
- Dental care
- Hospice services
- Durable medical equipment in excess of $300

CHAMPVA enrollees do not need to obtain nonavailability statements, since they are not eligible to receive service in military treatment facilities. A VA hospital is not considered a military treatment facility.

Participating Providers

For most services, CHAMPVA does not contract with providers. Beneficiaries may receive care from providers of their choice, as long as those providers are properly licensed to perform the services being delivered and are not on the Medicare exclusion list. For mental health treatment, CHAMPVA maintains a list of approved providers.

Providers who treat CHAMPVA patients are prohibited from charging more than the CHAMPVA allowable amounts. Providers agree to accept CHAMPVA payment and the patient's cost-share payment as payment in full for services. Figure 12.5 (on page 412) illustrates an online CHAMPVA provider newsletter, a resource for updating CHAMPVA information in the medical practice.

Costs

Most persons enrolled in CHAMPVA pay an annual deductible and a portion of their health care charges. Some services are exempt from the deductible and cost-share requirement. A patient's out-of-pocket costs are subject to a catastrophic cap of $3,000 per calendar year. Once the beneficiary has paid $3,000 in medical bills for the year, CHAMPVA pays claims for covered services at 100 percent for the rest of that year.

In most cases, CHAMPVA pays equivalent to Medicare/TRICARE rates. The maximum amount CHAMPVA will pay for a procedure is known as the CHAMPVA Maximum Allowable Charge (CMAC). CHAMPVA has an outpatient deductible ($50 per person up to $100 per family per calendar year) and a cost-share of 25%. The cost-share percentages were 75 percent for CHAMPVA and 25 percent for the beneficiary. Beneficiaries are also responsible for the costs of health care services not covered by CHAMPVA.

CHAMPVA and Other Health Insurance Plans

When the individual has other health insurance benefits in addition to CHAMPVA, CHAMPVA is almost always the secondary payer. Two exceptions are Medicaid and supplemental policies purchased to cover deductibles, cost-shares, and other services.

Insurance claims are first filed with the primary payer. When the remittance advice from the primary plan arrives, a copy is attached to the claim that is then filed with CHAMPVA.

Persons under age sixty-five who are eligible for Medicare benefits and who are enrolled in Parts A and B may also enroll in CHAMPVA.

CHAMPVA for Life

CHAMPVA for Life extends CHAMPVA benefits to spouses or dependents who are age sixty-five and over. Similar to TRICARE for Life, CHAMPVA for Life benefits are payable after payment by Medicare or other third-party payers. Eligible beneficiaries must be sixty-five or older and must be enrolled in Medicare Parts A and B. For services not covered by Medicare, CHAMPVA acts as the primary payer.

Filing Claims

The CHAMPVA program is covered by HIPAA regulations. Most CHAMPVA claims are filed by providers and are submitted to the centralized CHAMPVA claims processing center in Denver, Colorado. The information required on a claim is the same as the information required for TRICARE.

In instances in which beneficiaries are filing their own claims, CHAMPVA Claim Form (VA Form 10-7959A) must be used. The claim must always be accompanied by an itemized bill from the provider. Claims must be filed within one year of the date of service or discharge.

Billing Tip

Secondary Claims/COB
Chapters 14 and 15 discuss processing secondary claims for TRICARE and CHAMPVA.

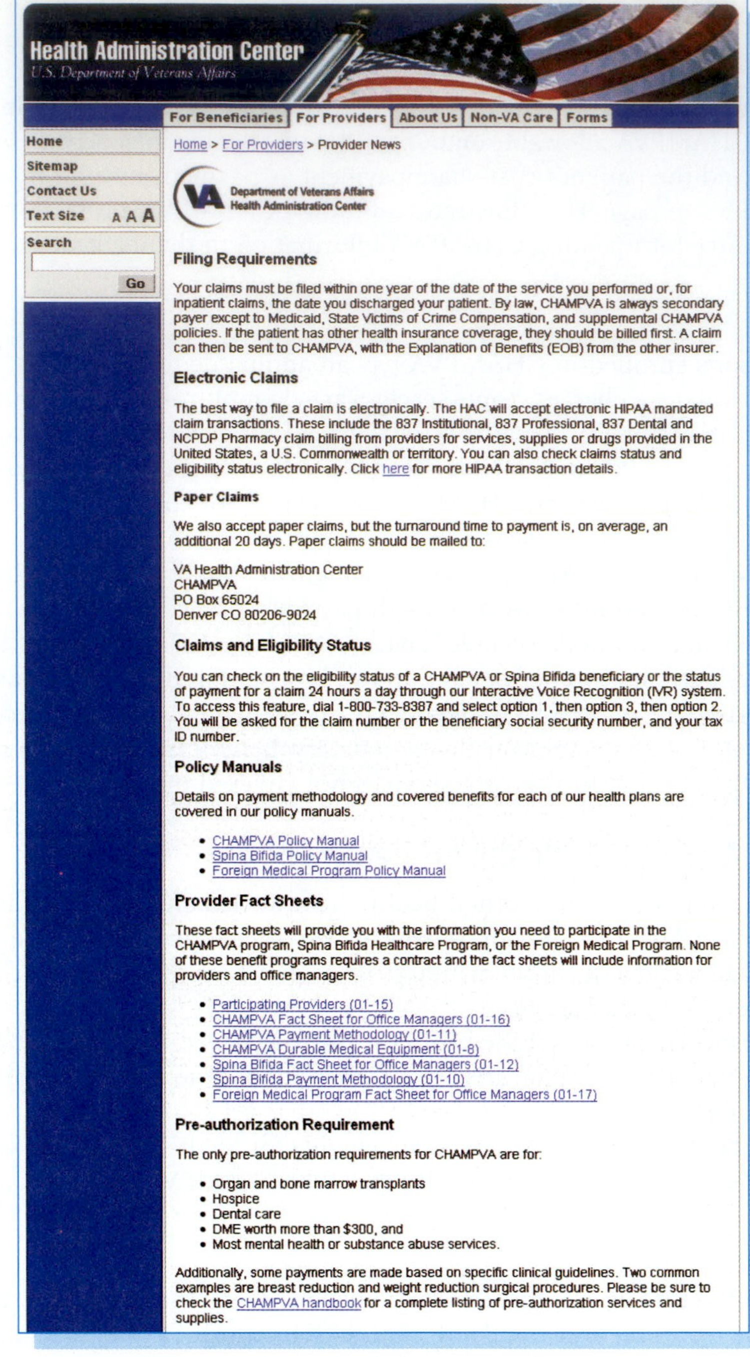

FIGURE 12.5 CHAMPVA Provider News

Review

Steps to Success

- ❒ Read this chapter and review the Key Terms and the Chapter Summary.
- ❒ Answer the Review Questions and Applying Your Knowledge in the Chapter Review.
- ❒ Access the chapter's websites and complete the Internet Activities to learn more about available professional resources.
- ❒ Complete the related chapter in the *Medical Insurance Workbook* to reinforce your understanding of TRICARE and CHAMPVA plans and billing procedures.

Chapter Summary

1. Members of the Army, Navy, Air Force, Marine Corps, Coast Guard, Public Health Service, and National Oceanic and Atmospheric Administration and their families are eligible for TRICARE. Reserve and National Guard personnel become eligible when on active duty for more than thirty consecutive days or on retirement from reserve status at age sixty.
2. Providers who participate accept the TRICARE allowable charge as payment in full for services. Participating providers are required to file claims on behalf of patients. Participating providers may appeal a decision. Nonparticipating providers may not charge more than 115 percent of the allowable charge and may not appeal a claims decision. The patient pays the provider, and TRICARE pays its portion of the allowable charges directly to the patient.
3. A nonavailability statement (NAS) is used to certify that a military treatment facility (MTF) cannot provide care for a TRICARE Standard beneficiary.
4. TRICARE Standard is a fee-for-service plan in which medical expenses are shared between TRICARE and the beneficiary. Most enrollees pay annual deductibles and cost-share percentages. TRICARE Prime is a managed care plan. After enrolling in the plan, each individual is assigned a Primary Care Manager (PCM) who coordinates and manages that patient's medical care. In addition to most of the benefits offered by TRICARE Standard, TRICARE Prime offers additional preventive care, including routine physical examinations. TRICARE Extra is also a managed care plan, but instead of services being provided primarily from military facilities, civilian facilities and physicians provide the majority of care. Individuals must receive health care services from a network of health care professionals.
5. Under the TRICARE for Life program, individuals age sixty-five and over who are eligible for both Medicare and TRICARE may continue to receive health care at military treatment facilities.
6. Individuals eligible for the CHAMPVA program include veterans who are totally and permanently disabled due to service-connected injuries, veterans who were totally and permanently disabled due to service-connected conditions at the time of death, and spouses or unmarried children of a veteran who is 100 percent disabled or who died as a result of a service-related disability in the line of duty. Under the CHAMPVA for Life program, CHAMPVA benefits are extended to individuals age sixty-five and over who are eligible for both Medicare and CHAMPVA.

Review Questions

Match the key terms with their definitions.

A. Military Treatment Facility (MTF)
B. cost-share
C. TRICARE
D. TRICARE Extra
E. TRICARE Standard
F. Defense Enrollment Eligibility Reporting System (DEERS)
G. TRICARE Prime
H. catastrophic cap
I. CHAMPUS
J. Primary Care Manager (PCM)
K. nonavailability statement
L. TRICARE for Life
M. Civilian Health and Medical Program of the Department of Veterans Affairs (CHAMPVA)
N. sponsor

____ 1. The amount of the provider charges for which the patient is responsible

____ 2. A program for individuals age sixty-five and over who are eligible for both Medicare and TRICARE that allows patients to receive health care at military treatment facilities

____ 3. A place where medical care is provided to members of the military service and their families

____ 4. The Department of Defense's new health insurance plan for military personnel and their families

____ 5. A government database that contains information about patient eligibility for TRICARE

____ 6. The government's health insurance program for veterans with 100 percent service-related disabilities and their families

____ 7. The uniformed services member whose status makes it possible for other family members to be eligible for TRICARE coverage

____ 8. An electronic document stating that the service the patient requires is not available at the local military treatment facility

____ 9. A fee-for-service program that covers medical services provided by a civilian physician when the individual cannot receive treatment from a Military Treatment Facility (MTF)

____ 10. A managed care plan in which most services are provided at civilian facilities

____ 11. A provider who coordinates and manages a patient's medical care under a managed care plan

____ 12. A managed care plan in which most services are provided at military treatment facilities

____ 13. The Department of Defense's health insurance plan for military personnel and their families that was replaced in 1998

____ 14. An annual limit on the total medical expenses that may be paid by an individual or family in one year

Decide whether each statement is true or false.

____ 1. National Guard personnel are eligible for TRICARE whether on active duty or not.

____ 2. Providers may elect to participate in TRICARE on a claim-by-claim basis.

____ 3. Providers confirm an individual's eligibility for TRICARE by accessing the Defense Enrollment Eligibility Reporting System (DEERS).

____ 4. TRICARE Standard pays a portion of charges provided by a civilian provider when treatment is not available at a military treatment facility.

____ 5. *Cost-share* is the term TRICARE uses to describe a patient's coinsurance responsibility.

____ 6. Under TRICARE Standard, preauthorization for treatment is not required.

____ 7. TRICARE Prime is more expensive than TRICARE Extra.

____ 8. Individuals enrolled in TRICARE become eligible for TRICARE for Life once they reach age sixty-five, provided they have Medicare Part A or Part B coverage.

____ 9. In most cases, CHAMPVA does not contract with providers to offer services.

____ 10. A CHAMPVA beneficiary must select a physician from a network of participating physicians.

Select the letter that best completes the statement or answers the question.

____ 1. The TRICARE plan that is an HMO and requires a PCM is
A. TRICARE Prime
B. TRICARE for Life
C. TRICARE Extra
D. TRICARE Standard

____ 2. ____ enrollees receive priority at military treatment facilities.
A. Active-duty service members
B. TRICARE Prime enrollees
C. TRICARE Extra enrollees
D. TRICARE Standard enrollees

____ 3. A TRICARE for Life beneficiary must be at least ____ years old.
A. seventy
B. twenty-one
C. sixty-five
D. thirty

____ 4. If a TRICARE Prime enrollee visits a provider outside the network, TRICARE pays _____ percent of the covered charges.
A. 80
B. 100
C. 20
D. 50

____ 5. The TRICARE health care program is a covered entity and subject to privacy rules under
A. NAS
B. HIPAA
C. TCS
D. CHAMPVA

____ 6. A person enrolled in CHAMPVA is responsible for _____ percent of covered charges.
A. 20
B. 25
C. 50
D. 60

____ 7. Nonparticipating TRICARE providers cannot bill for more than _____ percent of allowable charges.
A. 80
B. 50
C. 100
D. 115

____ 8. Active-duty service members are automatically enrolled in
A. TRICARE Prime
B. TRICARE Extra
C. CHAMPUS
D. TRICARE Standard

____ 9. For individuals enrolled in TRICARE for Life, the primary payer is
A. TRICARE
B. CHAMPVA
C. a supplementary plan
D. Medicare

____ 10. Decisions about an individual's eligibility for TRICARE are made by the
A. military treatment facility
B. provider
C. Defense Enrollment Eligibility Reporting System
D. branch of military service

Answer the following questions.

1. What is the purpose of the TRICARE program?

2. What is the priority of treatment in a military treatment facility?

Applying Your Knowledge

The objective of these exercises is to correctly complete TRICARE claims, applying what you have learned in the chapter. Following the information about the provider for the cases are two sections. The first section contains information about the patient, the insurance coverage, and the current medical condition. The second section is an encounter form for Valley Associates, P.C.

If you are using Medisoft to complete the cases, read the *Guide to Medisoft* before beginning. Information from the first section, the patient information form, has already been entered in the program for you. You must enter information from the second section, the encounter form, to complete the claim. If you are gaining experience by completing a paper CMS-1500 claim form, use the blank claim form supplied to you (from the back of the book or printed from the Student Data Template CD ROM) and follow the instructions on page 407.

The following provider information, which is also preloaded in the Medisoft database, should be used for the case studies in this chapter.

Provider Information

Name	Nancy Ronkowski, M.D.
Practice Name	Valley Associates, P.C.
Address	1400 West Center Street Toledo, OH 43601-0213
Phone	555-321-0987
Employer ID Number	06-7890123
NPI	9475830260
TRICARE PIN	TC4567
Assignment	Accepts
Signature	On File (1-1-2008)

Case 12.1

From the Patient Information Form:

Name	Robyn Janssen
Sex	F
Birth Date	02/12/1978
Marital Status	M
Employment	Part-time student; not employed
Address	310 Wilson Ave. Brooklyn, OH 44144-3456
Telephone	555-312-6649
SSN	334-62-5079
Health Plan	TRICARE
Signature	On File 01/01/08

Information About the Insured:

Insured	Lee Janssen
Patient Relationship to Insured	Spouse
Date of Birth	01/05/1978
Sex	M
Address	Box 404 Fort Dix, NJ 08442-3456
Phone	555-442-3600
SSN	602-37-0442
Insurance Plan	TRICARE
Insurance ID Number	602370442
Signature	*On File*

VALLEY ASSOCIATES, PC

Nancy Ronkowski, MD - Obstetrics & Gynecology
555-321-0987
FED I.D. #06-7890123

PATIENT NAME	APPT. DATE/TIME
Janssen, Robyn	10/13/2008 10:00 am
PATIENT NO.	**DX**
JANSSRO0	1. 626.0 absence of menstruation 2. 3. 4.

DESCRIPTION	✓	CPT	FEE	DESCRIPTION	✓	CPT	FEE
OFFICE VISITS				**PROCEDURES**			
New Patient				Artificial Insemination		58322	
LI Problem Focused		99201		Biopsy, Cervix		57500	
LII Expanded		99202		Biopsy, Endometrium		58100	
LIII Detailed		99203		Biopsy, Needle Asp., Breast		19100	
LIV Comp./Mod.		99204		Colposcopy		57452	
LV Comp./High		99205		Cyro of Cervix		57511	
Established Patient				Diaphragm Fitting		57170	
LI Minimum		99211		Endocervical Currettage		57505	
LII Problem Focused		99212		Hysteroscopy		58558	
LIII Expanded	✓	99213	62	IUD Insertion		58300	
LIV Detailed		99214		IUD Removal		58301	
LV Comp./High		99215		Mammography (Bilateral)		76092	
				Marsup. of Bartholin Cyst		56440	
CONSULTATION: OFFICE/OP				Norplant Insertion		11975	
Requested By:				Norplant Removal		11976	
LI Problem Focused		99241		Pap Smear		88150	
LII Expanded		99242		Paracervical Block		64435	
LIII Detailed		99243		Pessary Insertion		57160	
LIV Comp./Mod.		99244		Pessary Washing		57150	
LV Comp./High		99245		Polypectomy		57500	
CULTURES				**ULTRASOUND**			
Chlamydia		87072		USG, Preg Uterus, Comp.		76805	
GC Culture		87081		USG, Preg Uterus, REPT.		76815	
Herpes Culture		87250		USG, Gyn Complete		76856	
Mycoplasma/Ureoplasm		87109		USG, Gyn Limited		76857	
Urinalysis		81000		USG, Transvaginal		76830	
Urine Culture		87088					
				MISCELLANEOUS			
				Wet Mount		87210	
				Specimen Handling		99002	
				TOTAL FEES			

Case 12.2

From the Patient Information Form

Name	Sylvia Evans	*Telephone*	555-229-3614
Birth Date	06/10/1929	*SSN*	140-39-6602
Marital Status	M	*Health Plan*	TRICARE
Employment	Retired	*ID Number*	140396602
Address	13 Ascot Way Sandusky, OH 44870-1234	*Signature*	On File 06/01/08

VALLEY ASSOCIATES, PC
Nancy Ronkowski, MD - Obstetrics & Gynecology
555-321-0987
FED I.D. #06-7890123

PATIENT NAME	APPT. DATE/TIME
Evans, Sylvia	10/13/2008 3:00 pm
PATIENT NO.	**DX**
EVANSSYØ	1. 627.1 postmenopausal bleeding 2. 3. 4.

DESCRIPTION	✓	CPT	FEE	DESCRIPTION	✓	CPT	FEE
OFFICE VISITS				**PROCEDURES**			
New Patient				Artificial Insemination		58322	
LI Problem Focused		99201		Biopsy, Cervix		57500	
LII Expanded		99202		Biopsy, Endometrium		58100	
LIII Detailed		99203		Biopsy, Needle Asp., Breast		19100	
LIV Comp./Mod.		99204		Colposcopy		57452	
LV Comp./High		99205		Cyro of Cervix		57511	
Established Patient				Diaphragm Fitting		57170	
LI Minimum		99211		Endocervical Currettage		57505	
LII Problem Focused	✓	99212	46	Hysteroscopy		58558	
LIII Expanded		99213		IUD Insertion		58300	
LIV Detailed		99214		IUD Removal		58301	
LV Comp./High		99215		Mammography (Bilateral)		76092	
				Marsup. of Bartholin Cyst		56440	
CONSULTATION: OFFICE/OP				Norplant Insertion		11975	
Requested By:				Norplant Removal		11976	
LI Problem Focused		99241		Pap Smear	✓	88150	29
LII Expanded		99242		Paracervical Block		64435	
LIII Detailed		99243		Pessary Insertion		57160	
LIV Comp./Mod.		99244		Pessary Washing		57150	
LV Comp./High		99245		Polypectomy		57500	
CULTURES				**ULTRASOUND**			
Chlamydia		87072		USG, Preg Uterus, Comp.		76805	
GC Culture		87081		USG, Preg Uterus, REPT.		76815	
Herpes Culture		87250		USG, Gyn Complete		76856	
Mycoplasma/Ureoplasm		87109		USG, Gyn Limited		76857	
Urinalysis		81000		USG, Transvaginal		76830	
Urine Culture		87088					
				MISCELLANEOUS			
				Wet Mount		87210	
				Specimen Handling		99002	
				TOTAL FEES			

Case 12.3

From the Patient Information Form

Name	Eunice Walker	*Telephone*	555-772-9203
Sex	F	*SSN*	704-62-9930
Birth Date	11/03/1936	*Health Plan*	TRICARE
Marital Status	S	*ID Number*	704629930140396602
Employment	Retired	*Signature*	On File 01/01/08
Address	693 River Rd. Toledo, OH 43601-1234		

VALLEY ASSOCIATES, PC
Nancy Ronkowski, MD - Obstetrics & Gynecology
555-321-0987
FED I.D. #06-7890123

PATIENT NAME	APPT. DATE/TIME
Walker, Eunice	10/13/2008 1:00 pm
PATIENT NO.	**DX**
WALKEEU0	1. 611.72 lump in breast 2. 3. 4.

DESCRIPTION	✓	CPT	FEE	DESCRIPTION	✓	CPT	FEE
OFFICE VISITS				**PROCEDURES**			
New Patient				Artificial Insemination		58322	
LI Problem Focused		99201		Biopsy, Cervix		57500	
LII Expanded		99202		Biopsy, Endometrium		58100	
LIII Detailed		99203		Biopsy, Needle Asp., Breast		19100	
LIV Comp./Mod.		99204		Colposcopy		57452	
LV Comp./High		99205		Cyro of Cervix		57511	
Established Patient				Diaphragm Fitting		57170	
LI Minimum		99211		Endocervical Currettage		57505	
LII Problem Focused	✓	99212	46	Hysteroscopy		58558	
LIII Expanded		99213		IUD Insertion		58300	
LIV Detailed		99214		IUD Removal		58301	
LV Comp./High		99215		Mammography (Bilateral)	✓	76092	134
				Marsup. of Bartholin Cyst		56440	
CONSULTATION: OFFICE/OP				Norplant Insertion		11975	
Requested By:				Norplant Removal		11976	
LI Problem Focused		99241		Pap Smear		88150	
LII Expanded		99242		Paracervical Block		64435	
LIII Detailed		99243		Pessary Insertion		57160	
LIV Comp./Mod.		99244		Pessary Washing		57150	
LV Comp./High		99245		Polypectomy		57500	
CULTURES				**ULTRASOUND**			
Chlamydia		87072		USG, Preg Uterus, Comp.		76805	
GC Culture		87081		USG, Preg Uterus, REPT.		76815	
Herpes Culture		87250		USG, Gyn Complete		76856	
Mycoplasma/Ureoplasm		87109		USG, Gyn Limited		76857	
Urinalysis		81000		USG, Transvaginal		76830	
Urine Culture		87088					
				MISCELLANEOUS			
				Wet Mount		87210	
				Specimen Handling		99002	
				TOTAL FEES			

Internet Activities

1. Access the official government website for TRICARE: http://www.tricare.osd.mil. In the beneficiary section, select the link for information on claims. Read through the information displayed. Where do you file a claim if you live in Philadelphia, Pennsylvania? Review the information about TRICARE Prime. In particular, study any changes in beneficiaries' cost-share requirements.

2. Visit one of the regional contractors' websites, such as Humana. Click Military on the home page and then review the provider transactions that can be handled online. Is it possible to check a member deductible and catastrophic cap limit information through that site?

3. Visit the CHAMPVA home page at the Department of Veterans Affairs Health Administration Center website: http://www.va.gov/hac/. Select the link on how to file a claim, and read through the general claim filing instructions

Chapter 13

Workers' Compensation and Disability

CHAPTER OUTLINE

Occupational Safety and Health Administration

Federal Workers' Compensation Plans

State Workers' Compensation Plans

Classification of Injuries

Workers' Compensation Terminology

Workers' Compensation and the HIPAA Privacy Rule

Claim Process

Billing and Claim Management

Disability Compensation Programs

Government Programs

Preparing Disability Reports

Learning Outcomes

After studying this chapter, you should be able to:

1. **List the four federal workers' compensation plans.**
2. **Describe the two types of workers' compensation benefits that are offered by states.**
3. **List the criteria an injury must meet to be considered a covered injury or illness.**
4. **List the five classifications of work-related injuries.**
5. **List three responsibilities of the physician of record in a workers' compensation case.**
6. **Explain the difference between workers' compensation insurance and disability compensation programs.**
7. **Explain the difference between Social Security Disability Insurance (SSDI) and Supplemental Security Income (SSI).**

Key Terms

Admission of Liability
disability compensation programs
Federal Employees' Compensation Act (FECA)
Federal Insurance Contribution Act (FICA)
final report
first report of injury
independent medical examination (IME)
Notice of Contest
occupational diseases or illnesses
Occupational Safety and Health Administration (OSHA)
Office of Workers' Compensation Programs (OWCP)
physician of record
progress report
Social Security Disability Insurance (SSDI)
Supplemental Security Income (SSI)
vocational rehabilitation

Workers' compensation was developed to benefit both the employer and the employee. It provides employees who are injured on the job with compensation for their injuries, and it protects employers from liability for employees' injuries. Before workers' compensation was established in the United States in the early 1900s, injured workers' only recourse was to pursue legal action against the employer. To be successful, the employee had to prove that the employer was negligent. Cases were often difficult to prove and took years to settle. By 1947, all states required employers to purchase workers' compensation insurance.

Occupational Safety and Health Administration

The **Occupational Safety and Health Administration (OSHA)** was created by Congress in 1970 to protect workers from health and safety risks on the job. OSHA sets standards to guard against known dangers in the workplace, such as toxic fumes, faulty machinery, and excess noise. Businesses must meet health and safety standards set by OSHA. If they do not, they are subject to significant fines. Almost all employers are governed by OSHA legislation; the few exceptions include independent contractors, churches, domestic workers in private home settings, and federal employees (whose health and safety is the responsibility of the Federal Agency Programs.)

If an employee believes that the work environment is unhealthy or unsafe, the employee may file a complaint directly with OSHA. The employer is prohibited from treating the employee adversely for filing a complaint with OSHA.

Federal Workers' Compensation Plans

Work-related illnesses or injuries suffered by civilian employees of federal agencies, including occupational diseases acquired by them, are covered under various programs administered by the **Office of Workers' Compensation Programs (OWCP)**. The OWCP is part of the U.S. Department of Labor. The programs are:

- The Federal Employees' Compensation Program, which provides workers' compensation benefits to individuals employed by the federal government under the **Federal Employees' Compensation Act (FECA)**
- The Longshore and Harbor Workers' Compensation Program, which provides coverage for individuals employed in the maritime field under the Longshore and Harbor Workers' Compensation Act and for certain other classes of workers covered by extensions of the act

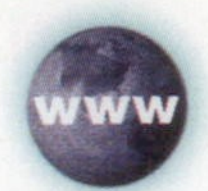

FECA Program Information

http://www.dol.gov/esa/regs/compliance/owcp/fecacont.htm

Compliance Guideline

Patient Rights
A federal worker injured on the job may select a physician from among those authorized by the OWCP. Payment is made directly to the provider based on the Medicare Fee Schedule. The patient may not be billed for excess charges beyond the allowed charge.

- The Federal Black Lung Program, under the administration of the Division of Coal Mine Workers' Compensation, which provides benefits to individuals working in coal mines under the Black Lung Benefits Act
- The Energy Employees Occupational Illness Compensation Program, which went into effect on July 31, 2001, and provides benefits under the Energy Employees Occupational Illness Compensation Program Act for workers who have developed cancer and other serious diseases because of exposure to radiation, beryllium, or silica at atomic weapons facilities or at certain federally owned facilities in which radioactive materials were used

Each program provides medical treatment, cash benefits for lost wages, vocational rehabilitation, and other benefits to workers of the employee group or industry it represents who have sustained workplace injuries or acquired occupational diseases.

State Workers' Compensation Plans

Each state administers its own workers' compensation program and has its own statutes that govern workers' compensation, so coverage varies from state to state. However, all states provide two types of workers' compensation benefits. One pays the employee's medical expenses that result from the work-related injury, and the other compensates the employee for lost wages while he or she is unable to return to work. Workers' compensation pays for all reasonable and necessary medical expenses resulting from the work-related injury.

Employers obtain workers' compensation insurance from one of the following sources: (1) a state workers' compensation fund, (2) a private plan, or (3) directly with a self-insured fund (as described in Chapter 9). Under a state fund, companies pay premiums into a central state insurance fund from which claims are paid. Many employers contract with private insurance carriers, which provide access to their networks of providers (primary care physicians, occupational medical centers, urgent care centers, physical therapy providers, chiropractors, radiology centers, orthopedists, and orthopedic surgeons and facilities).When a firm self-insures, it sets money aside in a fund that is to be used to pay workers' compensation claims. Most states require a company to obtain authorization before choosing to self-insure. Regardless of the source of workers' compensation insurance, the money that funds workers' compensation insurance is fully paid by the employer; no money is withdrawn from an employee's pay.

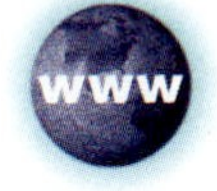

Links to States' Workers Compensation Agencies

http://www.workerscompensation.com

Employers or their insurance carriers must file proof of workers' compensation insurance with the state Workers' Compensation Board. In some states, this proof may be filed electronically through a Web-based data-entry application. In addition, the employer must post a Notice of Workers' Compensation Coverage in a place accessible to all employees. This notice must list the name, address, and telephone number of the administrator of the company's workers' compensation program.

Eligibility

Most states require public and private companies to provide workers' compensation coverage to all full-time and part-time employees, including minors. Companies that are required to carry workers' compensation insurance but fail to do so are subject to legal penalties.

The following categories of employee–employer relationships are generally not covered by state workers' compensation insurance:

- Federal employees (because they are covered under a federal program)
- Railroad employees (because they are covered under a federal program)
- Self-employed individuals
- Real estate agents working on commission
- For-hire domestic, maintenance, or repair workers hired to perform a job for a homeowner on less than a full-time basis
- Drivers under a lease agreement with a carrier, such as some long-haul truck drivers
- Prison inmates employed by the prison
- Volunteers
- Independent contractors
- Clergy and members of religious orders
- Agricultural laborers

Billing Tip

Workers' Compensation Fees
Some states have mandated the use of RVS (see Chapter 7) unit values as the schedule of fees for workers' compensation services. These states have often also set a conversion factor. Many, however, do not use RVS or the CPT codes for their fee schedules. The office may have to crosswalk from the CPT code to the workers' compensation fee schedule.

Benefits

Workers' compensation insurance covers injuries, illnesses, and job-related deaths. Injuries are not limited to on-the-job occurrences. An injury may occur while performing an off-site service for the company, such as driving to the post office on its behalf. Accidents such as falls in the company parking lot are also covered under workers' compensation rules.

Occupational diseases or illnesses develop as a result of workplace conditions or activities. These include lung disorders caused by poor air quality, repetitive motion illnesses such as carpal tunnel syndrome, and occupational hearing loss, among others. Illnesses may develop rapidly or over the course of many years.

Medical benefits are payable from the first day of the injury. Cash benefits vary from state to state and are generally not paid for the first seven days of disability. In most states, a worker must be disabled for more than seven calendar days before benefits are payable. However, if the disability extends beyond fourteen days, a worker may become retrospectively eligible for cash benefits for the first seven days. Different states have different methods of determining wage-loss benefits. Usually, the benefits are a percentage of the worker's salary before the injury. For example, it is not uncommon for workers to be compensated at two-thirds of their average weekly wage, up to a weekly maximum. The weekly maximums differ among states, as do the formulas for determining workers' average weekly wages.

When an individual is fatally injured on the job, workers' compensation pays death benefits to the employee's survivors. Funeral expenses may also be paid.

Covered Injuries and Illnesses

States determine the types of injuries that are covered under workers' compensation. Generally, an injury is covered if it meets all of the following criteria:

- It results in personal injury or death.
- It occurs by accident.
- It arises out of employment.
- It occurs during the course of employment.

An accident can be either an immediate event or the unexpected result of an occurrence over time. A worker who cuts a finger while using a box cutter is an example of an immediate accident. An employee who suffers a repetitive stress injury that developed over the course of several years is an example of an unexpected result over time.

Thinking It Through — 13.1

Joe Marino works in the mailroom of a large telecommunications company. His job requires lifting packages in excess of eighty pounds. Over the course of his employment with the company, Joe has been out on temporary disability several times because of back pain. On his way home from work last Friday, Joe stopped by the post office to drop off some personal mail. As he was walking into the post office, he slipped on an icy patch on the sidewalk and injured his back. After an examination by his physician, Joe was ordered to stay out of work for a minimum of two weeks.

Would this injury be covered under workers' compensation insurance? Provide an argument to support your position.

The following are examples of covered injuries:

- Back injuries due to heavy lifting or falls
- Repetitive stress injuries such as carpal tunnel syndrome
- Parking lot injuries such as falls
- Heat-related injuries such as heat stroke or heat exhaustion if the job requires a lot of work time in the hot sun
- Hernias if they are related to a work injury
- Personal time injuries, such as injuries that occur in the cafeteria or restroom

Some generally covered injuries may be excluded from workers' compensation, or benefits may be reduced if certain conditions were present at the time of the injury. Examples include the following:

- Employee intoxication by alcohol or illegal drugs led to the injury.
- The injury was intentionally self-inflicted.
- The employee violated the law.
- The employee failed to use safety equipment.
- The employee failed to obey safety procedures.
- The employee is also a recipient of Social Security disability benefits.
- The employee is also a recipient of unemployment insurance.
- The employee receives an employer-paid pension or disability benefit.

Classification of Injuries

Work-related injuries are grouped into five categories.

Injury Without Disability

A worker is injured on the job and requires treatment, but is able to resume working within several days. All medical expenses are paid by workers' compensation insurance.

Injury with Temporary Disability

A worker is injured on the job, requires treatment, and is unable to return to work within several days. All medical expenses are paid by workers' compensation insurance, and the employee receives compensation for lost wages. Compensation varies from state to state and is usually a percentage of the worker's salary before injury. Before an injured employee can return to work, the physician must file a doctor's **final report** indicating that he or she is fit to return to work and resume normal job activities.

Injury with Permanent Disability

A worker is injured on the job, requires treatment, is unable to return to work, and is not expected to be able to return to his or her regular job in the future. Usually this employee has been on temporary disability for an extended period of time and is still unable to resume work. When that is the case, the physician of record files a report stating that the individual is permanently disabled. The state workers' compensation office or the insurance carrier may request an additional medical opinion before a final determination is made. An impartial physician is called in to provide an **independent medical examination (IME)**. Once the IME report is submitted, a final determination of disability is made, and a settlement is reached. The length of coverage varies from state to state.

When an employee is rated as having a permanent disability, all medical expenses are paid by workers' compensation insurance, and the worker receives compensation for lost wages. The amount of compensation depends on a number of factors, including whether the disability is partial or total, the age of the employee, and the job performed before the injury. Partial disability is generally classified by percentage and varies by severity. For example, a worker who has lost the use of a hand would receive less compensation than a worker paralyzed from the waist down.

Injury Requiring Vocational Rehabilitation

A worker is injured on the job, requires treatment, and is unable to return to work without vocational rehabilitation. All medical expenses are paid by workers' compensation insurance, as are the costs of the vocational rehabilitation program. **Vocational rehabilitation** is the process of retraining an employee to return to the workforce, although not necessarily in the same position as before the injury. For example, an employee who injured his or her back working in a job that required heavy lifting may be trained for work that does not involve lifting.

Injury Resulting in Death

A worker dies as a result of an injury on the job. Death benefits are paid to survivors based on the worker's earning capacity at the time of the injury.

Workers' Compensation Terminology

Physicians who examine patients under workers' compensation coverage use a set of standardized terms to describe the effects of work-related injuries and illnesses. These widely accepted terms are used by most states and insurance carriers. Different terminology is used to describe levels of pain and the effects of injuries or illnesses.

Pain Terminology

Pain is classified as minimal, slight, moderate, or severe:

- Minimal pain is annoying but does not interfere with the individual's ability to perform the job.
- Slight pain is tolerable, but the performance of some work assignments may be impaired.

- Moderate pain is tolerable, but the performance of some work assignments will show marked impairment.
- Severe pain requires avoiding activities that lead to pain.

Disability Terminology

Disabilities due to spinal injuries, heart disease, pulmonary disease, or abdominal weakness are classified as follows:

- *Limitation to light work*: Individual may work in an upright or walking position as long as no greater than minimal effort is required.
- *Precluding heavy work*: Individual has lost 50 percent or more of the ability to lift, push, pull, bend, stoop, and climb.
- *Precluding heavy lifting, repeated bending, and stooping*: Individual has lost 50 percent of the ability to perform these activities.
- *Precluding heavy lifting*: Individual has lost 50 percent of heavy lifting ability (categorization limited to lifting and does not include bending and stooping).
- *Precluding very heavy work*: Individual has lost 25 percent of the ability to lift, push, pull, bend, stoop, and climb.
- *Precluding very heavy lifting*: Individual has lost 25 percent of the ability for very heavy lifting.

Disabilities due to lower extremity injuries are described as follows:

- *Limitation to sedentary work*: Individual is able to work while in a sitting position with minimal physical effort required. Some walking and standing is possible.
- *Limitation to semisedentary work*: Individual is able to work in a job that allows 50 percent sitting and 50 percent standing or walking, with minimal physical effort demanded.

Workers' Compensation and the HIPAA Privacy Rule

Workers' compensation cases are one of the few situations in which a health care provider may disclose a patient's protected health information (PHI) to an employer without the patient's authorization. Workers' compensation claim information is not subject to the same confidentiality rules as other medical records.

Most states allow claims adjusters and employers unrestricted access to the workers' compensation files. Likewise, at the federal level, the HIPAA Privacy Rule permits disclosures of PHI for workers' compensation purposes without the patient's authorization. Disclosure for any judicial or administrative proceeding in response to a court order, subpoena, or similar process is also allowed. Following the minimum necessary standard, covered entities can disclose information to the full extent authorized by state or other law. In addition, where PHI is requested by a state workers' compensation or other public official for such purposes, covered entities are permitted to reasonably rely on the official's representations that the information requested is the minimum necessary for the intended purpose.

Individuals do not have a right under the Privacy Rule to request that a physician restrict a disclosure of their PHI for workers' compensation purposes when that disclosure is required by law or authorized by, and necessary to comply with, a workers' compensation or similar law. However, for the physician to disclose information about a previous condition that is not directly related to the claim to an employer or insurer requires the individual's written authorization.

Claim Process

When an employee is injured on the job, the injury must be reported to the employer within a certain time period. Most states require notification in writing. Once notified, the employer must notify the state workers' compensation office and the insurance carrier, also within a certain period of time. In some cases, the employee is given a medical service order to take to the physician who provides treatment.

In most instances, the injured employee must be treated by a provider selected by the employer or insurance carrier. Some employers contract with a managed care organization for services. In these cases, the patient must be examined and treated by a physician in the managed care plan's network. If the employee refuses to comply with the request, benefits may not be granted.

Responsibilities of the Physician of Record

The physician who first treats the injured or ill employee is known as the **physician of record.** This physician is responsible for treating the patient's condition and for determining the percentage of disability and the return-to-work date. A sample workers' compensation physician's report form is displayed in Figure 13.1 on page 430.

The physician of record also files a **progress report** with the insurance carrier every time there is a substantial change in the patient's condition that affects disability status or when required by state rules and regulations (see Figure 13.2 on page 431 for a sample physician's progress report).

Providers submit their charges to the workers' compensation insurance carrier and are paid directly by the carrier. Charges are limited to an established fee schedule. Patients may not be billed for any medical expenses. In addition, the employer may not be billed for any amount that exceeds the established fee for the service provided.

Responsibilities of the Employer and Insurance Carrier

The **first report of injury** form must be filed by either the employer or the physician (under state law) within a certain time period. The amount of time varies among states; the range is normally from twenty-four hours to ten days. The form contains information about the patient, the employer, and the injury or illness. Depending on the insurance carrier, the report may be filed electronically or mailed to the carrier. A first report of injury form is displayed in Figure 13.3 on page 432.

The insurance carrier assigns a claim number to the case, determines whether the claim is eligible for workers' compensation, and notifies the employer. This determination is either an **Admission of Liability**, stating that the employer is responsible for the injury, or a **Notice of Contest**, which is a denial of liability. The worker must be informed of the outcome within a given number of days.

If the employee is eligible for compensation for lost wages, checks are sent directly to him or her, and no income taxes are withheld from the payments. If the claim is denied, the employee must pay all medical bills associated with the accident. These charges may be submitted to the individual's own health insurance carrier for payment.

Billing Tip

Workers' Compensation Diagnoses Coding
The ICD-9-CM coding must include an E code (secondary, never primary) to report the cause of the accident, such as transport, falls, and fire/flames.

HIPAA Tip

First Report of Injury Transaction Standard

The first report of injury transaction will be one of the HIPAA EDI standard transactions. The format and rules for the first report must be HIPAA-compliant after the uniform transaction standard is mandated under federal law.

Billing Tip

Workers' Compensation Global Periods
Many workers' compensation plans do not follow Correct Coding Initiative global periods. Contact the carrier to learn its global periods, and get instructions on using modifiers.

FLORIDA DEPT. OF LABOR & EMPLOYMENT SECURITY
DIVISION OF WORKERS' COMPENSATION
2728 Centerview Drive, 202 Forrest Building
Tallahassee, Florida 32399-0685

FIRST REPORT OF INJURY OR ILLNESS

For assistance call 1-800-342-1741
or contact your local EAO Office
Report all deaths within 24 hours 800-219-8953

RECEIVED BY CARRIER	SENT TO DIVISION	DIVISION REC'D DATE

PLEASE PRINT OR TYPE

EMPLOYEE INFORMATION

NAME (First, Middle, Last) | Social Security Number | Date of Accident (Month/Day/Year) | Time of Accident ☐ AM ☐ PM

HOME ADDRESS
Street/Apt #: ______
City: ______ State: ______ Zip: ______

EMPLOYEE'S DESCRIPTION OF ACCIDENT (Include Cause of Injury)

TELEPHONE Area Code Number

OCCUPATION

INJURY/ILLNESS THAT OCCURRED | PART OF BODY AFFECTED

DATE OF BIRTH ____/____/____ | SEX ☐ M ☐ F

EMPLOYER INFORMATION

COMPANY NAME: ______
D. B. A.: ______
Street: ______
City: ______ State: ______ Zip: ______

FEDERAL I.D. NUMBER (FEIN) | DATE FIRST REPORTED (Month/Day/Year)

NATURE OF BUSINESS | POLICY/MEMBER NUMBER

TELEPHONE Area Code Number

DATE EMPLOYED ____/____/____ | PAID FOR DATE OF INJURY ☐ YES ☐ NO

EMPLOYER'S LOCATION ADDRESS (If different)
Street: ______
City: ______ State: ______ Zip: ______
LOCATION # (If applicable) ______

LAST DATE EMPLOYEE WORKED ____/____/____

WILL YOU CONTINUE TO PAY WAGES INSTEAD OF WORKERS' COMP? ☐ YES

RETURNED TO WORK ☐ YES ☐ NO
IF YES, GIVE DATE ____/____/____

LAST DAY WAGES WILL BE PAID INSTEAD OF WORKERS' COMP ____/____/____

PLACE OF ACCIDENT (Street, City, State, Zip)
Street: ______
City: ______ State: ______ Zip: ______
COUNTY OF ACCIDENT ______

DATE OF DEATH (If applicable) ____/____/____

RATE OF PAY ☐ HR ☐ WK
$ ______ PER ☐ DAY ☐ MO

AGREE WITH DESCRIPTION OF ACCIDENT? ☐ YES ☐ NO

Number of hours per day ______
Number of hours per week ______
Number of days per week ______

Any person who, knowingly and with intent to injure, defraud, or deceive any employer or employee, insurance company, or self-insured program, files a statement of claim containing any false or misleading information is guilty of a felony of the third degree. I have reviewed, understand and acknowledge the above statement.

NAME, ADDRESS AND TELEPHONE OF PHYSICIAN OR HOSPITAL

______ EMPLOYEE SIGNATURE (If available to sign) ______ DATE

______ EMPLOYER SIGNATURE ______ DATE

AUTHORIZED BY EMPLOYER ☐ YES ☐ NO

CARRIER INFORMATION

☐ 1. Case Denied - DWC-12, Notice of Denial Attached ☐ 2. Medical Only which became Lost Time Case (Complete all info in #3)

☐ 3. Lost Time Case - 1st day of disability ____/____/____ Salary continued in lieu of comp? ☐ YES Salary End Date ____/____/____

Date First Payment Mailed ____/____/____ AWW ______ Comp Rate ______

☐ T.T. ☐ T.T. - 80% ☐ T.P. ☐ I.B. ☐ P.T. ☐ DEATH

REMARKS:

CARRIER NAME, ADDRESS & TELEPHONE

CARRIER CODE #	EMPLOYEE'S RISK CLASS CODE	EMPLOYER'S SIC CODE
SERVICE CO/TPA CODE #	CARRIER FILE #	

Is employer self-insured? ☐ YES ☐ NO

LES Form DWC-1 (11/94)

FIGURE 13.1 Sample Workers' Compensation First Report of Injury or Illness: Florida

State of California
Division of Workers' Compensation

Additional pages attached ❑

PRIMARY TREATING PHYSICIANS PROGRESS REPORT (PR-2)

Check the box(es) which indicate why you are submitting a report at this time. If the patient is "Permanent and Stationary" (i.e., has reached maximum medical improvement), do not use this form. You may use DWC Form PR-3 or IMC Form 81556.

❑ Periodic Report (required 45 days after last report) ❑ Change in treatment plan ❑ Discharged
☒ Change in work status ❑ Need for referral or consultation ❑ Info. requested by: ________
❑ Change in patient's condition ❑ Need for surgery or hospitalization ❑ Other:

Patient:
Last *McDonald* First *James* M.I.____ Sex *M* D.O.B *11/29/1964*
Address *3209 Ridge Rd* City *Cleveland* State *OH* Zip *44101-2345*
Occupation *Truck driver* SS # *602 - 39 - 4408* Phone *(555) 432-6049*

Claims Administrator:
Name *Janice Brown* Claim Number *WC*
Address *312 East King St* City *Toledo* State *OH* Zip *43601-1234*
Phone *(555) 999-1000* FAX *(555) 999-1001*

Employer name: *JV Trucking* Employer Phone *(555) 555-5000*

The information below must be provided. You may use this form or you may substitute or append a narrative report.

Subjective complaints:

Lower back pain

Objective findings: (Include significant physical examination, laboratory, imaging, or other diagnostic findings.)

Lower back pain when bending or lifting >10 lbs.

Diagnoses:
1. *overexertion from lifting* ICD-9 *E927*
2. ________ ICD-9 ________
3. ________ ICD-9 ________

Treatment Plan: (Include treatment rendered to date. List methods, frequency and duration of planned treatment(s). Specify consultation/referral, surgery, and hospitalization. **Identify each physician and non-physician provider.** Specify type, frequency and duration of physical medicine services (e.g., physical therapy, manipulation,acupuncture). Use of CPT codes is encouraged. Have there been any **changes** in treatment plan? If so, why?

Exam, x-rays, physical therapy, advised restricted activity.

Work Status: this patient has been instructed to:
❑ Remain off-work until ________.
☒ Return to modified work on *10/27/2008* with the following limitations or restrictions
(List all specific restrictions re: standing, sitting, bending, use of hands, etc.):
No bending
No lifting >10 lbs.
❑ Return to full duty on ________ with no limitations or restrictions.

Primary Treating Physician: (original signature, do not stamp) Date of exam: *10/24/2008*

I declare under penalty of perjury that this report is true and correct to the best of my knowledge and that I have not violated Labor Code § 139.3.

Signature: *Sarah Jamison, M.D.* Cal. Lic. # *16-1234567*
Executed at: *Valley Medical Associates* Date: *10/24/2008*
Name: *Sarah Jamison, M.D.* Specialty: *orthopedics*
Address: *1400 West Center St., Toledo, OH 43601-0123* Phone: *555-321-0987*
Next report due no later than *11/17/2008*

DWC Form PR-2 (Rev.1/1/99) **(Use additional pages, if necessary)**

FIGURE 13.2 Sample Physician's Progress Report Form: California

NEW HAMPSHIRE WORKERS' COMPENSATION MEDICAL FORM

This form must be completed at each health professional visit (MD, DO, DC or DDS) and must be filed with the worker's compensation insurance carrier within 10 days of the treatment (first aid excluded). Failure to comply and complete this form shall result in the provider not being reimbursed for services rendered and may result in a civil penalty of up to $2,500.

In compliance with RSA 281-A:23-b, the employer with 5 or more employees must provide temporary alternative/transitional work opportunities to all employees temporarily disabled by a work related injury or illness.

Employee ____________________ Employer ____________________

SS # ____________________ Work telephone # ____________________

Occupation ____________________ Employer contact ____________________

Date last worked ____________________ Employer address ____________________

W.C. insurer ____________________ ____________________

HEALTH PROFESSIONAL TO COMPLETE

☐ Initial visit ☐ Follow-up visit Date of injury ____________________ Time __________

Worker's statement of the incident ____________________

Worker's complaints ____________________

Diagnosis/Prognosis ____________________

Treatment plan ____________________

____

In your opinion is this injury and disability as a result of injury described above? ☐ Yes ☐ No ☐ Unclear

EMPLOYEE WORK CAPABILITY

☐ Continue Working Can return to work: ☐ Yes Date __________ ☐ No

☐ Full Duty ☐ With Modification. If so, for what duration? ____________________

Employee can	No Restrictions	Frequently	Occasionally	Unable to
bend				
kneel				
squat				
climb				
stand				
walk				
sit				
reach				
drive				
do fine motor				

No repetitive motions		Wrist	Elbow	Shoulder	Ankle
	Right				
	Left				

Employee can lift/carry maximally ______ lbs.

Employee can lift/carry frequently ______ lbs.

Employee can work a maximum of #___ hours/day, #___days /wk.

What special accommodations are required? ____________________

____

Other ____________________

Has employee reached maximum medical improvement?
☐ Yes ☐ No

Has injury caused permanent impairment?
☐ Yes ☐ No ☐ Undetermined

ALL MEDICAL NOTES MUST BE ATTACHED TO BILL

I certify that the narrative descriptions of the principal and secondary diagnosis and the major procedures performed are accurate and complete to the best of my knowledge.

____________________ Provider's signature ____________________ Provider's Printed name ____________________ Provider's telephone#

____________________ Federal ID# ____________________ Date of visit

MEDICAL AUTHORIZATION: The act of the worker in applying for workers' compensation benefits constitutes authorization to any physician, hospital, chiropractor, or other medical vendor to supply all relevant medical information regarding the worker's occupational injury or illness to the insurer, the worker's employer, the worker's representative, and the department. Medical information relevant to a claim includes a past history of complaints of, or treatment of, a condition similar to that presented in the claim. [281-A:23 V(a)]

75 WCA-1 (06/94) White - Insurer/Managed Care Yellow - Provider Pink - Employee/Employer

FIGURE 13.3 Sample First Report of Injury Form: New Hampshire

Termination of Compensation and Benefits

Temporary partial and temporary total disability benefits cease when one of the following occurs:

- The employee is given a physician's release authorizing a return to his or her regular job.

- The employee is offered a different job by the employer (not the same job as before the injury) and either returns to work or refuses to accept the new assignment.
- The employee has exhausted the maximum workers' compensation benefits for the injury or illness.
- The employee cannot work due to circumstances other than the work-related injury (for example, the individual is injured in an automobile accident that results in an unrelated disability).
- The employee does not cooperate with request for a medical examination. (Medical examinations determine the type and duration of the disability and the relationship of the injury to the patient's condition.)
- The employee has returned to work.
- The employee has died. (Death benefits go to survivors, however.)

Billing Tip

Turnaround Times
Track the date a workers' compensation claim is filed. Insurance carriers must pay workers' compensation claims within an amount of time, usually thirty to forty-five days, depending on the state. If the claim is not paid within the time specified, the claimant may be eligible for interest on the payment, or a late fee may apply.

Appeals

Individuals may appeal workers' compensation decisions. The first step in the appeal process is to request mediation. A mediator is an impartial individual who works with both parties to obtain a satisfactory resolution.

If mediation efforts on behalf of the injured employee fail, a hearing may be requested. A hearing is a formal legal proceeding. A judge listens to both sides and renders a decision, referred to as an order. If the employee is not satisfied with the judge's decision, the claim may be appealed at higher levels, for example, at a workers' compensation appeals board or, after that, at a state supreme court.

Compliance Guideline

Maintain Separate Files
A separate file or case number should be maintained for each workers' compensation case, even if the individual is an established patient.

Billing and Claim Management

Workers' compensation claims require special handling. The first medical treatment report on the case must be exact. If it is not, future treatments may appear unrelated to the original injury and may be denied.

When a patient makes an appointment for an injury that could have occurred on the job, the scheduler asks whether the visit is work-related. If the answer is yes, pertinent information should be collected before the office visit:

- Date of injury
- Workers' compensation carrier
- Employer at time of injury
- Patient's other insurance

The medical insurance specialist contacts the workers' compensation carrier for authorization to treat the patient before the initial visit. Note that the practice management program (PMP) captures workers' compensation and injury-related information when the patient's injury case record is created and updated.

There are no universal rules for completing a claim form. Some plans use the HIPAA 837 or the CMS-1500, while other plans have their own claim forms. Although the specific procedures vary depending on the state and the insurance carrier, the following are some general guidelines:

- Payment from the insurance carrier must be accepted as payment in full. Patients or employers may not be billed for any of the medical expenses.
- A separate file must be established when a provider treats an individual who is already a patient of the practice. Information in the patient's regular medical record (non-workers' compensation) must not be released to the insurance carrier.

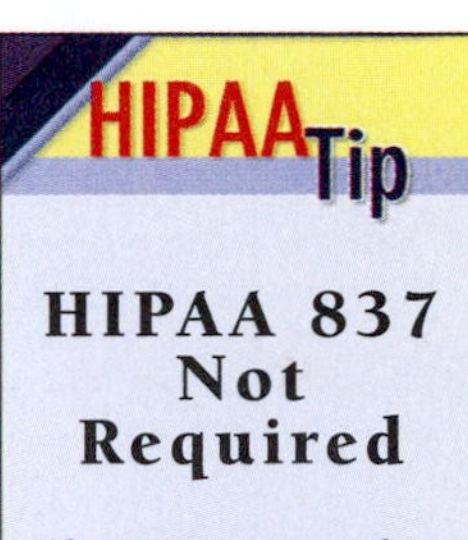

HIPAA 837 Not Required

The HIPAA mandate to file claims electronically does not cover workers' compensation plans.

Thinking It Through — 13.2

Anna Ferraro has an accident at work when the arm of her office chair gives way. She is covered by her employer's insurance. She is also a Medicare beneficiary. Should the claim connected with the accident be filed with her employer's workers' compensation carrier or with Medicare?

- The patient's signature is not required on any billing forms.
- The workers' compensation claim number should be included on all forms and correspondence.
- Use the eight-digit format when reporting dates such as the date last worked.

Disability Compensation Programs

Disability compensation programs do not provide policyholders with reimbursement for health care charges. Instead, they provide partial reimbursement for lost income when a disability—whether work-related or not—prevents the individual from working. Benefits are paid in the form of regular cash payments. Workers' compensation coverage is a type of disability insurance, but most disability programs do not require an injury or illness to be work-related in order to pay benefits.

To receive compensation under a disability program, an individual's medical condition must be documented in his or her medical record. The medical record often serves as substantiation for the disability benefits, and an inadequate or incomplete medical record may result in a denial of disability benefits. The more severe the disability, the greater the standard of medical documentation required. For this reason, an accurate and thorough medical record is of primary significance in disability cases.

Employers are not required to provide disability insurance. Many companies provide employees with disability coverage and pay a substantial amount of the premiums, but others do not. Federal or state government employees are eligible for a public disability program. Individuals not covered by employer- or government-sponsored plans may purchase disability policies from private insurance carriers.

Many individuals covered by employer-sponsored plans or private policies are also covered by a government program, such as Social Security Disability Insurance (SSDI). In these cases, the employer or private program supplements the government-sponsored coverage.

Government Programs

The federal government provides disability benefits to individuals through several different programs. The major government disability programs are:

- Workers' compensation (covered earlier in the chapter)
- Social Security Disability Insurance (SSDI)
- Supplemental Security Income (SSI)
- Federal Employees Retirement System (FERS) or Civil Service Retirement System (CSRS)
- Department of Veterans Affairs disability programs

Social Security Disability Insurance (SSDI)

The **Social Security Disability Insurance** (SSDI) program is funded by workers' payroll deductions and matching employer contributions. It provides compensation for lost wages due to disability. The employee payroll deductions are known as **Federal Insurance Contribution Act** (FICA) deductions.

The definition of disability used by the SSDI program and found in Section 223(d) of the Social Security Act lists the specific criteria that must be met:

> The inability to engage in any substantial gainful activity by reason of any medically determinable physical or mental impairment which can be expected to result in death, or, which has lasted or can be expected to last for a continuous period of not less than twelve months.

The SSDI program defines the categories of disability that are eligible for coverage. These are:

- Presumptive legal disability, which includes cases that are specifically listed in the Social Security disability manual
- Cases with more than one condition that together meet the disability standards
- Cases in which individuals cannot return to their former positions and also cannot obtain employment in the local area

Individuals also have to meet certain other criteria to be eligible for disability benefits from the SSDI program. The following individuals are eligible:

- A disabled employed or self-employed individual who is under age sixty-five and has paid Social Security taxes for a minimum number of quarters that varies according to age
- An individual disabled before reaching age twenty-two who has a parent receiving Social Security benefits who retires, becomes disabled, or dies
- A disabled divorced spouse over age fifty whose former spouse paid into Social Security for a minimum of ten years and is deceased
- A disabled widow or widower age fifty years or older whose deceased spouse paid into Social Security for at least ten years
- An employee who is blind or whose vision cannot be corrected to more than 20/200 in the better eye, or whose visual field is 20 degrees or less, even with a corrective lens

After an application for SSDI has been filed, there is a five-month waiting period before payments begin. Individuals receiving SSDI may apply for additional Medicare disability benefits twenty-four months after they become disabled.

Supplemental Security Income (SSI)

Supplemental Security Income (SSI) is a welfare program. SSI provides payments to individuals in need, including aged, blind, and disabled individuals. Eligibility is determined using nationwide standards. A person whose income and resources are under certain limits can qualify even if he or she has never worked or paid taxes under FICA. Children under age eighteen who are disabled or blind and in need may also qualify. The basic benefit is the same nationwide. Many states add money to the basic benefit.

Federal Worker Disability Programs

The Federal Employees Retirement System (FERS) provides disability coverage to federal workers hired after 1984. Employees hired before 1984 enrolled in the Civil Service Retirement System (CSRS). The FERS program consists of a federal disability program and the Social Security disability program. The two parts of the program have different eligibility rules, and some workers qualify for FERS benefits but not for SSDI benefits. If a worker is eligible for both, the amount of the SSDI payment is reduced based on the amount of the FERS payment.

The CSRS criteria of disability are not as strict as the SSDI criteria. CSRS determines that a worker is disabled if he or she is unable "because of disease or injury, to render useful and efficient service in the employee's current position and is not qualified for reassignment to a similar position elsewhere in the agency." Unlike the SSDI criteria, the CSRS criteria do not specifically mention the duration of the medical condition, although it may be expected to continue for at least a year. To qualify, a worker must have become disabled during the course of his or her federal career and must have completed at least five years of federal civilian service. Employees who are eligible for CSRS benefits are able to retain their health insurance coverage through the Federal Employee Health Benefit Program.

Veterans Programs

The Department of Veterans Affairs (VA) provides former armed services members with two disability programs: the Veteran's Compensation Program and the Veteran's Pension Program. Certain veterans may qualify to receive benefits from both. The Veteran's Compensation Program provides coverage for individuals with permanent and total disabilities that resulted from service-related illnesses or injuries. In order for a veteran to be eligible for benefits, the disability must affect his or her earning capacity.

The Veteran's Pension Program provides benefits to veterans who are not and will not be able to obtain gainful employment. The disability must be service-related and must be permanent and total.

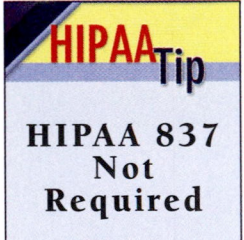

HIPAA 837 Not Required

The HIPAA mandate to file claims electronically does not cover disability claims.

Preparing Disability Reports

When a request is made for a medical report to support a disability claim, the physician or a member of the staff prepares the report by abstracting information from the patient's medical record. It is important to thoroughly document each examination by the physician. In many cases, an incomplete or inadequate medical report leads to denial of a disability claim.

The report for a disability claim should include the following medical information:

- Medical history
- Subjective complaints
- Objective findings
- Diagnostic test results
- Diagnosis
- Treatment
- Description of patient's ability to perform work-related activities

Supporting documents, such as X-rays, pulmonary function tests, range of motion tests, and ECGs, should also be included when appropriate.

Disability claim forms must be completed fully and accurately and must be supported by thorough and accurate medical reports.

Two possible ways of billing the time spent on preparing disability and workers' compensation claims are as follows:

1. Bill CPT code 99080 with the correct evaluation and management (E/M) office visit code. This code, which must be reported in conjunction with another service, covers the time required to complete insurance forms that convey more than a standard reporting form.
2. Bill CPT codes 99455–99456. In addition to covering medical disability examinations (initial and interval) these codes include the time required to complete corresponding reports and documentation. If this service is mandated, the use of a –32 modifier is appropriate.

Billing Tip

Do not report 99455 or 99456 together with 99080 for completion of workers' compensation claims.

Review

Steps to Success

- ❒ Read this chapter and review the Key Terms and the Chapter Summary.
- ❒ Answer the Review Questions and Applying Your Knowledge in the Chapter Review.
- ❒ Access the chapter's websites and complete the Internet Activities to learn more about available professional resources.
- ❒ Complete the related chapter in the *Medical Insurance Workbook* to reinforce your understanding of workers' compensation and disability plans and billing procedures.

Chapter Summary

1. The workers' compensation plans that provide coverage to federal government employees are the Federal Employees' Compensation Program, the Longshore and Harbor Workers' Compensation Program, the Federal Black Lung Program, and the Energy Employees Occupational Illness Compensation Program.
2. States provide two types of workers' compensation benefits. One pays the worker's medical expenses that result from work-related illness or injury, and the other pays for lost wages while the worker is unable to return to work.
3. For an injury to be covered under a workers' compensation plan, it must (a) result in personal injury or death, (b) occur by accident, (c) arise out of employment, and (d) occur during the course of employment.
4. Work-related injuries are classified as (a) injury without disability, (b) injury with temporary disability, (c) injury with permanent disability, (d) injury requiring vocational rehabilitation, and (e) injury resulting in death.
5. The physician of record in a workers' compensation case is responsible for treating the injured worker, determining the percentage of disability, determining the return-to-work date, and filing progress notes.
6. Workers' compensation insurance pays an employee's medical bills that result from a job-related injury; disability compensation programs do not pay medical expenses. Workers' compensation insurance provides coverage for illnesses and injuries that are job-related. Most disability compensation programs provide benefits for injuries or illnesses that are not work-related.
7. Social Security Disability Insurance (SSDI) provides compensation for lost wages to individuals who have contributed to Social Security through FICA payroll taxes. Supplemental Security Income (SSI) is a welfare program that provides financial assistance to individuals in need, including aged, blind, and disabled individuals.

Review Questions

Match the key terms with their definitions.

A. Federal Insurance Contribution Act (FICA)

B. Notice of Contest

C. occupational diseases or illnesses

____ 1. Employee payroll deductions that are used to partially fund Social Security Disability Insurance (SSDI)

____ 2. The government agency that administers workers' compensation programs for civilian employees of federal agencies

____ 3. Programs that provide reimbursement for lost income that occurs due to a disability that prevents the individual from working, whether the injury is work-related or not

D. Office of Workers' Compensation Programs (OWCP)

E. Social Security Disability Insurance (SSDI)

F. final report

G. Federal Employees' Compensation Act (FECA)

H. Occupational Safety and Health Administration (OSHA)

I. first report of injury

J. Admission of Liability

K. Supplemental Security Income (SSI)

L. disability compensation programs

M. physician of record

N. progress reports

____ 4. Legislation that provides workers' compensation benefits to individuals employed by the federal government

____ 5. Determination that the employer is responsible for the worker's injury or illness

____ 6. Agency set up by Congress in 1970 to protect workers from health and safety risks on the job

____ 7. Program funded by workers' payroll deductions and matching employer contributions that provides compensation for lost wages due to disability

____ 8. Illnesses that develop as a result of workplace conditions or activities

____ 9. A document indicating that an individual is fit to return to work and resume normal job activities

____10. The physician who first treats an injured or ill employee

____11. A welfare program that provides financial assistance to individuals in need, including aged, blind, and disabled individuals

____12. Documents filed with the insurance carrier when there is a substantial change in the patient's condition that affects the status of an occupational illness

____13. A determination that the employer is not liable for the worker's injury or illness

____14. A document that contains information about the patient, the employer, and the injury or illness that must be filed by the employer, often within twenty-four hours of the incident

Decide whether each statement is true or false.

____ 1. A physician who treats a patient covered by workers' compensation insurance may not charge the patient for any amount of the medical expenses.

____ 2. Social Security Disability Insurance (SSDI) is a welfare program.

____ 3. The Federal Employees' Compensation Act (FECA) was created to protect workers from health and safety risks on the job.

____ 4. A disability classified as a limitation to semisedentary work allows an individual to work at a position that requires 50 percent standing and 50 percent walking.

____ 5. Federal Insurance Contribution Act (FICA) payroll deductions provide partial funding for Social Security Disability Insurance (SSDI).

____ 6. Most states require corporations that meet established financial standards to obtain authorization to become self-insured against workers' compensation claims.

____ 7. Workers' compensation insurance does not cover injuries that occur in the company parking lot or cafeteria.

____ 8. Individuals classified as permanently disabled receive compensation for lost wages and paid medical treatment for the work-related illness or injury.

____ 9. The physician of record is the provider who initially treats the injured or ill worker.

____ 10. Occupational illnesses that develop over time are generally not covered by workers' compensation insurance.

Select the letter that best completes the statement or answers the question.

____ 1. Once an application for Social Security Disability Insurance (SSDI) is filed, there is a ______ waiting period before benefits begin.
A. thirty day
B. five month
C. fourteen day
D. one month

____ 2. A ______ is a denial of employer liability issued by the workers' compensation insurance carrier.
A. First Report of Liability
B. Notice of Contest
C. No-Fault Notice
D. Denial of Finding

____ 3. An individual with a disability described as precluding heavy work has lost ______ of the capacity to push, pull, bend, stoop, and climb.
A. 20 percent
B. 25 percent
C. 90 percent
D. 50 percent

____ 4. Before an injured employee can return to work, a physician must write
A. a progress report
B. a doctor's final report
C. an admission of liability report
D. a final report of injury

____ 5. ______ provides workers' compensation insurance coverage to employees of the federal government.
A. Office of Workers' Compensation Programs (OWCP)
B. Federal Insurance Contribution Act (FICA)
C. Supplemental Security Income (SSI)
D. Federal Employees' Compensation Act (FECA)

____ 6. The classifications of pain used in workers' compensation claims are
A. minimal, moderate, severe
B. slight, moderate, major, severe
C. minimal, slight, moderate, severe
D. minimal, slight, major, severe

____ 7. A disability that limits a worker to jobs that are performed in an upright or standing position and that require no greater than minimal effort are classified as
A. precluding very heavy work
B. limitation to light work
C. limitation to semisedentary work
D. precluding heavy lifting, repeated bending, and stooping

____ 8. Vocational rehabilitation programs provide ______ for individuals with job-related disabilities.
A. physical therapy
B. compensation for lost wages
C. training in a different job
D. payment for medical expenses

____ 9. For a disabled widow or widower age fifty years or older to qualify for Social Security Disability Insurance (SSDI), his or her spouse must have paid into Social Security for at least
A. six months
B. one year
C. five years
D. ten years

____10. An employee who believes the work environment to be dangerous may file a complaint with the
A. Office of Workers' Compensation Programs
B. local Social Security office
C. Occupational Safety and Health Administration
D. Workers' Compensation Board in the state in which the company is headquartered

Answer the following questions.

1. How do the criteria for disability differ in the Social Security Disability Insurance (SSDI) program and the Civil Service Retirement System (CSRS) program?

2. What criteria does an injury or illness have to meet to be eligible for workers' compensation coverage?

Applying Your Knowledge

The objective of these exercises is to correctly complete workers' compensation claims, applying what you have learned in the chapter. Each case has two sections. The first section contains information about the patient, the insurance coverage, and the current medical condition. The second section is an encounter form for Valley Associates, P.C.

If you are using Medisoft to complete the cases, read the *Guide to Medisoft* before beginning. Information from the first section, the patient information form, has already been entered in the program for you. You must enter information from the second section, the encounter form, to complete the claim. If you are gaining experience by completing a paper CMS-1500 claim form, use the blank claim form supplied to you (from the back of the book or printed from the Student Data Template CD ROM) and follow the billing notes on pages 433–434.

The following provider information, which is also available in the Medisoft database, should be used for Cases 13.1 and 13.2.

Provider Information

Name	Sarah Jamison, M.D.
Practice Name	Valley Associates, P.C.
Address	1400 West Center Street Toledo, OH 43601-0213
Telephone	555-321-0987
Employer ID Number	07-2345678
NPI	5544882211
Commercial PIN	CP1234
Assignment	Accepts
Signature	On File (1-1-2008)

Case 13.1

From the Patient Information Form

Name	Frank Puopolo
Sex	M
Birth Date	05/17/1963
Marital Status	M
Address	404 Belmont Place Sandusky, OH 44870-8901
Telephone	555-330-6467
SSN	239-04-9372
Health Plan	CarePlus Workers' Compensation
Insurance ID Number	2090462-37
Group Number	OH111
Employment Status	Full-time
Employer	JV Trucking
Condition Related to:	
Employment?	Yes
Auto Accident?	No
Other Accident?	No
Date of Current Illness, Injury, LMP	6/2/2008
Dates Patient Unable to Work	6/2/2008
Date of Hospitalization	6/2/2008

VALLEY ASSOCIATES, PC
Sarah Jamison, MD - Orthopedic Medicine
555-321-0987
FED I.D. #07-2345678

PATIENT NAME	APPT. DATE/TIME
Puopolo, Frank	06/02/2008 12:00 pm
PATIENT NO.	**DX**
PUOPOFRØ	1. 823.22 fracture, shaft, closed, tibia 2. and fibula 3. 4.

DESCRIPTION	✓	CPT	FEE	DESCRIPTION	✓	CPT	FEE
OFFICE VISITS				**FRACTURES**			
New Patient				Clavicle		23500	
LI Problem Focused		99201		Scapula		23570	
LII Expanded		99202		Humerus, proximal		23600	
LIII Detailed		99203		Humerus, shaft		24500	
LIV Comp./Mod.		99204		Radial, colles w/manip		25605	
LV Comp./High		99205		Radial, h or n w/out manip		24650	
Established Patient				Ulna, proximal		24670	
LI Minimum		99211		Radius & Ulna		25560	
LII Problem Focused		99212		Radius, colles, distal		25600	
LIII Expanded		99213		Ulna, styloid		25650	
LIV Detailed		99214		Hand MC		26600	
LV Comp./High		99215		Finger/Thumb		26720	
				Coccyx		27200	
CONSULTATION: OFFICE/OP				Femur, distal		27508	
Requested By:				Tibia prox/plateua		27530	
LI Problem Focused		99241		Tibia & Fibula, shaft	✓	27750	681
LII Expanded		99242		Fibula, prox/shaft		27780	
LIII Detailed		99243		Foot, MT		28470	
LIV Comp./Mod.		99244		Toe, great		28490	
LV Comp./High		99245		Toe, others		28510	
				X-RAY			
EMG STUDIES				Clavicle		73000	
EMG - 1 extremity		95860		Humerus		73060	
EMG - 2 extremities		95861		Forearm		73090	
EMG - 3 extremities		95863		Hand, 2 views		73120	
Nerve Conduct, M w/out F		95900		Hand, 3 views		73130	
Nerve Conduct, M w/ F		95903		Fingers		73140	
Nerve Conduct, sensory		95904		Femur		73550	
				Tibia & Fibula	✓	73590	89
				Foot, 2 views		73620	
				Foot, 3 views		73630	
				Toes		73660	
				TOTAL FEES			

Case 13.2

From the Patient Information Form

Name	Marilyn Grogan
Sex	F
Birth Date	03/21/1959
Marital Status	M
Address	23 Brookside Drive Alliance, OH 44601-1234
Telephone	555-729-4416
SSN	139-46-0589
Health Plan	CarePlus Workers' Compensation
Insurance ID Number	627422-19
Group Number	OH6319
Employment Status	Full-time
Employer	Microtech, Inc.
Condition Related to:	
Employment?	Yes
Auto Accident?	No
Other Accident?	No
Date of Current Illness, Injury, LMP	3/6/2008
Dates Patient Unable to Work	3/6/2008–3/10/2008 (no hospitalization)

VALLEY ASSOCIATES, PC

Sarah Jamison, MD - Orthopedic Medicine
555-321-0987
FED I.D. #07-2345678

PATIENT NAME	APPT. DATE/TIME
Grogan, Marilyn	03/06/2008 10:30 am
PATIENT NO.	**DX**
GROGAMA0	1. 810.0 fracture, closed, clavicle 2. 3. 4.

DESCRIPTION	✓	CPT	FEE	DESCRIPTION	✓	CPT	FEE
OFFICE VISITS				**FRACTURES**			
New Patient				Clavicle	✓	23500	1349
LI Problem Focused		99201		Scapula		23570	
LII Expanded		99202		Humerus, proximal		23600	
LIII Detailed		99203		Humerus, shaft		24500	
LIV Comp./Mod.		99204		Radial, colles w/manip		25605	
LV Comp./High		99205		Radial, h or n w/out manip		24650	
Established Patient				Ulna, proximal		24670	
LI Minimum		99211		Radius & Ulna		25560	
LII Problem Focused		99212		Radius, colles, distal		25600	
LIII Expanded		99213		Ulna, styloid		25650	
LIV Detailed		99214		Hand MC		26600	
LV Comp./High		99215		Finger/Thumb		26720	
				Coccyx		27200	
CONSULTATION: OFFICE/OP				Femur, distal		27508	
Requested By:				Tibia prox/plateua		27530	
LI Problem Focused		99241		Tibia & Fibula, shaft		27750	
LII Expanded		99242		Fibula, prox/shaft		27780	
LIII Detailed		99243		Foot, MT		28470	
LIV Comp./Mod.		99244		Toe, great		28490	
LV Comp./High		99245		Toe, others		28510	
				X-RAY			
EMG STUDIES				Clavicle	✓	73000	82
EMG - 1 extremity		95860		Humerus		73060	
EMG - 2 extremities		95861		Forearm		73090	
EMG - 3 extremities		95863		Hand, 2 views		73120	
Nerve Conduct, M w/out F		95900		Hand, 3 views		73130	
Nerve Conduct, M w/ F		95903		Fingers		73140	
Nerve Conduct, sensory		95904		Femur		73550	
				Tibia & Fibula		73590	
				Foot, 2 views		73620	
				Foot, 3 views		73630	
				Toes		73660	
				TOTAL FEES			

Internet Activities

1. Using a search engine, locate the home page of the federal Office of Workers' Compensation Programs. Click the link for OWCP Press Releases, and read some of the latest information. Click the link for Information About OWCP to read more about the Office of Workers' Compensation Programs.

2. Search for the workers' compensation website for your state. If you prefer, you may try entering the URL for your state: http://www.state.oh.us where "oh" is the two-letter abbreviation for your state (in this example, Ohio), and then locate workers' compensation information from there. What are your state's requirements for workers' compensation coverage? Try to locate a sample claim form for your state.

3. Research the Social Security Administration's online publications that are located at http://www.ssa.gov/pubs. Read the material in Part 1—General Information of an electronic booklet entitled "If You Are Blind or Have Low Vision—How We Can Help" under the heading Disability Benefits to learn about the differences between SSDI and SSI.

Part 5 Payment Processing

Chapter 14
Payments (RAs/EOBs), Appeals, and Secondary Claims

Chapter 15
Patient Billing and Collections

5

Chapter 14

Payments (RAs/EOBs), Appeals, and Secondary Claims

CHAPTER OUTLINE

Claim Adjudication

Monitoring Claim Status

The Remittance Advice/Explanation of Benefits (RA/EOB)

Reviewing and Processing RAs/EOBs

Appeals, Postpayment Audits, Overpayments, and Grievances

Billing Secondary Payers

Learning Outcomes

After studying this chapter, you should be able to:

1. Describe the steps payers follow to adjudicate claims.
2. List ten checks that automated medical edits perform.
3. Describe the procedures for following up on claims after they are sent to payers.
4. Identify the types of codes and other information contained on an RA/EOB.
5. List the points that are reviewed on an RA/EOB.
6. Explain the process for posting payments and managing denials.
7. Describe the purpose and general steps of the appeal process.
8. Discuss how appeals, postpayment audits, and overpayments may affect claim payments.
9. Describe the procedures for filing secondary claims.
10. Discuss procedures for complying with the Medicare Secondary Payer (MSP) program.

Key Terms

adjudication
aging
appeal
appellant
autoposting
claim adjustment group codes (GRP)
claim adjustment reason codes (RC)
claimant
claim status category codes
claim status codes
claim turnaround time
concurrent care
determination
development
electronic funds transfer (EFT)
explanation of benefits (EOB)
grievance
HIPAA X12 835 Health Care Payment and Remittance Advice (HIPAA 835)
HIPAA X12 276/277 Health Care Claim Status Inquiry/Response (HIPAA 276/277)
insurance aging report
medical necessity denial
Medicare Outpatient Adjudication remark codes (MOA)
Medicare Redetermination Notice (MRN)
Medicare Secondary Payer (MSP)
overpayments
pending
prompt-pay laws
RA/EOB
reconciliation
redetermination
remittance advice (RA)
remittance advice remark codes (REM)
suspended

Claim follow-up and payment processing are important procedures in billing and reimbursement. Medical insurance specialists track claims that are due, process payments, check that claims are correctly paid, and file claims with secondary payers. These procedures help generate maximum appropriate reimbursement from payers for providers.

Claim Adjudication

When the payer receives claims, it issues an electronic response to the sender showing that the transmission has been successful. Each claim then undergoes a process known as **adjudication**, made up of steps designed to judge how it should be paid:

1. Initial processing
2. Automated review
3. Manual review
4. Determination
5. Payment

Initial Processing

Each claim's data elements are checked by the payer's front-end claims processing system. Paper claims and any paper attachments are date-stamped and entered into the payer's computer system, either by data-entry personnel or by the use of a scanning system. Initial processing might find such problems as the following:

- The patient's name, plan identification number, or place of service code is wrong.
- The diagnosis code is missing or is not valid for the date of service.
- The patient is not the correct sex for a reported gender-specific procedure code.

Claims with errors or simple mistakes are rejected, and the payer transmits instructions to the provider to correct errors and/or omissions and to re-bill the

Billing Tip

Minor Errors on Transmitted Claims
When the practice finds or is notified about a minor error—such as a data-entry mistake or an incorrect place of service—it can usually be corrected by asking the payer to re-open the claim and make the changes.

Billing Tip

Proof of Timely Filing

- Payers may reduce payment for or deny claims filed after their deadline. Different payers may have different timelines; be familiar with the rules of each payer. Usually, providers cannot bill patients if they have missed the payer's submission deadline.
- Practice management programs create a tamper-proof record of the filing date of every claim that can be used to prove timely filing.

service. The medical insurance specialist should respond to such a request as quickly as possible by supplying the correct information and, if necessary, submitting a clean claim that is accepted by the payer for processing.

Automated Review

Payers' computer systems then apply edits that reflect their payment policies. For example, a Medicare claim is subject to the Correct Coding Initiative (CCI) edits (see Chapters 7 and 10). The automated review checks for the following:

1. *Patient eligibility for benefits:* Is the patient eligible for the services that are billed?
2. *Time limits for filing claims:* Has the claim been sent within the payer's time limits for filing claims? The time limit is generally between 90 and 180 days from the date of service.
3. *Preauthorization and referral:* Are valid preauthorization or referral numbers present as required under the payer's policies? Some authorizations are for specific dates or number of service, so these data will be checked, too.
4. *Duplicate dates of service:* Is the claim billing for a service on the same date that has already been adjudicated?
5. *Noncovered services*: Are the billed services covered under the patient's policy?
6. *Valid code linkages*: Are the diagnosis and procedure codes properly linked for medical necessity?
7. *Bundled codes:* Have surgical code bundling rules and global periods been followed?
8. *Medical review:* Are the charges for services that are not medically necessary or that are over the frequency limits of the plan? The payer's medical director and other professional medical staff have a medical review program to ensure that providers give patients the most appropriate care in the most cost-effective manner. The basic medical review edits that are done at this stage are based on its guidelines.
9. *Utilization review:* Are the hospital-based health care services appropriate? Are days and services authorized consistent with services and dates billed?
10. *Concurrent care*: If concurrent care is being billed, was it medically necessary? **Concurrent care** refers to medical situations in which a patient receives extensive care from two or more providers on the same date of service. For example, both a nephrologist and a cardiologist would attend a hospitalized patient with kidney failure who has had a myocardial infarction. Instead of one provider's working under the direction of another, such as the relationship between a supervising surgeon and an anesthesiologist, in concurrent care each provider has an independent role in treating the patient. When two providers report services as attending physicians, rather than as one attending and one consulting provider, a review is done to determine whether the concurrent care makes sense given the diagnoses and the providers' specialties.

Manual Review

If problems result from the automated review, the claim is **suspended** and set aside for **development**—the term used by payers to indicate that more information is needed for claim processing. These claims are sent to the medical review department, where a claims examiner reviews the claim. The examiner may ask the provider for clinical documentation to check:

- Where the service took place
- Whether the treatments were appropriate and a logical outcome of the facts and conditions shown in the medical record
- That services provided were accurately reported

Claims examiners are trained in the payer's payment policies, but they usually have little or no clinical medical background. When there is insufficient guidance on the point in question, examiners may have it reviewed by staff medical professionals—nurses or physicians—in the medical review department. This step is usually followed, for example, to review the medical necessity of an unlisted procedure.

Compliance Guideline

Documentation is Essential
If proper and complete documentation is not provided on time when requested during a manual review, claim denial or downcoding may result, with the risk for an investigation or audit. Supply both the date-of-service record and any applicable patient or treatment information to support the facts that the service was provided as billed, was medically necessary, and has been correctly coded.

Example

As an example, the following table shows the benefit matrix—a grid of benefits and policies—for a preferred provider organization's coverage of mammography.

BENEFIT MATRIX		
FEMALE PATIENT AGE GROUP	**IN-NETWORK**	**OUT-OF-NETWORK**
35–39 One baseline screening	No charge	20 percent per visit after deductible
40–49 One screening every two years, or more if recommended	No charge	20 percent per visit after deductible
50 and older One screening every year	No charge	10 percent per visit after deductible

- *Initial processing*: The payer's initial claim processing checks that the patient for whom a screening mammogram is reported is a female over age thirty-five.
- *Automated review*: The payer's edits reflect its payment policy for female patients in each of the three age groups. If a claim reports a single screening mammogram for a forty-five-year-old in-network patient within a twenty-four-month period, it passes the edit. If the claim contains two mammograms in fewer than twenty-four months, the edit would flag the claim for manual review by the claims examiner.
- *Manual review*: If two mammograms are reported within a two-year period for a patient in the forty- to forty-nine-year age range, the claims examiner would require documentation that the extra procedure was recommended and then review the reason for the recommendation. If an X-ray is included as a claim attachment, the claims examiner would probably ask a staff medical professional to evaluate the patient's condition and judge the medical necessity for the extra procedure.

Billing Tip

Medical Necessity Denials
Understand payers' regulations on medical necessity denials. Often, when claims are denied for lack of medical necessity, fees cannot be recovered from patients. For example, the participation contract may prohibit balance billing when a claim is denied for lack of medical necessity unless the patient agreed in advance to pay.

Determination

For each service line on a claim, the payer makes a payment **determination**—a decision whether to (1) pay it, (2) deny it, or (3) pay it at a reduced level. If the service falls within normal guidelines, it will be paid. If it is not reimbursable, the item on the claim is denied. If the examiner determines that the service was at too high a level for the diagnosis, a lower-level code is assigned. When the level of service is reduced, the examiner has downcoded the service (see also Chapter 7). A **medical necessity denial** may result from a lack of clear, correct linkage between the diagnosis and procedure. A medical necessity denial can also happen when a higher level of service was provided without first trying a lower, less invasive procedure. Some payers or polices require a patient to fail less invasive or more conservative treatment before more intense services are covered.

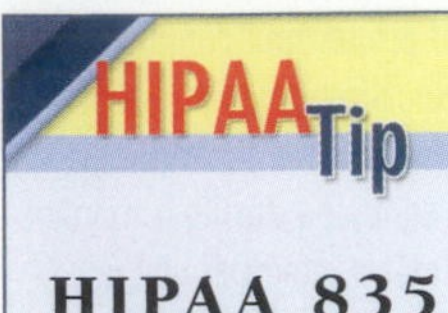

HIPAA 835

The HIPAA X12 835 Health Care Payment and Remittance Advice (HIPAA 835) is the HIPAA-mandated electronic transaction for payment explanation.

Payment

If payment is due, the payer sends it to the provider along with a **remittance advice (RA)** or electronic remittance advice (ERA), a transaction that explains the payment decisions to the provider. In most cases, if the claim has been sent electronically, this transaction is also electronic; but it may sometimes be paper. An older term that now usually refers to the paper document is **explanation of benefits (EOB)**. When the general term **RA/EOB** is used in this text, it means both formats.

Thinking It Through — 14.1

A payer's utilization guidelines for preventive care and medical services benefits are shown below.

SERVICE	*UTILIZATION*
Pediatric:	
Birth–1 year	Six exams
1–5 years	Six exams
6–10 years	One exam every two years
11–21 years	One exam
Adult:	
22–29 years	One exam every 5 years
30–39 years	One exam every 3 years
40–49 years	One exam every 2 years
+50 years	One exam every year
Vision Exam	Covered once every 24 months
Gynecological	Covered once every year
Medical Office Visit	No preset limit
Outpatient Therapy	60 consecutive days per condition/year
Allergy Services	Maximum benefit: 60 visits in 2 years

If a provider files claims for each of the following cases, what is the payer's likely response? (Research the CPT codes in the current CPT before answering.) Explain your answers. An example is provided.

PATIENT	AGE	CPT CODE	DOS	PAYER RESPONSE?
Case Example: Patient X	*45*	*99212*	*11/09/2008*	*Pay the claim, because unlimited medical office visits are covered.*
1. Guy Montrachez	25	92004	11/08/2008	
2. Carole Regalle	58	99385	12/04/2008	
3. Mary Hiraldo	25	99385 and 88150 88150	11/08/2008 12/10/2008	
4. George Gilbert	48	99386 99386	10/20/2007 11/02/2008	

Monitoring Claim Status

Practices closely track their accounts receivable (A/R)—the money that is owed for services rendered—using the practice management program (PMP). The accounts receivable is made up of payments due from payers and from patients. For this reason, after claims have been accepted for processing by payers, medical insurance specialists monitor their status.

Claim Status

Monitoring claims during adjudication requires two types of information. The first is the amount of time the payer is allowed to take to respond to the claim, and the second is how long the claim has been in process.

> **Billing Tip**
>
> **Prompt-Pay Laws for States**
> The websites of states' insurance commissions or departments cover their prompt-pay laws. Research the law in the state where claims are being sent to determine the payment time frames and the penalty for late payers.

Claim Turnaround Time

Just as providers have to file claims within a certain number of days after the date of service, payers also have to process clean claims within the **claim turnaround time**. The participation contract often specifies a time period of thirty to sixty days from claim submission. States have **prompt-pay laws** that obligate state-licensed carriers to pay clean claims for both participating and nonparticipating providers within a certain time period, or incur interest penalties, fines, and lawyers' fees. ERISA (self-funded) plans' claims are under federal prompt-pay rules.

Aging

The other factor in claim follow-up is **aging**—how long a payer has had the claim. The practice management program is used to generate an **insurance aging report** that lists the claims transmitted on each day and shows how long they have been in process with the payer. A typical report, shown in Figure 14.1 on page 454, lists claims that were sent fewer than thirty days ago, between thirty and sixty days ago, and so on.

HIPAA Health Care Claim Status Inquiry/Response

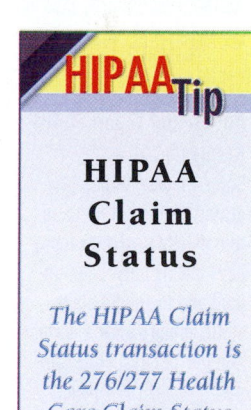

HIPAA Claim Status

The HIPAA Claim Status transaction is the 276/277 Health Care Claim Status Inquiry/Response.

The medical insurance specialist examines the insurance aging report and selects claims for follow-up. Most practices follow up on claims that are aged less that thirty days in seven to fourteen days. The **HIPAA X12 276/277 Health Care Claim Status Inquiry/Response** is the standard electronic transaction to obtain information on the current status of a claim during the adjudication process. The inquiry is the **HIPAA 276**, and the response returned by the payer is the **HIPAA 277**. Figure 14.2 shows how this exchange is sent between provider and payer.

The HIPAA 277 transaction from the payer uses **claim status category codes** for the main types of responses:

- *A* codes indicate an acknowledgment that the claim has been received.
- *P* codes indicate that a claim is **pending**; that is, the payer is waiting for information before making a payment decision.
- *F* codes indicate that a claim has been finalized.
- *R* codes indicate that a request for more information has been sent.
- *E* codes indicate that an error has occurred in transmission; usually these claims need to be re-sent.

These codes are further detailed in **claim status codes**, as shown in Table 14.1.

Valley Associates, P.C.

Primary Insurance Aging

As of 11/30/2008

Date of Service	Procedure	-- Past -- 0 - 30	-- Past -- 31 - 60	-- Past -- 61 - 90	-- Past -- 91 - 120	-- Past -- 121 ---->	Total Balance
Aetna Choice (AET00)							**(555)777-1000**
WILLIWA0	**Walter Williams**		**SS: 401-26-9939**		**Policy: ABC103562239**		**Group: BDC1001**
Birthdate: 9/4/1936							
Claim: 53	Initial Billing Date: 10/8/2008		Last Billing Date: 10/8/2008				
10/1/2008	99212		46.00				46.00
10/1/2008	93000		70.00				70.00
		0.00	116.00	0.00	0.00	0.00	116.00
	Insurance Totals	$0.00	$116.00	$0.00	$0.00	$0.00	$116.00
Anthem BCBS PPO (ANT01)							**(555)888-1000**
CARUTRO0	**Robin Caruthers**		**SS: 331-24-0789**		**Policy: GH331240789**		**Group: OH4071**
Birthdate: 3/29/1979							
Claim: 49	Initial Billing Date: 10/6/2008		Last Billing Date: 10/6/2008				
10/6/2008	99212		46.00				46.00
		0.00	46.00	0.00	0.00	0.00	46.00
	Insurance Totals	$0.00	$46.00	$0.00	$0.00	$0.00	$46.00
Cigna HMO Plus (CIG00)							**(555)666-3001**
PEREZCA0	**Carmen Perez**		**SS: 140-24-6113**		**Policy: 140603312X**		
Birthdate: 5/15/1934							
Claim: 52	Initial Billing Date: 10/8/2008		Last Billing Date: 10/8/2008				
10/1/2008	99213		62.00				62.00
		0.00	62.00	0.00	0.00	0.00	62.00
	Insurance Totals	$0.00	$62.00	$0.00	$0.00	$0.00	$62.00

FIGURE 14.1 Example of an Insurance Aging Report

> **Billing Tip**
>
> **Automated Claim Status Requests**
>
> Some medical billing programs can be set up to automatically track how many days claims have been unpaid and to send a claim status inquiry after a certain number of days. For example, if a particular payer pays claims on the twentieth day, the program transmits a 276 for unpaid claims aged day twenty-one.

Working with Payers

In order to have claims processed as quickly as possible, medical insurance specialists must be familiar with the payers' claim-processing procedures, including:

- The timetables for submitting corrected claims and for filing secondary claims. The latter is usually a period of time from the date of payment by the primary payer.
- How to resubmit corrected claims that are denied for missing or incorrect data. Some payers have online or automated telephone procedures that can be used to resubmit claims after missing information has been supplied.
- How to handle requests for additional documentation if required by the payer.

Requests for information should be answered as quickly as possible, and the answers should be courteous and complete. Medical insurance specialists use correct terms to show that they understand what the payer is asking. For example, a payer often questions an office visit (E/M) service that is reported on the same date of service as a procedure or a preventive physical examination on the grounds that the E/M should not be reimbursed separately. Saying "well, the doctor did do both" is less persuasive than saying "the patient's presenting problems required both the level of E/M as indicated as well as the reported procedure; note that we attached the modifier–25 to indicate the necessity for this separate service."

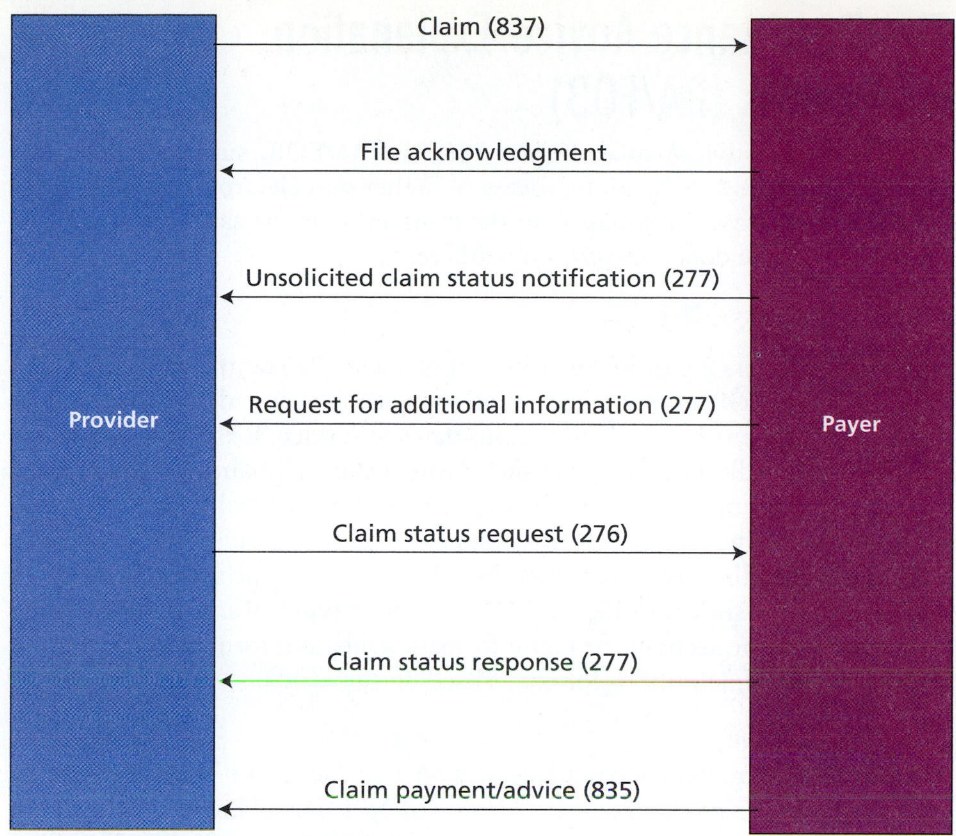

FIGURE 14.2 General Claim Status Request/Response Information Flow

Table 14.1 Selected Claim Status Codes

1	For more detailed information, see remittance advice.
2	More detailed information in letter.
3	Claim has been adjudicated and is awaiting payment cycle.
4	This is a subsequent request for information from the original request.
5	This is a final request for information.
6	Balance due from the subscriber.
7	Claim may be reconsidered at a future date.
9	No payment will be made for this claim.
12	One or more originally submitted procedure codes have been combined.
15	One or more originally submitted procedure codes have been modified.
16	Claim/encounter has been forwarded to entity.
29	Subscriber and policy number/contract number mismatched.
30	Subscriber and subscriber ID mismatched.
31	Subscriber and policyholder name mismatched.
32	Subscriber and policy number/contract number not found.
33	Subscriber and subscriber ID not found.

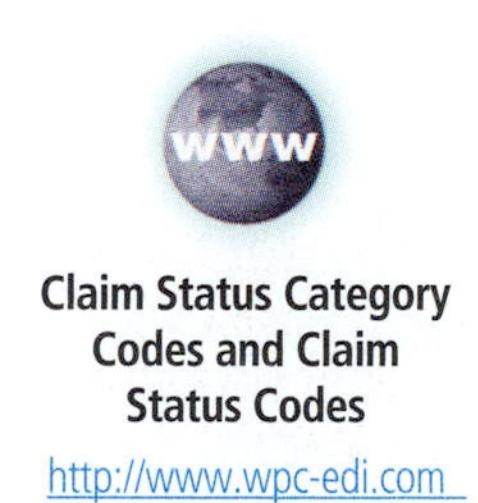

Claim Status Category Codes and Claim Status Codes

http://www.wpc-edi.com

A payer may fail to pay a claim on time without providing notice that the claim has problems, or the payer may miscalculate payments due. If the problem is covered in the participation contract, the recommended procedure is to send a letter pointing this out to the payer. This notice should be sent to the plan representative identified in the contract.

> **Billing Tip**
>
> **Medicare Professional Versus Institutional RAs**
> A provider that submits claims to Medicare carriers or DMERCS receives a professional RA; one that submits claims to fiscal intermediaries receives an institutional RA.

The Remittance Advice/Explanation of Benefits (RA/EOB)

The remittance advice/explanation of benefits (RA/EOB) summarizes the results of the payer's adjudication process. Whether sent electronically or in a paper format, the basic information in the transaction is the same, although the appearance of the documents is often different.

Content of RAs/EOBs

An RA/EOB covers a group of claims, not just a single claim. The claims paid on a single RA/EOB are not consecutive or logically grouped; they are usually for different patients' claims and various dates of service. RAs/EOBs list claims that have been adjudicated within the payment cycle alphanumerically by the patient account number assigned by provider, alphabetically by client name, or numerically by the internal control number. A corresponding EOB sent to the patient, on the other hand, lists just the information for the recipient.

RAs/EOBs, as shown in Figure 14.3, have four types of information, often located in separate sections: header information, claim information, totals, and a glossary (list of definitions for codes used on the form).

Header Information

The header information section (see section 1 in Figure 14.3) contains payer name and address; provider name, address, and NPI; date of issue; and the check or electronic funds transfer (EFT, see page 462) transaction number. There is a place for "bulletin board" information, made up of notes to the provider.

Claim Information

For each claim, section 2 contains the patient's name, plan identification number, account number, and claim control number, and whether the provider accepts assignment (using the abbreviations ASG = Y or N) if this information applies. Under column headings, these items are shown:

COLUMN HEADING	*MEANING*
PERF PROF	Performing provider
SERV DATE	Date(s) of service
POS	Place of service code
NOS	Number of services rendered
PROC	CPT/HCPCS procedure code
MODS	Modifiers for the procedure code
BILLED	Amount provider billed for the service
ALLOWED	Amount payer allows
DEDUCT	Any deductible the beneficiary must pay to the provider
COINS	Any coinsurance the beneficiary must pay to the provider
GRP/RC	Group (GRP) and reason (RC) adjustment codes (explained below)
AMT	Amount of adjustments due to GRP/RC codes
PROV PD	Total amount provider is paid for the service
PT RESP	Total amount that the beneficiary owes the provider for the claim
CLAIM TOTALS	Total amount for each of these columns: BILLED, ALLOWED, DEDUCT, COINS, AMT, and PROV PD

```
1
EXAMPLE MEDICARE CARRIER
1000 SOMEPLACE LANE
FAIRFAX, VA 22033-0000                                        MEDICARE
1-877-555-1234                                                REMITTANCE
                                                              NOTICE

EXAMPLE MEDICARE PROVIDER                                     PROVIDER #:999999
200 DOCTORS DRIVE                                             PAGE #:  1 OF 2
SUITE 200                                                     DATE:  01/28/08
SOMEWHERE, NJ   16666-0200                                    CHECK/EFT #:  000234569
*****************************************************************************************
*                                                                                       *
*              WELCOME TO THE MEDICARE PART B STANDARD PAPER REMITTANCE                 *
*                                                                                       *
*                                                                                       *
*                                                                                       *
*                                                                                       *

2
PERF PROV   SERV DATE  POS NOS  PROC  MODS  BILLED  ALLOWED  DEDUCT  COINS  GRP/RC  AMT  PROV PD

NAME FISCHER, BENNY      HIC 9999999999 ACNT  FISC6123133-01  ICN 0202199306840  ASG Y      MOA MA01
123456ABC  0225 022502 11  1  99213             66.00    49.83    0.34    9.97  PR-96  16.17   39.52
PT RESP    10.31              CLAIM TOTALS     66.00    49.83    0.34    9.97         16.17
                                                                                 NET   39.52

NAME FISCHER, BENNY      HIC 9999999999 ACNT  FISC6123133-01  ICN 0202199306850  ASG Y  MOA MA01 MA07
123456ABC  0117 011702 11  1 99213              66.00    49.83    0.00    9.97  PR-96  16.17   39.86
PT RESP     9.97              CLAIM TOTALS     66.00    49.83    0.00    9.97         16.17   39.86
CLAIM INFORMATION FORWARDED TO:  NEW JERSEY MEDICAID                             NET   39.86

NAME HURT, I. M.         HIC 9999999999 ACNT  HURT5-329       ICN 0202199306860  ASG Y      MOA MA01
123456ABC  0117 011702 11  1  90659             25.00     3.32    0.00    0.00  CO-42  21.68    3.32
123456ABC  0117 011702 11  1  G0008             10.00     4.46    0.00    0.00  CO-42   5.54    4.46
PT RESP     0.00              CLAIM TOTALS     35.00     7.78    0.00    0.00         27.22    7.78
                                                                                 NET    7.78

NAME MARLOWE, PHILIP     HIC 9999999999 ACNT  MARLO861-316    ICN 0202199306870  ASG Y  MOA MA01 MA07
123456ABC  0209 020902 11  1  99213             66.00    49.83    0.00    9.97  PR-96  16.17   39.86
PT RESP     9.97              CLAIM TOTALS     66.00    49.83    0.00    9.97         16.17   39.86
ADJ TO TOTALS:  PREV PD  10.00   INT  0.00        LATE FILING CHARGE  0.00
CLAIM INFORMATION FORWARDED TO:  NEW JERSEY MEDICAID                             NET   29.86
NAME RAP, JACK           HIC 9999999999 ACNT  RAP33-721       ICN 0202199306880  ASG Y  MOA MA01 MA07
123456ABC  0314 031402 11  1  99213             66.00    49.83    0.00    9.97  PR-96  16.17   39.86
123456ABC  0314 031402 11  1  82962             10.00     4.37    0.00    0.00  CO-42   5.63    4.37
123456ABC  0314 031402 11  1  94760             12.00     0.00    0.00    0.00  CO-B15 12.00    0.00
REM: M80
PT RESP     9.97              CLAIM TOTALS     88.00    54.20    0.00    9.97         33.80   44.23
                                                                                 NET   44.23

3
TOTALS:  # of     BILLED   ALLOWED   DEDUCT    COINS    TOTAL     PROV PD     PROV      CHECK
         CLAIMS      AMT       AMT      AMT      AMT   RC AMT         AMT   ADJ AMT       AMT
           5      321.00   211.47     0.34    39.88   109.53     161.25     31.25    108.75
  PROVIDER ADJ DETAILS:        PLB REASON CODE      FCN            HIC           AMOUNT
                                     50                                          15.44
                                     FB           0202199306770  9999999999       5.81

4
GROUP CODES:
PR       Patient Responsibility
CO       Contractual Obligation
OA       Other Adjustment

GLOSSARY:  Group, Reason, MOA, Remark and Adjustment Codes
CO       Contractual Obligation.  Amount for which the provider is financially liable.  The patient may
         not be billed for this amount.
PR       Patient Responsibility.  Amount that may be billed to a patient or another payer.
42       Charges exceed our fee schedule or maximum allowable amount.
96       Non-covered charge(s)
B15      Claim/service denied/reduced because this procedure/service is not paid separately.
         Charges exceed our fee schedule or maximum allowable amount.
M80      We cannot pay for this when performed during the same session as another approved procedure for
         this beneficiary
MA01     (Initial Part B determination, carrier or intermediary)  If you do not agree with what we
         approved for these services, you may appeal our decision.  To make sure that we are fair to you,
         we require another individual that did not process your initial claim to conduct the review.
         However, in order to be eligible for a review, you must write to us within 6 months of the date
         of this notice, unless you have a good reason for being late.  (An institutional provider, e.g.,
         hospital, SNF, HHA may appeal only if the claim involves a medical necessity denial, a SNF
         recertified bed denial, or a home health denial because the patient was not homebound or was not
         in need of intermittent skilled nursing services, and either the patient or the provider is
         liable under 1879 of the Social Security Act, and the patient chooses not to appeal.)  NOTE:  If
         you are a member of the telephone review demonstration, or if telephone reviews are expanded,
         add the following to the end of the description for MA01.  If you meet the criteria for a
         telephone review, you may phone to request a telephone review.
MA07     The claim information has also been forwarded to Medicaid for review.
MA28     Receipt of this notice by a physician who did not accept assignment is for information only and
         does not make the physician a party to the determination.  No additional rights to appeal this
         decision, above those rights already provided for by regulation/instruction, are conferred by
         receipt of this notice
50       Late Filing Reduction
FB       Forwarding Balance
```

FIGURE 14.3 Sections of the RA/EOB

Totals

The third part (see section 3 in Figure 14.3) shows the totals for all the claims on the RA/EOB. At the end, the CHECK AMT field contains the amount of the check or EFT payment that the provider receives.

Glossary

The glossary section is the fourth area (see section 4 in Figure 14.3) of an RA/EOB. It lists the adjustment codes shown on the transaction with their meanings.

Adjustments

An adjustment on the RA/EOB means that the payer is paying a claim or a service line differently than billed. The adjustment may be that the item is:

- Denied
- Zero pay (if accepted as billed but no payment is due)
- Reduced amount paid (most likely paid according to the allowed amount)
- Less because a penalty is subtracted from the payment

To explain the determination to the provider, payers use a combination of codes: (1) claim adjustment group code, (2) claim adjustment reason code, and (3) remittance advice remark code. Each of these is a HIPAA administrative code set, like place of service (POS) codes and taxonomy codes.

Billing Tip

Code Updates
Claim adjustment reason codes and remark codes are updated three times each year. Access the website (http:www.wpc-edi.com/codes) for updated lists.

Claim Adjustment Group Codes

Claim adjustment group codes (group codes, abbreviated **GRP**) are:

- *PR—Patient Responsibility:* Appears next to an amount that can be billed to the patient or insured. This group code typically applies to deductible and coinsurance/copayment adjustments.
- *CO—Contractual Obligations:* Appears when a contract between the payer and the provider resulted in an adjustment. This group code usually applies to allowed amounts. CO adjustments are not billable to patients under the contract.
- *CR—Corrections and Reversals:* Appears to correct a previous claim.
- *OA—Other Adjustments*: Used only when neither PR nor CO applies, as when another insurance is primary.
- *PI—Payer Initiated Reduction:* Appears when the payer thinks the patient is not responsible for the charge but there is no contract between the payer and the provider that states this. It might be used for medical review denials.

Billing Tip

Patient Balance Billing
A group code PR with an associate reason code indicates whether a provider may or may not bill a beneficiary for the unpaid balance of the furnished services.

Claim Adjustment Reason Codes
http://www.wpc-edi.com/codes/claimadjustment

Claim Adjustment Reason Codes

Payers use **claim adjustment reason codes** (reason codes, abbreviated **RC**) to provide details about adjustments. Examples of these codes and their meanings are provided in Table 14.2.

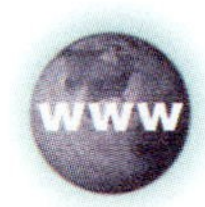

Remittance Advice Remark Codes
http://www.wpc-edi.com/codes/remittanceadvice

Remittance Advice Remark Codes

Payers may also use **remittance advice remark codes** (remark codes, **REM**) for more explanation. Remark codes are maintained by CMS but can be used by all payers. Codes that start with *M* are from a Medicare code set that was in place before HIPAA but that is still used, including **Medicare Outpatient Adjudication remark codes (MOA)**. Codes that begin with *N* are new. Table 14.3 on page 461 shows selected remark codes.

Table 14.2	Selected Claim Adjustment Reason Codes
1	Deductible amount
2	Coinsurance amount
3	Copayment amount
4	The procedure code is inconsistent with the modifier used, or a required modifier is missing.
5	The procedure code/bill type is inconsistent with the place of service.
6	The procedure/revenue code is inconsistent with the patient's age.
7	The procedure/revenue code is inconsistent with the patient's gender.
8	The procedure code is inconsistent with the provider type/specialty (taxonomy).
9	The diagnosis is inconsistent with the patient's age.
10	The diagnosis is inconsistent with the patient's gender.
11	The diagnosis is inconsistent with the procedure.
12	The diagnosis is inconsistent with the provider type.
13	The date of death precedes the date of service.
14	The date of birth follows the date of service.
15	Payment adjusted because the submitted authorization number is missing, is invalid, or does not apply to the billed services or provider.
16	Claim/service lacks information that is needed for adjudication. Additional information is supplied using remittance advice remarks codes whenever appropriate.
17	Payment adjusted because requested information was not provided or was insufficient/incomplete. Additional information is supplied using the remittance advice remarks codes whenever appropriate.
18	Duplicate claim/service.
19	Claim denied because this is a work-related injury/illness and thus the liability of the workers' compensation carrier.
20	Claim denied because this injury/illness is covered by the liability carrier.
21	Claim denied because this injury/illness is the liability of the no-fault carrier.
22	Payment adjusted because this care may be covered by another payer per coordination of benefits.
23	Payment adjusted due to the impact of prior payer(s) adjudication including payments and/or adjustments.
24	Payment for charges adjusted. Charges are covered under a capitation agreement/managed care plan.
25	Payment denied. Your stop loss deductible has not been met.
26	Expenses incurred prior to coverage.
27	Expenses incurred after coverage terminated.
29	The time limit for filing has expired.
31	Claim denied as patient cannot be identified as our insured.
32	Our records indicate that this dependent is not an eligible dependent as defined.
33	Claim denied. Insured has no dependent coverage.
36	Balance does not exceed copayment amount.
37	Balance does not exceed deductible.
38	Services not provided or authorized by designated (network/primary care) providers.
39	Services denied at the time authorization/precertification was requested.
40	Charges do not meet qualifications for emergency/urgent care.
41	Discount agreed to in preferred provider contract.
42	Charges exceed our fee schedule or maximum allowable amount.
45	Charges exceed your contracted/legislated fee arrangement.
49	These are noncovered services because this is a routine exam or screening procedure done in conjunction with a routine exam.
50	These are noncovered services because this is not deemed a medical necessity by the payer.

(continued on next page)

Table 14.2 Selected Claim Adjustment Reason Codes *(continued)*

51	These are noncovered services because this is a preexisting condition.
55	Claim/service denied because procedure/treatment is deemed experimental/investigational by the payer.
56	Claim/service denied because procedure/treatment has not been deemed "proven to be effective" by the payer.
57	Payment denied/reduced because the payer deems that the information submitted does not support this level of service, this many services, this length of service, this dosage, or this day's supply.
58	Payment adjusted because treatment was deemed by the payer to have been rendered in an inappropriate or invalid place of service.
62	Payment denied/reduced for absence of, or exceeded, precertification/authorization.
63	Correction to a prior claim.
65	Procedure code was incorrect. This payment reflects the correct code.
96	Noncovered charge(s).
97	Payment is included in the allowance for another service/procedure.
109	Claim not covered by this payer/contractor. You must send the claim to the correct payer/contractor.
110	Billing date predates service date.
111	Not covered unless the provider accepts assignment.
112	Payment adjusted as not furnished directly to the patient and/or not documented.
114	Procedure/product not approved by the Food and Drug Administration.
115	Payment adjusted as procedure postponed or canceled.
123	Payer refund due to overpayment.
124	Payer refund amount—not our patient.
125	Payment adjusted due to a submission/billing error(s). Additional information is supplied using the remittance advice remarks codes whenever appropriate.
138	Claim/service denied. Appeal procedures not followed or time limits not met.
140	Patient/insured health identification number and name do not match.
145	Premium payment withholding.
146	Payment denied because the diagnosis was invalid for the date(s) of service reported.
150	Payment adjusted because the payer deems that the information submitted does not support this level of service.
151	Payment adjusted because the payer deems that the information submitted does not support this many services.
152	Payment adjusted because the payer deems that the information submitted does not support this length of service.
155	This claim is denied because the patient refused the service/procedure.
160	Payment denied/reduced because injury/illness was the result of an activity that is a benefit exclusion.
A0	Patient refund amount.
A1	Claim denied charges.
B5	Claim/service denied/reduced because coverage guidelines were not met.
B12	Services not documented in patients' medical records.
B13	Previously paid. Payment for this claim/service may have been provided in a previous payment.
B14	Payment denied because only one visit or consultation per physician per day is covered.
B15	Payment adjusted because this procedure/service is not paid separately.
B16	Payment adjusted because "new patient" qualifications were not met.
B18	Payment denied because this procedure code and modifier were invalid on the date of service.
B22	This payment is adjusted based on the diagnosis.
D7	Claim/service denied. Claim lacks date of patient's most recent physician visit.
D8	Claim/service denied. Claim lacks indicator that "X-ray is available for review."
D21	This (these) diagnosis(es) is (are) missing or invalid.
W1	Workers' Compensation State Fee Schedule adjustment.

Table 14.3	Selected Remark Codes
M11	DME, orthotics, and prosthetics must be billed to the DME carrier who services the patient's ZIP code.
M12	Diagnostic tests performed by a physician must indicate whether purchased services are included on the claim.
M37	Service not covered when the patient is under age 35.
M38	The patient is liable for the charges for this service, as you informed the patient in writing before the service was furnished that we would not pay for it, and the patient agreed to pay.
M39	The patient is not liable for payment for this service, as the advance notice of noncoverage you provided the patient did not comply with program requirements.
N14	Payment based on a contractual amount or agreement, fee schedule, or maximum allowable amount.
N15	Services for a newborn must be billed separately.
N16	Family/member out-of-pocket maximum has been met. Payment based on a higher percentage.
N210	You may appeal this decision.
N211	You may not appeal this decision.

Thinking It Through — 14.2

Review the RA/EOB from Medicare for assigned claims shown in Figure 14.4, locating the highlighted claims that contain these data:

A. **GRP/RC AMT CO-42 $18.04**

B. **GRP/RC AMT PR-96 $162.13**

1. **What do the adjustment codes mean in the first claim?**
2. **What do the adjustment codes mean in the second claim?**
3. **In the second claim, the modifier –GY is appended to the E/M code 99397. What does this modifier mean? Check Chapter 10, Medicare, if necessary to interpret this information. Who is responsible for payment?**

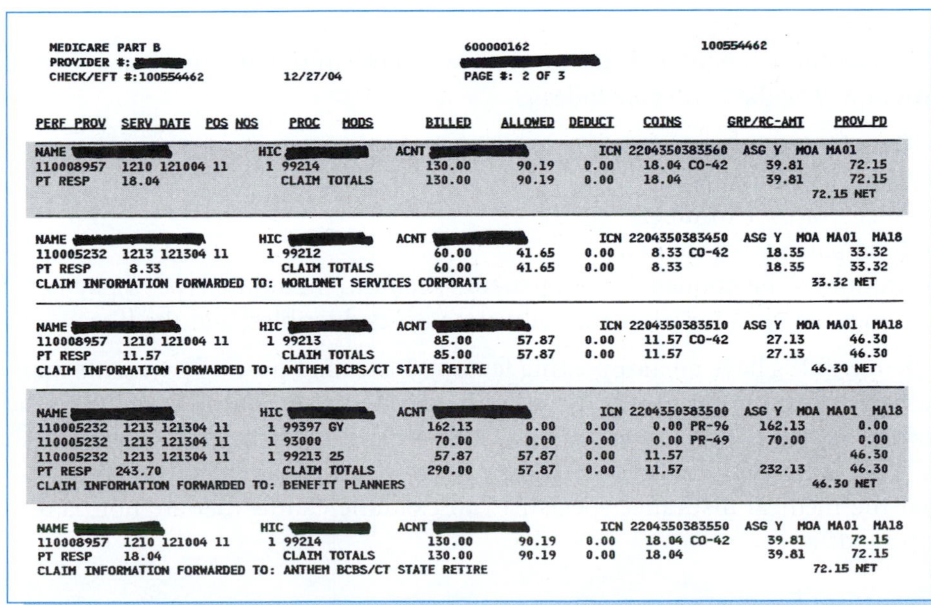

```
MEDICARE PART B                                    600000162                 100554462
PROVIDER #:
CHECK/EFT #:100554462          12/27/04            PAGE #: 2 OF 3

PERF PROV  SERV DATE  POS NOS   PROC   MODS     BILLED    ALLOWED  DEDUCT   COINS        GRP/RC-AMT    PROV PD

NAME                       HIC             ACNT                  ICN 2204350383560  ASG Y  MOA MA01
110008957  1210 121004 11   1 99214         130.00     90.19    0.00   18.04 CO-42    39.81        72.15
PT RESP    18.04              CLAIM TOTALS  130.00     90.19    0.00   18.04          39.81        72.15
                                                                                            72.15 NET

NAME                       HIC             ACNT                  ICN 2204350383450  ASG Y  MOA MA01  MA18
110005232  1213 121304 11   1 99212          60.00     41.65    0.00    8.33 CO-42    18.35        33.32
PT RESP     8.33              CLAIM TOTALS   60.00     41.65    0.00    8.33          18.35        33.32
CLAIM INFORMATION FORWARDED TO: WORLDNET SERVICES CORPORATI                                 33.32 NET

NAME                       HIC             ACNT                  ICN 2204350383510  ASG Y  MOA MA01  MA18
110008957  1210 121004 11   1 99213          85.00     57.87    0.00   11.57 CO-42    27.13        46.30
PT RESP    11.57              CLAIM TOTALS   85.00     57.87    0.00   11.57          27.13        46.30
CLAIM INFORMATION FORWARDED TO: ANTHEM BCBS/CT STATE RETIRE                                 46.30 NET

NAME                       HIC             ACNT                  ICN 2204350383500  ASG Y  MOA MA01  MA18
110005232  1213 121304 11   1 99397 GY      162.13      0.00    0.00    0.00 PR-96   162.13         0.00
110005232  1213 121304 11   1 93000          70.00      0.00    0.00    0.00 PR-49    70.00         0.00
110005232  1213 121304 11   1 99213 25       57.87     57.87    0.00   11.57                       46.30
PT RESP   243.70              CLAIM TOTALS  290.00     57.87    0.00   11.57         232.13        46.30
CLAIM INFORMATION FORWARDED TO: BENEFIT PLANNERS                                            46.30 NET

NAME                       HIC             ACNT                  ICN 2204350383550  ASG Y  MOA MA01  MA18
110008957  1210 121004 11   1 99214         130.00     90.19    0.00   18.04 CO-42    39.81        72.15
PT RESP    18.04              CLAIM TOTALS  130.00     90.19    0.00   18.04          39.81        72.15
CLAIM INFORMATION FORWARDED TO: ANTHEM BCBS/CT STATE RETIRE                                 72.15 NET
```

FIGURE 14.4 Medicare RA

Reviewing and Processing RAs/EOBs

An RA/EOB repeats the unique claim control number that the provider assigned to the claim when sending it. This number is the resource needed to match the payment to a claim. To process the RA/EOB, each claim is located in the practice management program—either manually or automatically by the computer system. The remittance data are reviewed and then posted to the PMP.

Reviewing RAs/EOBs

This procedure is followed to double-check the remittance data:

1. Check the patient's name, account number, insurance number, and date of service against the claim.
2. Verify that all billed CPT codes are listed.
3. Check the payment for each CPT against the expected amount, which may be an allowed amount or a percentage of the usual fee. Many practice management programs build records of the amount each payer has paid for each CPT code as the data are entered. When another RA/EOB payment for the same CPT is posted, the program highlights any discrepancy for review.
4. Analyze the payer's adjustment codes to locate all unpaid, downcoded, or denied claims for closer review.
5. Decide whether any items on the RA/EOB need clarifying with the payer, and follow up as necessary.

Billing Tips

Paper Check Processing

- Because payments may be mailed, the practice's mail should be opened daily and checks deposited according to the office's guidelines.
- All checks that come into the practice should be routed through the staff member who processes claims.

Procedures for Posting

Many practices that receive RAs/EOBs authorize the payer to provide an **electronic funds transfer (EFT)** of the payment. Payments are deposited directly into the practice's bank account. Otherwise, the payer sends a check to the practice, and the check is taken to the practice's bank for deposit.

Posting and Applying Payments and Adjustments

Payment and adjustment transactions are entered in the practice management program. The data entry includes:

- Date of deposit.
- Payer name and type.
- Check or EFT number.
- Total payment amount.
- Amount to be applied to each patient's account, including type of payment. Codes are used for payments, adjustments, deductibles, and the like.

Some PMPs have an **autoposting** feature. Instead of posting payments manually, this feature automatically posts the payment data in the RA/EOB to the correct account. The software allows the user to establish posting rules, such as "post a payment automatically only if the claim is paid at 100 percent," so that the medical insurance specialist can examine claims that are not paid as expected.

Reconciling Payments

The process of **reconciliation** means making sure that the totals on the RA/EOB check out mathematically. The total amount billed minus the adjustments (such as for allowed amounts and patient responsibility to pay) should equal the total amount paid. For example, study this report for an assigned claim:

POS	PROC MODS	BILLED	ALLOWED	DEDUCT	COINS	GRP/RC-AMT	PROV PD
11	99213	85.00	57.87	0.00	11.57	CO-42 27.13	46.30

RECONCILIATION

Amount Billed	$85.00
(Coinsurance)	–11.57
(GRP/RC Amount)	–27.13
Payment	$46.30

In this case, the allowed amount (ALLOWED) of $57.87 is made up of the coinsurance (COINs) to be collected from the patient of $11.57 plus the amount the payer pays to the provider (PROV PD) of $46.30. The difference between the billed amount (BILLED) of $85.00 and the allowed amount of $57.87 is $27.13. This amount is written off unless it can be billed to the patient under the payer's rules.

Billing Tip

Auditing Payments per Contract Terms
Verify that payments are correct according to payers' participation contracts. This double-check is particularly important if payments are autoposted. In this case, periodically post a representative number of RAs/EOBs manually as an audit to uncover any payment problems.

Denial Management

Typical problems and solutions are:

- *Rejected claims:* A claim that is not paid due to incorrect information must be corrected and sent to the payer according to its procedures.
- *Procedures not paid*: If a procedure that should have been paid on a claim was overlooked, another claim is sent for that procedure.
- *Partially paid, denied, or downcoded claims*: If the payer has denied payment, the first step is to study the adjustment codes to determine why. If a procedure is not a covered benefit or if the patient was not eligible for that benefit, typically the next step will be to bill the patient for the noncovered amount. If the claim is denied or downcoded for lack of medical necessity, a decision about the next action must be made. The options are to bill the patient, write off the amount, or challenge the determination with an appeal, as discussed on page 464. Some provider contracts prohibit billing the patient if an appeal or necessary documentation has not been submitted to the payer.

Billing Tip

Organize Before Calling
Before calling a payer to question a claim determination, prepare by gathering the RA/EOB, the patient's medical record, and the claim data. Be ready to explain the situation and to politely ask to speak to a supervisor if necessary.

To improve the rate of paid claims over time, medical insurance specialists track and analyze each payer's reasons for denying claims. This record may be kept in a denial log or by assigning specific denial-reason codes for the practice management program to store and report on. Denials should be grouped into categories, such as:

- Coding errors (incorrect unbundling, procedure codes not payable by plan with the reported diagnosis codes)
- Registration mistakes, such as incorrect patient ID numbers
- Billing errors, such as failure to get required preauthorizations or referral numbers
- Payer requests for more information or general delays in claims processing

The types of denials should be analyzed to find out what procedures can be implemented to fix the problems. For example, educating the staff members responsible for getting preauthorizations about each payer's requirements may be necessary.

Thinking It Through — 14.3

Based on the following RA/EOB:

1. What is the total amount paid by check? (Fill in the "amount paid provider" column before calculating the total.)
2. Were any procedures paid at a rate lower than the claim charge? If so, which?
3. Why do you think there is no insurance payment for services for Gloria Vanderhilt?
4. Was payment denied for any claim? For what reason?

Date prepared: 6/22/2008 **Claim number:** 0347914

Patient's name	Dates of service from - thru	POS	Proc	Qty	Charge amount	Eligible amount	Patient liability	Amt paid provider
Kavan, Gregory	04/15/04 - 04/15/04	11	99213	1	$48.00	$48.00	$4.80	______
Ferrara, Grace	05/11/04 - 05/11/04	11	99212	1	$35.00	$35.00	$3.50	______
Cornprost, Harry	05/12/04 - 05/12/04	11	99214	1	$64.00	$54.00	-0-	______
Vanderhilt, Gloria	05/12/04 - 05/12/04	11	99212	1	$35.00	$35.00	$35.00	-0-
Dallez, Juan	05/13/04 - 05/13/04	11	99212	1	$35.00	*	*	-0-

* * * * * * * * *Check #1039242 is attached in the amount of* ________ * * * * * * * *

*** Procedure not covered under Medicaid**

Appeals, Postpayment Audits, Overpayments, and Grievances

After RAs/EOBs are reviewed and processed, events that may follow can alter the amount of payment. When a claim has been denied or payment reduced, an appeal may be filed with the payer for reconsideration, possibly reversing the nonpayment. Postpayment audits by payers may change the initial determination. Under certain conditions, refunds may be due to either the payer or the patient. In some cases, the practice may elect to file a complaint with the state insurance commissioner.

The General Appeal Process

An **appeal** is a process that can be used to challenge a payer's decision to deny, reduce, or otherwise downcode a claim. A provider may begin the appeal process by asking for a review of the payer's decision. Patients, too, have the right to request appeals. The person filing the appeal is the **claimant** or the **appellant**, whether that individual is a provider or a patient.

Basic Steps

Each payer has consistent procedures for handling appeals. These procedures are based on the nature of the appeal. The practice staff reviews the appropriate procedure before starting an appeal and plans its actions according to the rules. Appeals must be filed within a specified time after the claim determination. Most payers have an escalating structure of appeals, such as (1) a complaint, (2) an appeal, and (3) a grievance. The claimant must move through the three levels in pursuing an appeal, starting at the lowest and continuing to the highest, final level. Some payers also set a minimum amount that must be involved in an appeal process, so that a lot of time is not spent on a small dispute.

Options After Appeal Rejection

A claimant can take another step if the payer has rejected all the appeal levels on a claim. Because they license most types of payers, state insurance commissions have the authority to review appeals that payers reject. If a claimant decides to pursue an appeal with the state insurance commission, copies of the complete case file—all documents that relate to the initial claim determination and the appeal process—are sent, along with a letter of explanation.

Medicare Appeals

Medicare participating providers have appeal rights. Note, though, that there is no need to appeal a claim if it has been denied for minor errors or omissions. The provider can instead ask the Medicare carrier to reopen the claim so the error can be fixed, rather than going through the appeals process. However, if a claim is denied because of untimely submission (it was submitted after the timely filing deadline), it cannot be appealed.

The current Medicare appeals process is the result of changes in the law; the Medicare, Medicaid, and SCHIP Benefits and Improvement Act of 2000, known as BIPA, and the Medicare Modernization Act significantly changed these procedures. The Medicare appeal process involves five steps:

1. *Redetermination*: The first step, called **redetermination**, is a claim review by an employee of the Medicare carrier who was not involved in the initial claim determination. The request, which must be made within 120 days of receiving the initial claim determination, is made by completing a form (Figure 14.5 on page 466) or writing a letter and attaching supporting medical documentation. If the decision is favorable, payment is sent. If the redetermination is either partially favorable or unfavorable, the answer comes as a letter (see Figure 14.6 on page 467) called the **Medicare Redetermination Notice (MRN)**. The decision must be made within 60 days; and the letter is sent to both the provider and the patient.
2. *Reconsideration*: The next step is a reconsideration request. This request must be made within 180 days of receiving the redetermination notice. At this level, the claim is reviewed by qualified independent contractors (QIC).
3. *Administrative law judge*: The third level is a hearing by an administrative law judge. The amount in question must be over $110, and the hearing must be requested within 60 days of receiving the reconsideration notice.
4. *Department appeals board*: The fourth level must be requested within 60 days of receiving the response from the hearing by the administrative law judge. No monetary amount is specified.
5. *Federal court (judicial) review:* The fifth and final Medicare appeal level is a hearing in federal court. The amount in dispute must be at least $1,090, and the hearing must be requested within 60 days of receiving the department appeals board decision.

Billing Tip

Late Claims Not Appealable
A claim that is denied because it was not timely filed is not subject to appeal.

Billing Tip

Calendar Days, Not Working Days
Note that the timelines for each appeal level are calendar days (including weekends), not working days.

DEPARTMENT OF HEALTH AND HUMAN SERVICES
CENTERS FOR MEDICARE & MEDICAID SERVICES

MEDICARE REDETERMINATION REQUEST FORM

1. Beneficiary's Name: ____________________
2. Medicare Number: ____________________
3. Description of Item or Service in Question: ____________________
4. Date the Service or Item was Received: ____________________
5. I do not agree with the determination of my claim. MY REASONS ARE: ____________________
6. Date of the initial determination notice ____________________
   (If you received your initial determination notice more than 120 days ago, include your reason for not making this request earlier.)
7. Additional Information Medicare Should Consider: ____________________
8. Requester's Name: ____________________
9. Requester's Relationship to the Beneficiary: ____________________
10. Requester's Address: ____________________
11. Requester's Telephone Number: ____________________
12. Requester's Signature: ____________________
13. Date Signed: ____________________
14. ❑ I have evidence to submit. (Attach such evidence to this form.)
    ❑ I do not have evidence to submit.

NOTICE: Anyone who misrepresents or falsifies essential information requested by this form may upon conviction be subject to fine or imprisonment under Federal Law.

Form CMS-20027 (05/05) EF 05/2005

FIGURE 14.5 Medicare Request for Redetermination Form

Compliance Guideline

Patients' Rights Under Medicare
A beneficiary may request an itemized statement from the provider. A provider who does not comply within thirty days may be fined $100 per outstanding request. The beneficiary may examine the itemized statement and request review of questionable or unclear charges. The provider is required to work with the enrollee to explain discrepancies.

Postpayment Audits

Most postpayment reviews are used to build clinical information. Payers use their audits of practices, for example, to study treatments and outcomes for patients with similar diagnoses. The patterns that are determined are used to confirm or alter best practice guidelines.

At times, however, the postpayment audit is done to verify the medical necessity of reported services or to uncover fraud and abuse. The audit may be based on the detailed records about each provider's services that are kept by payers' medical review departments. Some payers keep records that go back

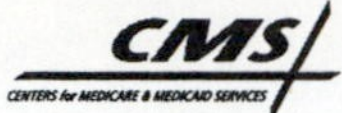

MODEL

Medicare Number of Beneficiary:
111-11-1111 A

MEDICARE APPEAL DECISION

Contact Information
If you questions, write or call:
Contractor Name
Street Address
City, State Zip
Phone Number

MONTH, DATE, YEAR

APELLANT'S NAME
ADDRESS
CITY, STATE ZIP

Dear *Appellant's Name*:

This letter is to inform you of the decision on your Medicare Appeal. An appeal is a new and independent review of a claim. You are receiving this letter because you made an appeal for *(insert: name of item or service)*.

The appeal decision is
*(Insert either: **unfavorable.** Our decision is that your claim in not covered by Medicare and over/under $100 remains in controversy.*
*OR **partially favorable**. Our decision is that your claim is partially covered by Medicare. and over/under $100 remains in controversy)*

More information on the decision is provided below. You are not required to take any action. However, if you disagree with the decision, you may appeal to *(insert: an Administrative Law Judge (for Part A), a Hearing Officer (for part B))*. You must file your appeal, in writing, within *(insert: 6 months (for Part B) or 60 days (for Part A)* of receiving this letter.

A copy of this letter was also sent to *(Insert: Beneficiary Name or Provider Name)*. *(Insert: Contractor Name)* was contracted by Medicare to review your appeal. For more information on how to appeal, see the section titled "Important Information About Your Appeal Rights."

Summary of the Facts
Instructions: You may present this information in this format, or in paragraph form.

Provider	Dates of Service	Type of Service
Insert: Provider Name	*Insert: Dates of Service*	*Insert: Type of Service*

- A claim was submitted for *(insert: kind of services and specific number)*.
- An initial determination on this claim was made on *(insert: Date)*.
- The *(insert: service(s)/item(s) were/was)* denied because *(insert: reason)*.
- On *(insert: date)* we received a request for a redetermination.
- *(Insert: list of documents)* was submitted with the request.

Decision
Instructions: Insert a brief statement of the decision, for example "We have determined that the above claim is not covered by Medicare. We have also determined that you are responsible for payment for this service."

Explanation of the Decision
Instructions: This is the most important element of the redetermination. Explain the logic/reasons that led to your final determination. Explain what policy (including local medical review policy, regional medical review policy, and/or national coverage policy), regulations and/or laws were used to make this determination. Make sure that the explanation contained in this paragraph is clear and that it included an explanation of why the claim can or cannot be paid. Statements such as "not medically reasonable and necessary under Medicare guidelines" or "Medicare does not pay for X" provide conclusions instead of explanation, and are not sufficient to meet the requirement of this paragraph.

Who is Responsible for the Bill?
Instructions: Include information on limitation of liability, waiver of recovery, and physician/supplier refund requirements as applicable.

What to Include in Your Request for an Independent Appeal
Instruction: If the denial was based on insufficient documentation or if specific types of documentation are necessary to issue a favorable decision, please indicate what documentation would be necessary to pay the claim.

Sincerely,

Reviewer Name
Contractor Name
A Medicare Contractor

FIGURE 14.6 Medicare Redetermination Notice

for many months or years. The payer analyzes these records to assess patterns of care from individual providers and to flag outliers—those that differ from what other providers do. A postpayment audit might be conducted to check the documentation of the provider's cases or, in some cases, to check for fraudulent practices (see Chapters 2 and 7).

Thinking It Through 14.4

In a large practice of forty providers, the staff responsible for creating claims and billing is located in one building, and the staff members who handle RAs/EOBs work at another location. In your opinion, what difficulties might this separation present? What strategies can be used to ensure the submission of complete and compliant claims?

Billing Tip

Medicare Beneficiaries and Overpayments
Medicare beneficiaries are notified when their providers receive overpayment notices from Medicare. Patients may be given the choice of receiving refund checks from the provider or credits on their accounts.

Compliance Guideline

Finding Overpayments Proactively
Part of the practice's compliance plan is a regular procedure to self-audit and discover whether overbilling has occurred—and to send the payer a notice of the situation and a refund.

Refunds of Overpayments

From the payer's point of view, **overpayments** (also called credit balances) are improper or excessive payments resulting from billing errors for which the provider owes refunds. Examples are:

- A payer may mistakenly overpay a claim.
- A payer's postpayment audit may find that a claim that has been paid should be denied or downcoded because the documentation does not support it.
- A provider may collect a primary payment from Medicare when another payer is primary.

In such cases, reimbursement that the provider has received is considered an overpayment, and the payer will ask for a refund (with the addition of interest for Medicare). If the audit shows that the claim was for a service that was not medically necessary, the provider also must refund any payment collected from the patient.

Often, the procedure is to promptly refund the overpayment. Many states require the provider to make the refund payment unless the overpayment is contested, which it may be if the provider thinks it is erroneous. A refund request may also be challenged because:

- Many practices set a time period beyond which they will not automatically issue a refund.
- State law may also provide for a reasonable time limit during which payers can recoup overpayments. For example, Missouri gives insurance companies twelve months from the date they processed the claim to request refunds; Maryland's period is six months.

Grievances

If a medical practice believes that it has been treated unfairly by an insurance company, it has the right to file a **grievance** with the state insurance commission. The law requires the state to investigate the complaint, and the state can require the insurance company to answer. Grievances, like appeals, require a good deal of staff time and effort. They should be filed when repeated unresolved problems cannot otherwise be worked out with payers. The state insurance commission sets the requirements and steps for pursuing this option.

Billing Secondary Payers

If a patient has additional insurance coverage, after the primary payer's RA/EOB has been posted, the next step is billing the second payer. The primary claim, of course, gave that payer information about the patient's secondary insurance policy. The secondary payer now needs to know what the primary payer paid on the claim in order to coordinate benefits. The primary claim crosses over automatically to the secondary payer in many cases—Medicare-Medicaid and Medicare-Medigap claims, as well as others—and no additional claim is filed. For non-crossover claims, the medical insurance specialist prepares an additional claim for the secondary payer and sends it with a copy of the RA/EOB.

Electronic Claims

The medical insurance specialist transmits a claim to the secondary payer with the primary RA/EOB, sent either electronically or on paper, according to the payer's procedures. The secondary payer determines whether additional benefits are due under the policy's coordination of benefits (COB) provisions and sends payment with another RA/EOB to the billing provider. This flow is shown in Figure 14.7(a).

The practice does not send a claim to the secondary payer when the primary payer handles the coordination of benefits transaction. In this case, the primary payer electronically sends the COB transaction, which is the same HIPAA 837 that reports the primary claim, to the secondary payer. This flow is shown in Figure 14.7(b).

When the primary payer forwards the COB transaction, a message appears on the primary payer's RA/EOB. For example, on the Medicare RA shown in Figure 14.4 on page 461, COB is indicated by the phrase "CLAIM INFORMATION FORWARDED TO," followed by the name of the secondary payer, such as Worldnet Services Corporation, Anthem BCBS/CT State Retirement, Benefit Planners, and so forth. Medicare has a consolidated claims crossover process that is managed by a special coordination of benefits contractor (COBC). Plans that are supplemental to Medicare sign one national crossover agreement.

Billing Tip

Coordination of Benefits (COB)
Many health plans receive Medicare claims automatically when they are the secondary payer. Do not send a paper claim to the secondary payer upon receipt of the RA/EOB; it will be coded as a duplicate claim and rejected.

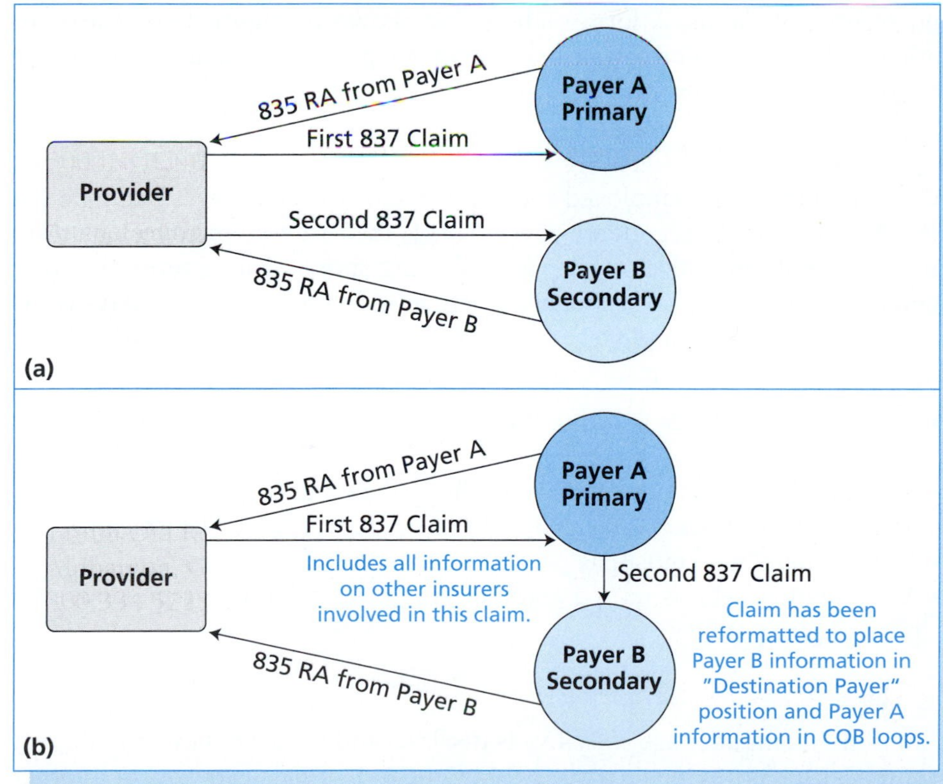

FIGURE 14.7 (a) Provider-to-Payer COB Model, (b) Provider-to-Payer-to-Payer COB Model

HIPAA Tip

PHI on RAs/EOBs

Black out other patients' protected health information (PHI) on printed RAs/EOBs being sent to secondary payers.

Paper Claims

If a paper RA/EOB is received, the procedure is to use the CMS-1500 to bill the secondary health plan that covers the beneficiary. The medical insurance specialist completes the claim form and sends it with the primary RA/EOB attached.

The Medicare Secondary Payer (MSP) Program, Claims, and Payments

Benefits for a patient who has both Medicare and other coverage are coordinated under the rules of the **Medicare Secondary Payer (MSP)** program. The Medicare Coordination of Benefits department receives inquiries regarding Medicare as second payer and has information on a beneficiary's eligibility for benefits and the availability of other health insurance that is primary to Medicare.

If Medicare is the secondary payer to one primary payer, the claim must be submitted using the HIPAA 837 transaction unless the practice is excluded from electronic transaction rules. The 837 must report the amount the primary payer paid for the claim or for a particular service line (procedure) in the Allow Amount field. Claims for which more than one plan is responsible for payment prior to Medicare, however, should be submitted using the CMS-1500 claim form. The other payers' RAs/EOBs must be attached when the claim is sent to Medicare for processing.

Billing Tip

Submit MSP Claims for Zero Balances
Send an MSP claim to Medicare even when the primary payer has fully paid the bill and the patient owes nothing so that the amount paid can be credited to the patient's Medicare Part B annual deductible.

Following MSP Rules

The medical insurance specialist is responsible for identifying the situations where Medicare is the secondary payer and for preparing appropriate primary and secondary claims. A form such as that shown in Figure 14.8 is used to gather and validate information about Medicare patients' primary plans during the patient check-in process.

Over Age Sixty-Five and Employed

When an individual is employed and is covered by the employer's group health plan, Medicare is the secondary payer. This is the case for employees who are on leaves of absence, even if they are receiving short- or long-term disability benefits. Medicare is also secondary when an individual over age sixty-five is covered by a spouse's employer (even if the spouse is younger than sixty-five). On the other hand, Medicare is the primary carrier for:

- An individual who is working for an employer with twenty employees or fewer
- An individual who is covered by another policy that is not a group policy
- An individual who is enrolled in Part B but not Part A of the Medicare program
- An individual who must pay premiums to receive Part A coverage
- An individual who is retired and receiving coverage under a previous employer's group policy

Disabled

If an individual under age sixty-five is disabled and is covered by an employer group health plan (which may be held by the individual, a spouse, or another family member), Medicare is the secondary payer. If the individual or family

Patient's Name ______________________ Medicare # ________________

▪ Medicare Secondary Payer Screening Questionnaire

1.	Are you covered by the Veterans Administration, the Black Lung Program, or Workers Compensation? If so which one? - ____________	( ) Yes	( ) No
2.	Is this illness or injury due to any type of accident?	( ) Yes	( ) No
3.	Are you age 65 or older?	( ) Yes	( ) No
	a. Are you currently employed?	( ) Yes	( ) No
	b. Is your spouse currently employed?	( ) Yes	( ) No
4.	Are you age 65 or under?	( ) Yes	( ) No
	a. Are you covered by any employer Group Health Plan?	( ) Yes	( ) No
	b. Or another large Group Health Plan?	( ) Yes	( ) No

▪ Authorization Statement and Payment Agreement

I declare under penalty of perjury that I do not have another primary insurance carrier to pay for medical care rendered to me by ______________________, and that all information with regard to residence, employment, and income is correct to the best of my knowledge.

I request that payment of authorized Medicare Benefits be made to this health center for any services furnished to me by its physicians or suppliers.

I understand that my signature requests that payment be made and that it authorizes release of medical information necessary to pay the claim(s). If a secondary insurance carrier is involved my signature also authorizes releasing information to the insurer or agency shown.

In Medicare assigned cases, the physician or supplier agrees to accept the charge determined by the Medicare Carrier as full charge, and the patient is responsible only for the deductible (Excluding UGS/Medicare) coinsurance and noncovered services. Coinsurance and deductible are based upon charge determined by the Medicare carrier.

______________________________ ______________

Signature of Patient or Authorized Representative Date

______________________________ ______________

Witnessed by Date

FIGURE 14.8 Medicare Secondary Payer Screening Questionnaire

member is not actively employed, Medicare is the primary payer. Medicare is also the primary payer for:

- An individual and family members who are retired and receiving coverage under a group policy from a previous employer
- An individual and family members who are working for an employer with a hundred employees or fewer
- An individual and family members receiving coverage under the Consolidated Omnibus Budget Reconciliation Act of 1985 (COBRA; see Chapter 9)
- An individual who is covered by another policy that is not a group policy

End-Stage Renal Disease (ESRD)

During a coordination-of-benefits period, Medicare is the secondary payer for individuals who are covered by employer-sponsored group health plans and who fail to apply for ESRD-based Medicare coverage. The coordination-of-benefits period begins the first month the individual is eligible for or entitled to Part A benefits based on an ESRD diagnosis. This rule is in effect regardless of whether the individual is employed or retired.

Workers' Compensation

If an individual receives treatment for a job-related injury or illness, Medicare coverage (and private insurance) is secondary to workers' compensation coverage (see Chapter 13). Included in this category is the Federal Black Lung Program, a government program that provides insurance coverage for coal miners. When an individual suffers from a lung disorder caused by working in a mine, Medicare is secondary to the Black Lung coverage. If the procedure or diagnosis is for something other than a mining-related lung condition, Medicare is the primary payer.

Automobile, No-Fault, and Liability Insurance

Medicare (and private insurance) is always the secondary payer when treatment is for an accident-related claim, whether automobile, no-fault (injuries that occur on private property, regardless of who is at fault), or liability (injuries that occur on private property when a party is held responsible).

Veterans' Benefits

If a veteran is entitled to Medicare benefits, he or she may choose whether to receive coverage through Medicare or through the Department of Veterans Affairs.

MSP Claims and Payments

Table 14.4 provides details for completing an MSP CMS-1500. Three formulas are used to calculate how much of the patient's coinsurance will be paid by Medicare under MSP. Of the three amounts, Medicare will pay the lowest. The formulas use Medicare's allowable charge, the primary insurer's allowable charge, and the actual amount paid by the primary payer. Medicare, as the secondary payer, pays 100 percent of most coinsurance payments if the patient's Part B deductible has been paid. See Figure 14.9 on page 475.

The three formulas are:

1. Primary payer's allowed charge minus payment made on claim
2. What Medicare would pay (80 percent of Medicare allowed charge)
3. Higher allowed charge (either primary payer or Medicare) minus payment made on the claim

Compliance Guideline

Patient Coinsurance When Medicare Is Secondary
Medicare patients should not be charged for the primary insurance coinsurance until the RA is received and examined, because the patient is entitled to have Medicare pay these charges. A patient who has not met the deductible is, however, responsible for the coinsurance, and that amount is applied toward the deductible.

Example

A patient's visit allowed charge from the primary payer is $100, and the primary payer pays $80, with a $20 patient coinsurance. Medicare allows $80 for the service. The patient has met the Part B deductible. The calculations using the three formulas result in amounts of (1) $100 - $80 = $20, (2) $80 × 80 percent = $64, and (3) $100 - $80 = $20. Medicare will pay $20, since this is the lowest dollar amount from the three calculations.

Medicare pays up to the higher of two allowable amounts when another plan is primary. But if the primary payer has already paid more than the Medicare allowed amount, no additional payment is made.

Table 14.4 Medicare Secondary Payer (MSP) CMS-1500 (08/05) Claim Completion

Item Number	*Content*
1	Check both Medicare and either Group Health Plan or Other as appropriate for the patient's primary insurance.
1a	Enter the Medicare health insurance claim number that appears on the patient's Medicare card.
2	Record the patient's name *exactly* as it appears on the Medicare card, entering it in last name, first name, middle initial order.
3	Enter the patient's date of birth in eight-digit format; select male or female.
4	Enter the name of the insured person who has the primary coverage. If the insured is the patient, enter SAME.
5	Enter the patient's mailing address.
6	Select the appropriate box for the relationship: Self, spouse, child, or other.
7	If the patient and the insured are the same person, leave blank. If the insured's address is the same as the patient's, enter SAME. If the insured's address is different, enter the mailing address.
8	Select the appropriate boxes for marital status and employment status.
9a-d	Leave blank.
10a–10c	Choose the appropriate box to indicate whether the patient's condition is the result of a work injury, an automobile accident, or another type of accident.
10d	Leave blank.
11	Enter the insured's policy/group number.
11a	Enter the insured's date of birth and sex if they differ from the information in IN 3.
11b	If the policy is obtained through an employer or a school, enter the name in IN 11b; otherwise leave it blank. If the patient's employment status has changed—for example, if the patient has retired— enter RETIRED followed by the retirement date.
11c	Name or plan ID of the primary insurance.
11d	Leave blank.
12	Enter "Signature on File,""SOF," or a legal signature per practice policy.
13	Enter"Signature on File," "SOF," or a legal signature to indicate that there is a signature on file assigning benefits to the provider from the primary insurance.
14	Enter the date that symptoms first began for the current illness, injury, or pregnancy.
15	Leave blank.
16	Enter the dates the patient is employed but unable to work in the current occupation.
17	Enter the name (first name, middle initial, last name) and credentials of the professional who referred or ordered the services or supplies on the claim.
17a	Enter the appropriate identifying number (either NPI or non-NPI/qualifier) for the referring physician.
18	If the services provided are needed because of a related inpatient hospitalization, the admission and discharge dates are entered. For patients still hospitalized, the admission date is listed in the From box, and the To box is left blank.
19	Complete according to the carrier's instructions.
20	Complete if billing for outside lab services.
21	Enter up to four ICD-9-CM codes in priority order. At least one code must be reported.
22	Leave blank.
23	Enter the preauthorization number assigned by the payer or a CLIA number.
24A	Enter the date(s) of service.
24B	Enter the place of service (POS) code.
24C	Check with the payer to determine whether this element (emergency indicator) is necessary. If required, enter Y (yes) or N (no) in the unshaded bottom portion of the field.
24D	Enter the CPT/HCPCS codes and applicable modifiers for services provided. Do not use hyphens.
24E	Using the numbers (1, 2, 3, 4) listed to the left of the diagnosis codes in IN 21, enter the diagnosis for the each service listed in IN 24D.

(continued on next page)

Table 14.4 Medicare Secondary Payer (MSP) CMS-1500 (08/05) Claim Completion *continued*

Item Number	*Content*
24F	For each service listed in IN 24D, enter charges without dollar signs or decimals. If the claim reports an encounter with no charge, such as a capitated visit, a value of zero (0) may be used.
24G	Enter the number of days or units, as applicable.
24H	Leave blank.
24I–24J	Enter the NPI or non-NPI/qualifier.
25	Enter the physician's or supplier's federal tax identification number and check the appropriate box for SSN or EIN.
26	Enter the patient account number used by the practice's accounting system.
27	If the physician accepts assignment for the primary payer and Medicare, select Yes.
28	Enter the total of all charges in IN 24F.
29	Enter the amount of the payments received for the services listed on this claim from the patient. Attach the RA/EOB to show what the primary payer paid.
30	Leave blank.
31	Enter the provider's signature, the date of the signature, and credentials or SOF.
32	Enter the name, address, city, state, and ZIP code of the location where the services were rendered if other than the physician's office or the patient's home, or enter SAME.
33	Enter the provider name, address, ZIP code, telephone number, NPI, non-NPI number, and appropriate qualifier. The NPI should be placed in FL 33a. Enter the identifying non-NPI number and qualifier in FL 33b.

TRICARE CMS-1500 Secondary Claims

When TRICARE is the secondary payer, six item numbers on a paper claim are filled in differently than when TRICARE is the primary payer:

Item Number	Content
11	Policy number of the primary insurance plan
11a	Birth date and gender of the primary plan policyholder
11b	Employer of the primary plan policyholder if the plan is a group plan through an employer
11c	Name of the primary insurance plan
11d	Select Yes or No as appropriate.
29	Enter all payments made by other insurance carriers. Do not include payments made by the patient.

Medicare and Medicaid

If a patient is covered by both Medicare and Medicaid (a Medi-Medi beneficiary), Medicare is primary. The claim that is sent to Medicare is automatically crossed over to Medicaid for secondary payment. In this case, if a paper claim is completed, the Item Numbers are as indicated in Table 14.5 on pages 476–477.

1500

HEALTH INSURANCE CLAIM FORM

APPROVED BY NATIONAL UNIFORM CLAIM COMMITTEE 08/05

PICA | PICA | CARRIER

1. MEDICARE [X] (Medicare #) MEDICAID [ ] (Medicaid #) TRICARE CHAMPUS [ ] (Sponsor's SSN) CHAMPVA [ ] (Member ID#) GROUP HEALTH PLAN [X] (SSN or ID) FECA BLK LUNG [ ] (SSN) OTHER [ ] (ID)

1a. INSURED'S I.D. NUMBER (For Program in Item 1): 123455669A

2. PATIENT'S NAME (Last Name, First Name, Middle Initial): RAMOS CARLA D

3. PATIENT'S BIRTH DATE MM DD YY: 05 13 1933 SEX M [ ] F [X]

4. INSURED'S NAME (Last Name, First Name, Middle Initial): SAME

5. PATIENT'S ADDRESS (No., Street): 28 PARK STREET

6. PATIENT RELATIONSHIP TO INSURED: Self [X] Spouse [ ] Child [ ] Other [ ]

7. INSURED'S ADDRESS (No., Street)

CITY: KANSAS CITY STATE: MO

8. PATIENT STATUS: Single [X] Married [ ] Other [ ]

CITY STATE

ZIP CODE: 64111 TELEPHONE (Include Area Code): (816) 555 2185

Employed [X] Full-Time Student [ ] Part-Time Student [ ]

ZIP CODE TELEPHONE (INCLUDE AREA CODE) ( )

9. OTHER INSURED'S NAME (Last Name, First Name, Middle Initial)

10. IS PATIENT'S CONDITION RELATED TO:

11. INSURED'S POLICY GROUP OR FECA NUMBER: G2IX

a. OTHER INSURED'S POLICY OR GROUP NUMBER

a. EMPLOYMENT? (CURRENT OR PREVIOUS) [ ] YES [X] NO

a. INSURED'S DATE OF BIRTH MM DD YY SEX M [ ] F [ ]

b. OTHER INSURED'S DATE OF BIRTH MM DD YY SEX M [ ] F [ ]

b. AUTO ACCIDENT? [ ] YES [X] NO PLACE (State)

b. EMPLOYER'S NAME OR SCHOOL NAME: CORELLI INC

c. EMPLOYER'S NAME OR SCHOOL NAME

c. OTHER ACCIDENT? [ ] YES [X] NO

c. INSURANCE PLAN NAME OR PROGRAM NAME: PLAINS HEALTH PLAN

d. INSURANCE PLAN NAME OR PROGRAM NAME

10d. RESERVED FOR LOCAL USE

d. IS THERE ANOTHER HEALTH BENEFIT PLAN? [ ] YES [ ] NO *If yes,* return to and complete item 9 a-d.

READ BACK OF FORM BEFORE COMPLETING & SIGNING THIS FORM.

12. PATIENT'S OR AUTHORIZED PERSON'S SIGNATURE I authorize the release of any medical or other information necessary to process this claim. I also request payment of government benefits either to myself or to the party who accepts assignment below.

SIGNED SOF DATE

13. INSURED'S OR AUTHORIZED PERSON'S SIGNATURE I authorize payment of medical benefits to the undersigned physician or supplier for services described below.

SIGNED SOF

PATIENT AND INSURED INFORMATION

14. DATE OF CURRENT: MM DD YY ILLNESS (First symptom) OR INJURY (Accident) OR PREGNANCY(LMP)

15. IF PATIENT HAS HAD SAME OR SIMILAR ILLNESS. GIVE FIRST DATE MM DD YY

16. DATES PATIENT UNABLE TO WORK IN CURRENT OCCUPATION FROM MM DD YY TO MM DD YY

17. NAME OF REFERRING PHYSICIAN OR OTHER SOURCE

17a.

17b. NPI

18. HOSPITALIZATION DATES RELATED TO CURRENT SERVICES FROM MM DD YY TO MM DD YY

19. RESERVED FOR LOCAL USE

20. OUTSIDE LAB? [ ] YES [X] NO $ CHARGES

21. DIAGNOSIS OR NATURE OF ILLNESS OR INJURY. (Relate Items 1,2,3 or 4 to Item 24e by Line)

1. 388.31

2. 477.9

3. ___ . ___

4. ___ . ___

22. MEDICAID RESUBMISSION CODE ORIGINAL REF. NO.

23. PRIOR AUTHORIZATION NUMBER

	24. A. DATE(S) OF SERVICE From MM DD YY	To MM DD YY	B. PLACE OF SERVICE	C. EMG	D. PROCEDURES, SERVICES, OR SUPPLIES (Explain Unusual Circumstances) CPT/HCPCS	MODIFIER	E. DIAGNOSIS POINTER	F. $ CHARGES	G. DAYS OR UNITS	H. EPSDT Family Plan	I. ID. QUAL.	J. RENDERING PROVIDER ID. #
1	10 01 2008		11		99204		1,2	128 00	1		NPI	
2	10 01 2008		11		92557		1	95 00	1		NPI	
3	10 01 2008		11		92567		1	10 00	1		NPI	
4											NPI	
5											NPI	
6											NPI	

25. FEDERAL TAX I.D. NUMBER: 016778002 SSN [ ] EIN [X]

26. PATIENT'S ACCOUNT NO.: RAM04

27. ACCEPT ASSIGNMENT? (For govt. claims, see back) [X] YES [ ] NO

28. TOTAL CHARGE: $ 313 00

29. AMOUNT PAID: $ 20 00

30. BALANCE DUE: $

31. SIGNATURE OF PHYSICIAN OR SUPPLIER INCLUDING DEGREES OR CREDENTIALS (I certify that the statements on the reverse apply to this bill and are made a part thereof.)

SIGNED SOF DATE

32. SERVICE FACILITY LOCATION INFORMATION: SAME

a. NPI b.

33. BILLING PROVIDER INFO & PHONE # ( )

RONALD R BERGEN
96 YORK AVE
KANSAS CITY MO 64112

a. NPI 0175328865 b.

PHYSICIAN OR SUPPLIER INFORMATION

NUCC Instruction Manual available at: www.nucc.org

FIGURE 14.9 CMS-1500 (08/05) Completion for Medicare Secondary Payer (MSP) Claims

Table 14.5 Medicare/Medicaid CMS-1500 (08/05) Claim Completion

Item Number	*Content*
1	Indicate Medicare and Medicaid.
1a	Enter the Medicare health insurance claim number that appears on the patient's Medicare card.
2	Record the patient's name *exactly* as it appears on the Medicare card, entering it in last name, first name, middle initial order.
3	Enter the patient's date of birth in eight-digit format; make the appropriate selection for male or female.
4	Enter the name of the insured if not the patient.
5	Enter the patient's mailing address.
6	Select the appropriate box for the relationship: Self, spouse, child, or other.
7	If the insured's address is the same as the patient's, enter SAME. If it is different, enter the mailing address.
8	Select the appropriate boxes for marital status and employment status.
9	Enter Medicaid patient's full name.
9a	Enter the Medicaid number here or in IN 10d, according to the payer.
9b	Medicaid insured's date of birth if different than patient's.
9c	Leave blank.
9d	Leave blank.
10a–10c	Choose the appropriate box to indicate whether the patient's condition is the result of a work injury, an automobile accident, or another type of accident.
10d	Varies with the insurance plan; complete if instructed.
11	Enter NONE.
11a-d	Leave blank.
12	Enter "Signature on File," "SOF," or a legal signature, per practice policy.
13	Leave blank.
14	Enter the date that symptoms first began for the current illness, injury, or pregnancy.
15	Leave blank.
16	Enter the dates the patient is employed but unable to work in the current occupation.
17	Enter the name and credentials of the professional who referred or ordered the services or supplies on the claim.
17a	Enter the appropriate identifying number (either NPI or non-NPI/qualifier) for the referring physician.
18	If the services provided are needed because of a related inpatient hospitalization, the admission and discharge dates are entered. For patients still hospitalized, the admission date is listed in the From box, and the To box is left blank.
19	Complete according to the carrier's instructions.
20	Complete if billing for outside lab services.
21	Enter up to four ICD-9-CM codes in priority order.
22	Leave blank.
23	Enter the preauthorization number assigned by the payer or a CLIA number.
24A	Enter the date(s) of service, from and to.
24B	Enter the place of service (POS) code that describes the location at which the service was provided.
24C	Check with the payer to determine whether this element (emergency indicator) is necessary. If required, enter Y (yes) or N (no) in the unshaded bottom portion of the field.
24D	Enter the CPT/HCPCS codes and applicable modifiers for services provided. Do not use hyphens.
24E	Using the numbers (1, 2, 3, 4) listed to the left of the diagnosis codes in IN 21, enter the diagnosis for the each service listed in IN 24D.
24F	For each service listed in IN 24D, enter charges without dollar signs or decimals. If the claim reports an encounter with no charge, such as a capitated visit, a value of zero (0) may be used.
24G	Enter the number of days or units, as applicable. If only one service is performed, the numeral 1 must be entered.

(continued on next page)

Table 14.5 Medicare/Medicaid CMS-1500 (08/05) Claim Completion *continued*

Item Number	Content
24H	Leave blank.
24I–24J	Enter NPI or non-NPI/qualifier.
25	Enter the physician's or supplier's federal tax identification number and check the appropriate box for SSN or EIN.
26	Enter the patient account number used by the practice's accounting system.
27	Select Yes. 28 Enter the total of all charges in IN 24F.
29	Amount of the payments received for the services listed on this claim. If no payment was made, enter "none" or "0.00."
30	Leave blank.
31	Enter the provider's or supplier's signature, the date of the signature, and the provider's credentials (such as MD).
32	Enter the name, address, city, state, and ZIP code of the location where the services were rendered if not the physician's office or the patient's home, or enter SAME.
	The supplier's NPI is entered in IN 32a. Enter the payer-assigned identifying non-NPI number and qualifier of the service facility in IN 32b.
33	Enter the billing provider's or supplier's name, address, ZIP code, telephone number, NPI, non-NPI number, and appropriate qualifier. The NPI should be placed in IN 33a. Enter the identifying non-NPI number and qualifier of the billing provider in IN 33b.

Thinking It Through — 14.5

Ron Polonsky is a seventy-one-year-old retired distribution manager. He and his wife Sandra live in Lincoln, Nebraska. Sandra is fifty-seven and is employed as a high-school science teacher. She has family coverage through a group health insurance plan offered by the state of Nebraska. Ron is covered as a dependent on her plan. The Medicare Part B carrier for Nebraska is Blue Cross and Blue Shield of Kansas.

Which carrier is Ron's primary insurance carrier? Why?

Review

Steps to Success

- ❒ Read this chapter and review the Key Terms and the Chapter Summary.
- ❒ Answer the Review Questions and Applying Your Knowledge in the Chapter Review.
- ❒ Access the chapter's websites and complete the Internet Activities to learn more about available professional resources.
- ❒ Complete the related chapter in the *Medical Insurance Workbook* to reinforce your understanding of processing payments from payers, handling appeals, and completing secondary claims.

Chapter Summary

1. Payers first perform initial processing checks on claims, rejecting those with missing or clearly incorrect information. During the adjudication process that follows, claims are processed through the payer's automated medical edits; a manual review is done if required; the payer makes a determination of whether to pay, deny, or reduce the claim; and payment is sent with a remittance advice/explanation of benefits (RA/EOB).
2. Automated edits check for (a) patient eligibility for benefits, (b) time limits for filing claims, (c) preauthorization and referral requirements, (d) duplicate dates of service, (e) noncovered services, (f) code linkage, (g) correct bundling, (h) medical review to confirm that services were appropriate and necessary, (i) utilization review, and (j) concurrent care.
3. Medical insurance specialists monitor claims by reviewing the insurance aging report and following up at properly timed intervals based on the payer's promised turnaround time. The HIPAA X12 276/277 Heath Care Claim Status Inquiry/Response (276/277) is used to track claim progress through the adjudication process.
4. The HIPAA X12 835 Health Care Payment and Remittance Advice (HIPAA 835) is the standard transaction payers use to transmit adjudication details and payments to providers. Electronic and paper RAs/EOBs contain the same essential data: (a) a heading with payer and provider information, (b) payment information for each claim, including adjustment codes, (c) total amounts paid for all claims, and (d) a glossary that defines the adjustment codes that appear on the document. These administrative code sets are claim adjustment group codes, claim adjustment reason codes, and remittance advice remark codes.
5. The unique claim control number reported on the RA/EOB is first used to match up claims sent and payments received. Then basic data are checked against the claim; billed procedures are verified; the payment for each CPT is checked against the expected amount; adjustment codes are reviewed to locate all unpaid, downcoded, or denied claims; and items are identified for follow up.
6. Payments are deposited in the practice's bank account, posted in the practice management program, and applied to patients' accounts. Rejected claims must be corrected and re-sent. Missed procedures are billed again. Partially paid, denied, or downcoded claims are analyzed and appealed, billed to the patient, or written off.
7. An appeal process is used to challenge a payer's decision to deny, reduce, or otherwise downcode a claim. Each payer has a graduated level of appeals, deadlines for requesting them, and medical review programs to answer them. In some cases, appeals may be taken beyond the payer to an outside authority, such as a state insurance commission.
8. Filing an appeal may result in payment of a denied or reduced claim. Postpayment audits are usually used to gather information about treat-

ment outcomes, but they may also be used to find overpayments, which must be refunded to payers. Refunds to patients may also be required.

9. Claims are sent to patients' additional insurance plans after the primary payer has adjudicated claims. Sometimes the medical office prepares and sends the claims; in other cases, the primary payer has a coordination of benefits (COB) program that automatically sends the necessary data to secondary payers.
10. Under the Medicare Secondary Payer program, Medicare is the secondary payer when (a) the patient is covered by an employer group health insurance plan or is covered through an employed spouse's plan; (b) the patient is disabled, under age sixty-five, and covered by an employee group health plan; (c) the patient is diagnosed with ESRD but is covered by an employer-sponsored group health plan; (d) the services are covered by workers' compensation insurance; (e) the services are for injuries in an automobile accident; or (f) the patient is a veteran who chooses to receive services through the Department of Veterans Affairs.

Review Questions

Match the key terms with their definitions.

A. medical necessity denial
B. adjudication
C. Medicare Redetermination Notice (MRN)
D. insurance aging report
E. adjustment
F. accounts receivable (A/R)
G. development
H. electronic funds transfer
I. concurrent care
J. determination

____ 1. Analysis of how long a payer has held submitted claims
____ 2. Payer paying a service at a different amount than billed
____ 3. Medical situation in which a patient receives extensive independent care from two or more attending physicians on the same date of service
____ 4. A payer's refusal to pay for a reported procedure that does not meet its medical necessity criteria
____ 5. Payer process to review claims
____ 6. Letter from Medicare to an appellant regarding a first-level appeal
____ 7. A payer's decision regarding payment of a claim
____ 8. A banking service for directly transmitting funds from one bank to another
____ 9. Money that is due to the practice from payers and patients
____ 10. Payer action to gather clinical documentation and study a claim before payment

Decide whether each statement is true or false.

____ 1. A claim may be rejected by a payer because the patient has not paid the premium for the reported date of service.
____ 2. The medical review program is created by the provider's practice manager to adjudicate claims.
____ 3. A payer's claims examiners are trained medical professionals.
____ 4. If a patient's medical record clearly documents a high level of evaluation and management service, the associated procedure code is not likely to be reduced by the payer.
____ 5. The claim turnaround time is often specified by state regulations.
____ 6. The insurance aging report shows when patients received their statements.
____ 7. The EFT summarizes the results of the payer's adjudication process.

____ 8. An appeal can be filed if the provider disagrees with the payer's determination.

____ 9. The RA/EOB shows the patient's financial responsibility, which is subtracted from the allowed charge to calculate the amount the provider is paid.

____ 10. The Medicare Secondary Payer program requires Medicaid to cost-share crossover claims.

Select the letter that best completes the statement or answers the question.

____ 1. A payer's initial processing of a claim screens for
   A. utilization guidelines
   B. medical edits
   C. basic errors in claim data or missing information
   D. claims attachments

____ 2. Some automated edits are for
   A. patient eligibility, duplicate claims, and noncovered services
   B. valid identification numbers
   C. medical necessity reduction denials
   D. clinical documentation

____ 3. A claim may be downcoded because
   A. the claim does not list a charge for every procedure code
   B. the claim is for noncovered services
   C. the documentation does not justify the level of service
   D. the procedure code applies to a patient of the other gender

____ 4. Payers should comply with the required
   A. insurance aging report
   B. claim turnaround time
   C. remittance advice
   D. retention schedule

____ 5. A person filing an appeal is called a
   A. guarantor
   B. claims examiner
   C. medical director
   D. claimant

____ 6. Appeals must always be filed
   A. within a specified time
   B. by the provider for the patient
   C. by patients on behalf of relatives
   D. with the state insurance commissioner

____ 7. If a postpayment audit determines that a paid claim should have been denied or reduced
   A. the provider is subject to civil penalties
   B. the provider must refund the incorrect payment
   C. the provider bills the patient for the denied amount
   D. none of the above

____ 8. If a patient has secondary insurance under a spouse's plan, what information is needed before transmitting a claim to the secondary plan?
   A. RA/EOB data
   B. 271 data
   C. PPO data
   D. none of the above

____ 9. The HIPAA standard transaction that is used to inquire and answer about the status of a claim is
   A. 837
   B. 835
   C. 276/277
   D. 980

____10. Which of the following appears only on secondary claims?
   A. primary insurance group policy number
   B. primary insurance employer name
   C. primary plan name
   D. primary payer payment

Define the following abbreviations.

1. RA ____________________
2. EOB ____________________
3. MSP ____________________
4. EFT ____________________

Applying Your Knowledge

Case 14.1 Auditing Claim Data

The following data elements were submitted to a third-party payer. Using the ICD-9-CM, the CPT/HCPCS, and the place of service codes in Appendix B, audit the information in each case and advise the payer about the correct action.

A. Dx 783.2
   CPT 80048
   POS 60

B. Dx 518.83
   CPT 99241-22

C. Dx 662.30
   CPT 54500

Case 14.2 Calculating Insurance Math

Patient ID	Patient Name	Plan	Date of Service	Procedure	Provider Charge	Allowed Amount	Patient Payment (Coinsurance and Deductible)	Claim Adjustment Reason Code	PROV PAY
537-88-5267	Ramirez, Gloria B.	R-1	02/13/2008–2/13/2008	99214	$105.60	$59.00	$8.85	2	$50.15
348-99-2537	Finucula, Betty R.	R-1	01/15/2008–1/15/2008	99292	$88.00	$50.00	$7.50	2	$42.50
537-88-5267	Ramirez, Gloria B.	R-1	02/14/2008–2/14/2008	90732	$38.00	0	$38.00	49	0
760-57-5372	Jugal, Kurt T.	R-1	02/16/2008–2/16/2008	93975 99204	$580.00 $178.00	$261.00 $103.00	$139.15 $15.45	12	$121.8 $87.55
875-17-0098	Quan, Mary K.	PPO-3	02/16/2008–2/16/2008	20004	$192.00	$156.00	$31.20	2	$124.80
								TOTAL	$426.85

The RA/EOB shown above has been received by a provider.

A. What is the patient coinsurance *percentage* required under plan R-1?

____

B. What is the patient coinsurance *percentage* required under plan PPO-3?

____

C. What is Gloria Ramirez's *balance due* for the two dates of service listed?

____

D. Kurt Jugal's first visit of the year is the encounter shown for DOS 2/16/2008. What is the patient *deductible* under plan R-1? (*Hint:* Since the deductible was satisfied by the patient's payment for the first charge, that payment was made up of the deductible and the coinsurance under the plan.)

____

Case 14.3 Using Insurance Terms

Read this information from a Medicare carrier and answer the questions that follow.

Noridian Administrative Services (*a Medicare Carrier*) denies Q4054 (Darbepoetin Alfa) and Q4055 (Epoetin alfa) services when coverage guidelines are not met using the adjustment reason code B5. In the past, we denied these services as beneficiary responsibility. It has now been determined that these denials are a medical necessity denial. As such, the Advance Beneficiary Notice (ABN) rules apply.

Effective for claims received on/after (*date*), when these services are billed with a –GA modifier, the beneficiary will be held liable for noncovered services. Claims submitted without a –GA modifier will be denied as provider responsibility.

A. Based on Table 14.2 on page 459, what is the meaning of adjustment reason code B5?

B. Based on the information on ABNs in Chapter 10, what is the meaning of ABN modifier –GA?

C. If a –GA modifier is attached to HCPCS codes Q4054 and Q4055 on a claim, can the patient be billed?

D. If a –GA modifier is *not* attached to the HCPCS codes Q4050 and Q4055 on a claim, can the provider balance-bill the patient?

Internet Activities

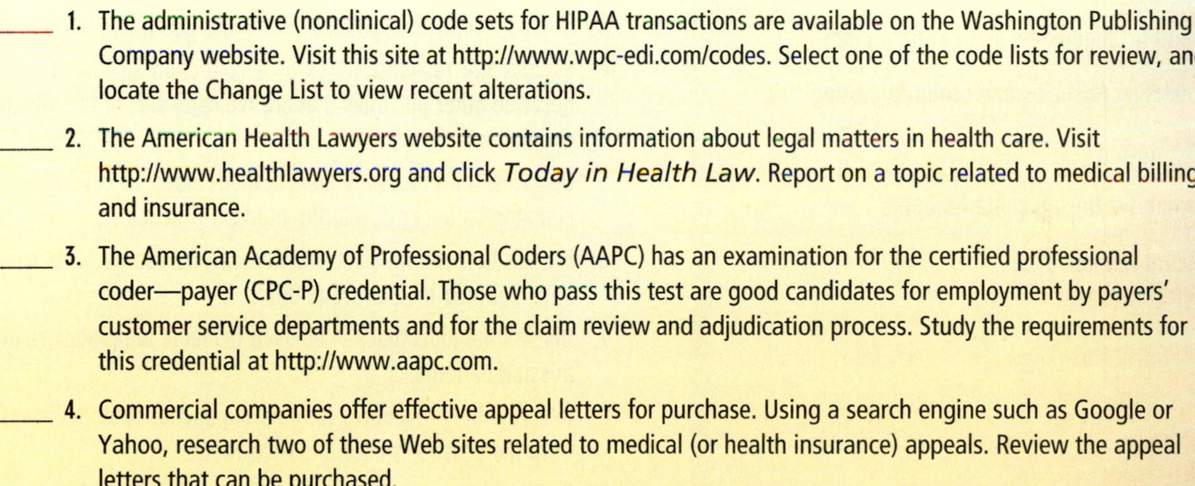

____ 1. The administrative (nonclinical) code sets for HIPAA transactions are available on the Washington Publishing Company website. Visit this site at http://www.wpc-edi.com/codes. Select one of the code lists for review, and locate the Change List to view recent alterations.

____ 2. The American Health Lawyers website contains information about legal matters in health care. Visit http://www.healthlawyers.org and click *Today in Health Law*. Report on a topic related to medical billing and insurance.

____ 3. The American Academy of Professional Coders (AAPC) has an examination for the certified professional coder—payer (CPC-P) credential. Those who pass this test are good candidates for employment by payers' customer service departments and for the claim review and adjudication process. Study the requirements for this credential at http://www.aapc.com.

____ 4. Commercial companies offer effective appeal letters for purchase. Using a search engine such as Google or Yahoo, research two of these Web sites related to medical (or health insurance) appeals. Review the appeal letters that can be purchased.

Chapter 15

Patient Billing and Collections

CHAPTER OUTLINE

Patient Billing

Organizing for Effective Collections

Collection Regulations and Procedures

Credit Arrangements and Payment Plans

Collection Agencies and Credit Reporting

Skip Tracing

Writing Off Uncollectible Accounts

Record Retention

Learning Outcomes

After studying this chapter, you should be able to:

1. Discuss the ways practices explain their financial policies to patients.
2. Describe the purpose and content of patients' statements and the procedures for working with them.
3. Compare individual patient billing and guarantor billing.
4. Discuss the responsibilities of a collection specialist, and describe other positions that are typically part of the billing and collections function.
5. Describe the processes and methods used to collect outstanding balances due to the medical practice.
6. Explain how the medical practice can pursue patients who have not paid their overdue bills.
7. Discuss the tools that can be used to locate unresponsive or missing patients.
8. Describe the procedures for clearing uncollectible balances from the practice's accounts receivable.
9. Explain the purpose of a retention schedule and the requirements for retaining patient information.

Key Terms

bankruptcy
bad debt
collection agency
collections
collections specialist
credit bureaus
credit reporting
cycle billing
day sheet
embezzlement
Fair and Accurate Credit Transaction Act (FACTA)
Fair Credit Reporting Act (FCRA)
Fair Debt Collection Practices Act of 1977 (FDCPA)
guarantor billing
means test
patient aging report
patient refunds
patient statement
payment plan
prepayment plan
retention schedule
skip trace
Telephone Consumer Protection Act of 1991
Truth in Lending Act
uncollectible account

"Patients are responsible for payment of all medical treatment and services provided. Let's discuss your bill and see if we can set up a payment plan that works for you."

Patient billing and collections, the last steps in the billing and reimbursement process, involves:

- Generating and mailing patient statements to show the balances that patients owe
- Posting patients' payments
- Examining aging reports for patients' accounts and handling collections

Medical practices have financial policies to regulate the billing of patients and the procedures used to collect money they are owed. Each administrative staff member contributes to effective patient collections and thus to the financial viability of the practice. All the money owed, though, cannot always be collected. Some patients do not pay their bills, and special circumstances cause a practice to write off the accounts of others. However, in all cases, the practice must comply with state and federal laws during collection activities and by maintaining patient records and information.

Patient Billing

Effective patient billing begins with sound financial policies and procedures that clearly explain patients' responsibilities for payment. These activities set the stage for the billing and reimbursement steps that follow, sending patient statements and following up on patient payments.

Financial Policies and Procedures

A good financial policy is one that both staff members and patients can follow. Practices must clearly explain their financial policies so that patients understand their obligations and administrative staff members know what is expected of the patients. Financial policies address all possible scenarios, including financial arrangements and payment plans, payments not covered by insurance, and various special circumstances. The policy should tell patients how the practice will handle the following:

- Collection of copayments, deductibles, and past-due balances
- Financial arrangements for unpaid balances
- Charity care or use of a sliding scale for patients with low incomes

- Payments for services not covered by insurance
- Prepayment for services
- Day-of-service discounts or discounts to patients with financial need
- Acceptance of cash, checks, money orders, and credit or debit cards
- Special circumstances for automobile accidents and nonassigned insurance

Policies are supported by clear office procedures that can be consistently applied by both professional and administrative staff members. A sample financial policy is shown in Figure 15.1. Figure 15.2 on page 488 shows the supporting office procedures that appear in the practice's procedure manual.

Effective patient billing also includes educating patients from the start of the billing and reimbursement process. Most practices mail brochures to patients that cover billing, post signs in the reception area with this information, and tell patients about the policies when they register. The patient information form that is completed and signed by new patients often presents a statement about patient payment responsibility, as shown in Figure 3.3 on page 79. On this example of a patient information form, the patient or insured is asked to sign this statement:

> I authorize treatment and agree to pay all fees and charges for the person named above. I agree to pay all changes shown by statements, promptly upon their presentation, unless credit arrangements are agreed upon in writing. I authorize payment directly to VALLEY ASSOCIATES of insurance benefits otherwise payable to me. I hereby authorize the release of any medical information necessary in order to process a claim for payment in my behalf.

Preauthorized credit card forms (see Figure 3.14 on page 100) and forms to arrange payments for professional services rendered (see Figure 3.13 on page 99) are also completed by patients for payment purposes.

Patients' Statements

To review: After an encounter, the transactions for the visit (charges and payments) are entered in the patient ledger (the record of a patient's financial transactions; also called the patient account record), and the patient's balance is updated. A claim is filed, and the resulting payment from the patient's insurance carrier is posted, based on the RA/EOB:

1. The payer's payment for each reported procedure is entered.
2. The amount the patient owes for each reported procedure is calculated.
3. If any part of a charge must be written off due to a payer's required adjustment, this amount is also entered.

Thinking It Through — 15.1

Study Figure 15.1 and Figure 15.2 (pages 487–488), and then answer the following questions:

1. **Who is responsible for any copayments, and when must they be paid?**
2. **What is a self-pay patient's financial responsibility for the initial visit? Under what circumstances can a self-pay patient be billed after the visit?**
3. **Whose job is it to explain the situation to patients when planned services are not covered by their insurance?**

VALLEY ASSOCIATES FINANCIAL POLICY

Our objective is to provide you with the highest health care in the most cost-effective manner. However the ability of Valley Associations, P. C. to achieve this objective depends greatly on your understanding of our financial policy. If you have medical insurance, we will file insurance claim forms on your behalf. We do this as courtesy to our patients and are anxious to help you receive the maximum allowable benefits from you insurer. Even though we file insurance claims for you, we need your active participation in the insurance claims process.

MEDICARE PATIENTS

As a participating provider of Medicare Part B* (physician Services), Valley Associates, P.C., will only bill you for your Medicare coinsurance, deductible, and any services rendered but not covered by Medicare. All other services will be billed directly to Medicare.

NOTE: You will be informed of services not covered by Medicare before they are rendered. Your signature upon the appropriate Medicare waiver form represents your authorization for the physician to perform these services and your acceptance of the financial responsibility for them. If you have Medicare Part A only, then the services you receive from our practice will not be covered by Medicare.

COMMERCIAL INSURANCE PATIENTS

Remember that your insurance contract is between you and your insurer. If your insurance company pays only part of your bill or rejects your claim, you are financially responsible for the balance and are to pay it upon receipt of your statement. You will be required to pay the co-pay for authorized services at the time of service.

HMO/MANAGED CARE INSURANCE PATIENTS

Many HMO/Managed Care plans require that you obtain a referral in order to receive care from a specialist. It is your responsibility for obtaining this referral if required. Unauthorized services will be the financial responsibility of the patient. Please have your referral forms and membership card handy when you check in. You will be required to pay the co-pay for authorized services at the time of service.

PATIENTS WITH NO INSURANCE

Generally, patients with no insurance are required to pay for the office/provider portion of their visit in full at the time of service. The cost of additional services, including but not limited to medications or injections, medical procedures, etc., will be calculated and billed after the office visit. If special financial arrangements are deemed necessary, you will be given information regarding whom to contact at the time of your visit. It is imperative you follow these instructions immediately to satisfy your financial responsibility with Valley Associates, P.C..

We accept cash, checks, and Visa/MasterCard/Discover/American Express payments.

________________________ ________________

Patient/ Guarantor Signature Date

FIGURE 15.1 Financial Policy

The practice management program (PMP) uses this information to update the **day sheet**, which is a summary of the financial transactions that occur each day. The patient ledger is also updated. These data are used to generate **patient statements**, printed bills that show the amount each patient owes. Patient statements are called patient ledger cards when billing is done manually rather than by computer. Patients may owe coinsurance, deductibles, and fees for noncovered services.

VALLEY ASSOCIATES, PC	SECTION: PATIENT SERVICES
PROCEDURE MANUAL	
APPROVED BY:	PAYMENT BEFORE SERVICE
Stan Mongin, Administrator	
EFFECTIVE DATE: January 2007	Page 1 of 1

PROCEDURE

1. All patients with insurance co-pays are expected to pay their co-pay in full at registration prior to seeing a provider. Our contracts with the insurer require that we collect this amount. The patient's agreement with his or her insurance company also requires payment of this fee by the patient at the time of service.

2. Patients with insurance seeking care for services that may be noncovered by their insurance shall be required to sign an "Advance Beneficiary Notice" or "Notice of Noncoverage" as appropriate to the situation. These patients are responsible for the cost of these services. Nursing personnel are responsible for explaining and obtaining these forms prior to delivery of services.

3. New patients without insurance or unable to provide evidence of insurance coverage are expected to pay for their visits in full at the time of service. Once these individuals have established themselves as patients of the Practice with a positive payment history, they may be billed for services after the fact as well.

4. Established Practice patients who lose insurance coverage may continue to be seen without payment required at each visit. These patients will be billed accordingly.

5. Patients involved in a motor vehicle accident (MVA) and seeking treatment related to injuries sustained in the accident, shall be required to pay for services in full at the time of service unless confirmation for payment of services can be obtained from the auto insurer prior to treatment. Health insurance typically does not cover injuries sustained in a motor vehicle accident.

6. Should a patient fail to keep his or her balance current, the Practice may employ various methods of collection of past due amounts including placing the patient on a cash only basis for future appointments.

7. Patients unable to meet their financial obligations at the time of registration should either be rescheduled for another appointment or referred to the emergency room if they believe their condition warrants immediate care. Appointments that are not rescheduled should be noted as cancelled by the patient in the practice management program.

8. We will provide, on request, any additional information requested by the patient to file a claim with his or her insurance.

9. Parents are responsible for the costs associated with the treatment of minor children. The parent accompanying the minor child shall be responsible for any co-pay regardless of custodial rights.

FIGURE 15.2 Patient Payment Procedures

The Content of Statements

Statements are mailed to patients for payment. They must be easy for the patient to read, and they must be accurate. They contain all necessary information so that there is no confusion about the amount owed:

- The name of the practice and the patient's name, address, and account number
- A cost breakdown of all services provided
- An explanation of the costs covered by the patient's payer(s)
- The date of the statement (and sometimes the due date for the payment)
- The balance due (if a previous balance was due on the account, the sum of the old balance and the new charges)
- In some cases, the payment methods the practice offers

For example, review this section taken from a patient statement. The policy is a high-deductible PPO that does not cover preventive services.

DATE	CODE	DESCRIPTION			CHARGES	CREDITS
09/10/07	99396	Prev Check up, Est. 40–64 Yr			169.00	
09/10/07	85018	Hemoglobin Count, Colorimetric			6.10	
09/10/07	81002	Urinalysis, Non-automated, w/o s			4.20	
09/11/07		Golden Rule Ins. Co. #31478			Filed	
10/17/07		Denied Golden Rule Ins. Co. #31478				00.00
10/17/07		Repriced Golden Rule Inc. Co. #31478				51.80—
10/17/07		$127.50 = deductible for 9/10/07 visit				
Current	30 – 60	60 – 90	>90	TOTAL	INS PENDING	TOTAL DUE FROM PATIENT
127.50	0.00	0.00	0.00	127.50	0.00	127.50

This section summarizes the following information for the patient:

- The patient had a preventive checkup with a hemoglobin level check and urinalysis on September 10, for which the provider's usual charges are shown.
- On the next day, the claim for the visit was sent to the payer, Golden Rule Insurance Company.
- On October 17, the RA/EOB for the claim was posted. The payer did not pay the claim ("denied it") because the patient's plan does not cover these preventive services. The payer repriced the charges according to the PPO's in-network allowed amount for the service. The PPO total allowed amount for the visit is $127.50.
- The patient has not met the annual deductible, so the repriced charge of $127.50 is being billed to the patient.

Relating Statements to the Practice Management Program

Clear and accurate statements help ensure that most patients will pay on time. Study parts a, b and c of Figure 15.3 on pages 490–491 to observe the connection between the practice management program's data entry screen, the patient ledger, and the patient statement.

Example

Patient: Karen Giroux

Date of Service: 10/7/08

Date of RA: 10/8/08

Billing Tip

Credit Cards

- When a credit card is accepted in advance for payments billed after treatment, the practice sends the patient a zero-balance statement showing the amount that was charged to the card.
- Practices may use online bill paying systems that let patients use credit cards online when statements are received.
- The American Medical Association (AMA) does not permit physicians to increase their charges to capture credit card processing fees the practice pays.

Billing Tip

Return Service Requested

Write or stamp "Return Service Requested" on envelopes containing patients' statements, so that the U.S. Postal Service will return the bill with the new address if the patient has moved and left a forwarding address.

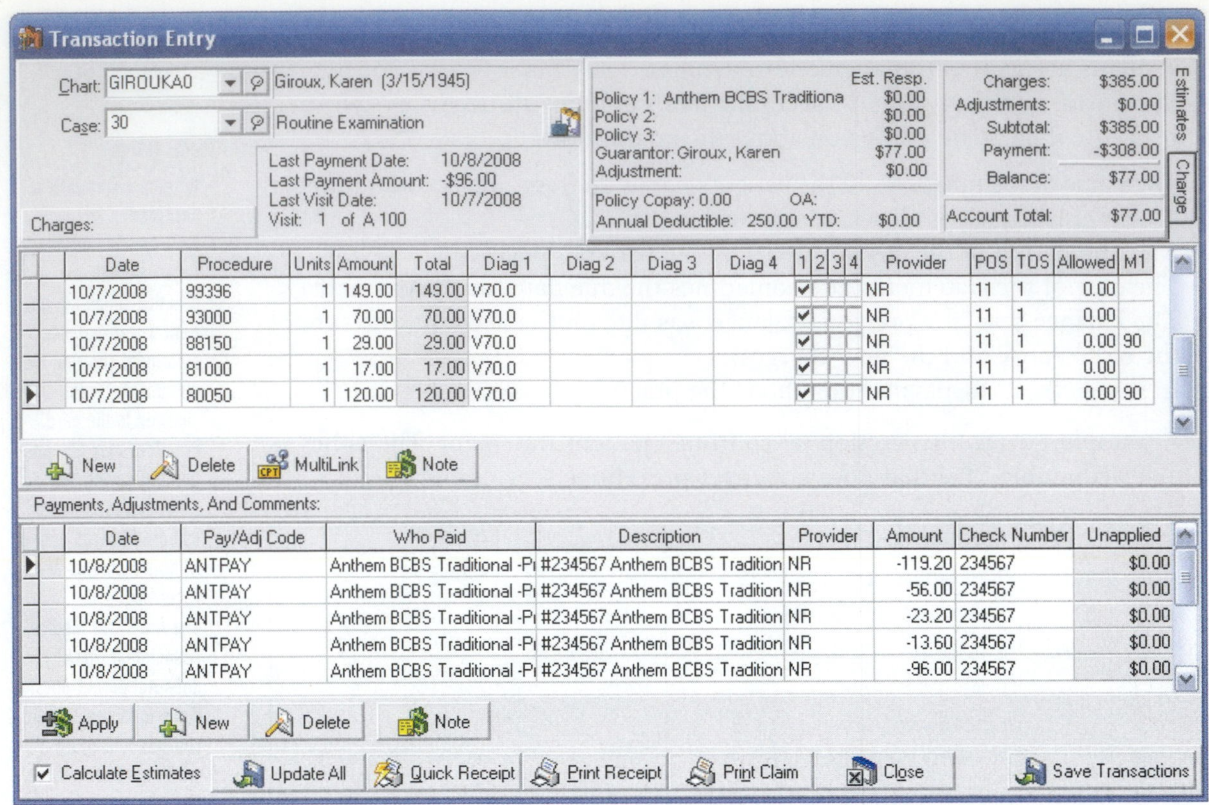

FIGURE 15.3 (a) Patient Transaction Data Entry Screen

The computer screen above illustrates the entry of the charges for Karen Giroux's office visit on October 7, 2008, and a payment received from the health plan on October 8, 2008. The patient ledger below shows each charge and each payment. The patient statement on page 491 is sent to the patient or guarantor and shows the balance that is owed. Compare the statement to the ledger to check the amounts charged and paid.

Valley Associates, P.C.

Patient Account Ledger

As of October 31, 2008

Entry	Date	POS	Description	Procedure	Document	Provider	Amount
GIROUKA0	**Karen Giroux**			(555)683-5364			
	Last Payment: -96.00		On: 10/8/2008				
6	10/7/2008			99396	0310060000	NR	149.00
7	10/7/2008			93000	0310060000	NR	70.00
8	10/7/2008			88150	0310060000	NR	29.00
9	10/7/2008			81000	0310060000	NR	17.00
10	10/7/2008			80050	0310060000	NR	120.00
40	10/8/2008		#234567 Anthem BCBS Traditiona	ANTPAY	0310060000	NR	-119.20
41	10/8/2008		#234567 Anthem BCBS Traditiona	ANTPAY	0310060000	NR	-56.00
42	10/8/2008		#234567 Anthem BCBS Traditiona	ANTPAY	0310060000	NR	-23.20
43	10/8/2008		#234567 Anthem BCBS Traditiona	ANTPAY	0310060000	NR	-13.60
44	10/8/2008		#234567 Anthem BCBS Traditiona	ANTPAY	0310060000	NR	-96.00
	Patient Totals						77.00
	Ledger Totals						77.00

FIGURE 15.3 (b) Patient Account Ledger

Valley Associates, P.C.
1400 West Center Street
Toledo, OH 43601-0123
(555)321-0987

Statement Date	Chart Number	Page
10/31/2008	**GIROUKA0**	**1**

Karen Giroux
14A West Front St
Brooklyn, OH 44144-1234

Make Checks Payable To:
Valley Associates, P.C.
1400 West Center Street
Toledo, OH 43601-0123
(555)321-0987

Date of Last Payment: 10/8/2008 Amount: -96.00 Previous Balance: 0.00

Patient: Karen Giroux Chart Number: GIROUKA0 Case: Routine Examination

Dates	Procedure	Charge	Paid by Primary	Paid By Guarantor	Adjustments	Remainder
10/07/08	99396	149.00	-119.20		0.00	29.80
10/07/08	93000	70.00	-56.00		0.00	14.00
10/07/08	88150	29.00	-23.20		0.00	5.80
10/07/08	81000	17.00	-13.60		0.00	3.40
10/07/08	80050	120.00	-96.00		0.00	24.00

Amount Due
77.00

FIGURE 15.3 (c) Patient Statement

The Billing Cycle

Instead of generating all statements at the end of a month, practices follow some kind of billing cycle to spread out the workload. **Cycle billing** is used to assign patient accounts to a specific time of the month and to standardize the times when statements will be mailed and payments will be due. If the billing cycle is weekly, for example, the patient accounts are divided into four groups—usually alphabetically—so that 25 percent of the bills go out each week.

Individual Patient Billing Versus Guarantor Billing

Practices may send statements to each individual patient, as shown in Figure 15.3c, or they may send one statement to the guarantor of a number of different accounts, called **guarantor billing**, shown in Figure 15.4 on page 492. For example, if a patient is responsible for his own bill as well as the bills of his wife and children, all of the family's recent charges can be categorized and sent together on one statement. Guarantor billing offers the following advantages:

- It reduces the amount of time and money spent on billing by reducing paper and mailing costs and by reducing time spent on billing follow-up for patients with overdue bills.
- It allows the practice to efficiently prioritize its accounts receivable and collection efforts by combining several small bills into one large bill.
- It improves patient satisfaction because the practice will not be making multiple phone calls to the patient or sending multiple follow-up letters and statements.

Valley Associates, PC
1400 West Center Street
Toledo, OH 43601-0123
(555)321-0987

Statement Date	Chart Number	Page
10/17/2008	SHAHRAJ0	1

Raj Shah
1433 Third Avenue
Cleveland, OH 44101-1234

Make Checks Payable To:
Valley Associates, PC
1400 West Center Street
Toledo, OH 43601-0123
(555)321-0987

Date of Last Payment: Amount: 0.00 Previous Balance: 0.00

Patient: Kalpesh Shah Chart Number: SHAHKAL0 Case: Cerumen in Ear

Dates	Procedure	Charge	Paid by Primary	Paid By Guarantor	Adjustments	Remainder
10/13/08	69210	63.00	0.00		0.00	63.00

Amount Due
63.00

FIGURE 15.4 Example of Guarantor Billing

Guarantor billing is advantageous and is usually used when parents are responsible for minor children who are living with them. However, when different health plans and policies apply for various family members and/or a secondary payer covers some members of the group, guarantor billing is not always possible to manage effectively. In those cases, it is simpler to bill each individual patient.

Organizing for Effective Collections

The term **collections** refers to all the activities that are related to patient accounts and follow-up. Collection activities should achieve a suitable balance between maintaining patient satisfaction and generating cash flow. While most patients pay their bills on time, every medical practice has patients who do not pay their monthly statements when they receive them. Many simply forget to pay the bills and need a reminder, but others require more attention and effort. A patient may not pay a bill for several reasons:

- The patient thinks the bill is too high.
- The patient thinks that the care rendered was not appropriate or not effective.
- The patient has personal financial problems.
- The bill was sent to an inaccurate address.
- There is a misunderstanding about the amount the patient's insurance pays on the bill.

A great deal of accounts receivable can be tied up in unpaid bills, and these funds can mean the difference between a successful and an unsuccessful practice.

Staff Assignments

Each practice's billing and collections effort must be organized for greatest efficiency. Because practice size varies widely from an office with one physician and a small support staff to practices with hundreds of providers and staff members, staff assignments vary, too. Small offices may assign collections duties to coders or billers on certain days of the week. Large practices may have separate collections departments with these typical job functions:

- Billing/collections manager
- Bookkeeper
- Collections specialist

Billing/Collections Manager

Either a physician, a practice administrator, an office manager, or a collections manager handles these tasks:

- Create and implement the practice's collections policies for all involved employees
- Monitor the results of the collections activities by creating and analyzing reports based on the financial statistics
- Organize the accounts and develop strategies to be used by the collections specialists
- Assist the collections specialists with difficult phone calls and other questions or concerns
- Train the collections specialists for success in their jobs
- Supervise and evaluate the efforts of the collections specialists

The Bookkeeper

Managing the finances of the medical practice is a complicated task, and most practices choose to dedicate an employee to this responsibility. The bookkeeper makes sure that all the funds coming into and owed to the practice are accurately recorded. An outside accountant usually audits this work periodically.

The Collections Specialists

Collections specialists are trained to work directly with the practice's patients to resolve overdue bills. Not every contact with a patient ends with an agreement to pay, but collections specialists are held accountable for their results against standards or goals that they are expected to achieve. Some practices provide incentives such as additional pay, prizes, or paid time away from work to encourage success. Collections specialists must always remember to act ethically and professionally as they represent the practice in their contact with patients.

Avoiding Opportunities for Fraud

A common organizing principle when finances are involved is to divide the tasks among several people with different responsibilities to reduce the chances of employee errors or **embezzlement** (stealing funds). If one person is solely responsible for maintaining the practice's finances, opportunities for fraud exist. Most practices have at least two or more people involved in the process. One employee might open incoming mail, and another might be responsible for posting payments. The practice will generally deposit the funds daily and have two people responsible for closing out the day's financial records. Bond or theft insurance is usually purchased to ensure against loss if embezzlement occurs.

Thinking It Through — 15.2

1. **Patient statements may be prepared using a spreadsheet format. The AMT DUE column is a running total; that is, the charge for each service line is added to the previous AMT DUE figure. The total due on the statement can be cross-checked by comparing the AMT DUE in the last box with the total of all CHARGES. These amounts should be the same. For example:**

SERVICE DATE	PT NAME	PROC CODE	DIAG. CODE	SERVICE DESCRIPTION	CHARGES	INS. PAID	ADJ.	PT PAID	AMT DUE
10/14/2008	Lund, Alan.	99384	V70.3	NP preventive visit	182.00	-0-	-0-	-0-	182.00
		81001		UA	10.00	-0-	-0-	-0-	192.00
					192.00				***192.00***

   A. If for the 10/14/2008 charges, the patient made a payment of $50 and the third-party payer paid $20, what balance would be due?

   B. What balance would be due if the patient and payer made these payments but the previous statement showed a $235 balance?

2. **Because of the nature of the contact between collections specialists and patients, phone calls can sometimes be difficult, and collections specialists may need to involve their managers. In your opinion, should all patient requests to speak with a manager be honored?**

Collection Regulations and Procedures

Collections from patients are classified as consumer collections and are regulated by federal and state laws. The Federal Trade Commission enforces the **Fair Debt Collection Practices Act of 1977 (FDCPA)** and the **Telephone Consumer Protection Act of 1991** that regulate collections to ensure fair and ethical treatment of debtors. The following guidelines apply:

- Contact patients once daily only, and leave no more than three messages per week.
- Do not call a patient before 8 A.M. or after 9 P.M.
- Do not threaten the patient or use profane language.
- Identify the caller, the practice, and the purpose of the call; do not mislead the patient.
- Do not discuss the patient's debt with another person, such as a neighbor.
- Do not leave a message on an answering machine that indicates that the call is about a debt or send an e-mail message stating that the topic is debt.
- If a patient requests that all phone calls cease and desist, do not call the patient again, but instead contact the patient via mail.
- If a patient wants calls to be made to an attorney, do not contact the patient directly again unless the attorney says to or cannot be reached.

State law may not permit contacting debtors at their place of employment, so this aspect needs to be checked. In addition to state and federal laws, the practice's policies for dealing with patients need to be followed. If the practice chooses to add late fees or finance charges to patient's accounts, it must do so in accordance with these laws. Often, it is required to disclose these at the time services are rendered.

Valley Associates, P.C.

Patient Aging Applied Payment

As of November 30, 2008

Chart	Name	Birthdate	Current 0 - 30	Past 31 - 60	Past 61 - 90	Past 91 --->	Total Balance
ESTEPWI0	**Wilma Estephan**	**3/14/1940**		5.60			5.60
Last Pmt: -22.40	On: 10/8/2008	(555)683-5272					
GIROUKA0	**Karen Giroux**	**3/15/1945**		77.00			77.00
Last Pmt: -96.00	On: 10/8/2008	(555)683-5364					
PEREZCA0	**Carmen Perez**	**5/15/1934**			62.00		62.00
Last Pmt: -20.00	On: 10/1/2008	(555)692-3314					
PORCEJE0	**Jennifer Porcelli**	**7/5/1970**		76.00			76.00
Last Pmt: -15.00	On: 10/13/2008	(555)709-0388					
WILLIWA0	**Walter Williams**	**9/4/1936**			116.00		116.00
Last Pmt: -15.00	On: 10/1/2008	(555)936-0216					
	Report Aging Totals		$0.00	$158.60	$178.00	$0.00	336.60
	Percent of Aging Total		0.0 %	47.1 %	52.9 %	0.0 %	100.00 %

FIGURE 15.5 Example of a Patient Aging Report

Procedures

The medical office tracks overdue bills by reviewing the **patient aging report**. Like the insurance aging report, it is analyzed to determine which patients are overdue on their bills and to group them into categories for efficient collection efforts (see Figure 15.5). Aging begins on the date of the bill. The patient aging report includes the patient's name, the most recent payment, and the remaining balance. It divides the information into these categories based on each statement's beginning date:

1. *Current or up to date:* Thirty days
2. *Past due:* Thirty-one to sixty days
3. *Past due:* Sixty-one to ninety days
4. *Past due:* More than ninety days

For example, Figure 15.5 shows that Rachel Atchely owes two charges. The $43 charge is current, and the $82 charge is thirty-one to sixty days past due.

Each practice sets its own procedures for the collections process. Large bills have priority over smaller ones. Usually, an automatic reminder notice and a second statement are mailed when a bill has not been paid thirty days after it was issued. Some practices phone a patient with a thirty-day overdue account. If the bill is not then paid, a series of collection letters is generated at intervals, each more stringent in its tone and more direct in its approach.

Following is an example of one practice's collection timetable; different guidelines are used in other practices.

30 days	Bill patient
45 days	Call patient regarding bill
60 days	Letter 1
75 days	Letter 2 and call
80 days	Letter 3
90 days	Turn over to collections

Billing Tip

Claims Under Appeal
If a denied claim is being appealed by the provider or the patient, the provider may not convert the account to past-due status until the final appeal decision has been received.

Collections Letters

For most patients, the collections letter is the first notice that their bill is past due. Collections letters are generally professional, courteous, brief, and to the point. They remind the patient of the practice's payment options and the patient's responsibility to pay the debt. Practices decide what types of letters should be sent to accounts in the various past-due stages. Accounts that are farther past due will receive more aggressive letters. For example, Figure 15.6 shows the differences in the tone of these three letters.

Collections Calls

Once the patient's account is past due, collections specialists begin calling to set up payment arrangements. The first call is used to verify that the patient has received a bill, and most collections are resolved easily at this point. However, some patients are unable or unwilling to pay. Each patient's situation is unique, and collections specialists treat each patient carefully. While it is important to be professional and polite, collections specialists are calling to collect money owed to the practice.

Collections Call Strategies

Collections specialists cannot follow a set formula when placing phone calls. They must react to situations and use effective methods to pursue payment arrangements. The following are general strategies that collections specialists use when talking to patients on the phone:

- Be straightforward and honest, and inform patients of the status of their accounts and of what needs to be accomplished.
- Maintain a professional attitude.
- Allow time for the patient to respond, and use appropriate pauses. Do not provide patients with excuses for not paying their bills.

Date:
Patient:
Acct. #:
Balance Due: $

Dear

Your insurance company has paid its portion of your bill. You are now responsible for the remaining balance. Full payment is due, or you must contact this office within 10 days to make suitable payment arrangements. As an added payment option, you may pay by credit card, using the payment form below.

Sincerely,

<Employee signature>
Employee Name and Title

(a) First Letter

FIGURE 15.6 (a–c) Samples of Collection Letters

Date:
Patient:
Acct. #:
Balance Due: $

Dear

This is a reminder that your account is overdue. If there are any problems we should know about, please telephone or stop in at the office. A statement is attached showing your past account activity.

Your prompt payment is requested.

Sincerely,

<Employee signature>
Employee Name and Title

(b) Second Letter

Date:
Patient:
Acct. #:
Balance Due: $

Dear

Your account is seriously past due and has been placed with our in-house collection department. Immediate payment is needed to keep an unfavorable credit rating from being reported on this account. If you are unable to pay in full, please call to make acceptable arrangements for payment. Failure to respond to this notice within 10 days will precipitate further collection actions.

Sincerely,

<Employee signature>
Employee Name and Title

(c) Third Letter

- Stay in control of the conversation, and do not allow a patient to get too far off topic.
- Assure patients that their unpaid bills will not affect the quality of the treatment they receive.
- Do not intimidate the patient, yell, or treat the patient with disrespect.

Collections specialists train to be ready for any scenario that could arise on the phone, and to have responses to common occurrences. However, it is important that they do not sound robotic to the patient, and that they show emotion and understanding when appropriate. When a person answers the phone who is not the patient, collections specialists remain professional, do not reveal the nature of the call or discuss the patient's debt, or mislead the person to secure information about the patient.

Common Collections Call Scenarios

Although collections calls are unique and patients have many different reasons for nonpayment, collections specialists can be prepared for common responses. The following are statements a patient might make and a collections specialist's possible replies.

Patient: "The check's in the mail."
Response: "May I please have the check number, the amount of the check, and the date it was mailed?"

Patient: "I can pay the bill at the end of the month."
Response: "Let's schedule the payment for that time."

Patient: "I can't pay this bill now."
Response: "How are you paying your other bills? Are you employed? The practice can set up payment arrangements if necessary, but the bill does need to be paid."

Patient: "My insurance company has already paid this bill."
Response: "Your insurance company paid the part of the bill covered by your policy. The remaining balance is currently unpaid and is your responsibility."

Documentation

After a collections specialist has completed a phone call, the conversation is documented. To quickly and effectively document phone calls, the collections specialist uses abbreviations for common results and situations:

TB	Telephoned business	PD	Phone disconnected
TR	Telephoned residence	LB	Line busy
TT	Talked to	PT	Patient
NA	No answer	UE	Unemployed
HU	Hung up	DNK	Did not know
PTP	Promise to pay	EOM	End of month
RP	Refused payment	EOW	End of week
LM	Left message	NLE	No longer employed
SD	Said	EDU	Educated

Thinking It Through — 15.3

How would a collections specialist document these results? Try out your note-taking skills:

1. Telephoned residence and talked to the patient. He promised to pay by the end of the week and said he did not know the bill was unpaid.
2. Telephoned business, but there was no answer.
3. Telephoned residence and talked to patient. She said that she was no longer employed and refused to pay. Educated the patient that she needed to pay by the end of the month, but the patient hung up the phone.

Credit Arrangements and Payment Plans

A practice may decide to extend credit to patients through a **payment plan** that lets patients pay bills over time, rather than in a single payment. At times, practices charge interest on these plan payments.

Credit and Truth in Lending Act

Both the patient and the practice must agree to all the terms before the arrangement is finalized. Patients agree to make set monthly payments; if no finance charges are applied to the account, the arrangement is not regulated by law. However, if the practice applies finance charges or late fees, or if payments are scheduled for more than four installments, the payment plan is governed by the **Truth in Lending Act**, which is part of the Consumer Credit Protection Act. Patients must sign off on the terms on a truth-in-lending form that the collections specialist negotiates.

Credit Counseling

Consumer credit counseling services and debt management programs are nonprofit organizations that can assist patients who are struggling to pay their bills or who have a great number of different bills. These companies collect information about income and unpaid bills from patients and contact creditors to work out payment plans at reduced costs to the patients. A patient is required to make only one monthly payment to the service, which will then divide it and pay the separate creditors as agreed.

Designing Payment Plans

Practices have guidelines for appropriate time frames and minimum payment amounts for payment plans. For example, the following schedule might be followed:

- *$50 balance or less:* Entire balance due the first month
- *$51–$500 balance due:* $50 minimum monthly payment
- *$501–$1,000 balance due:* $100 minimum monthly payment
- *$1,001–$2,500 balance due:* $200 minimum monthly payment
- *Over $2,500 balance due:* 10 percent of the balance due each month

Thinking It Through — 15.4

A patient owes $1,200 to the physician for a surgical procedure. Based on the payment schedule shown above, what monthly payment is the collections specialist likely to set up?

HIPAA Tip

Collection Agencies and PHI

- Collection agencies are business associates of practices and must agree to follow their security and privacy policies to protect patients' PHI.
- Employees of collection agencies should sign confidentiality agreements to ensure that PHI is not inappropriately released.

Collections specialists work out payment plans using patient information such as the amount of the bill, the date of the payday, the amount of disposable income the patient has, and any other contributing factors.

Setting Up Prepayment Plans

When patients are scheduled to have major, expensive procedures, the practice policy may be to set up **prepayment plans.** The insurance carrier is contacted for an estimate of the patient's financial responsibility. The patient then makes a down payment or makes arrangements for preprocedure and possibly postprocedure monthly payments.

Collection Agencies and Credit Reporting

Internal office collections are not always successful, and when they are not the practice may use a **collection agency.** Collection agencies are external companies that perform specialized collection efforts on difficult debtors. Once a patient's account has been forwarded to a collection agency, the practice must discontinue all other attempts to collect on the balance. Collection agencies must also follow the guidelines of the Fair Debt Collection Practices Act.

When to Use a Collection Agency

Collection agencies are often hired to handle cases in which the practice has failed in its attempts to collect money owed by a debtor. Often, the providers approve the list of overdue accounts before they are sent to outside collections. Accounts are referred to collection agencies when they are overdue an amount of time specified by the practice, such as 120 days, but they can be sent earlier if necessary. The following reasons could force the practice to send patients' bills to a collection agency early:

- All attempts to contact a patient have been unsuccessful, and the patient has not responded to any letters or phone calls.
- A patient has declared that he of she will not pay a bill.
- A patient's check has been returned for lack of funds in the checking account, and the patient has not attempted to resolve the problem.
- A patient has not met the requirements of an established payment plan for an unexplained or invalid reason and has thereby not honored a promise to pay.
- A patient has received a payment for the services from an insurance company and has withheld it from the practice.
- The contact information for a patient is outdated or incorrect, and attempts to locate the patient have failed.

The practice must be careful when sending accounts to a collection agency earlier than normal. Prematurely forwarding an account could negatively affect the patient's desire to pay. Not all unpaid bills are sent out; accounts with small balances and those for patients experiencing extreme circumstances might be forgiven, according to practice policy.

Selecting a Collection Agency

Several key factors need to be considered when choosing a collection agency for the practice. The most important thing to remember is that the selected agency will represent the practice. For this reason, a reputable agency with a history of fair and ethical collection practices should be chosen.

Collection agencies that specialize in handling medical office accounts are generally preferred. Practices usually review references and collection statistics before choosing an agency. Good collection agencies can clearly explain their procedures. Carefully reviewing this information helps the practice avoid using an agency that does not actively pursue payment. Some agencies send simple letters only, assuming that a good percentage of patients will immediately pay upon receiving a letter from an agency outside of the practice, and are not effective at further follow-up.

Types of Collection Agencies

Practices can choose among collection agencies that operate on a local, regional, or national scale. Local and regional agencies usually have a better understanding of a patient's surroundings and economic status, and are thus better able to relate to the patient. However, national agencies incorporate more advanced tools to contact and locate debtors, often at less cost.

Analyzing the Cost of a Collection Agency

Most practices use collection agencies because they are cost-efficient and are able to retrieve enough of the unpaid balances to cover their service fees. Nevertheless, effectively analyzing and comparing the cost of using different agencies can save the practice a good deal of money. Agencies usually retain a percentage of the funds they collect, but the agency with the lowest rate is not necessarily the best one to choose.

For example, the practice may compare the results of two agencies given $50,000 worth of unpaid balances to collect. If one agency charges 20 percent of the funds it collects but collects only $1,000 it would be less efficient than an agency that retains 80 percent of the $10,000 it manages to collect. The practice will consider all of this information when choosing the agency to best meet its needs.

Credit Reporting

One of the advantages of using a collection agency is its ability to use **credit reporting** as a collection tool. Through this process, unpaid medical bills can be viewed on a person's record by other potential creditors in the future. This financial information is obtained through **credit bureaus**, which gather credit information and make it available to members at a cost. Patients who do not want their credit information to be adversely affected by unpaid medical bills may be more motivated to pay. Credit reporting processes are regulated by law under the **Fair Credit Reporting Act (FCRA)**, and the **Fair and Accurate Credit Transaction Act (FACTA)** of 2003, which amended the FCRA. These laws are designed to protect the privacy of credit report information and to

HIPAA Tip

The NPP and Collections

The Notice of Privacy Practices should explain the practice's policy on when accounts are sent to an outside collector. Patients' acknowledgement of receiving this document protects the practice from liability under HIPAA.

Thinking It Through — 15.5

1. Which of the following collection agencies would be the best choice to represent the practice based on financial statistics? Why?

   Company A: Collection rate of 30 percent, charges 50 percent of the funds it collects.

   Company B: Collection rate of 20 percent, charges 30 percent of the funds it collects.

   (Hint: Work out the results based on $100.)

2. Assume that the practice has sent $10,000 worth of unpaid balances to Company B. How much money would the practice expect to receive based on the listed percentages?

guarantee that information supplied by consumer reporting agencies is as accurate as possible. Practices must act appropriately with regard to these services and must be sure that the billing services and collection agencies they employ do so as well.

Skip Tracing

When the standard attempts to contact a patient are unsuccessful, it may become necessary to **skip trace** the debtor. This term refers to the process of locating a patient with an outstanding balance through additional methods of contact. Sometimes the patient has moved, has forgotten about the bill, and will gladly pay when reached. However, a patient may attempt to avoid a debt by moving away without notification or by not responding to attempted contacts. Regardless of the reason the patient cannot be reached, action must be taken, and practices have policies to handle these situations.

A statement returned to the practice through the mail without a known forwarding address causes suspicion. The envelopes is usually marked "Return to Sender" and often indicates that a forwarding address is not known. In these cases, contacting the patient by telephone may be difficult as well. People can disconnect their phone lines, get unlisted phone numbers, use cell phones, or simply not answer the phone to avoid contact.

Tracing a Debtor

Before extensive skip tracing begins, an employee double-checks the address written on the returned envelope to be sure that it matches the address on file. Accurately gathering billing information (see Chapter 3) can greatly decrease the number of skip traces needed. Once it is determined that a patient cannot be reached by mail or at the telephone numbers on file, the skip tracing process begins. The following methods can all be used to locate a debtor:

- Contact the post office to find a new address for the patient, or clear up any errors in the address on file.
- Search telephone directories for relatives with the same last name.
- Run a search on the Internet at one of the free person-finding services.
- Examine publicly available state and federal records for contact information.

Professional Skip Tracing Assistance

Larger practices or those that perform a large number of skip traces often consider hiring a specialized external agency. Most of these companies allow the practice to specify the type or depth of skip tracing done on each patient, which corresponds to the cost of the service. Before making a decision, the practice should analyze the time and money required for effective internal skip tracing and compare it to the cost of using a specialized agency. Some collection agencies include skip tracing in their charges.

Computerized Skip Tracing

A less expensive method of skip tracing is to use online directories and databases. The practice can elect to pay a fee for access to information provided electronically by a company that creates these resources. The price includes access to the information only, so administrative staff members need to be trained to search for debtors. The databases are extensive, and many different types of searches can be performed, including the following:

- *Name search:* Use a person's first or last name or any partial combination of letters in case the person is using an alias.
- *Address search:* Enter an address to verify a resident, or search for an unknown or partially incorrect address.
- *Telephone number search:* View the names of all the people listed at a phone number.
- *Relatives search:* Names, addresses, and phone numbers for possible relatives of a person are displayed.
- *Neighbor search:* Find the names, addresses, and phone number of people living on the same street or in the same apartment building.

Different combinations of information can return very useful results from these databases. When searching, employees can be creative and can follow up on the returned information. Searches on a state or national level and for business names may also be available.

Effective Skip Tracing Calls

When making a phone call based on the results gathered from skip tracing, the caller must be cautious. While information provided by the Internet, professional companies, electronic directories, and other methods can be extremely useful, it is not always correct. Patient information should not be revealed, and the nature of the call should remain confidential. Not exposing the purpose of the call may enhance results, but deception and lies are still inappropriate, especially if contacting the debtor's neighbor. The FDCPA guidelines that regulate all other collection calls still apply.

Writing Off Uncollectible Accounts

After the practice has exhausted all of its collection efforts and a patient's balance is still unpaid, the account may be labeled as an **uncollectible account**, also known as a write-off account. Uncollectible accounts are those with unpaid balances that the practice does not expect to be able to collect and that are not worth the time and cost to pursue. Also, accounts over a year old have a little chance of collection.

The practice must determine which debts to write off in the practice management program and whether to continue to treat the patients. Practice management programs can be set to automatically write off small balances, such as less than $5.00. After an account is determined to be uncollectible, it is removed from the practice's expected accounts receivable and classified as **bad debt**.

Common Types of Uncollectible Accounts

The most common reason an account becomes uncollectible is that a patient cannot pay the bill. Under federal and state laws, there are **means tests** that help a practice decide whether patients are indigent. The patient completes a form that is used to evaluate ability to pay. A combination of factors, such as income level (verified by recent federal tax returns) as compared to the federal poverty level, other expenses, and the practice's policies, are used to determine what percentage of the bill will be forgiven and written off.

Another reason that an account is uncollectible is that the patient cannot be located through skip tracing, so the account must be written off. Accounts of patients who have died are often marked as uncollectible. Large unpaid balances of deceased patients may be pursued by filing an estate claim or by working—considerately—with the deceased patient's family members.

Another reason for a write-off is a patient's **bankruptcy.** Debtors may choose to file for bankruptcy when they determine that they will not be able to repay the money they owe. When a patient files for bankruptcy, the practice, which is considered to be an unsecured creditor, must file a claim in order to join the group of creditors that may receive some compensation for unpaid bills. Claims must be filed by the date specified by the bankruptcy court so as not to forfeit the right to any money.

Practices only rarely sue individuals to collect money they are owed. Usually, unpaid balances are deemed uncollectible to avoid going through the expense of a court case with uncertain results.

Dismissing Patients Who Do Not Pay

A physician has the right to terminate the physician-patient relationship for any reason under the regulations of each state. The doctor also has the right to be paid for care provided. The physician may decide to dismiss a patient who does not pay medical bills. If the patient is to be dismissed, this action should be documented in a letter to the patient that:

- Offers to continue care for a specific period of time after the date of the dismissal letter, so that the patient is never endangered
- Provides referrals to other physicians and offers to send copies of the patients' records
- Does not state a specific reason for the dismissal; the letter must be tactful and carefully worded

The letter should be signed by the physician and mailed certified, return receipt requested, so there will be proof that the patient received it.

Patient Refunds

The medical office focuses on accounts receivable, but at times the practice may need to issue **patient refunds.** Money needs to be refunded to patients when the practice has overcharged a patient for a service. Note that the balance due must be refunded promptly if the practice has completed the patient's care. However, if the practice is still treating the patient, the credit balance resulting

Compliance Guideline

Avoid Deleting Posted Data
Transactions should not be deleted from the PMP, because this could be interpreted by an auditor as fraud. Instead, corrections, changes, and write-offs are made with adjustments to the existing transactions. Adjustments maintain a history of events in case there should be a billing inquiry or an audit.

Billing Tip

Means Test Forms
Retain the forms patients complete in determining write-offs in the event of an audit.

Compliance Guideline

Avoid Fraudulently Writing Off Accounts
A practice must follow strict guidelines and the established office policy for write-offs. Both Medicare and Medicaid require a practice to follow a specific series of steps before an account can be written off. Writing off some accounts and not others could be considered fraud if there are discrepancies between charges for the same services.

Thinking It Through — 15.6

The following patient bill has been in collections and is going to be written off:

DATE	CODE	DESCRIPTION			CHARGES	CREDITS
09/10/07	99396	Prev Check up, Est. 40 – 64 Yr			169.00	
09/10/07	85018	Hemoglobin Count, Colorimetric			6.10	
09/10/07	81002	Urinalysis, Non-automated, w/o s			4.20	
09/11/07		Golden Rule Ins. Co. #31478 Filed				
10/17/07		Denied Golden Rule Ins. Co. #31478				00.00
10/17/07		Repriced Golden Rule Ins. Co. #31478				51.80–
10/17/07		$127.50 = deductible for 9/10/07 visit				
Current	30 – 60	60 – 90	>90	TOTAL	INS PENDING	TOTAL DUE FROM PATIENT
0.00	0.00	0.00	127.50	127.50	0.00	127.50

1. **What amount has previously been written off as an adjustment due to the payer's allowed charge?**
2. **What amount must now be deemed bad debt?**

from a patient's overpayment may be noted on the patient's statement and account and applied to charges at the next visit.

Record Retention

Patients' medical records and financial records are retained according to the practice's policy. The practice manager or providers set the retention policy after reviewing the state regulations that apply. Any federal laws, such as HIPAA and FACTA regulations, are also taken into account.

The practice's policy about keeping records is summarized in a **retention schedule,** a list of the items from a record that are retained and for how long. The retention schedule usually also covers the method of retention. For example, a policy might state that all established patients' records are stored in the practice's files for three years and then microfilmed and removed to another storage location for another four years.

The retention schedule protects both the provider and the patient. Continuity of care is the first concern: the record must be available for anyone within or outside of the practice who is caring for the patient. Also, records must be kept in case of legal proceedings. For example, a provider might be asked to justify the level and nature of treatment when a claim is investigated or challenged, requiring access to documentation.

Although state guidelines cover medical information about patients, most do not specifically cover financial records. Financial records are generally saved according to federal business records retention requirements. Under HIPAA, covered entities must keep records of HIPAA compliance for six years. In general, the storage method chosen and the means of destroying the records when the retention period ends must strictly adhere to the same confidentiality requirements as patient medical records.

HIPAA Tip

Disposing of Electronic Protected Health Information

The HIPAA security rule requires covered entities to implement policies and procedures to address the final disposition of electronic PHI and/or the hardware or electronic media on which it is stored. The practice must have procedures for reasonably ensuring that electronic PHI cannot be recovered from a device or medium such as a hard disk, floppy disk, CD, Zip disk,

Compliance Guideline

Retention Advice
The American Health Information Management Association (AHIMA) publishes guidelines called "Practice Briefs" on many topics, including retention of health information and of health care business records, available at http://www.ahima.org Under the HIM Resources tab.

Review

Steps to Success

- ❒ Read this chapter and review the Key Terms and the Chapter Summary.
- ❒ Answer the Review Questions and Applying Your Knowledge in the Chapter Review.
- ❒ Access the chapter's websites and complete the Internet Activities to learn more about available professional resources.
- ❒ Complete the related chapter in the *Medical Insurance Workbook* to reinforce your understanding of patient billing and collections.

Chapter Summary

1. Medical practices use multiple methods to inform patients of their financial policies and procedures. Payment policies are explained in brochures and on signs in the reception area as well as orally by registration staff. Patients are often asked to read and sign a statement that they understand and will comply with the payment policy.
2. Updated patient ledgers reflecting all charges, adjustments, and previous payments to patients' accounts are used to generate patient statements, printed bills that show the amount each patient owes. Patients may owe coinsurance, deductibles, and fees for noncovered services. The statements are mailed according to the billing cycle that is followed. They are designed to be direct and easy to read, clearly stating the services provided, balances owed, due dates, and accepted methods of payment.
3. Under individual patient billing, each patient who has a balance receives a mailed patient statement. Under guarantor billing, statements are grouped by guarantor and cover all patient accounts that are guaranteed by that individual. Guarantor billing produces fewer bills to track but can become unwieldy when family members have various health plans and/or secondary payers.
4. The process of bill collecting in the medical office is usually governed by set policies and overseen by a manager. Several employees may assist in this part of the business, including managers, bookkeepers, and collections specialists. Managers are responsible for establishing office policies and enabling collections specialists to successfully perform their jobs. Bookkeepers record funds coming into and going out of the practice. Collections specialists study aging reports and follow up on patient accounts that are due.
5. Efforts to collect past-due patient balances are strictly regulated by law and by office policy. Both collection letters and phone calls are integral parts of the collections process. Collections specialists maintain a professional attitude while being straightforward. They must be prepared for difficult situations and ready to work out credit arrangements and payment plans.
6. When patients have not met their financial obligations and collection activities need to be assigned to an agency for further efforts, practices use collection agencies. The practice chooses an agency that best fits its needs. Credit reporting can be a valuable collection tool and is enforced on debtors who have not paid their bills.
7. When patients cannot be reached or do not respond to letters and phone calls, it often becomes necessary to skip trace. There are several inexpensive ways to locate a missing patient, and specialized agencies or electronic databases are effective methods at a cost. Phone calls to possible contacts must be handled carefully.
8. Not all balances due to the practice will be paid. Patients sometimes die, file for bankruptcy, are unable to pay their bills, or cannot be traced. Knowing when to write off an account is im-

portant, and using caution when doing so to avoid possible fraud is a top priority. Likewise, it is important to pay a refund if a patient has been overcharged.

9. The retention of medical records follows office policy and is also regulated by law. Retention schedules are followed to ensure records will be available for proper patient care. Medical practices must be ready to answer patient requests for information and records and to defend any claims that are questioned.

Review Questions

Match the key terms with their definitions.

A. guarantor billing
B. skip trace
C. patient aging report
D. retention schedule
E. patient refunds
F. uncollectible account
G. payment plan
H. cycle billing
I. credit reporting
J. collection agency

____ 1. Summarizes the practice's policies about keeping records, including the type of information that is retained and the length of time it is kept

____ 2. Consists of sending one statement to the guarantor of a number of different accounts

____ 3. Shows which patients are overdue on their bills, and groups them into distinct categories for efficient collection efforts

____ 4. Patient balance that the practice has not collected and does not expect to be able to collect

____ 5. Occur when the practice has overcharged a patient for a service and must return the extra amount

____ 6. Refers to the process of locating a patient with an outstanding balance through additional methods of contact

____ 7. Through this process, unpaid medical bills can be viewed on a person's record by potential creditors

____ 8. Programs set up to accommodate the patient's schedule and ability to pay while ensuring that the practice receives the money it is owed

____ 9. An external company that performs specialized collection efforts on difficult debtors

____10. Assigns patient accounts to a specific time of the month and standardizes the times when statements will be mailed and payments will be due

Decide whether each statement is true or false.

____ 1. Guarantor billing generally reduces the number of phone calls made to a patient.

____ 2. The practice does not have to issue patient refunds under $50.00.

____ 3. Collections specialists can keep their identities secret when talking to patients to obtain more information.

____ 4. External skip tracing agencies may provide online databases that allow people to search for debtors by their addresses.

____ 5. A statement usually contains the balance due and a cost breakdown of all the services the practice provided.

____ 6. The patient aging report helps the practice track its accounts receivable.

____ 7. If a patient is deceased, the practice has no chance to collect any funds from the account.

____ 8. The practice's retention schedule policies are affected by state and federal laws.

____ 9. An unpaid bill is considered past due thirty-one days after the date of the bill.

____ 10. Practices always choose the collection agency that charges the lowest percentage of the funds it collects.

Select the letter that best completes the statement or answers the question.

____ 1. When talking with someone other than the patient about an overdue bill, collection specialists will
   A. reveal the purpose of the phone call
   B. mislead the person they are talking with
   C. be unprofessional
   D. not discuss the patient's debt

____ 2. The day sheet produced by the practice management program shows
   A. what each patient owes the practice as of that date
   B. what each payer owes the practice as of that date
   C. the payments and charges that occurred on that date
   D. the overdue accounts on that date

____ 3. During collections, most practices use
   A. letters and calls
   B. audit reports and tax returns
   C. e-mail messages and faxes
   D. local police and state police

____ 4. Credit bureaus keep records about a patient's
   A. medical history
   B. credit information
   C. disposable income
   D. salary

____ 5. Collection calls are regulated by the guidelines set by
   A. FCRA
   B. FACTA
   C. HIPAA
   D. FDCPA

____ 6. Accounts might be considered uncollectible when a patient
   A. files for bankruptcy
   B. directs phone calls to an attorney
   C. needs a payment plan
   D. has not responded to the first bill

____ 7. Skip tracing increases the practice's chances of
   A. avoiding embezzlement
   B. locating a patient with an overdue bill
   C. following FDCPA guidelines
   D. successfully using the patient aging report

____ 8. The practice will need to pay patient refunds if it has
   A. only received a payment from a third-party payer
   B. miscalculated its accounts receivable
   C. overcharged the patient for a service
   D. used information from a credit bureau

____ 9. The patient aging report is used to
   A. enter payments in the patient billing system
   B. enter write-offs to a patient's account
   C. track overdue claims from payers
   D. collect overdue accounts from patients

____ 10. Bad debt is defined as
   A. payer refunds
   B. patient refunds
   C. uncollectible A/R
   D. collectible A/R

Define these abbreviations.

1. FACTA ______________________________

2. FCRA ______________________________

Applying Your Knowledge

Case 15.1 Calculating Insurance math

A. Alan Lund is responsible for his medical bills and for those of his daughter, Alana, and he receives a guarantor statement. Complete the AMT DUE column by adding each charge to the previous total to find the running total. What amount is due for Alan, and what amount for Alana? What total amount is due on the October statement?

SERVICE DATE	PT NAME	PROC CODE	DIAG. CODE	SERVICE DESCRIPTION	CHARGE	INS.PAID	ADJ.	PT PAID	AMT DUE
10/14/2008	Lund, Alana.	99384	V70.3	NP preventive visit	182.00	-0-	-0-	-0-	
		81001		UA	10.00	-0-	-0-	-0-	
		85018		HBG	4.50	-0-	-0-	-0-	
10/28/2008	Lund, Alana	99201	599.0	NP OV	54.10	-0-	-0-	-0-	
		81001		UA	10.00	-0-	-0-	-0-	
		87088		UC	32.33	-0-	-0-	-0-	

B. Gail Ferrar's statement is shown below. Gail is responsible for a 20 percent coinsurance. Calculate the total amount due.

SERVICE DATE	PT NAME	PROC CODE	DIAG. CODE	SERVICE DESCRIPTION	CHARGE	INS. PAID	ADJ.	PT PAID	AMT DUE
									DUE: APRIL STATEMENT $245.00
05/26//2008	Ferrar, Gail	99213	625.3	EP OV	100.00	80.00	-0-	-0-	
		88150		Pap Smear	30.00	24.00	-0-	-0-	

Case 15.2 Preparing Insurance Communications

Andrea Martini owes $400 to Valley Associates, P.C., for her son Ben's visit last month. Her account number is RR109. Ben is a dependent on her insurance, Amerigo Health Plan, which has paid on the account. The account is at more than thirty days. Draft a collection letter requesting payment.

Internet Activities

1. Using a search engine such as Google or Yahoo, research collection agencies. Are you able to find out how to compare their costs?

2. Locate the Federal Trade Commission's website on credit and research the topic of credit scoring. How are credit scores determined?

Part 6 Hospital Services

Chapter 16
Hospital Billing and Reimbursement

Chapter 16

Hospital Billing and Reimbursement

CHAPTER OUTLINE

Health Care Facilities: Inpatient Versus Outpatient

Hospital Claim Processing

Inpatient (Hospital) Coding

Payers and Payment Methods

Claims and Follow-up

Learning Outcomes

After studying this chapter, you should be able to:

1. Distinguish between inpatient and outpatient hospital services.
2. List the major steps relating to hospital billing and reimbursement.
3. Describe two differences in coding diagnoses for hospital inpatient cases and physician services.
4. Describe the classification system used for coding hospital procedures.
5. Describe the factors that affect the rate that Medicare pays for inpatient services.
6. Discuss the important items that are reported on the hospital health care claim.

KeyTerms

admitting diagnosis (ADX)
ambulatory care
ambulatory patient classification (APC)
ambulatory surgical center (ASC)
ambulatory surgical unit (ASU)
at-home recovery care
attending physician
case mix index
charge master
CMS-1450
comorbidities
complications
diagnosis-related groups (DRGs)
837I
emergency
grouper
health information management (HIM)
home health agency (HHA)
home health care
hospice care
inpatient
Inpatient Prospective Payment System (IPPS)
master patient index
observation services
Outpatient Prospective Payment System (OPPS)
principal diagnosis (PDX)
principal procedure
registration
skilled nursing facility (SNF)
UB-92
UB-04
Uniform Hospital Discharge Data Set (UHDDS)

Although this text focuses on billing and reimbursement in medical practices, medical insurance specialists should be aware of the coding systems and billing process used in hospitals. There are many financial agreements between physicians and hospitals; physicians in practices may have staff privileges at hospitals or be associated with hospitals as medical specialists. Physician practice staff members also must bill for the procedures physicians perform in the hospital environment. It is important to distinguish between hospital and physician services for accurate billing.

This chapter provides a brief overview of the types of inpatient and outpatient facilities, the various methods used by payers to pay for these services, and the coding systems that are used to report diagnoses and procedures for reimbursement.

Health Care Facilities: Inpatient Versus Outpatient

There are more than 6,500 primarily nonprofit facilities that are known as acute care hospitals. Other kinds of health care facilities include psychiatric hospitals, rehabilitation facilities, clinics, nursing homes, subacute hospitals, and home health care agencies. Hospital size is measured by the number of beds. Hospitals are also classified by the type of facility and services they provide, such as teaching hospital or burn center. These classifications have a direct relationship to the payments hospitals receive.

Inpatient Care

Inpatient facilities are equipped for patients to stay overnight. In addition to hospitals, inpatient care may be provided for special populations:

- *Skilled nursing facilities:* A **skilled nursing facility** (SNF) provides skilled nursing and/or rehabilitation services to help with recovery after a hospital stay. Skilled nursing care includes care given by licensed nurses under the direction of a physician, such as intravenous injections, tube feeding, and changing sterile dressings on a wound.

- *Long-term care facilities*: This term describes facilities such as nursing homes that provide custodial care for patients with chronic disabilities and prolonged illnesses.

Outpatient or Ambulatory Care

Hospital emergency rooms (ER) or departments are the most familiar type of outpatient service. **Emergency** care involves a situation in which a delay in treatment would lead to a significant increase in the threat to a patient's life or body part. (Emergency care differs from urgently needed care, in which the condition must be treated right away but is not life-threatening.) Patients treated in an emergency room are either discharged or admitted as inpatients to the hospital after treatment or observation.

Many hospitals have expanded beyond inpatient and ER services to offer a variety of outpatient services. Outpatient care, often called **ambulatory care**, covers all types of health services that do not require an overnight hospital stay. Most hospitals, for example, have outpatient departments that provide these services. Same-day surgery is performed in two types of facilities where patients do not stay overnight: a separate part of a hospital called an **ambulatory surgical unit (ASU)** and a free-standing facility called an **ambulatory surgical center** (ASC).

Different types of outpatient services are also provided in patients' home settings. **Home health care** services include care given at home, such as physical therapy or skilled nursing care. Home health care is provided by a **home health agency (HHA)**, an organization that provides home care services, including skilled nursing, physical therapy, occupational therapy, speech therapy, and care by home health aides. **At-home recovery care** is a different category; it includes help with the activities of daily living (ADLs), such as bathing and eating. **Hospice care** is a special approach to caring for people with terminal illnesses—that is, people who are not expected to live longer than six months—in a familiar and comfortable place, either a special hospice facility or the patient's home.

Integrated Delivery Systems

An important trend is the development of patient-centered integrated health care delivery systems, which are also called integrated networks. Health care providers from various specialties and health care facilities join together to provide patient services. At the center of the system is a single administration. Most integrated systems are locally organized, such as through the merger of local hospitals into large multi-facility systems.

Integrated delivery systems change the focus of care from acute care to the continuum of care the patient needs. For example, an acute care hospital, a rehabilitation hospital, a long-term care facility, and a home care program might merge to form one system that can provide services for a stroke patient from the time of the stroke until the resumption of normal activities. The network is set up to move the patient and the patient's record from facility to facility as the patient's treatment and condition require.

Hospital Claim Processing

Hospitals generally have large departments that are responsible for major business functions. The admissions department records the patient's personal and financial information. In some hospitals, a separate insurance verification department is responsible for double-checking the patient's identity and confirming insurance coverage. The patient accounting department handles billing, and there is often a separate collections department. Organizing and maintaining patient medical records in hospitals are the duties of the **health information management (HIM)** department. Hospitals are also structured into departments for patient care. For example, there are professional services departments, such as laboratory, radiology, and surgery, as well as food service and housekeeping.

The three major steps in a patient's hospital stay from the insurance perspective are:

1. Admission, for creating or updating the patient's medical record, verifying patient insurance coverage, securing consent for release of information to payers, and collecting advance payments as appropriate
2. Treatment, during which the various departments' services are provided and charges are generated
3. Discharge from the hospital or transfer to another facility, at which point the patient's record is compiled, claims and/or bills are created, and payment is followed up on

HIPAA Tip

Verifying Insurance Coverage

The HIPAA standard transaction used to verify patients' insurance is the 270/271 Eligibility for a Health Plan Inquiry/Response.

Admission

Inpatients are admitted to hospitals in a process called **registration.** Like physician practices, hospitals must keep clear, accurate records of patients' diagnoses and treatments. The record begins at a patient's first admission to the facility or, in some facilities, during a preadmission process used to gather information before actual admission. Having a preadmission process gives staff members time to verify insurance coverage, calculate patients' likely financial responsibilities, work out payment plans if necessary, and also to handle any ordered preadmission tests.

The HIM department keeps a health record system that permits storage and retrieval of clinical information by patient name or number, by physician, and by diagnosis and procedure. At almost every facility, part or all of the records are computerized (each with a different computer system; the systems are not standardized). Each patient is listed in a patient register under a unique number. These numbers make up the **master patient index**—the main database that identifies patients. This index contains the patient's:

- Last name, first name, and middle name or initial
- Birth date (eight-digit format)
- Sex
- Address
- Admission and/or treatment date
- Admitting physician
- **Attending physician**—the clinician primarily responsible for the care of the patient from the beginning of the hospital episode
- Health record number

More information is gathered for a hospital admission than is required for a visit to a physician practice. For example, in addition to hospital insurance, a patient may have long-term coverage. Special points about the patient's care, such as language requirements, religion, or disabilities, are also entered in the record.

Outpatient department and emergency room insurance claims are often delayed because verifying insurance coverage is difficult in these settings. The

HIPAA Tip

Treatment, Payment, and Operations (TPO)

In hospital work as well as in physician offices, patients' protected health information (PHI) can be released as necessary for treatment, payment, and operations (TPO).

HIPAA Tip

Notice of Privacy Practices

Under the HIPAA Privacy Rule, a hospital must also present a patient with a copy of its privacy practices at registration and have the patient sign an acknowledgment that he or she has received this notice.

emergency department may have its own registration system because people who come for emergency and urgent treatment must receive care by the nursing staff first. Both outpatient and emergency room procedures must be set up to collect the minimum information. Many admissions departments join online insurance verification systems so that payers can be contacted during the registration process and verification received in seconds.

Consent

As in medical practices, the admission staff in hospitals must be sure patients give written consent for the medical treatments and procedures they will receive. Figure 16.1 is an example of a consent form used in hospitals. It includes the same kinds of items that patients sign in practices (the consent for medical treatment, acceptance of responsibility for payment, and assignment of benefits) as well as three unique items:

1. A statement covering the conditions under which the facility is responsible for the patient's personal possessions.
2. Advance directives, also called living wills, that cover how patients want to receive health care, including routine treatments and life-saving methods, if they become incapacitated. A patient may also appoint another person to make such decisions if the patient cannot with a medical power of attorney.
3. Acknowledgment that Medicare patients have received a copy of the one-page "An Important Message from Medicare." The printout, which CMS requires hospitals to give Medicare patients on registration, explains the beneficiary's rights as a hospital patient as well as his or her appeal rights regarding hospital discharge (see Figure 16.2 on page 518).

Medicare as a Secondary Payer

As is the case for office visits, health plans require coordination of benefits when more than one insurance policy is in effect for a patient. As an example, many patients are classified as Medicare Secondary Payer (MSP) accounts. These patients are Medicare beneficiaries, but Medicare is the secondary payer. For example, if a patient or a patient's spouse has medical insurance through an employer's plan, that coverage is primary to Medicare. In these cases, the MSP information must be taken at registration to avoid delays in claim processing. The form used to determine the primary payer is shown in Figure 16.3 (on pages 519–522). If the patient does not know what insurance company covered the other person involved in the accident, the hospital may request a police accident report to obtain the information needed to bill the accident insurance that is primary to Medicare.

Pretreatment Patient Payment Collection

Most facilities set up pretreatment payment plans to collect at least a deposit before admission and treatment. The following types of payments may be collected in advance:

- Medicare Part A and Part B/private payer deductibles, coinsurance, copayments, and noncovered services.
- Medicare lifetime reserve (LTR) day amounts. Medicare pays for sixty days (over a person's lifetime) when a patient is in the hospital for more than ninety days. For each lifetime reserve day, Medicare pays all covered costs ex-

CONSENT FOR MEDICAL TREATMENT

I, the undersigned, acknowledge and understand that, in presenting myself for voluntary registration, Inpatient, Outpatient, or Emergency Services at Memorial Hospital, authorize and consent to such diagnostic procedures, tests, or treatments as may be ordered by my physician(s) and/or emergency department physician and carried out by members of the medical staff and hospital associates. I voluntarily consent to such health care, medical and surgical, including anesthesia, X-ray, and lab procedures as may be conduced, requested, directed by delegate, or designated in the judgment of the attending physician or consulting physician. Administrative fluids, blood, and blood products/components, medications, and radiology procedures are included in this consent.

RELEASE OF MEDICAL INFORMATION

I authorize Memorial Hospital to release medical information or copies from my medical record from my date of admission through my date of discharge to insurance companies, third-party payers or authorized paying agent, or claims review organizations in order to process a claim for payment in my behalf. This information may be disseminated to any and all employers, insurance companies, or their designees present in the Hospital by the patient or the patient's representative that may provide coverage for the health care organization's charges, and to comply with the requirement of any Professional Review Organization for Joint Commission on Accreditation of Healthcare Organizations for Utilization Review and Medical Audit. I also authorize release of information to agencies that may be involved in my continuity of care. I authorize any health care provider including my physician and consulting physicians to provide to the hospital or its designee, upon request, information concerning my care, condition, and treatment for quality assurance and risk management purposes.

VALUABLES: RELEASE FROM RESPONSIBILITY

I understand that Memorial Hospital does not assume responsibility for personal possessions unless they are registered in the hospital safe. This opportunity has been offered to me.

ADVANCE DIRECTIVES

Has a living will or health care power of attorney been prepared?	Yes	No	N/A
I have provided Memorial Hospital with the most current copy.	Yes	No	N/A
I have received advance directives information.	Yes	No	N/A
The Patient's Bill of Rights has been presented to me.	Yes	No	N/A

Courtesy of Illini Hospital, Silvis, Illinois

FINANCIAL AGREEMENT AND ASSIGNMENT OF INSURANCE BENEFITS

I hereby assign, transfer, and convey all my rights, title, and interest to medical reimbursement under by insurance policy(s) to Memorial Hospital. It is understood, whether I sign as agent, patient, or as guarantor, that I am directly responsible and will pay for service rendered and not paid by insurance agency. An assignment of benefits by any insurance policy or medical reimbursement plan shall not be deemed a waiver of Memorial Hospital's right to require payment directly from the undersigned or the patient. Memorial Hospital expressly reserves the right to require such payment. Should the account be referred to any agency for collection (collection agency or attorney), the undersigned shall pay all reasonable attorney fees, collection costs, and interest. All delinquent accounts may bear a late payment penalty of not more than 10 1/2% per month thereafter charged from the date of service. I assign payment of all insurance benefits to physicians providing professional services at Memorial Hospital in conjunction with hospital services.

BILLING OF PROFESSIONAL SERVICES

I understand that I am financially responsible for professional services of the radiologist(s), pathologist(s), anesthesiologist(s), emergency department physician, and other physician charges that are not billed by the hospital. I acknowledge that the physicians providing professional services, including consultants and on-call physicians, are an independent medical staff who are not employees or agents of Memorial Hospital. I hereby authorize release of information requested by insurance/billing agencies to the aforementioned parties.

AN IMPORTANT MESSAGE FROM MEDICARE

I acknowledge that I have received a copy of *An Important Message from Medicare* and have been directed to read this brochure.

I have read this form that consists of six important areas and understand its contents. I have had an opportunity to ask questions that have been answered to my satisfaction. I voluntarily sign immediately below.

MR#________ Date of Admission/Service ________

PA# ________ Signature: ______________________

Witness (name and relation) __________________

Hospital Representative: ______________________

UCF0004 Rev: 3/97

FIGURE 16.1 Hospital Consent Form

cept for a daily coinsurance. Patients without additional coverage may be required to make arrangements for paying this daily amount before admission.

- Estimated amounts for noncovered services.
- Private room differential and fees for extras, such as telephone and television services. Most payers do not pay for any item that is considered a convenience rather than a medical necessity.

IMPORTANT MESSAGE FROM MEDICARE

YOUR RIGHTS AS A HOSPITAL PATIENT

- You have the right to receive necessary hospital services covered by Medicare, or covered by your Medicare Health Plan ("your Plan") if you are a Plan enrollee.
- You have the right to know about any decisions that the hospital, your doctor, your Plan, or anyone else makes about your hospital stay and who will pay for it.
- Your doctor, your Plan, or the hospital should arrange for services you will need after you leave the hospital. Medicare or your Plan may cover some care in your home (home health care) and other kinds of care, if ordered by your doctor or by your Plan. You have a right to know about these services, who will pay for them, and where you can get them. If you have any questions, talk to your doctor or Plan, or talk to other hospital personnel.

YOUR HOSPITAL DISCHARGE & MEDICARE APPEAL RIGHTS

Date of Discharge: When your doctor or Plan determines that you can be discharged from the hospital, you will be advised of your planned date of discharge. You may appeal if you think that you are being asked to leave the hospital too soon. If you stay in the hospital after your planned date of discharge, it is likely that your charges for additional days in the hospital will not be covered by Medicare or your Plan.

Your Right to an Immediate Appeal without Financial Risk: When you are advised of your planned date of discharge, if you think you are being asked to leave the hospital too soon, you have the right to appeal to your Quality Improvement Organization (also known as a QIO). The QIO is authorized by Medicare to provide a second opinion about your readiness to leave. You may call Medicare toll-free, 24 hours a day, at 1-800-MEDICARE (1-800-633-4227), or TTY/TTD: 1-877-486-2048, for more information on asking your QIO for a second opinion. If you appeal to the QIO by noon of the day after you receive a noncoverage notice, you are not responsible for paying for the days you stay in the hospital during the QIO review, even if the QIO disagrees with you. The QIO will decide within one day after it receives the necessary information.

Other Appeal Rights: If you miss the deadline for filing an immediate appeal, you may still request a review by the QIO (or by your Plan, if you are a Plan enrollee) before you leave the hospital. However, you will have to pay for the costs of your additional days in the hospital if the QIO (or your Plan) denies your appeal. You may file for this review at the address or telephone number of the QIO (or of your Plan).

OMB Approval No. 0938-0692. Form No. CMS-R-193 (January 2003)

FIGURE 16.2 Printout Entitled "An Important Message from Medicare"

Billing Tip

Electronic Medical Records
Hospitals are leading the way in the implementation of electronic medical records. Although this progress affects the collection, storage, and dissemination of health information, including PHI, the content of the health record remains the same.

Records of Treatments and Charges during the Hospital Stay

Standards for hospital patient medical records are set by the Joint Commission on Accreditation of Healthcare Organizations (JCAHO). The hospital's own bylaws and Medicare regulations for participating hospitals also influence medical record standards. The medical record contains (1) notes of the attending physician and other treating physicians, such as operative reports; (2) ancillary documents like nurses' notes and pathology, radiology, and laboratory reports; (3) patient data, including insurance information for patients who have been in the hospital before; and (4) a correspondence section that contains signed consent forms and other documents. In line with HIPAA security requirements, the confidentiality and security of patients' medical records are guarded by all hospital staff members. Both technical means, such as passwords and encryption, and legal protections, such as requiring staff members to sign confidentiality pledges, are used to ensure privacy.

Patients are usually charged by hospitals for the following services:

The following chart lists questions that can be used to ask Medicare beneficiaries upon each inpatient and outpatient admission. Providers use this chart as a guide to help identify other payers that may be primary to Medicare. If you choose to use this questionnaire, please note that it was developed to be used in sequence. Instructions are listed after the questions to facilitate transition between questions. The instructions will direct them to the next appropriate question to determine Medicare Secondary Payer situations.

Part I

1. Are you receiving Black Lung (BL) Benefits?
   _____Yes; Date benefits began: CCYY/MM/DD
   BL IS PRIMARY ONLY FOR CLAIMS RELATED TO BL.
   _____No.
2. Are the services to be paid by a government program such as a research grant?
   _____Yes; Government Program will pay primary benefits for these services
   _____No.
3. Has the Department of Veterans Affairs (DVA) authorized and agreed to pay for care at this facility?
   _____Yes.
   DVA IS PRIMARY FOR THESE SERVICES.
   _____No.
4. Was the illness/injury due to a work related accident/condition?
   _____Yes; Date of injury/illness: CCYY/MM/DD
   Name and address of WC plan:
   ____
   Policy or identification number: ______________
   Name and address of your employer:
   ____
   WC IS PRIMARY PAYER ONLY FOR CLAIMS RELATED TO WORK RELATED INJURIES OR ILLNESS, GO TO PART III.
   _____No. **GO TO PART II.**

Part II

1. Was illness/injury due to a non-work related accident?
   _____Yes; Date of accident: CCYY/MM/DD
   _____No: **GO TO PART III**
2. What type of accident caused illness/injury?
   _____Automobile.
   _____Non-Automobile.
   Name and address of no-fault or liability insurer:
   ____
   ____
   ____
   Insurance claim number: _____________
   NO-FAULT INSURER IS PRIMARY PAYER ONLY FOR THOSE CLAIMS RELATED TO THE ACCIDENT. GO TO PART III.
   _____Other

FIGURE 16.3 Medicare Secondary Payer Determination Form

- Room and board
- Medications
- Ancillary tests and procedures, such as laboratory workups
- Equipment/supplies used during surgery or therapy
- The amount of time spent in an operating room, recovery room, or intensive care unit

3. Was another party responsible for this accident?
_____Yes;
Name and address of any liability insurer:
____
____
____
Insurance claim number: _____________
LIABILITY INSURER IS PRIMARY PAYER ONLY FOR THOSE CLAIMS RELATED TO THE ACCIDENT. GO TO PART III.
_____No. **GO TO PART III**

PART III

1. Are you entitled to Medicare based on:
_____Age. **GO TO PART IV.**
_____Disability. **GO TO PART V.**
_____ESRD. **GO TO PART VI.**

PART IV–Age

1. Are you currently employed?
_____Yes.
Name and address of your employer:
____
____
____
_____No. Date of retirement: CCYY/MM/DD
_____No. Never Employed
2. Is your spouse currently employed?
_____Yes.
Name and address of spouse's employeer:
____
____
____
_____No. Date of retirement: CCYY/MM/DD
_____No. Never Employed
IF THE PATIENT ANSWERED NO TO BOTH QUESTIONS 1 AND 2, MEDICARE IS PRIMARY UNLESS THE PATIENT ANSWERED YES TO QUESTIONS IN PART I OR II. DO NOT PROCEED FURTHER.
3. Do you have group health plan (GHP) coverage based on your own, or a spouse's current employment?
_____Yes.
_____No. **STOP. MEDICARE IS PRIMARY PAYER UNLESS THE PATIENT ANSWERED YES TO THE QUESTIONS IN PART I OR II.**
4. Does the employer that sponsors your GHP employ 20 or more employees?
_____Yes. **STOP. GROUP HEALTH PLAN IS PRIMARY. OBTAIN THE FOLLOWING INFORMATION.**
Name and address of GHP:
____
____
____
Policy identification number: _____________
Group identification number: _____________
Name of policyholder: _____________
Relationship to patient: _____________
_____No. **STOP. MEDICARE IS PRIMARY PAYER UNLESS THE PATIENT ANSWERED YES TO QUESTIONS IN PART I OR II.**

FIGURE 16.3 Medicare Secondary Payer Determination Form *(continued)*

PART V–Disability

1. Are you currently employed?

   _____Yes.

   Name and address of your employer:

   ____

   ____

   ____

   _____No. Date of retirement: CCYY/MM/DD

2. Is a family member currently employed?

   _____Yes.

   Name and address of your employer:

   ____

   ____

   ____

   _____No.

   IF THE PATIENT ANSWERED NO TO BOTH QUESTIONS 1 AND 2, MEDICARE IS PRIMARY UNLESS THE PATIENT ANSWERED YES TO QUESTIONS IN PART I OR II. DO NOT PROCEED FURTHER.

3. Do you have group health plan (GHP) coverage based on your own, or a family member's current employment?

   _____Yes.

   _____No. **STOP. MEDICARE IS PRIMARY PAYER UNLESS THE PATIENT ANSWERED YES TO THE QUESTIONS IN PART I OR II.**

4. Does the employer that sponsors your GHP employ 100 or more employees?

   _____Yes. **STOP. GROUP HEALTH PLAN IS PRIMARY. OBTAIN THE FOLLOWING INFORMATION.**

   Name and address of GHP:

   ____

   ____

   ____

   Policy identification number: ____________

   Group identification number: ____________

   Name of policyholder: ____________

   Relationship to patient: ____________

   Membership number: ____________

   _____No. **STOP. MEDICARE IS PRIMARY PAYER UNLESS THE PATIENT ANSWERED YES TO QUESTIONS IN PART I OR II.**

PART VI–ESRD

1. Do you have group health plan (GHP) coverage?

   Name and address of GHP:

   ____

   ____

   ____

   Policy identification number: ____________

   Group identification number: ____________

   Name of policyholder: ____________

   Relationship to patient: ____________

   Name and address of employer, if any, from which you receive GHP coverage:

   ____

   ____

   ____

   _____No. **STOP. MEDICARE IS PRIMARY.**

FIGURE 16.3 Medicare Secondary Payer Determination Form *(continued)*

2. Have you received a kidney transplant?
   _____Yes. Date of transplant: CCYY/MM/DD
   _____No.
3. Have you received maintenance dialysis treatments?
   _____Yes. Date dialysis began: CCYY/MM/DD
   If you participated in a self-dialysis training program, provide date training started: CCYY/MM/DD
   _____No
4. Are you within the 30-month coordination period?
   _____Yes
   _____No. **STOP. MEDICARE IS PRIMARY.**
5. Are you entitled to Medicare on the basis of either ESRD and age or ESRD and disability?
   _____Yes.
   _____No. **STOP. GHP IS PRIMARY DURING THE 30 MONTH COORDINATION PERIOD.**
6. Was your initial entitlement to Medicare (including simultaneous entitlement) based on ESRD?
   _____Yes. **STOP. GHP CONTINUES TO PAY PRIMARY DURING THE 30 MONTH COORDINATION PERIOD.**
   _____No. **INITIAL ENTITLEMENT BASED ON AGE OR DISABILITY.**
7. Does the working aged or disability MSP provision apply (i.e., is the GHP primarily based on age or disability entitlement?
   _____Yes. **STOP. GHP CONTINUES TO PAY PRIMARY DURING THE 30-MONTH COORDINATION PERIOD.**
   _____No. **MEDICARE CONTINUES TO PAY PRIMARY.**

Applies to the states of: AK, AZ, CO, IA, HI, ND, NV, OR, SD, WA, & WY.

Source: Change request 3504, dated January 21, 2005.

FIGURE 16.3 Medicare Secondary Payer Determination Form *(continued)*

Patients are charged according to the type of accommodations and services they receive. For example, the rate for a private room is higher than the rate for a semiprivate room, and intensive care unit or recovery room charges are higher than charges for standard rooms. When patients are transferred to these services, the activity is tracked. In an outpatient or an emergency department encounter, there is no room and bed charge; instead, there is a visit charge. **Observation services** are provided in a hospital room but are billed as an outpatient service. These stays are charged by the hour, rather than a per diem charge. Observation services normally do not extend beyond 23 hours.

Discharge and Billing

By the time patients are discharged from the hospital, their accounts usually have been totaled and insurance claims or bills created. The goal in most cases is to file a claim or bill within seven days after discharge. A typical bill for a patient contains many items. The items are recorded on the hospital's charge description master file, usually called the **charge master**, which is the equivalent of a medical practice encounter form. This master list contains the following information for each item:

- The hospital's code for the service and a brief description of it
- The charge for the service
- The hospital department (such as laboratory)
- The hospital's cost to provide the service
- A procedure code for the service

The hospital's computer system tracks the services in various departments. For example, if the patient is sent to the intensive care (IC) unit after surgery, the IC billing group reports the specific services received by the patient, and these charges are entered on the patient's account.

> **Billing Tip**
>
> **Physician's Fees**
> The professional fee for the physician's services, such as surgeon's fee, is charged by the physician rather than by the hospital.

Inpatient (Hospital) Coding

Coding is done by inpatient medical coders as soon as a patient is discharged. Some inpatient coders are generalists; others may have special skills in a certain area, like surgical coding or Medicare. ICD-9-CM Volumes 1 and 2 are used to code inpatient diagnoses, and Volume 3 is used to code procedures performed during the hospitalization.

Hospital Diagnostic Coding

Different rules apply for assigning inpatient codes than for physician office diagnoses. These rules, found in the *Coding Clinic for ICD-9-CM,* a publication of the American Hospital Association's (AHA) Central Office on ICD-9-CM, were developed by the four groups that are responsible for the ICD-9-CM: the AHA, the American Health Information Management Association (AHIMA), the Centers for Medicare and Medicaid Services (CMS), and the National Center for Health Statistics (NCHS). The rules are based on the requirements for sequencing diagnoses and reporting procedures that are part of the **Uniform Hospital Discharge Data Set (UHDDS).** Medicare, Medicaid, and many private payers require the UHDDS rules to be followed for reimbursement of hospital services. The rules are extensive. Three of them are briefly described below to illustrate some of the major differences between inpatient and outpatient coding.

Thinking it Through — 16.1

What are some of the differences between working for a hospital facility and for a physician practice? Which employment setting is more likely to have specialized job functions?

Principal Diagnosis

For diagnostic coding in medical practices, the first code listed is the primary diagnosis, defined as the main reason for the patient's encounter with the provider. Under hospital inpatient rules, the **principal diagnosis (PDX)** is listed first. The principal diagnosis is the condition established *after study* to be chiefly responsible for the admission. This principal diagnosis is listed even if the patient has other, more severe diagnoses. In some cases, the **admitting diagnosis (ADX)**—the condition identified by the physician at admission to the hospital—is also reported.

Example

Inpatient principal diagnosis after surgery: Acute appendicitis (540)
Inpatient admitting diagnosis: Severe abdominal pain (789.00)

Suspected or Unconfirmed Diagnoses

When the patient is admitted for workups to uncover the cause of a problem, inpatient medical coders can also use suspected or unconfirmed conditions (rule-outs) if they are listed as the admitting diagnosis. The admitting diagnosis may not match the principal diagnosis once a final decision has been made.

Example

Inpatient principal diagnosis: Diverticulosis of the small intestine (562.00)
Inpatient admitting diagnosis: Probable acute appendicitis (540)

Comorbidities and Complications

The inpatient coder also lists all the other conditions that have an effect on the patient's hospital stay or course of treatment. A patient's other conditions at admission that affect care during the hospitalization being coded are called **comorbidities**, meaning coexisting conditions. Conditions that develop as problems related to surgery or other treatments are coded as **complications.** Comorbidities and complications are shown in the patient medical record with the initials *CC*.

Examples

Comorbidity: The physician's discharge summary stated that the patient needed additional care because of chronic obstructive pulmonary disease (COPD) with emphysema.

Code: 492.8

Complication: The physician's discharge summary indicates a diagnosis of postoperative hypertension as a postoperative complication.

Codes: Hypertension, 402.90, and 997.1, Cardiac Complications

Coding CCs is important, because their presence may increase the hospital's reimbursement level for the care. The hospital insurance claim form discussed later in this chapter allows for up to eight additional conditions to be reported.

Hospital Procedural Coding

The UHDDS requires significant procedures to be reported along with the principal diagnosis, comorbidities, and complications. Significant procedures have any of these characteristics (F. Brown, *ICD-9-CM Coding Handbook,* 2002, 47):

- They involve surgery.
- Anesthesia (other than topical) is administered.
- The procedure involves a risk to the patient.
- The procedure requires specialized training.

In inpatient coding, the ICD's Volume 3, *Procedures,* is used to assign procedure codes. Reporting Volume 3 codes when appropriately documented may increase the hospital's reimbursement because some procedures require more hospital time for recovery. For example, codes in range 93.31 to 93.39 are assigned when patients require physical therapy procedures such as whirlpool therapy.

Volume 3 Organization

Volume 3 of the ICD-9-CM has an Alphabetic Index and a Tabular List, similar to Volumes 1 and 2. The Alphabetic Index is used to locate the procedure, and the Tabular List is used to confirm the code selection. Codes are either three or four digits. The fourth digit must be assigned if available.

The organization of the Tabular List and the range of codes are shown in Table 16.1.

Principal Procedure

The **principal procedure** assigned by the inpatient medical coder is the procedure that is most closely related to the treatment of the principal diagnosis. It

TABLE 16.1 ICD-9-CM Volume 3 Tabular List Organization

CHAPTER	RANGE
1 Operations on the Nervous System	01–05
2 Operations on the Endocrine System	06–07
3 Operations on the Eye	08–17
4 Operations on the Ear	18–20
5 Operations on the Nose, Mouth, and Pharynx	21–29
6 Operations on the Respiratory System	30–34
7 Operations on the Cardiovascular System	35–39
8 Operations on the Hemic and Lymphatic System	40–41
9 Operations on the Digestive System	42–54
10 Operations on the Urinary System	55–59
11 Operations on the Male Genital Organs	60–64
12 Operations on the Female Genital Organs	65–71
13 Obstetrical Procedures	72–75
14 Operations on the Musculoskeletal System	76–84
15 Operations on the Integumentary System	85–86
16 Miscellaneous Diagnostic and Therapeutic Procedures	87–99

Thinking it Through — 16.2

In which chapter of the ICD-9-CM Volume 3 would you expect to find codes for

1. an appendectomy?
2. injection into a ganglion?
3. dilation and curettage (D & C)?
4. replacement of heart valve?

is usually a surgical procedure. If no surgery is performed, the principal procedure may be a therapeutic procedure. Here is an example:

Inpatient principal diagnosis: Chronic tonsillitis 474.00 (ICD-9-CM code from Volume 1, the Tabular list)
Inpatient principal procedure: Tonsillectomy 28.2 (ICD-9-CM code from Volume 3, Procedures, the Tabular List)

Compliance Guideline

Inpatient Versus Outpatient Diagnosis Coding
The UHDDS inpatient rules apply only to inpatient services. Hospital-based outpatient services and physician-office services are reported using ICD-9-CM Volumes 1 and 2, following the outpatient rules (see Chapter 4) and CPT/HCPCS.

American Hospital Association Clearing House—Information on HCPCS Coding for Outpatient Billing

http://www.ahacentraloffice.org

Payers and Payment Methods

Medicare and Medicaid both provide coverage for eligible patients' hospital services. Medicare Part A, known as hospital insurance, helps pay for inpatient hospital care, skilled nursing facilities, hospice care, and home health care. Private payers also offer hospitalization insurance. Most employees have coverage for hospital services through employers' programs.

Medicare Inpatient Prospective Payment System

Diagnosis-Related Groups

CMS's actions to control the cost of hospital services began with the implementation of **diagnosis-related groups (DRGs)** in 1983. Under the DRG classification system, hospital stays of patients who had similar diagnoses were studied. Groupings were created based on the relative value of the resources that hospitals used nationally for patients with similar conditions.

The ICD-9-CM diagnosis and procedure codes are used to calculate the DRG. The calculations combine data about the patient's diagnosis and procedures with factors that affect the outcome of treatment, such as age, gender, comorbidities, and complications. DRGs are ranked by weight. Higher-weight DRGs use resources more intensively and are therefore paid more. Each hospital's **case mix index** is an average of the DRG weights handled for a specific period of time.

Figure 16.4 shows the DRGs for conditions related to the circulatory system.

Billing Tip

DRG Grouper
A computer program called a grouper calculates the DRG to be paid based on the codes assigned to the patient's stay.

Inpatient Prospective Payment System

At the same time the DRG system was created, CMS changed the way hospitals were paid. Payment for institutional services moved from a fee-for-service to a prospective payment approach. The Medicare **Inpatient Prospective Payment System (IPPS)** determines the number of hospital days and the hospital services that are reimbursed. If a patient has a principal diagnosis accompanied by comorbidities or complications, such as coma or convulsions,

DRG 103, Heart Transplant
DRG 104, Cardiac Valve Procedures with Cardiac Catheterization
DRG 105, Cardiac Valve Procedures without Cardiac Catheterization
DRG 106, Coronary Bypass with PTCA
DRG 107, Coronary Bypass without PTCA
DRG 108, Other Cardiothoracic Procedures
DRG 109, Coronary Bypass without PTCA or Cardiac Catheterization
DRG 110, Major Cardiovascular Procedures with Comorbidity or Complication
DRG 111, Major Cardiovascular Procedures without Cormorbidity or Complication
DRG 112, Percutaneous Cardiovascular Procedures
DRG 113, Amputation for Circulatory System Disorders Except Upper Limb and Toe
DRG 114, Upper Limb and Toe Amputation for Circulatory System Disorders
DRG 115, Permanent Cardiac Pacemaker Implant with Acute Myocardial Infarction, Heart Failure, or Shock
DRG 116, Other Permanent Cardiac Pacemaker Implant or Generator Procedure
DRG 117, Cardiac Pacemaker Revision Except Device Replacement
DRG 118, Cardiac Pacemaker Device Replacement
DRG 119, Vein Ligation and Stripping
DRG 120, Other Circulatory System Operating Room Procedures
DRG 121, Circulatory Disorders with Acute Myocardial Infarction and Cardiovascular Complication, Discharged Alive
DRG 122, Circulatory Disorders with Acute Myocardial Infarction without Cardiovascular Complication, Discharged Alive
DRG 123, Circulatory Disorders with Acute Myocardial Infarction, Expired
DRG 124, Circulatory Disorders Except Acute Myocardial Infarction with Cardiac Catheterization and Complex Diagnosis
DRG 125, Circulatory Disorders Except Acute Myocardial Infarction with Cardiac Catheterization without Complex Diagnosis
DRG 126, Acute and Subacute Endocarditis
DRG 127, Heart Failure and Shock
DRG 128, Deep Vein Thrombophlebitis
DRG 129, Cardiac Arrest, Unexplained
DRG 130, Peripheral Vascular Disorders with Cormorbidity or Complication
DRG 131, Peripheral Vascular Disorders without Comorbidity or Complication
DRG 132, Atherosclerosis with Cormorbidity or Complication
DRG 133, Atherosclerosis without Cormorbidity or Complication
DRG 134, Hypertension
DRG 135, Cardiac Congenital and Valvular Disorders, Age Greater than 17 with Comorbidity or Complication
DRG 136, Cardiac Congenital and Valvular Disorders, Age Greater than 17 without Comorbidity or Complication
DRG 137, Cardiac Congenital and Valvular Disorders, Age 0-17
DRG 138, Cardiac Arrhythmia and Conduction Disorders with Comorbidity or Complication
DRG 139, Cardiac Arrhythmia and Conduction Disorders without Comorbidity or Complication
DRG 140, Angina Pectoris
DRG 141, Syncope and Collapse with Comorbidity or Complication
DRG 142, Syncope and Collapse without Comorbidity or Complication
DRG 143, Chest Pain
DRG 144, Other Circulatory System Diagnoses with Comorbidity or Complication
DRG 145, Other Circulatory System Diagnoses without Comorbidity or Complication
DRG 479, Other Vascular Procedures with Comorbidity or Complication
DRG 480, Other Vascular Procedures without Comorbidity or Complication

FIGURE 16.4 Diagnosis-Related Groups for Diseases and Disorders of the Circulatory System

these additional signs are evidence of a more difficult course of treatment, and the DRG reimbursement is raised. If, however, the hospital holds the patient for longer than the DRG specifies without such circumstances, it still receives only the allowed amount and must write off the difference between the reimbursement and its actual costs. Each hospital negotiates a rate for each

DRG with CMS based on its geographic location, labor and supply costs, and teaching costs.

Quality Improvement Organizations and Utilization Review

When DRGs were established, CMS also set up peer review organizations (PROs), which were later renamed Quality Improvement Organizations (QIOs). As noted in Chapter 10, QIOs are made up of practicing physicians and other health care experts who are contracted by CMS in each state to review Medicare and Medicaid claims for the appropriateness of hospitalization and clinical care.

QIOs aim to ensure that payment is made only for medically necessary services. In many circumstances, Medicare requires precertification for inpatient or outpatient surgery, as do many private payers. While the admission or the procedure may be approved, the amount of payment is usually not determined until the QIO reviews the services. When reviewing submitted claims, QIOs may take one of the following actions:

- Review and fully approve a claim
- Review and deny portions of a claim
- Review a claim for a patient's inpatient services, and decide that no stay was medically necessary
- Decide to conduct a postpayment audit

QIOs are also resources for investigating quality of care. They review patients' complaints about the quality of care provided by inpatient hospitals, hospital outpatient departments, hospital emergency rooms, skilled nursing facilities, home health agencies, Medicare managed care plans, and ambulatory surgical centers. They also contract with private payers to perform these services.

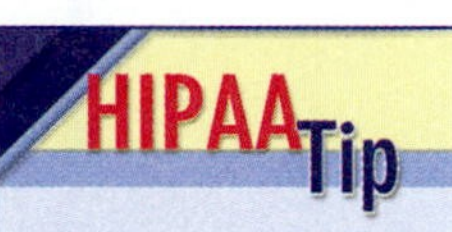

HCPCS/ CPT Code Set for APCs

The HCPCS/CPT code set along with selected modifiers is mandated for APCs. E/M codes are used according to a crosswalk the provider develops for its emergency department services.

Medicare Outpatient Prospective Payment Systems

The use of DRGs under a prospective payment system proved to be very effective in controlling costs. In 2000, CMS implemented this type of approach for outpatient hospital services, which previously were paid on a fee-for-service basis. These payment systems are in place:

- *Outpatient Prospective Payment System (OPPS):* The Balanced Budget Act of 1997 authorized Medicare to begin paying for hospital outpatient services under a prospective payment system called the **Outpatient Prospective Payment System (OPPS)**. In place of DRGs, patients are grouped under an **ambulatory patient classification (APC)** system. Reimbursement is made according to preset amounts based on the value of each APC group to which the service is assigned.
- *Ambulatory surgical centers (ASC):* CMS also sets prospective APC rates for facility services provided by Medicare-participating ASCs.
- *Skilled nursing facility (SNF) Prospective Payment System:* The Balanced Budget Act of 1997 also requires SNFs to be paid under a prospective payment system; patients are classified under the Resource Utilization Group (RUG) system.

Private Payers

Because of the expense involved with hospitalization, private payers encourage providers to minimize the number of days patients stay in the hospital. Most private payers establish the standard number of days allowed for various conditions (called the estimated length of stay, or ELOS), and compare the ELOS to the patient's actual stay as a way to control costs.

Many private payers have also adopted the UHDDS format and the DRG method of setting prospective payments for hospital services. Hospitals and the payers, which may include Blue Cross and Blue Shield or other managed care plans, negotiate the rates for each DRG.

A number of private payers use the DRG to negotiate the fees they pay hospitals. Two other payment methods are used by managed care plans. Preferred provider organizations (PPOs) often negotiate a discount from the DRG with the hospital and its affiliated physicians. The hospital may have discounted fee structures with a number of PPOs and other managed care plans—each different, depending on what was agreed to. Health maintenance organizations (HMOs) negotiate capitated contracts with hospitals, too. The hospital agrees to provide care for a set population of prospective patients who are plan members. The HMO in turn pays the hospital a flat rate—a single set fee for each member. This rate may be a per diem (per day) rate that is paid for each day the patient is in the hospital regardless of the specific services. Like the DRG model, when a patient is held in the hospital for longer than is stated in the agreement between the HMO and the hospital, the hospital has to write off the extra cost.

Claims and Follow-up

Hospitals must submit claims for Medicare Part A reimbursement to Medicare fiscal intermediaries using the HIPAA health care claim called **837I.** This electronic data interchange (EDI) format, similar to the 837 claim (Chapter 8), is called *I* for *Institutional;* the physicians' claim is called 837P *(Professional).*

In some situations, a paper claim form called the **UB-04** (uniform billing 2004), also known as the **CMS-1450,** is also accepted by most other payers. The UB-04 is maintained by the National Uniform Billing Committee. This form was previously called the **UB-92.**

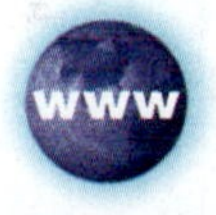

National Uniform Billing Committee (NUBC)

http://www.nubc.org

837I Health Care Claim Completion

The 837I, like the 837P, has sections requiring data elements for the billing and the pay-to provider, the subscriber and patient, and the payer, plus claim and service level details. Most of the data elements report the same information as summarized below for the paper claim.

Billing Tip

UB-04 versus UB-92
UB-04, a replacement for claim form UB-92, is mandated for use as of March 1, 2007. Providers can use the old UB-92 until May 22, 2007, but not after. The reason is that the new form has a field for reporting NPIs, as required under HIPAA.

UB-04 Claim Form Completion

The UB-04 claim form has eighty-one data fields, some of which require multiple entries (see Figure 16.5 on page 530). The information for the form locators often requires choosing from a list of codes. Table 16.2 on pages 531–534 shows required information and possible choices for a Medicare claim. (In some cases, because the list of code choices is extensive, selected entries are shown as examples.) Private-payer-required fields may be slightly different, and other condition codes or options are often available. All dates should use the eight-digit format.

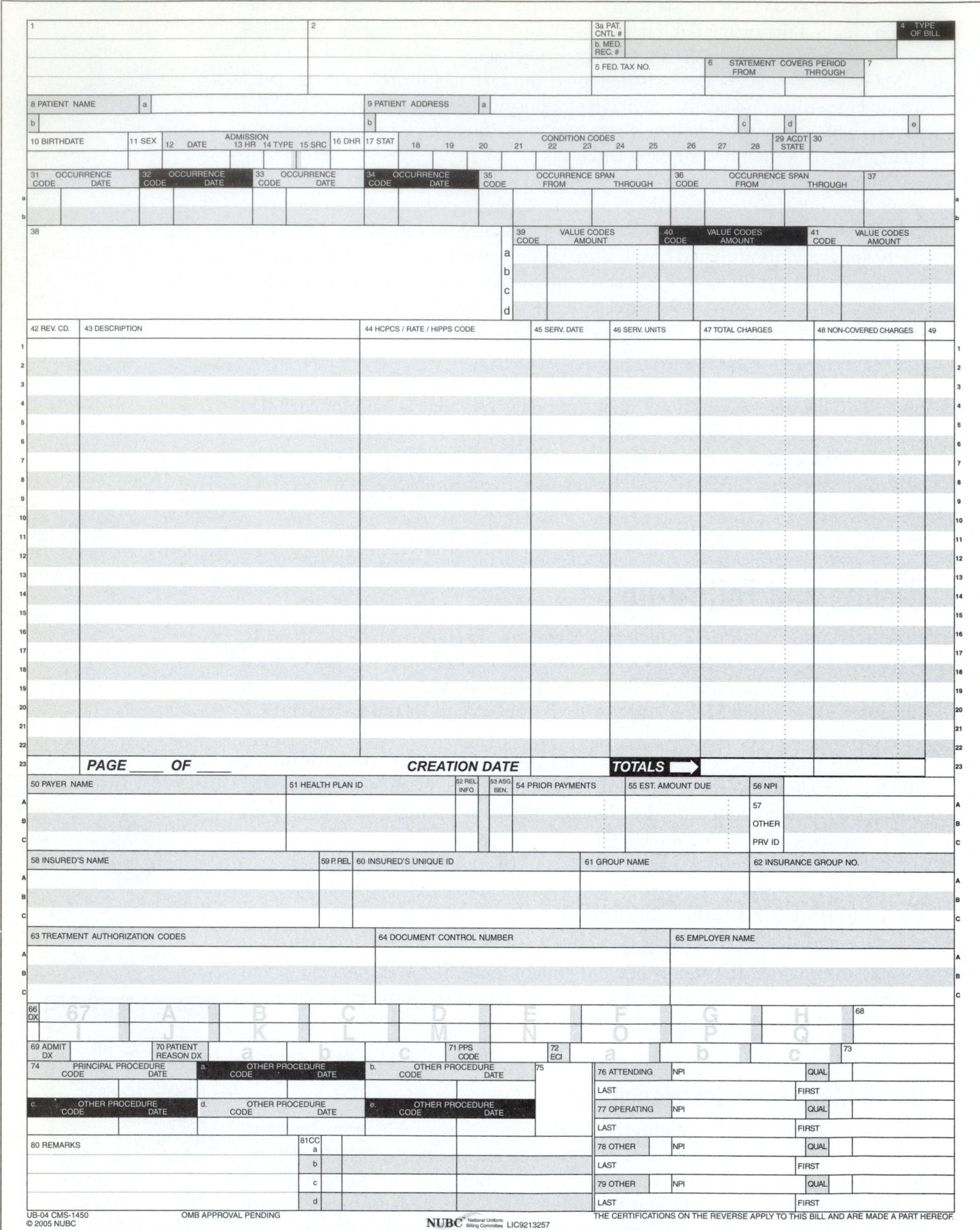

1 | 2 | 3a PAT. CNTL # | b. MED. REC. # | 4 TYPE OF BILL

5 FED. TAX NO. | 6 STATEMENT COVERS PERIOD FROM THROUGH | 7

8 PATIENT NAME a | b | 9 PATIENT ADDRESS a | b | c | d | e

10 BIRTHDATE | 11 SEX | ADMISSION 12 DATE | 13 HR | 14 TYPE | 15 SRC | 16 DHR | 17 STAT | CONDITION CODES 18 | 19 | 20 | 21 | 22 | 23 | 24 | 25 | 26 | 27 | 28 | 29 ACDT STATE | 30

31 OCCURRENCE CODE DATE | 32 OCCURRENCE CODE DATE | 33 OCCURRENCE CODE DATE | 34 OCCURRENCE CODE DATE | 35 OCCURRENCE SPAN CODE FROM THROUGH | 36 OCCURRENCE SPAN CODE FROM THROUGH | 37

a
b

38 | 39 VALUE CODES CODE AMOUNT | 40 VALUE CODES CODE AMOUNT | 41 VALUE CODES CODE AMOUNT

a
b
c
d

42 REV. CD.	43 DESCRIPTION	44 HCPCS / RATE / HIPPS CODE	45 SERV. DATE	46 SERV. UNITS	47 TOTAL CHARGES	48 NON-COVERED CHARGES	49
1							
2							
3							
4							
5							
6							
7							
8							
9							
10							
11							
12							
13							
14							
15							
16							
17							
18							
19							
20							
21							
22							
23	PAGE ____ OF ____	CREATION DATE		TOTALS			

50 PAYER NAME | 51 HEALTH PLAN ID | 52 REL. INFO | 53 ASG. BEN. | 54 PRIOR PAYMENTS | 55 EST. AMOUNT DUE | 56 NPI | 57 OTHER PRV ID

A
B
C

58 INSURED'S NAME | 59 P. REL | 60 INSURED'S UNIQUE ID | 61 GROUP NAME | 62 INSURANCE GROUP NO.

A
B
C

63 TREATMENT AUTHORIZATION CODES | 64 DOCUMENT CONTROL NUMBER | 65 EMPLOYER NAME

A
B
C

66 DX | 67 | A | B | C | D | E | F | G | H | 68
I | J | K | L | M | N | O | P | Q

69 ADMIT DX | 70 PATIENT REASON DX | a | b | c | 71 PPS CODE | 72 ECI | a | b | c | 73

74 PRINCIPAL PROCEDURE CODE DATE | a. OTHER PROCEDURE CODE DATE | b. OTHER PROCEDURE CODE DATE | 75

c. OTHER PROCEDURE CODE DATE | d. OTHER PROCEDURE CODE DATE | e. OTHER PROCEDURE CODE DATE

76 ATTENDING NPI QUAL
LAST FIRST

77 OPERATING NPI QUAL
LAST FIRST

80 REMARKS | 81CC a | b | c | d

78 OTHER NPI QUAL
LAST FIRST

79 OTHER NPI QUAL
LAST FIRST

UB-04 CMS-1450
© 2005 NUBC

OMB APPROVAL PENDING

NUBC™ National Uniform Billing Committee LIC9213257

THE CERTIFICATIONS ON THE REVERSE APPLY TO THIS BILL AND ARE MADE A PART HEREOF.

FIGURE 16.5 UB-04 Form

TABLE 16.2 UB-04 Form Completion

FORM LOCATOR	DESCRIPTION	MEDICARE-REQUIRED?
1 (untitled)	Provider name, address, and telephone no.	Yes
2 (untitled)	Unassigned; for state use.	No
3 Patient Control Number	Patient's unique number assigned by the facility.	Yes
4 Type of Bill	Three-digit alphanumeric code: First digit identifies the facility type (e.g., 1 = hospital, 2 = SNF). Second digit identifies the care type (e.g., 1 = inpatient Part A, 2 = inpatient Part B, 3 = outpatient). Third digit identifies the billing sequence in this episode of care (e.g., 1 = this bill encompasses entire inpatient confinement or course of outpatient treatment for which provider expects payment from the payer).	Yes
5 Federal Tax Number	Not required.	No
6 Statement Covers Period (From–Through)	The beginning and ending dates of the period included on the bill; dates before patient's entitlement are not shown. From date is used to determine timely filing.	Yes
Covered Days	The total number of covered days during the billing period, including lifetime reserve days elected for which Medicare payment is requested. Should be the total of units in form locator 46.	Yes
Noncovered Days	The total number of noncovered days during the billing period not billable to Medicare.	Yes
Coinsurance Days	The number of covered inpatient hospital days after the 60th day and before the 91st day, or the number of covered inpatient SNF days after the 20th day and before the 101st day.	Yes
Lifetime Reserve Days	Number of lifetime reserve days applicable.	Yes
7 (untitled)	Unassigned; for state use.	No
8 Patient's Name	Patient's last name, first name, and middle initial.	Yes
9 Patient's Address	Patient's full mailing address: street number and name, PO Box or RFD; city, state, and ZIP code.	Yes
10 Patient's Birthdate	Patient's birthdate; if unavailable, use zeroes.	Yes
11 Patient Sex	M for male; F for female.	Yes
12 Admission Date	Month, day, and year of inpatient admission.	Yes
13 Admission Hour	Time of day of admission.	No
14 Type of Admission	Required for inpatient bills: 1 = emergency, 2 = urgent, 3 = elective, 9 = information not available (rarely used).	Yes
15 Source of Admission	Source of admission: 1 = physician referral. 2 = clinic referral. 3 = HMO referral. 4 = transfer from a hospital. 5 = transfer from an SNF. 6 = transfer from another facility. 7 = emergency room. 8 = court/law enforcement. 9 = information not available. A = transfer from a rural primary care hospital.	Yes
16 Discharge Hour	Time of day of patient discharge.	No

TABLE 16.2 UB-04 Form Completion *continued*

FORM LOCATOR	DESCRIPTION	MEDICARE-REQUIRED?
17 Patient Status	For Part A inpatient, SNF, hospice, and outpatient hospital services: 01 = routine discharge to self or home. 02 = discharge to another short-term general hospital. 03 = discharge to SNF. 04 = discharge to ICF. 05 = discharge to another type of facility. 06 = discharge to home under care of home health organization. 07 = left against medical advice or discontinued care. 08 = discharge to home under care of home IV drug therapy provider. 09 = admitted as inpatient (after outpatient services). 20 = expired. 30 = still patient or expected to return for outpatient services. 40 = expired at home (hospice claims only). 41 = expired in a medical facility (hospice claims only). 42 = expired, place unknown (hospice claims only). 50 = hospice—home. 51 = hospice—medical facility.	Yes
18–28 Condition Codes*	Codes relating to bill that may affect processing; examples include: 02 = condition is employment-related. 04 = patient is HMO-enrollee. 05 = lien has been filed. 06 = ESRD patient in first eighteen months of employer group health insurance. 07 = treatment of nonterminal condition for hospice. 08 = beneficiary would not provide information about other insurance coverage. 09 = neither patient nor spouse is employed. 10 = patient and/or spouse employed, but no employer group health plan coverage exists. 31 = patient is student (full-time, day). 67 = beneficiary elects not to use lifetime reserve days.	Yes
29 (untitled) ACDT state.		
30 (untitled)	Unassigned.	No
31–36 Occurrence Codes and Dates (span)	Codes and date data that affect Medicare processing; examples include: 01 = auto accident. 04 = accident/employment related. 05 = other accident. 11 = onset of symptoms/illness. 17 = date occupational therapy plan established or reviewed. 18 = date of patient/beneficiary retirement. 19 = date of spouse retirement. 21 = utilization notice received. 24 = date insurance denied by primary payer. 25 = date benefits terminated by primary payer. 31 = date beneficiary notified of intent to bill for inpatient care accommodations. 32 = date beneficiary notified of intent to bill for Medicare medically unnecessary procedures or treatments. A1 = birthdate—insured A. A2 = effective date—insured A policy. A3 = benefits for insured A exhausted.	Yes

(continued)

TABLE 16.2 UB-04 Form Completion *continued*

FORM LOCATOR	DESCRIPTION	MEDICARE-REQUIRED?
37–38 (untitled)	For Medicare as secondary payer, the address of the primary payer may be shown here.	No
39, 40, 41 Value Codes and Amounts*	Codes and related dollar amounts required to process the claim; examples include: 08 = Medicare lifetime reserve amount for first calendar year in billing period. 09 = Medicare coinsurance amount for first calendar year in billing period. 14 = no-fault, including auto, when primary payer payments are being applied to covered Medicare charges on this bill. 31 = patient liability amount, the amount approved by hospital or the QIO to charge the beneficiary for noncovered services. A1, B1, C1 = amounts assumed by provider to be applied to the patient's deductible amount for payer A, B, or C. A2, B2, C2 = amounts assumed by provider to be applied to the patient's coinsurance amount involving payer A, B, or C. A3, B3, C3 = amount estimated by provider to be paid by payer A, B, or C.	Yes
42 Revenue Code*	For each Medicare cost center—such as rental or purchase of durable medical equipment (DME)—for which a separate charge is billed in form locator 47, the Medicare-assigned revenue code is listed. Code 001 is placed before the total charge amount.	Yes
43 Revenue Description	Narrative description for each revenue code used in form locator 42.	No
44 HCPCS/Rates	HCPCS codes for applicable procedures.	Yes
45 Service Date	Not required.	No
46 Service Units	Number of units for each applicable service provided, such as number of months of rental for DME.	Yes
47 Total Charges	Total charges for the billing period.	Yes
48 Noncovered Charges	Total noncovered charges of those shown in form locator 42.	Yes
49 (untitled)	Unassigned.	No
50 A, B, C Payer Identification	If Medicare is primary payer, Medicare is entered on line A. If Medicare is the secondary or tertiary payer, the primary payer is entered on line A, and Medicare information on lines B or C.	Yes
51 A, B, C Provider Number	The provider's six-digit Medicare-assigned number is entered on the line corresponding to Medicare in form locator 50.	Yes
52 A, B, C Release of Information	Y = provider has on file a signed statement permitting data release to other organizations in order to adjudicate the claim. R = release is limited or restricted. N = no release is on file.	Yes
53 A, B, C Assignment of Benefits Certification Indicator	Not required; the back of the CMS-1450 contains this certification.	No
54 A, B, C Prior Payments	For other than inpatient hospital and SNF services; amount patient has paid (deductible/coinsurance).	Yes
55 A, B, C Estimated Amount Due	Not required.	No
56 NPI	National Provider Identifier.	Yes
57	Other Provider ID.	Yes
58 A, B, C Insured's Name	Patient/insured's name on line corresponding to the Medicare line in form locator 50; form locators 59–66 pertain to this person.	Yes

(continued)

TABLE 16.2 UB-04 Form Completion *continued*

FORM LOCATOR	DESCRIPTION	MEDICARE-REQUIRED?
59 A, B, C Patient's Relationship to Insured	Code for patient's relationship to insured: 01 = self. 02 = spouse. 03 = natural child/insured has financial responsibility. 04 = natural child/insured does not have financial responsibility. 05 = stepchild. 06 = foster child. 08 = employee. 09 = unknown. 11 = organ donor. 12 = cadaver donor. 15 = injured plaintiff.	Yes
60 A, B, C Certificate/Social Security Number/HI Claim/Identification Number	Patient's Medicare number; if Medicare is primary, entered in line A.	Yes
61 A, B, C Group Name	For Medicare secondary, the primary payer's insurance group or plan name.	Yes
62 A, B, C Insurance Group Number	Number for insurance named in form locator 61.	Yes
63 Treatment Authorization Code	Whenever QIO review is performed for outpatient preadmission, preprocedure, or inpatient preadmission, authorization number is shown.	Yes
64 Document Control Number		Yes
65 Employer Name	Insured's employer's name.	Yes
66 Principal Diagnosis Code	ICD-9-CM diagnosis and procedure codes to highest level of specificity available.	Yes
67–68 Other Diagnoses Codes	Codes for up to fifteen additional conditions that coexisted at admission or developed and that had an effect on the treatment or the length of stay.	Yes
69 Admitting Diagnosis	The patient's admitting diagnosis is required if the claim is subject to QIO review.	Yes
70 Patient Reason Diagnosis		
71 PPS		
72 ECI		No
74 Principal Procedure Code and Date; Other Procedure Codes and Dates	ICD-9-CM procedure code most closely related to principal diagnosis code. Up to five additional ICD-9-CM procedure codes as reported by the provider.	Yes—inpatient only Yes—inpatient only
76 Attending	NPI and name of the attending or referring physician.	Yes
77 Operating	NPI and name of physician who also performed principal or surgical procedures.	Conditional
78 Other	NPIs and names of other providers	
79		
80 Remarks	Completed for DMEs and Medicare Secondary Payer.	Conditional
81 CC		

* Detailed information is provided in fiscal intermediary manuals.

Remittance Advice Processing

Hospitals receive a remittance advice (RA) when payments are transmitted by payers to their accounts. The patient accounting department and HIM check that appropriate payment has been received. Unless the software used for billing automatically reports that the billed code is not the same as the paid code, procedures to find and follow up on these exceptions must be set up between the two departments.

Similar to medical practices, hospitals set up schedules when accounts receivable are due and follow up on late payments. The turnaround time for electronic claims is usually from ten to fifteen days faster than for manual paper claims, so the follow-up procedures are organized according to each payer's submission method and usual turnaround time. Payers' requests for attachments such as emergency department reports may delay payment.

Hospital Billing Compliance

Both outpatient and inpatient facilities must comply with federal and state law. In the Medicare program, compliance is as important for Part A claims as it is for Part B claims. To uncover fraud and abuse in Part A payments, the Office of the Inspector General (see Chapter 2) directs part of its annual OIG Work Plan at institutional providers. For example, CMS's annual Medical Provider Analysis and Review (MedPar) data show national averages for each DRG group in hospitals. The OIG uses these figures in preparing the part of the OIG Work Plan that is directed at hospital coding. A major target has been upcoding of DRG groups. The OIG has sought to uncover fraud when a hospital too often reports codes that result in high-relative-value DRGs.

Example

A patient has a pulmonary edema (fluid in the lungs) that is due to the principal diagnosis of congestive heart failure. The correct ICD-9-CM code order leads to a DRG 127 classification. If the coder instead incorrectly reports pulmonary edema and respiratory failure, the patient is assigned DRG 87, which has a higher relative value, resulting in an improperly high payment.

> **Compliance Guideline**
>
> **OIG Guidance**
> **The OIG has issued both a 1998 Compliance Program Guidance for Hospitals and a Supplemental Compliance Program Guidance, together presenting effective compliance policies and programs for hospitals.**

The OIG has established lists of DRGs that are often the result of upcoding. Patterns of higher-than-normal reporting by a hospital of these DRGs may cause an investigation and possibly an audit of the hospital.

The OIG has also used MedPar data over the years to monitor other improper Medicare payments to hospitals. Two problem areas have been improper payments for nonphysician outpatient services and overpayments for patient transfers.

To safeguard against fraud, hospitals:

- Double-check registration information. The admissions department verifies that the patient is being admitted for a medically necessary diagnosis under the payer's rules. If items will not be covered under Medicare Part A, patients must sign the Hospital-Issued Notice of Noncoverage (HINN) (or an ABN for Part B; see Chapter 10) to acknowledge their responsibility for payment.

- Update their charge masters every year with current HCPCS, ICD-9-CM, and CPT codes.
- Compare clinical documentation with the patient's bill to make sure reported services are properly documented.
- Conduct postpayment audits to uncover patterns of denied or partially paid codes.

Thinking it Through — 16.3

How are the Medicare Prospective Payment System and the use of capitated rates in managed care organizations similar? How are they different?

Review

Steps to Success

- ❒ Read this chapter and review the Key Terms and the Chapter Summary.
- ❒ Answer the Review Questions and Applying Your Knowledge in the Chapter Review.
- ❒ Access the chapter's websites and complete the Internet Activities to learn more about available professional resources.
- ❒ Complete the related chapter in the *Medical Insurance Workbook* to reinforce your understanding of hospital coding and billing procedures.

Chapter Summary

1. Inpatient services, those involving an overnight stay, are provided by general and specialized hospitals, skilled nursing facilities, and long-term care facilities. Outpatient services are provided by ambulatory surgical centers or units, by home health agencies, and by hospice staff.
2. The first major step in the hospital claims processing sequence is admission, when the patient is registered. Personal and financial information is entered in the hospital's health record system; insurance coverage is verified; consent forms are signed by the patient; a notice of the hospital's privacy policy is presented to the patient; and some pretreatment payments are collected. In the second step, the patient's treatments and transfers among the various departments in the hospital are tracked and recorded. The third step, discharge and billing, follows the discharge of the patient from the facility and the completion of the patient's record.
3. Diagnostic coding for inpatient services follows the rules of the Uniform Hospital Discharge Data Set (UHDDS). Two ways in which inpatient coding differs from physician and outpatient diagnostic coding are that (1) the main diagnosis, called the principal rather than the primary diagnosis, is established after study in the hospital setting, and (2) coding an unconfirmed condition (rule-out) as the admitting diagnosis is permitted.
4. Volume 3 of the ICD-9-CM, *Procedures,* is used to report the procedures for inpatient services. It is organized by surgical procedures divided into body systems, followed by diagnostic and therapeutic procedures. The three- or four-digit codes are assigned based on the principal diagnosis.
5. Medicare pays for inpatient services under its Inpatient Prospective Payment System, which uses diagnosis-related groups (DRGs) to classify patients into similar treatment and length-of-hospital-stay units and sets prices for each classification group. A hospital's geographic location, labor and supply costs, and teaching costs also affect the per-DRG pay rate it negotiates with CMS.
6. The 837I—the HIPAA standard transaction for the facility claim—or, in some cases, the UB-04 form (CMS-1450) is used to report patient data, information on the insured, facility and patient type, the source of the admission, various conditions that affect payment, whether Medicare is the primary payer (for Medicare claims), the principal and other diagnosis codes, the admitting diagnosis, the principal procedure code, the attending physician, other key physicians, and charges.

Review Questions

Match the key terms with their definitions.

A. attending physician
B. principal diagnosis
C. charge master
D. inpatient
E. diagnosis-related groups (DRGs)
F. comorbidities
G. admitting diagnosis
H. principal procedure
I. ambulatory care
J. 837I

____ 1. A person admitted to a hospital for services that require an overnight stay

____ 2. The main service performed for the condition listed as the principal diagnosis for a hospital inpatient

____ 3. The clinician primarily responsible for the care of the patient from the beginning of the hospital episode

____ 4. Outpatient care

____ 5. HIPAA standard transaction for the facility claim

____ 6. A hospital's list of the codes and charges for its services

____ 7. The patient's condition identified by the physician at admission to the hospital

____ 8. A system of analyzing conditions and treatments for similar groups of patients used to establish Medicare fees for hospital inpatient services

____ 9. Conditions in addition to the principal diagnosis that the patient had at hospital admission which affect the length of the hospital stay or the course of treatment

____10. The condition that after study is established as chiefly responsible for a patient's admission to a hospital

Decide whether each statement is true or false.

____ 1. Skilled nursing facilities (SNF) are classified as outpatient facilities.

____ 2. Emergency care involves a life-threatening situation.

____ 3. An inpatient's insurance coverage is usually verified in the discharge process.

____ 4. The master patient index contains the name of each patient's attending physician.

____ 5. When a patient is covered by Medicare, the admissions staff must find out whether Medicare is the primary payer.

____ 6. The hospital's charge master serves the same purpose as a medical practice's encounter form.

____ 7. The principal diagnosis is based on the admitting diagnosis.

____ 8. Inpatient coding rules do not permit the reporting of suspected or unconfirmed diagnoses.

____ 9. ICD-9-CM, Volume 3, is used to report inpatient procedures.

____ 10. The UB-04 is a paper claim form that is sometimes used by hospitals.

Select the letter that best completes the statement or answers the question.

____ 1. When the hospital staff collects data on a patient who is being admitted for services, the process is called
A. health information management
B. registration
C. MSP
D. precertification

_____ 2. Which of the following hospital departments has different procedures for collecting patients' personal and insurance information?
  A. accounting department
  B. surgery department
  C. emergency department
  D. collections department

_____ 3. Patient charges in hospitals vary according to
  A. their accommodations only
  B. their services only
  C. their accommodations and services
  D. their age and gender

_____ 4. Which of these rules governs the reporting of hospital inpatient services on insurance claims?
  A. ASC
  B. HIM
  C. APC
  D. UHDDS

_____ 5. Conditions that arise during the patient's hospital stay as a result of treatments are called
  A. comorbidities
  B. admitting diagnoses
  C. complications
  D. correlates

_____ 6. In inpatient coding, the initials *CC* mean
  A. chief complaint
  B. comorbidities and complications
  C. cubic centimeters
  D. convalescent center

_____ 7. The code 76.23 is an example of which type of code?
  A. CPT-4
  B. ICD-9-CM Volume 1
  C. ICD-9-CM Volume 2
  D. ICD-9-CM Volume 3

_____ 8. Under a Prospective Payment System, payments for services are
  A. set in advance
  B. based on the provider's fees
  C. discounts to the provider's usual fees
  D. none of the above

_____ 9. The UB-04 form locator 4 requires the
  A. type of bill
  B. admission hour
  C. revenue code
  D. patient status

_____ 10. Under Medicare rules for patients in car accidents, the automobile insurance is
  A. primary
  B. secondary
  C. supplemental
  D. tertiary

Define the following abbreviations:

1. DRG ______________________________
2. PPS ______________________________
3. SNF ______________________________
4. ASC ______________________________
5. HHA ______________________________

Applying Your Knowledge

Case 16.1 Coding Hospital Services

Follow the inpatient coding guidelines for (1) identifying the principal diagnosis, (2) coding suspected conditions, and (3) differentiating between statements of admitting, principal, comorbidity, and complication diagnoses as you analyze these cases.

A. What is the principal diagnosis for this patient?

Discharge Date: 07/05/2008

Patient: Kellerman, Larry H.

Patient is a 59-year-old male who was recently found to have some evidence of induration of his prostate gland. He was referred for urologic evaluation and admitted to the hospital for further study and biopsy. Under general anesthesia, cystoscopy revealed early prostatic enlargement, and needle biopsy was accomplished. Pathological examination of the tissue removed confirmed the presence of adenocarcinoma of the prostate.

B. What is the admitting diagnosis for this patient?

Room: S-920

Patient: Koren, Sarah I.

Admission Date: 10/11/2008

Chief Complaint: Severe, right upper abdominal pain radiating to the back.

History of Present Illness: This 38-year-old female reports having this severe pain for two weeks. She has had some nausea and vomiting. Condition worsened by previous treatment with pain medication and Tagamet. Previous ultrasound of her gallbladder showed a very thickened gallbladder wall with a large stone, impacted at the neck of the cystic duct. Her family physician has admitted her to be taken to surgery for a cholecystectomy. She notes diarrhea a few days ago but no other change in bowel habits.

Impression: Probable acute cholecystitis.

C. Identify the principal diagnosis, the principal procedure, the comorbidity diagnosis, and the complication in the following discharge statement.

Flora Raniculli is a 65-year-old female admitted to the hospital with a three-month history of cough, yellow-sputum production, weight loss, and shortness of breath. Chest X-ray reveals probable bronchiectasis. Patient may also have pulmonary fibrosis. She underwent a bronchoscopy that showed thick secretions in both lower lobes. Post-bronchoscopy fever finally cleared up. She is now being discharged and will call me in one week for a progress report.

Case 16.2 Calculating Insurance Math

A hospital has a per diem payment arrangement with an HMO. The plan will pay the hospital $1,200 a day for inpatient care, regardless of the services the hospital provides. This month, one member has been hospitalized for three days for observation and tests. The hospital charges for the three days are $1,275, $1,330, and $1,200.

A. What is the total hospital fee for the three days? ______________________

B. How much will the HMO pay the hospital for this patient's care? ______________________

C. How is the balance handled? ______________________

Internet Activities

1. The Centers for Medicare and Medicaid (CMS) website contains a designated area for hospital information. To view this information, go to the CMS hospital website at http://www.cms.hhs.gov/center/hospital.asp. To view the range of topics available at the site, review the Important Links list and click on Hospitals. To learn more about the Acute Inpatient Prospective Payment System (PPS), click this subtopic, and then read the Overview. What did you learn about the role of DRGs in this payment system?

2. Go to the Medicare Quality Improvement Community's website at http://www.medqic.org/. Look up information about the Quality Improvement Organizations program. How many QIOs make up the national network? Who do these organizations represent?

Part 7 Claim Case Studies

Chapter 17
Primary Case Studies

Chapter 18
RA/EOB/Secondary Case Studies

Chapter 17

Primary Case Studies

CHAPTER OUTLINE

Method of Claim Completion

About the Practice

Claim Case Studies

Learning Outcomes

This chapter provides an opportunity to demonstrate the ability to complete correct primary claims. Twenty patient encounters with the Valley Associates, P.C., practice require the preparation of claims.

1. For the first ten encounters (claim case studies 1 – 10), completed patient information forms and encounter forms are supplied. Completion of a correct claim for each encounter based on abstracting information from these forms is required.
2. For the second ten encounters (claim case studies 11 – 20), patient information, a diagnostic statement, and a procedural statement are provided. To prepare correct claims requires selecting the correct ICD-9-CM and CPT codes for the encounter, abstracting the patient information, and completing a claim.

Method of Claim Completion

If you are using Medisoft to complete the cases, read the *Guide to Medisoft* on pages 593–616 before beginning. Information from the first section, patient information, has already been entered in the program for you. You must enter encounter information to complete the claim. If you are gaining experience by completing a paper CMS-1500 claim form, use the blank claim form supplied to you (from the back of the book or printed from the Student Data Template CD-ROM) and follow the instructions in the text chapter that is appropriate for the particular payer.

Patient Copayments

In Chapter 17, copayment information for each claim case is included in the patient information form. If the patient's plan requires a copay and you are completing a paper CMS-1500 claim form, assume that the patient has paid the copay at the time of the visit, and enter this amount in the Amount Paid box on the form (IN 29). If you are working in Medisoft, you will be prompted to enter the copay amount in the Transaction Entry dialog box when you enter a procedure charge. (Medisoft stores this information in the Transaction Entry dialog box rather than printing it on the claim form.)

About the Practice

The Valley Associates, P.C., practice has four physicians:

Christopher M. Connolly, M.D. – Internal Medicine
Telephone: 555-967-0303
NPI: 8877365552
FED I.D. #16-1234567, Medicaid I.D.: MCD0123/

David Rosenberg, M.D. – Dermatology
Telephone: 555-967-0303
NPI: 1288560027
FED I.D. #16-2345678, Medicaid I.D.: MCD0123/

Nancy Ronkowski, M.D. – OB/GYN
Telephone: 555-321-0987
NPI: 9475830260
FED I.D. #06-7890123

Sarah Jamison, M.D. – Orthopedic Medicine
Telephone: 555-321-0987
NPI: 5544882211
FED I.D. #07-2345678

All four physicians have signatures on file as of 1/1/2008 and all are Medicare-participating.

The address for the practice is:

Valley Associates, P.C.
1400 West Center Street
Toledo, OH 43601-0213

The fee schedule for Valley Associates, P.C., is shown in Table 17.1.

TABLE 17.1 FEE SCHEDULE for Valley Associates, P.C.

Code	*Description*	Price Code A: Provider's Usual Fee	Price Code B: Medicare and Medicaid
	OFFICE VISITS		
	New Patient		
99201	LI Problem Focused	$56	$32
99202	LII Expanded	75	50
99203	LIII Detailed	103	69
99204	LIV Comp./Mod	150	103
99205	LV Comp./High	194	128
	Established Patient		
99211	LI Minimum	30	14
99212	LII Problem Focused	46	28
99213	LIII Expanded	62	39
99214	LIV Detailed	91	59
99215	LV Comp./High	140	94
	PREVENTIVE VISIT		
	New Patient		
99384	Age 12-17	178	113
99385	Age 18-39	166	106
99386	Age 40-64	180	130
99387	Age 65+	200	142
	Established Patient		
99394	Age 12-17	149	101
99395	Age 18-39	137	95
99396	Age 40-64	149	106
99397	Age 65+	120	118
	CONSULTATION: OFFICE/OP		
99241	LI Problem Focused	95	48
99242	LII Expanded	127	75
99243	LIII Detailed	162	97
99244	LIV Comp./Mod.	219	136
99245	LV Comp./High	293	183
	CARE PLAN OVERSIGHT		
99339	Supervision, 15-29 min.	80	60
99340	Supervision, 30+ min.	110	80
	SURGERY		
10040	Acne Surgery	80	53
10060	I&D, Abscess, Smpl	98	57
10061	I&D, Abscess, Mult	215	106
10080	I&D, Pilonidal Cyst, Smpl	105	65
10081	I&D, Pilonidal Cyst, Compl	210	135
10120	I&R, Foreign Body, Smpl	119	60

TABLE 17.1	FEE SCHEDULE for Valley Associates, P.C. (Continued)		
Code	***Description***	**Price Code A: Provider's Usual Fee**	**Price Code B: Medicare and Medicaid**
10121	I&R, Foreign Body, Compl	225	140
10140	I&D Hematoma	85	71
10160	Puncture Aspiration	72	61
11000	Debride Skin, To 10%	89	36
11001	Each Addl 10%	84	25
11055	Pare Benign Skin Lesion	26	16
11056	Pare Benign Skin Lesion, 2-4	37	23
11057	Pare Benign Skin Lesion, 4+	40	25
11100	Skin Biopsy, Single Les.	111	47
11101	Skin Biopsy, Mult Les.	73	25
11200	Remove Skin Tags, 1-15	104	43
11201	Remove Skin Tags, Addl 10	55	21
11719	Trim Nails	9	7
11720	Debride Nails, 1-5	38	24
11721	Debride Nails, 6+	60	40
11730	Avulsion of Nail Plate, 1	107	56
11732	Avulsion of Nail Plate, Addl 1	54	32
11755	Nail Biopsy	167	91
11760	Repair Nail Bed	240	105
11765	Excision, Ingrown Toenail	113	52
11975	Norplant Insertion	238	98
11976	Norplant Removal	278	118
17000	Removal 1 Lesion	89	37
17003	Removal 2-14 Lesions	18	10
17004	Removal 15+ Lesions	313	184
19100	Biopsy, Needle Asp., Breast	216	71
23500	Clavicle	1349	521
23570	Scapula	345	147
23600	Humerus, proximal	501	221
24500	Humerus, shaft	432	214
24650	Radial, h or n w/out manip	396	167
24670	Ulna, proximal	466	175
25560	Radius & Ulna	509	208
25600	Radius, colles, distal	803	363
25605	Radial, colles w/manip	412	167
25650	Ulna, styloid	729	213
26600	Hand MC	315	131
26720	Finger/Thumb	241	102
27200	Coccyx	307	123
27508	Femur, distal	976	375
27530	Tibia prox/plateau	683	271
27750	Tibia & Fibula, shaft	681	252
27780	Fibula, prox/shaft	395	171

(Continued)

TABLE 17.1	FEE SCHEDULE for Valley Associates, P.C. (Continued)		
Code	***Description***	**Price Code A: Provider's Usual Fee**	**Price Code B: Medicare and Medicaid**
28470	Foot, MT	360	141
28490	Toe, great	207	73
28510	Toe, others	174	73
36415	Venipuncture	17	17
45330	Sigmoidoscopy, diag.	226	82
46600	Diagnostic Anoscopy	72	28
56440	Marsup. Of Bartholin Cyst	695	211
57150	Pessary Washing	75	30
57160	Pessary Insertion	88	41
57170	Diaphragm Fitting	127	45
57452	Colposcopy	251	62
57500	Biopsy, Cervix	181	58
57505	Endocervical Currettage	186	66
57511	Cyro of Cervix	248	101
58100	Biopsy, Endometrium	189	53
58300	IUD Insertion	222	67
58301	IUD Removal	117	62
58322	Artificial Insemination	260	69
58558	Hysteroscopy	706	201
64435	Paracervical Block	229	69
69210	Removal of Cerumen	63	34
	X-RAY		
73000	Clavicle	82	28
73060	Humerus	89	30
73090	Forearm	83	28
73120	Hand, 2 views	79	27
73130	Hand, 3 views	91	29
73140	Fingers	71	23
73550	Femur	94	30
73590	Tibia & Fibula	89	28
73620	Foot, 2 views	78	27
73630	Foot, 3 views	90	29
73660	Toes	70	23
76092	Mammography (Bilateral)	134	34
76805	USG, Preg Uterus, Comp.	344	31
76815	USG, Preg Uterus, REPT.	252	87
76830	USG, Transvaginal	296	94
76856	USG, Gyn Complete	290	94
76857	USG, Gyn Limited	212	59
80061	Lipid Panel	64	64
81000	Urinalysis	17	17

TABLE 17.1 FEE SCHEDULE for Valley Associates, P.C. (Continued)			
Code	***Description***	**Price Code A: Provider's Usual Fee**	**Price Code B: Medicare and Medicaid**
82270	Stool/Occult Blood	15	15
82948	Glucose Finger Stick	15	15
85008	Tine Test	14	14
85590	Tuberculin PPD	28	28
87072	Chlamydia	30	30
87081	Bacteria Culture	30	30
87088	Urine Culture	34	34
87101	Fungal Culture	35	35
87109	Mycoplasma/Ureoplasm	64	64
87210	Wet Mount	20	20
87250	Herpes Culture	100	100
88150	Pap Smear	29	29
	MEDICINE		
90471	Immun. Admin.	25	25
90472	Ea. Add'l.	13	13
90632	Hepatitus A Immun	74	74
90659	Influenza Immun	68	68
90732	Pneumovax	32	32
90746	Hepatitis B Immun	105	105
93000	ECG Complete	70	29
93040	Rhythm ECG w/Report	43	16
93041	Rhythm ECG w/Tracing	35	6
95860	EMG – 1 extremity	199	76
95861	EMG – 2 extremities	306	130
95863	EMG – 3 extremities	388	154
95900	Nerve Conduct, M w/out F	105	39
95903	Nerve Conduct, M w/ F	126	44
95904	Nerve Conduct, sensory	104	33
99000	Specimen Handling	21	21

Patient Account Numbers

On the CMS-1500 claim form, IN 26 is used to record the patient's account number, also known as a chart number. For Claim Case Studies 17.1 through 17.10, this number is listed on each patient's encounter form. For Claim Case Studies 17.11 through 17.20, since no encounter forms are provided, you will need to create this number. At Valley Associates, P.C., eight-digit account numbers are created by using the first five letters of the patient's last name, followed by the first two letters of the first name, followed by a zero. For example, Wendy Walker's patient account number is WALKEWE0.

If the patient's last name is less than five letters, additional letters are supplemented from the first name to create the eight digits. Therefore, Jean Ruff's patient account number would be RUFFJEA0. (Note: If you are using Medisoft to create claims, chart numbers are already entered in the database for each case.)

Claim Case Study 17.1

Patient: Wendy Walker

VALLEY ASSOCIATES, PC
1400 West Center Street
Toledo, OH 43601-0123
555-321-0987

PATIENT INFORMATION FORM

THIS SECTION REFERS TO PATIENT ONLY

Name: Wendy Walker	Sex: F	Marital Status: ☑S ☐M ☐D ☐W	Birth Date: 11/14/35
Address: 85 Woodmont Dr.	SS#: 321-69-0809		
City: Alliance State: OH Zip: 44601	Employer: Retired	Phone:	
Home Phone: 555-024-1689	Employer's Address:		
Work Phone:	City: State: Zip:		
Spouse's Name:	Spouse's Employer:		
Emergency Contact:	Relationship:	Phone #:	

FILL IN IF PATIENT IS A MINOR

Parent/Guardian's Name:	Sex:	Marital Status: ☐S ☐M ☐D ☐W	Birth Date:
Phone:	SS#:		
Address:	Employer:	Phone:	
City: State: Zip:	Employer's Address:		
Student Status:	City: State: Zip:		

INSURANCE INFORMATION

Primary Insurance Company: Medicare HMO	Secondary Insurance Company:
Subscriber's Name: Wendy Walker Birth Date: 11/14/35	Subscriber's Name: Birth Date:
Plan: SS#: 321-69-0809	Plan:
Policy #: 321690809A Group #:	Policy #: Group #:
Copayment/Deductible: $10 copay Price Code: B	

OTHER INFORMATION

Reason for visit: pain in hips	Allergy to Medication (list):
Name of referring physician:	If auto accident, list date and state in which it occurred:

I authorize treatment and agree to pay all fees and charges for the person named above. I agree to pay all charges shown by statements, promptly upon their presentation, unless credit arrangements are agreed upon in writing.

I authorize payment directly to VALLEY ASSOCIATES, PC of insurance benefits otherwise payable to me. I hereby authorize the release of any medical information necessary in order to process a claim for payment in my behalf.

Wendy Walker — 10/6/08

(Patient's Signature/Parent or Guardian's Signature) (Date)

I plan to make payment of my medical expenses as follows (check one or more):

____ Insurance (as above) ____ Cash/Check/Credit/Debit Card ✓ Medicare ____ Medicaid ____ Workers' Comp.

VALLEY ASSOCIATES, PC

Christopher M. Connolly, MD - Internal Medicine
555-967-0303
FED I.D. #16-1234567

PATIENT NAME	APPT. DATE/TIME
Walker, Wendy	10/6/2008 10:30 am
PATIENT NO.	**DX**
WALKEWE0	1. 719.45 pain in hips 2. 719.50 joint stiffness NEC 3. 780.6 fever and chills 4.

DESCRIPTION	✓	CPT	FEE	DESCRIPTION	✓	CPT	FEE
OFFICE VISITS				**PROCEDURES**			
New Patient				Diagnostic Anoscopy		46600	
LI Problem Focused		99201		ECG Complete		93000	
LII Expanded		99202		I&D, Abscess		10060	
LIII Detailed		99203		Pap Smear		88150	
LIV Comp./Mod.		99204		Removal of Cerumen		69210	
LV Comp./High		99205		Removal 1 Lesion		17000	
Established Patient				Removal 2-14 Lesions		17003	
LI Minimum		99211		Removal 15+ Lesions		17004	
LII Problem Focused		99212		Rhythm ECG w/Report		93040	
LIII Expanded		99213		Rhythm ECG w/Tracing		93041	
LIV Detailed	✓	99214	59	Sigmoidoscopy, diag.		45330	
LV Comp./High		99215					
				LABORATORY			
PREVENTIVE VISIT				Bacteria Culture		87081	
New Patient				Fungal Culture		87101	
Age 12-17		99384		Glucose Finger Stick		82948	
Age 18-39		99385		Lipid Panel		80061	
Age 40-64		99386		Specimen Handling		99000	
Age 65+		99387		Stool/Occult Blood		82270	
Established Patient				Tine Test		85008	
Age 12-17		99394		Tuberculin PPD		85590	
Age 18-39		99395		Urinalysis		81000	
Age 40-64		99396		Venipuncture		36415	
Age 65+		99397					
				INJECTION/IMMUN.			
CONSULTATION: OFFICE/OP				Immun. Admin.		90471	
Requested By:				Ea. Add'l.		90472	
LI Problem Focused		99241		Hepatitis A Immun		90632	
LII Expanded		99242		Hepatitis B Immun		90746	
LIII Detailed		99243		Influenza Immun		90659	
LIV Comp./Mod.		99244		Pneumovax		90732	
LV Comp./High		99245					
				TOTAL FEES			

Claim Case Study 17.2

Patient: Walter Williams

VALLEY ASSOCIATES, PC
1400 West Center Street
Toledo, OH 43601-0123
555-321-0987

PATIENT INFORMATION FORM

THIS SECTION REFERS TO PATIENT ONLY

Name: Walter Williams	Sex: M	Marital Status: ☐S ☑M ☐D ☐W	Birth Date: 9/4/36
Address: 17 Mill Road	SS#: 401-26-9939		
City: Brooklyn State: OH Zip: 44144	Employer: Retired		Phone:
Home Phone: 555-936-0216	Employer's Address:		
Work Phone:	City: State: Zip:		
Spouse's Name: Vareen Williams	Spouse's Employer: Brooklyn Day Care		
Emergency Contact:	Relationship:		Phone #:

FILL IN IF PATIENT IS A MINOR

Parent/Guardian's Name:	Sex:	Marital Status: ☐S ☐M ☐D ☐W	Birth Date:
Phone:	SS#:		
Address:	Employer:		Phone:
City: State: Zip:	Employer's Address:		
Student Status:	City: State: Zip:		

INSURANCE INFORMATION

Primary Insurance Company: Aetna Choice		Secondary Insurance Company: Medicare Nationwide	
Subscriber's Name: Vareen Williams	Birth Date: 7/14/45	Subscriber's Name: Walter Williams	Birth Date: 9/4/36
Plan:	SS#: 103-56-2239	Plan:	
Policy #: ABC103562239	Group #: BDC1001	Policy #: 401269939A	Group #:
Copayment/Deductible: $15 copay	Price Code: A		

OTHER INFORMATION

Reason for visit: hypertension	Allergy to Medication (list):
Name of referring physician:	If auto accident, list date and state in which it occurred:

I authorize treatment and agree to pay all fees and charges for the person named above. I agree to pay all charges shown by statements, promptly upon their presentation, unless credit arrangements are agreed upon in writing.

I authorize payment directly to VALLEY ASSOCIATES, PC of insurance benefits otherwise payable to me. I hereby authorize the release of any medical information necessary in order to process a claim for payment in my behalf.

Walter Williams
(Patient's Signature/Parent or Guardian's Signature)

1/1/08
(Date)

I plan to make payment of my medical expenses as follows (check one or more):

✓ Insurance (as above) ____ Cash/Check/Credit/Debit Card ____ Medicare ____ Medicaid ____ Workers' Comp.

VALLEY ASSOCIATES, PC

Christopher M. Connolly, MD - Internal Medicine
555-967-0303
FED I.D. #16-1234567

PATIENT NAME	APPT. DATE/TIME
Williams, Walter	10/3/2008 9:00 am
PATIENT NO.	**DX**
WILLIWA0	1. 401.1 benign essential hypertension 2. 780.79 fatigue 3. 4.

DESCRIPTION	✓	CPT	FEE	DESCRIPTION	✓	CPT	FEE
OFFICE VISITS				**PROCEDURES**			
New Patient				Diagnostic Anoscopy		46600	
LI Problem Focused		99201		ECG Complete		93000	
LII Expanded		99202		I&D, Abscess		10060	
LIII Detailed		99203		Pap Smear		88150	
LIV Comp./Mod.		99204		Removal of Cerumen		69210	
LV Comp./High		99205		Removal 1 Lesion		17000	
Established Patient				Removal 2-14 Lesions		17003	
LI Minimum		99211		Removal 15+ Lesions		17004	
LII Problem Focused		99212		Rhythm ECG w/Report		93040	
LIII Expanded		99213		Rhythm ECG w/Tracing		93041	
LIV Detailed		99214		Sigmoidoscopy, diag.		45330	
LV Comp./High		99215					
				LABORATORY			
PREVENTIVE VISIT				Bacteria Culture		87081	
New Patient				Fungal Culture		87101	
Age 12-17		99384		Glucose Finger Stick		82948	
Age 18-39		99385		Lipid Panel		80061	
Age 40-64		99386		Specimen Handling		99000	
Age 65+		99387		Stool/Occult Blood		82270	
Established Patient				Tine Test		85008	
Age 12-17		99394		Tuberculin PPD		85590	
Age 18-39		99395		Urinalysis		81000	
Age 40-64		99396		Venipuncture	✓	36415	17
Age 65+		99397					
				INJECTION/IMMUN.			
CONSULTATION: OFFICE/OP				Immun. Admin.		90471	
Requested By:				Ea. Add'l.		90472	
LI Problem Focused		99241		Hepatitis A Immun		90632	
LII Expanded		99242		Hepatitis B Immun		90746	
LIII Detailed		99243		Influenza Immun		90659	
LIV Comp./Mod.		99244		Pneumovax		90732	
LV Comp./High		99245					
				TOTAL FEES			

Claim Case Study 17.3

Patient: Donna Gaeta

VALLEY ASSOCIATES, PC
1400 West Center Street
Toledo, OH 43601-0123
555-321-0987

PATIENT INFORMATION FORM

THIS SECTION REFERS TO PATIENT ONLY

Name: Donna Gaeta	Sex: F — Marital Status: ☑S ☐M ☐D ☐W — Birth Date: 12/2/37
Address: 11 Brigade Hill Road	SS#: 138-46-2400
City: Toledo State: OH Zip: 43601	Employer: Retired Phone:
Home Phone: 555-402-0621	Employer's Address:
Work Phone:	City: State: Zip:
Spouse's Name:	Spouse's Employer:
Emergency Contact:	Relationship: Phone #:

FILL IN IF PATIENT IS A MINOR

Parent/Guardian's Name:	Sex: Marital Status: ☐S ☐M ☐D ☐W Birth Date:
Phone:	SS#:
Address:	Employer: Phone:
City: State: Zip:	Employer's Address:
Student Status:	City: State: Zip:

INSURANCE INFORMATION

Primary Insurance Company: Medicare Nationwide	Secondary Insurance Company:
Subscriber's Name: Donna Gaeta Birth Date: 12/2/37	Subscriber's Name: Birth Date:
Plan: SS#: 138-46-2400	Plan:
Policy #: 138462400A Group #:	Policy #: Group #:
Copayment/Deductible: $100 deductible, not met Price Code: B	

OTHER INFORMATION

Reason for visit: routine examination	Allergy to Medication (list):
Name of referring physician:	If auto accident, list date and state in which it occurred:

I authorize treatment and agree to pay all fees and charges for the person named above. I agree to pay all charges shown by statements, promptly upon their presentation, unless credit arrangements are agreed upon in writing.

I authorize payment directly to VALLEY ASSOCIATES, PC of insurance benefits otherwise payable to me. I hereby authorize the release of any medical information necessary in order to process a claim for payment in my behalf.

Donna Gaeta — 10/7/08

(Patient's Signature/Parent or Guardian's Signature) (Date)

I plan to make payment of my medical expenses as follows (check one or more):

____ Insurance (as above) ____ Cash/Check/Credit/Debit Card __✓__ Medicare ____ Medicaid ____ Workers' Comp.

VALLEY ASSOCIATES, PC

Christopher M. Connolly, MD - Internal Medicine
555-967-0303
FED I.D. #16-1234567

PATIENT NAME	APPT. DATE/TIME
Gaeta, Donna	10/7/2008 3:30 pm
PATIENT NO.	**DX**
GAETADO0	1. v70.0 routine medical exam 2. 3. 4.

DESCRIPTION	✓	CPT	FEE	DESCRIPTION	✓	CPT	FEE
OFFICE VISITS				**PROCEDURES**			
New Patient				Diagnostic Anoscopy		46600	
LI Problem Focused		99201		ECG Complete	✓	93000	29
LII Expanded		99202		I&D, Abscess		10060	
LIII Detailed		99203		Pap Smear	✓	88150	29
LIV Comp./Mod.		99204		Removal of Cerumen		69210	
LV Comp./High		99205		Removal 1 Lesion		17000	
Established Patient				Removal 2-14 Lesions		17003	
LI Minimum		99211		Removal 15+ Lesions		17004	
LII Problem Focused		99212		Rhythm ECG w/Report		93040	
LIII Expanded		99213		Rhythm ECG w/Tracing		93041	
LIV Detailed		99214		Sigmoidoscopy, diag.		45330	
LV Comp./High		99215					
				LABORATORY			
PREVENTIVE VISIT				Bacteria Culture		87081	
New Patient				Fungal Culture		87101	
Age 12-17		99384		Glucose Finger Stick		82948	
Age 18-39		99385		Lipid Panel		80061	
Age 40-64		99386		Specimen Handling		99000	
Age 65+	✓	99387	142	Stool/Occult Blood		82270	
Established Patient				Tine Test		85008	
Age 12-17		99394		Tuberculin PPD		85590	
Age 18-39		99395		Urinalysis	✓	81000	17
Age 40-64		99396		Venipuncture	✓	36415	17
Age 65+		99397					
				INJECTION/IMMUN.			
CONSULTATION: OFFICE/OP				Immun. Admin.		90471	
Requested By:				Ea. Add'l.		90472	
LI Problem Focused		99241		Hepatitis A Immun		90632	
LII Expanded		99242		Hepatitis B Immun		90746	
LIII Detailed		99243		Influenza Immun		90659	
LIV Comp./Mod.		99244		Pneumovax		90732	
LV Comp./High		99245					
				TOTAL FEES			

Claim Case Study 17.4

Patient: Lakshmi Prasad

VALLEY ASSOCIATES, PC
1400 West Center Street
Toledo, OH 43601-0123
555-321-0987

PATIENT INFORMATION FORM

THIS SECTION REFERS TO PATIENT ONLY

Name: Lakshmi Prasad	Sex: F	Marital Status: ☐S ☑M ☐D ☐W	Birth Date: 8/2/45
Address: 38 Mountain Ave.	SS#: 351-42-6798		
City: Alliance State: OH Zip: 44601	Employer: Towne Restaurant (part-time)	Phone:	
Home Phone: 555-492-3601	Employer's Address:		
Work Phone:	City:	State:	Zip:
Spouse's Name:	Spouse's Employer:		
Emergency Contact:	Relationship:	Phone #:	

FILL IN IF PATIENT IS A MINOR

Parent/Guardian's Name:	Sex:	Marital Status: ☐S ☐M ☐D ☐W	Birth Date:
Phone:	SS#:		
Address:	Employer:	Phone:	
City: State: Zip:	Employer's Address:		
Student Status:	City:	State:	Zip:

INSURANCE INFORMATION

Primary Insurance Company: Medicare Nationwide	Secondary Insurance Company:
Subscriber's Name: Lakshmi Prasad Birth Date: 8/2/45	Subscriber's Name: Birth Date:
Plan: SS#: 351-42-6798	Plan:
Policy #: 351426798A Group #:	Policy #: Group #:
Copayment/Deductible: $100 deductible, paid Price Code: B	

OTHER INFORMATION

Reason for visit: routine examination	Allergy to Medication (list):
Name of referring physician:	If auto accident, list date and state in which it occurred:

I authorize treatment and agree to pay all fees and charges for the person named above. I agree to pay all charges shown by statements, promptly upon their presentation, unless credit arrangements are agreed upon in writing.

I authorize payment directly to VALLEY ASSOCIATES, PC of insurance benefits otherwise payable to me. I hereby authorize the release of any medical information necessary in order to process a claim for payment in my behalf.

Lakshmi Prasad — 1-1-08

(Patient's Signature/Parent or Guardian's Signature) (Date)

I plan to make payment of my medical expenses as follows (check one or more):

____ Insurance (as above) ____ Cash/Check/Credit/Debit Card __✓__ Medicare ____ Medicaid ____ Workers' Comp.

VALLEY ASSOCIATES, PC

Christopher M. Connolly, MD - Internal Medicine
555-967-0303
FED I.D. #16-1234567

PATIENT NAME	APPT. DATE/TIME
Prasad, Lakshmi	10/9/2008 11:00 am
PATIENT NO.	**DX**
PRASALA0	1. v70.0 routine medical exam 2. 3. 4.

DESCRIPTION	✓	CPT	FEE	DESCRIPTION	✓	CPT	FEE
OFFICE VISITS				**PROCEDURES**			
New Patient				Diagnostic Anoscopy		46600	
LI Problem Focused		99201		ECG Complete		93000	
LII Expanded		99202		I&D, Abscess		10060	
LIII Detailed		99203		Pap Smear	✓	88150	29
LIV Comp./Mod.		99204		Removal of Cerumen		69210	
LV Comp./High		99205		Removal 1 Lesion		17000	
Established Patient				Removal 2-14 Lesions		17003	
LI Minimum		99211		Removal 15+ Lesions		17004	
LII Problem Focused		99212		Rhythm ECG w/Report		93040	
LIII Expanded		99213		Rhythm ECG w/Tracing		93041	
LIV Detailed		99214		Sigmoidoscopy, diag.		45330	
LV Comp./High		99215					
				LABORATORY			
PREVENTIVE VISIT				Bacteria Culture		87081	
New Patient				Fungal Culture		87101	
Age 12-17		99384		Glucose Finger Stick		82948	
Age 18-39		99385		Lipid Panel		80061	
Age 40-64		99386		Specimen Handling		99000	
Age 65+		99387		Stool/Occult Blood		82270	
Established Patient				Tine Test		85008	
Age 12-17		99394		Tuberculin PPD		85590	
Age 18-39		99395		Urinalysis		81000	
Age 40-64		99396		Venipuncture		36415	
Age 65+	✓	99397	118				
				INJECTION/IMMUN.			
CONSULTATION: OFFICE/OP				Immun. Admin.		90471	
Requested By:				Ea. Add'l.		90472	
LI Problem Focused		99241		Hepatitis A Immun		90632	
LII Expanded		99242		Hepatitis B Immun		90746	
LIII Detailed		99243		Influenza Immun	✓	90659	68
LIV Comp./Mod.		99244		Pneumovax		90732	
LV Comp./High		99245					
				TOTAL FEES			

Claim Case Study 17.5

Patient: Joseph Zylerberg

VALLEY ASSOCIATES, PC
1400 West Center Street
Toledo, OH 43601-0123
555-321-0987

PATIENT INFORMATION FORM

THIS SECTION REFERS TO PATIENT ONLY					
Name: Joseph Zylerberg			Sex: M	Marital Status: ☑S ☐M ☐D ☐W	Birth Date: 3/14/35
Address: 18 Alpine Dr.			SS#: 201-36-4413		
City: Alliance	State: OH	Zip: 44601	Employer: Retired		Phone:
Home Phone: 555-692-3417			Employer's Address:		
Work Phone:			City:	State:	Zip:
Spouse's Name:			Spouse's Employer:		
Emergency Contact:			Relationship:		Phone #:
FILL IN IF PATIENT IS A MINOR					
Parent/Guardian's Name:			Sex:	Marital Status: ☐S ☐M ☐D ☐W	Birth Date:
Phone:			SS#:		
Address:			Employer:		Phone:
City:	State:	Zip:	Employer's Address:		
Student Status:			City:	State:	Zip:
INSURANCE INFORMATION					
Primary Insurance Company: Medicare Nationwide			Secondary Insurance Company: Medicaid		
Subscriber's Name: Joseph Zylerberg		Birth Date: 3/14/35	Subscriber's Name: Joseph Zylerberg		Birth Date: 3/14/35
Plan:	SS#: 201-36-4413		Plan:		
Policy #: 201364413A	Group #:		Policy #: 201364413C	Group #:	
Copayment/Deductible: $100 deductible, paid	Price Code: B				
OTHER INFORMATION					
Reason for visit: angina			Allergy to Medication (list):		
Name of referring physician:			If auto accident, list date and state in which it occurred:		

I authorize treatment and agree to pay all fees and charges for the person named above. I agree to pay all charges shown by statements, promptly upon their presentation, unless credit arrangements are agreed upon in writing.

I authorize payment directly to VALLEY ASSOCIATES, PC of insurance benefits otherwise payable to me. I hereby authorize the release of any medical information necessary in order to process a claim for payment in my behalf.

Joseph Zylerberg (Patient's Signature/Parent or Guardian's Signature) — 10/9/08 (Date)

I plan to make payment of my medical expenses as follows (check one or more):

____ Insurance (as above) ____ Cash/Check/Credit/Debit Card ✓ Medicare ✓ Medicaid ____ Workers' Comp.

VALLEY ASSOCIATES, PC

Christopher M. Connolly, MD - Internal Medicine
555-967-0303
FED I.D. #16-1234567

PATIENT NAME	APPT. DATE/TIME
Zylerberg, Joseph	10/9/2008 4:30 pm
PATIENT NO.	**DX**
ZYLERJO0	1. 413.9 angina pectoris 2. 414.01 atherosclerotic heart disease 3. 4.

DESCRIPTION	✓	CPT	FEE	DESCRIPTION	✓	CPT	FEE
OFFICE VISITS				**PROCEDURES**			
New Patient				Diagnostic Anoscopy		46600	
LI Problem Focused		99201		ECG Complete	✓	93000	29
LII Expanded		99202		I&D, Abscess		10060	
LIII Detailed		99203		Pap Smear		88150	
LIV Comp./Mod.	✓	99204	103	Removal of Cerumen		69210	
LV Comp./High		99205		Removal 1 Lesion		17000	
Established Patient				Removal 2-14 Lesions		17003	
LI Minimum		99211		Removal 15+ Lesions		17004	
LII Problem Focused		99212		Rhythm ECG w/Report		93040	
LIII Expanded		99213		Rhythm ECG w/Tracing		93041	
LIV Detailed		99214		Sigmoidoscopy, diag.		45330	
LV Comp./High		99215					
				LABORATORY			
PREVENTIVE VISIT				Bacteria Culture		87081	
New Patient				Fungal Culture		87101	
Age 12-17		99384		Glucose Finger Stick		82948	
Age 18-39		99385		Lipid Panel		80061	
Age 40-64		99386		Specimen Handling		99000	
Age 65+		99387		Stool/Occult Blood		82270	
Established Patient				Tine Test		85008	
Age 12-17		99394		Tuberculin PPD		85590	
Age 18-39		99395		Urinalysis		81000	
Age 40-64		99396		Venipuncture		36415	
Age 65+		99397					
				INJECTION/IMMUN.			
CONSULTATION: OFFICE/OP				Immun. Admin.		90471	
Requested By:				Ea. Add'l.		90472	
LI Problem Focused		99241		Hepatitis A Immun		90632	
LII Expanded		99242		Hepatitis B Immun		90746	
LIII Detailed		99243		Influenza Immun		90659	
LIV Comp./Mod.		99244		Pneumovax		90732	
LV Comp./High		99245					
				TOTAL FEES			

Claim Case Study 17.6

Patient: Shih-Chi Yang

VALLEY ASSOCIATES, PC
1400 West Center Street
Toledo, OH 43601-0123
555-321-0987

PATIENT INFORMATION FORM

THIS SECTION REFERS TO PATIENT ONLY			
Name: Shih-Chi Yang	Sex: M	Marital Status: ☐S ☑M ☐D ☐W	Birth Date: 12/3/69
Address: 6 Sparrow Road	SS#: 334-72-9081		
City: Brooklyn State: OH Zip: 44144	Employer: J & M Manufacturing (full-time) Phone:		
Home Phone: 555-602-7779	Employer's Address:		
Work Phone:	City: State: Zip:		
Spouse's Name:	Spouse's Employer:		
Emergency Contact:	Relationship: Phone #:		

FILL IN IF PATIENT IS A MINOR			
Parent/Guardian's Name:	Sex:	Marital Status: ☐S ☐M ☐D ☐W	Birth Date:
Phone:	SS#:		
Address:	Employer: Phone:		
City: State: Zip:	Employer's Address:		
Student Status:	City: State: Zip:		

INSURANCE INFORMATION	
Primary Insurance Company: CarePlus Workers' Compensation	Secondary Insurance Company:
Subscriber's Name: Shih-Chi Yang Birth Date: 12/3/69	Subscriber's Name: Birth Date:
Plan: SS#: 334-72-9081	Plan:
Policy #: 1045891-22 Group #: OH3967	Policy #: Group #:
Copayment/Deductible: Price Code: A	

OTHER INFORMATION	
Reason for visit: hand fracture	Allergy to Medication (list):
Name of referring physician:	If auto accident, list date and state in which it occurred:

I authorize treatment and agree to pay all fees and charges for the person named above. I agree to pay all charges shown by statements, promptly upon their presentation, unless credit arrangements are agreed upon in writing.
I authorize payment directly to VALLEY ASSOCIATES, PC of insurance benefits otherwise payable to me. I hereby authorize the release of any medical information necessary in order to process a claim for payment in my behalf.

(Patient's Signature/Parent or Guardian's Signature) (Date)

I plan to make payment of my medical expenses as follows (check one or more):

____Insurance (as above) ____Cash/Check/Credit/Debit Card ____Medicare ____Medicaid _✓_Workers' Comp.

Workers' Compensation Notes

Condition Related to Employment?	Yes
Date of Current Illness, Injury, LMP	11/12/2008
First Consultation Date	11/12/2008
Dates Patient Unable to Work	11/12/2008 –

VALLEY ASSOCIATES, PC

Sarah Jamison, MD - Orthopedic Medicine
555-321-0987
FED I.D. #07-2345678

PATIENT NAME	APPT. DATE/TIME
Yang, Shih-Chi	11/12/2008 9:30 am
PATIENT NO.	**DX**
YANGSHIØ	1. 817.1 multiple open fractures of handbones 2. 3. 4.

DESCRIPTION	✓	CPT	FEE	DESCRIPTION	✓	CPT	FEE
OFFICE VISITS				**FRACTURES**			
New Patient				Clavicle		23500	
LI Problem Focused		99201		Scapula		23570	
LII Expanded		99202		Humerus, proximal		23600	
LIII Detailed		99203		Humerus, shaft		24500	
LIV Comp./Mod.		99204		Radial, colles w/manip		25605	
LV Comp./High		99205		Radial, h or n w/out manip		24650	
Established Patient				Ulna, proximal		24670	
LI Minimum		99211		Radius & Ulna		25560	
LII Problem Focused		99212		Radius, colles, distal		25600	
LIII Expanded		99213		Ulna, styloid		25650	
LIV Detailed		99214		Hand MC	✓	26600	315
LV Comp./High		99215		Finger/Thumb		26720	
				Coccyx		27200	
CONSULTATION: OFFICE/OP				Femur, distal		27508	
Requested By:				Tibia prox/plateua		27530	
LI Problem Focused		99241		Tibia & Fibula, shaft		27750	
LII Expanded		99242		Fibula, prox/shaft		27780	
LIII Detailed		99243		Foot, MT		28470	
LIV Comp./Mod.		99244		Toe, great		28490	
LV Comp./High		99245		Toe, others		28510	
				X-RAY			
EMG STUDIES				Clavicle		73000	
EMG - 1 extremity		95860		Humerus		73060	
EMG - 2 extremities		95861		Forearm		73090	
EMG - 3 extremities		95863		Hand, 2 views		73120	
Nerve Conduct, M w/out F		95900		Hand, 3 views	✓	73130	91
Nerve Conduct, M w/ F		95903		Fingers		73140	
Nerve Conduct, sensory		95904		Femur		73550	
				Tibia & Fibula		73590	
				Foot, 2 views		73620	
				Foot, 3 views		73630	
				Toes		73660	
				TOTAL FEES			

Claim Case Study 17.7

Patient: Andrea Spinelli

VALLEY ASSOCIATES, PC
1400 West Center Street
Toledo, OH 43601-0123
555-321-0987

PATIENT INFORMATION FORM

THIS SECTION REFERS TO PATIENT ONLY

Name: Andrea Spinelli	Sex: F	Marital Status: ☑S ☐M ☐D ☐W	Birth Date: 1/1/41
Address: 23 N. Brook Ave.	SS#: 701-69-4342		
City: Sandusky State: OH Zip: 44870	Employer: Retired		Phone:
Home Phone: 555-402-0396	Employer's Address:		
Work Phone:	City: State: Zip:		
Spouse's Name:	Spouse's Employer:		
Emergency Contact:	Relationship:		Phone #:

FILL IN IF PATIENT IS A MINOR

Parent/Guardian's Name:	Sex:	Marital Status: ☐S ☐M ☐D ☐W	Birth Date:
Phone:	SS#:		
Address:	Employer:		Phone:
City: State: Zip:	Employer's Address:		
Student Status:	City: State: Zip:		

INSURANCE INFORMATION

Primary Insurance Company: Medicare HMO	Secondary Insurance Company:
Subscriber's Name: Andrea Spinelli Birth Date: 1/1/41	Subscriber's Name: Birth Date:
Plan: SS#: 701-69-4342	Plan:
Policy #: 701694342A Group #:	Policy #: Group #:
Copayment/Deductible: $10 copay Price Code: B	

OTHER INFORMATION

Reason for visit: cerumen in ear	Allergy to Medication (list):
Name of referring physician:	If auto accident, list date and state in which it occurred:

I authorize treatment and agree to pay all fees and charges for the person named above. I agree to pay all charges shown by statements, promptly upon their presentation, unless credit arrangements are agreed upon in writing.
I authorize payment directly to VALLEY ASSOCIATES, PC of insurance benefits otherwise payable to me. I hereby authorize the release of any medical information necessary in order to process a claim for payment in my behalf.

Andrea Spinelli 1/1/08

(Patient's Signature/Parent or Guardian's Signature) (Date)

I plan to make payment of my medical expenses as follows (check one or more):

____ Insurance (as above) ____ Cash/Check/Credit/Debit Card __✓__ Medicare ____ Medicaid ____ Workers' Comp.

VALLEY ASSOCIATES, PC
Christopher M. Connolly, MD - Internal Medicine
555-967-0303
FED I.D. #16-1234567

PATIENT NAME	APPT. DATE/TIME
Spinelli, Andrea	10/9/2008 1:30 pm
PATIENT NO.	**DX**
SPINEANØ	1. 394.0 cerumen in ear 2. 3. 4.

DESCRIPTION	✓	CPT	FEE	DESCRIPTION	✓	CPT	FEE
OFFICE VISITS				**PROCEDURES**			
New Patient				Diagnostic Anoscopy		46600	
LI Problem Focused		99201		ECG Complete		93000	
LII Expanded		99202		I&D, Abscess		10060	
LIII Detailed		99203		Pap Smear		88150	
LIV Comp./Mod.		99204		Removal of Cerumen	✓	69210	34
LV Comp./High		99205		Removal 1 Lesion		17000	
Established Patient				Removal 2-14 Lesions		17003	
LI Minimum		99211		Removal 15+ Lesions		17004	
LII Problem Focused		99212		Rhythm ECG w/Report		93040	
LIII Expanded		99213		Rhythm ECG w/Tracing		93041	
LIV Detailed		99214		Sigmoidoscopy, diag.		45330	
LV Comp./High		99215					
				LABORATORY			
PREVENTIVE VISIT				Bacteria Culture		87081	
New Patient				Fungal Culture		87101	
Age 12-17		99384		Glucose Finger Stick		82948	
Age 18-39		99385		Lipid Panel		80061	
Age 40-64		99386		Specimen Handling		99000	
Age 65+		99387		Stool/Occult Blood		82270	
Established Patient				Tine Test		85008	
Age 12-17		99394		Tuberculin PPD		85590	
Age 18-39		99395		Urinalysis		81000	
Age 40-64		99396		Venipuncture		36415	
Age 65+		99397					
				INJECTION/IMMUN.			
CONSULTATION: OFFICE/OP				Immun. Admin.		90471	
Requested By:				Ea. Add'l.		90472	
LI Problem Focused		99241		Hepatitis A Immun		90632	
LII Expanded		99242		Hepatitis B Immun		90746	
LIII Detailed		99243		Influenza Immun		90659	
LIV Comp./Mod.		99244		Pneumovax		90732	
LV Comp./High		99245					
				TOTAL FEES			

Claim Case Study 17.8

Patient: Nancy Lankhaar

VALLEY ASSOCIATES, PC
1400 West Center Street
Toledo, OH 43601-0123
555-321-0987

PATIENT INFORMATION FORM

THIS SECTION REFERS TO PATIENT ONLY

Name: Nancy Lankhaar	Sex: F — Marital Status: ☑S ☐M ☐D ☐W — Birth Date: 8/12/35
Address: 44 Crescent Rd.	SS#: 109-36-5528
City: Cleveland State: OH Zip: 44101	Employer: Retired Phone:
Home Phone: 555-787-3424	Employer's Address:
Work Phone:	City: State: Zip:
Spouse's Name:	Spouse's Employer:
Emergency Contact:	Relationship: Phone #:

FILL IN IF PATIENT IS A MINOR

Parent/Guardian's Name:	Sex: — Marital Status: ☐S ☐M ☐D ☐W — Birth Date:
Phone:	SS#:
Address:	Employer: Phone:
City: State: Zip:	Employer's Address:
Student Status:	City: State: Zip:

INSURANCE INFORMATION

Primary Insurance Company: Medicare Nationwide	Secondary Insurance Company: AARP Medigap
Subscriber's Name: Nancy Lankhaar Birth Date: 8/12/35	Subscriber's Name: Nancy Lankhaar Birth Date: 8/12/35
Plan: SS#: 109-36-5528	Plan:
Policy #: 109365528A Group #:	Policy #: 109365528B Group #:
Copayment/Deductible: $100 deductible, paid Price Code: B	

OTHER INFORMATION

Reason for visit: rash	Allergy to Medication (list):
Name of referring physician:	If auto accident, list date and state in which it occurred:

I authorize treatment and agree to pay all fees and charges for the person named above. I agree to pay all charges shown by statements, promptly upon their presentation, unless credit arrangements are agreed upon in writing.

I authorize payment directly to VALLEY ASSOCIATES, PC of insurance benefits otherwise payable to me. I hereby authorize the release of any medical information necessary in order to process a claim for payment in my behalf.

Nancy Lankhaar — 1-1-08

(Patient's Signature/Parent or Guardian's Signature) (Date)

I plan to make payment of my medical expenses as follows (check one or more):

✓ Insurance (as above) ____ Cash/Check/Credit/Debit Card ✓ Medicare ____ Medicaid ____ Workers' Comp.

VALLEY ASSOCIATES, PC
Christopher M. Connolly, MD - Internal Medicine
555-967-0303
FED I.D. #16-1234567

PATIENT NAME	APPT. DATE/TIME
Lankhaar, Nancy	10/7/2008 11:00 am
PATIENT NO.	**DX**
LANKHNA0	1. 782.1 rash on leg 2. 3. 4.

DESCRIPTION	✓	CPT	FEE	DESCRIPTION	✓	CPT	FEE
OFFICE VISITS				**PROCEDURES**			
New Patient				Diagnostic Anoscopy		46600	
LI Problem Focused		99201		ECG Complete		93000	
LII Expanded		99202		I&D, Abscess		10060	
LIII Detailed		99203		Pap Smear		88150	
LIV Comp./Mod.		99204		Removal of Cerumen		69210	
LV Comp./High		99205		Removal 1 Lesion		17000	
Established Patient				Removal 2-14 Lesions		17003	
LI Minimum		99211		Removal 15+ Lesions		17004	
LII Problem Focused	✓	99212	28	Rhythm ECG w/Report		93040	
LIII Expanded		99213		Rhythm ECG w/Tracing		93041	
LIV Detailed		99214		Sigmoidoscopy, diag.		45330	
LV Comp./High		99215					
				LABORATORY			
PREVENTIVE VISIT				Bacteria Culture		87081	
New Patient				Fungal Culture		87101	
Age 12-17		99384		Glucose Finger Stick		82948	
Age 18-39		99385		Lipid Panel		80061	
Age 40-64		99386		Specimen Handling		99000	
Age 65+		99387		Stool/Occult Blood		82270	
Established Patient				Tine Test		85008	
Age 12-17		99394		Tuberculin PPD		85590	
Age 18-39		99395		Urinalysis		81000	
Age 40-64		99396		Venipuncture		36415	
Age 65+		99397					
				INJECTION/IMMUN.			
CONSULTATION: OFFICE/OP				Immun. Admin.		90471	
Requested By:				Ea. Add'l.		90472	
LI Problem Focused		99241		Hepatitis A Immun		90632	
LII Expanded		99242		Hepatitis B Immun		90746	
LIII Detailed		99243		Influenza Immun		90659	
LIV Comp./Mod.		99244		Pneumovax		90732	
LV Comp./High		99245					
				TOTAL FEES			

Claim Case Study 17.9

Patient: Donald Aiken

VALLEY ASSOCIATES, PC
1400 West Center Street
Toledo, OH 43601-0123
555-321-0987

PATIENT INFORMATION FORM

THIS SECTION REFERS TO PATIENT ONLY

Name: Donald Aiken	Sex: M	Marital Status: ☑S ☐M ☐D ☐W	Birth Date: 4/30/35
Address: 24 Beacon Crest Dr.	SS#: 138-02-1649		
City: Sandusky State: OH Zip: 44870	Employer: Retired		Phone:
Home Phone: 555-602-9947	Employer's Address:		
Work Phone:	City:	State:	Zip:
Spouse's Name:	Spouse's Employer:		
Emergency Contact:	Relationship:		Phone #:

FILL IN IF PATIENT IS A MINOR

Parent/Guardian's Name:	Sex:	Marital Status: ☐S ☐M ☐D ☐W	Birth Date:
Phone:	SS#:		
Address:	Employer:		Phone:
City: State: Zip:	Employer's Address:		
Student Status:	City:	State:	Zip:

INSURANCE INFORMATION

Primary Insurance Company: Medicare Nationwide		Secondary Insurance Company: AARP Medigap	
Subscriber's Name: Donald Aiken	Birth Date: 4/30/35	Subscriber's Name: Donald Aiken	Birth Date: 4/30/35
Plan:	SS#: 138-02-1649	Plan:	
Policy #: 138021649A	Group #:	Policy #: 138021649B	Group #:
Copayment/Deductible: $100 deductible, paid	Price Code: B		

OTHER INFORMATION

Reason for visit: anemia	Allergy to Medication (list):
Name of referring physician:	If auto accident, list date and state in which it occurred:

I authorize treatment and agree to pay all fees and charges for the person named above. I agree to pay all charges shown by statements, promptly upon their presentation, unless credit arrangements are agreed upon in writing.

I authorize payment directly to VALLEY ASSOCIATES, PC of insurance benefits otherwise payable to me. I hereby authorize the release of any medical information necessary in order to process a claim for payment in my behalf.

Donald Aiken — (Patient's Signature/Parent or Guardian's Signature)   10/10/08 — (Date)

I plan to make payment of my medical expenses as follows (check one or more):

✓ Insurance (as above)   ___ Cash/Check/Credit/Debit Card   ✓ Medicare   ___ Medicaid   ___ Workers' Comp.

VALLEY ASSOCIATES, PC

Christopher M. Connolly, MD - Internal Medicine
555-967-0303
FED I.D. #16-1234567

PATIENT NAME	APPT. DATE/TIME
Aiken, Donald	10/10/2008 10:30 am
PATIENT NO.	**DX**
AIKENDO0	1. 281.0 pernicious anemia 2. 782.4 jaundice 3. 4.

DESCRIPTION	✓	CPT	FEE	DESCRIPTION	✓	CPT	FEE
OFFICE VISITS				**PROCEDURES**			
New Patient				Diagnostic Anoscopy		46600	
LI Problem Focused		99201		ECG Complete		93000	
LII Expanded		99202		I&D, Abscess		10060	
LIII Detailed	✓	99203	69	Pap Smear		88150	
LIV Comp./Mod.		99204		Removal of Cerumen		69210	
LV Comp./High		99205		Removal 1 Lesion		17000	
Established Patient				Removal 2-14 Lesions		17003	
LI Minimum		99211		Removal 15+ Lesions		17004	
LII Problem Focused		99212		Rhythm ECG w/Report		93040	
LIII Expanded		99213		Rhythm ECG w/Tracing		93041	
LIV Detailed		99214		Sigmoidoscopy, diag.		45330	
LV Comp./High		99215					
				LABORATORY			
PREVENTIVE VISIT				Bacteria Culture		87081	
New Patient				Fungal Culture		87101	
Age 12-17		99384		Glucose Finger Stick		82948	
Age 18-39		99385		Lipid Panel		80061	
Age 40-64		99386		Specimen Handling		99000	
Age 65+		99387		Stool/Occult Blood		82270	
Established Patient				Tine Test		85008	
Age 12-17		99394		Tuberculin PPD		85590	
Age 18-39		99395		Urinalysis		81000	
Age 40-64		99396		Venipuncture	✓	36415	17
Age 65+		99397					
				INJECTION/IMMUN.			
CONSULTATION: OFFICE/OP				Immun. Admin.		90471	
Requested By:				Ea. Add'l.		90472	
LI Problem Focused		99241		Hepatitis A Immun		90632	
LII Expanded		99242		Hepatitis B Immun		90746	
LIII Detailed		99243		Influenza Immun		90659	
LIV Comp./Mod.		99244		Pneumovax		90732	
LV Comp./High		99245					
				TOTAL FEES			

Claim Case Study 17.10

Patient: Eric Huang

VALLEY ASSOCIATES, PC
1400 West Center Street
Toledo, OH 43601-0123
555-321-0987

PATIENT INFORMATION FORM

THIS SECTION REFERS TO PATIENT ONLY

Name: Eric Huang	Sex: M — Marital Status: ☐S ☑M ☐D ☐W — Birth Date: 3/13/40
Address: 1109 Bauer St.	SS#: 302-46-1884
City: Shaker Heights State: OH Zip: 44118	Employer: Retired Phone:
Home Phone: 555-639-1787	Employer's Address:
Work Phone:	City: State: Zip:
Spouse's Name:	Spouse's Employer:
Emergency Contact:	Relationship: Phone #:

FILL IN IF PATIENT IS A MINOR

Parent/Guardian's Name:	Sex: — Marital Status: ☐S ☐M ☐D ☐W — Birth Date:
Phone:	SS#:
Address:	Employer: Phone:
City: State: Zip:	Employer's Address:
Student Status:	City: State: Zip:

INSURANCE INFORMATION

Primary Insurance Company: Medicare Nationwide	Secondary Insurance Company:
Subscriber's Name: Eric Huang Birth Date: 3/13/40	Subscriber's Name: Birth Date:
Plan: SS#: 302-46-1884	Plan:
Policy #: 302-46-1884A Group #:	Policy #: Group #:
Copayment/Deductible: $100 deductible, not met Price Code: B	

OTHER INFORMATION

Reason for visit: weight loss	Allergy to Medication (list):
Name of referring physician:	If auto accident, list date and state in which it occurred:

I authorize treatment and agree to pay all fees and charges for the person named above. I agree to pay all charges shown by statements, promptly upon their presentation, unless credit arrangements are agreed upon in writing.

I authorize payment directly to VALLEY ASSOCIATES, PC of insurance benefits otherwise payable to me. I hereby authorize the release of any medical information necessary in order to process a claim for payment in my behalf.

Eric Huang — 1-1-08

(Patient's Signature/Parent or Guardian's Signature) (Date)

I plan to make payment of my medical expenses as follows (check one or more):

____ Insurance (as above) ____ Cash/Check/Credit/Debit Card _✓_ Medicare ____ Medicaid ____ Workers' Comp.

VALLEY ASSOCIATES, PC

Christopher M. Connolly, MD - Internal Medicine
555-967-0303
FED I.D. #16-1234567

PATIENT NAME	APPT. DATE/TIME
Huang, Eric	10/9/2008 9:00 am
PATIENT NO.	**DX**
HUANGERØ	1. 782.4 jaundice 2. 3. 4.

DESCRIPTION	✓	CPT	FEE	DESCRIPTION	✓	CPT	FEE
OFFICE VISITS				**PROCEDURES**			
New Patient				Diagnostic Anoscopy		46600	
LI Problem Focused		99201		ECG Complete		93000	
LII Expanded		99202		I&D, Abscess		10060	
LIII Detailed		99203		Pap Smear		88150	
LIV Comp./Mod.		99204		Removal of Cerumen		69210	
LV Comp./High		99205		Removal 1 Lesion		17000	
Established Patient				Removal 2-14 Lesions		17003	
LI Minimum		99211		Removal 15+ Lesions		17004	
LII Problem Focused		99212		Rhythm ECG w/Report		93040	
LIII Expanded		99213		Rhythm ECG w/Tracing		93041	
LIV Detailed		99214		Sigmoidoscopy, diag.		45330	
LV Comp./High		99215					
				LABORATORY			
PREVENTIVE VISIT				Bacteria Culture		87081	
New Patient				Fungal Culture		87101	
Age 12-17		99384		Glucose Finger Stick		82948	
Age 18-39		99385		Lipid Panel		80061	
Age 40-64		99386		Specimen Handling		99000	
Age 65+		99387		Stool/Occult Blood		82270	
Established Patient				Tine Test		85008	
Age 12-17		99394		Tuberculin PPD		85590	
Age 18-39		99395		Urinalysis		81000	
Age 40-64		99396		Venipuncture		36415	
Age 65+		99397					
				INJECTION/IMMUN.			
CONSULTATION: OFFICE/OP				Immun. Admin.		90471	
Requested By:				Ea. Add'l.		90472	
LI Problem Focused		99241		Hepatitis A Immun		90632	
LII Expanded		99242		Hepatitis B Immun		90746	
LIII Detailed	✓	99243	97	Influenza Immun		90659	
LIV Comp./Mod.		99244		Pneumovax		90732	
LV Comp./High		99245					
				TOTAL FEES			

Claim Case Study 17.11

Patient: Isabella Neufeld

From the Patient Information Form

Name	Isabella Neufeld
Sex	F
Birth Date	01/29/1980
Marital Status	Single
SSN	410-39-0648
Address	39 Brandywine Dr. Alliance, OH 44601
Telephone	555-239-7154
Employer	Not employed
Insured	Self
Health Plan	Medicaid
Insurance ID Number	410390648MC
Copayment/Deductible Amt.	$15 copay
Assignment of Benefits	Y
Signature on File	10/01/2008
Condition unrelated to Employment, Auto Accident, or Other Accident	
Physician	David Rosenberg, M.D.

Encounter Date: 10/01/2008

Diagnoses

The patient presents with urticaria following prolonged exposure to recent cold weather conditions.

Procedures

Saw this new patient in the office. Performed a problem-focused history and exam, with straightforward decision making.

Claim Case Study 17.12

Patient: Alan Harcar

From the Patient Information Form

Name	Alan Harcar
Sex	M
Birth Date	12/19/1942
Marital Status	Divorced
SSN	321-60-5549
Address	344 Wilson Ave. Brooklyn, OH 44144
Telephone	555-666-9283
Employer	Retired
Insured	Self
Health Plan	Medicare Nationwide
Insurance ID Number	321605549A
Copayment/Deductible Amt.	$100 deductible; not met
Assignment of Benefits	Y
Signature on File	10/01/2008

Condition unrelated to Employment, Auto Accident, or Other Accident

Physician	David Rosenberg, M.D.

Encounter Date: 10/01/2008

Diagnoses

The patient presents with an upper respiratory infection.

Procedures

Saw this new patient in the office. Performed an expanded problem-focused history and exam, with low-complexity decision making.

Claim Case Study 17.13

Patient: Jose Velaquez

From the Patient Information Form

Name	Jose Velaquez
Sex	M
Birth Date	06/21/1984
Marital Status	Single
SSN	514-62-7935
Address	63 Castle Ridge Dr.
	Shaker Heights, OH 44118
Telephone	555-624-7739
Employer	State Street Financial
Insured	Self
Health Plan	Anthem BCBS PPO
Insurance ID Number	YHU514627935
Group Number	G36479
Copayment/Deductible Amt.	$20 copay
Assignment of Benefits	Y
Signature on File	10/06/2008
Condition unrelated to Employment, Auto Accident, or Other Accident	
Physician	Christopher Connolly, M.D.

Encounter Date: 10/06/2008

Diagnoses

Following an office visit with further workup, the patient's diagnosis is mitral valve stenosis due to rheumatic heart disease.

Procedures

Saw this new patient in the office. Performed a comprehensive history and exam, with moderate-complexity decision making. Also completed a rhythm ECG with a report.

Claim Case Study 17.14

Patient: Wilma Estephan

From the Patient Information Form

Name	Wilma Estephan
Sex	F
Birth Date	03/14/1940
Marital Status	Widowed
SSN	140-32-4102
Address	109 River Rd. Cleveland, OH 44101
Telephone	555-683-5272
Employer	Retired
Insured	Self
Primary Health Plan	Medicare Nationwide
Insurance ID Number	140324102A
Copayment/Deductible Amt.	$100 deductible; not met
Secondary Health Plan	AARP Medigap
Insurance ID Number	099655820
Assignment of Benefits	Y
Signature on File	1/1/2008
Condition unrelated to Employment, Auto Accident, or Other Accident	
Physician	Christopher Connolly, M.D.

Encounter Date: 10/06/2008

Diagnoses

The patient presents for a checkup on her benign hypertension.

Procedures

Saw this established patient in the office for a second checkup on her blood pressure after a six-month prescription of an ACE inhibitor. The presenting problem was minimal.

Claim Case Study 17.15

Patient: John O'Rourke

From the Patient Information Form

Name	John O'Rourke
Sex	M
Birth Date	07/01/1985
Marital Status	Single
SSN	401-36-0228
Address	3641 Mountain Ave. Toledo, OH 43601
Telephone	555-649-3349
Employer	The Kaufman Group
Insured	Self
Health Plan	Anthem BCBS PPO
Insurance ID Number	GH401360228
Group Number	OH4071
Copayment/Deductible Amt.	$20 copay
Assignment of Benefits	Y
Signature on File	10/07/2008
Condition unrelated to Employment, Auto Accident, or Other Accident	
Physician	Christopher Connolly, M.D.

Encounter Date: 10/07/2008

Diagnoses

The patient presents with angina upon exertion; coronary atherosclerosis is diagnosed.

Procedures

Saw this new patient in the office; referred the patient for a treadmill test. Performed a comprehensive history and exam, with moderately complex decision making.

Claim Case Study 17.16

Patient: Sylvia Evans

From the Patient Information Form

Name	Sylvia Evans
Sex	F
Birth Date	06/10/1929
Marital Status	Married
SSN	140-39-6602
Address	13 Ascot Way
	Sandusky, OH 44870
Telephone	555-229-3614
Employer	Retired
Insured	Self
Health Plan	TRICARE
Insurance ID Number	140396602
Copayment/Deductible Amt.	$10 copay
Assignment of Benefits	Y
Signature on File	06/01/2008
Condition unrelated to Employment, Auto Accident, or Other Accident	
Physician	Nancy Ronkowski, M.D.

Encounter Date: 10/17/2008

Diagnoses

The patient presents with postmenopausal bleeding due to estrogen deficiency.

Procedures

Saw this established patient in the office for a follow-up visit on her postmenopausal bleeding. Performed a problem-focused history and exam, with straightforward decision making.

Medisoft Tip

Note that Sylvia Evans already has a set of transactions in the database for her visit on 10/13/2008. Enter the new transactions (for 10/17/2008) in the Transaction Entry dialog box under the previous transactions. When applying the $10 copayment for the second visit, make sure to apply it to the procedure code with the 10/17/2008 date.

Claim Case Study 17.17

Patient: Karen Giroux

From the Patient Information Form

Name	Karen Giroux
Sex	F
Birth Date	03/15/1955
Marital Status	Married
SSN	530-39-2903
Address	14A West Front St.
	Brooklyn, OH 44144
Telephone	555-683-5364
Employer	First USA Trust Company
Insured	Self
Primary Health Plan	Anthem BCBS Traditional
Insurance ID Number	YHA530392903
Group Number	G30017
Copayment/Deductible Amt.	$250 deductible; not met
Secondary Health Plan	Medicare Nationwide
Secondary Insured's Name	Jack Giroux
Birth Date	1/02/1944
Insurance ID Number	222306590A
Assignment of Benefits	Y
Signature on File	10/07/2008
Condition unrelated to Employment, Auto Accident, or Other Accident	
Physician	Nancy Ronkowski, M.D.

Encounter Date: 10/07/2008

Diagnoses

The patient presents for a routine annual physical.

Procedures

Saw this new patient in the office for her annual examination.

Claim Case Study 17.18

Patient: Jean Ruff

From the Patient Information Form

Name	Jean Ruff
Sex	F
Birth Date	04/09/1947
Marital Status	Married
SSN	224-36-0478
Address	436 River Rd. Cleveland, OH 44101
Telephone	555-904-1161
Employer	First USA Trust Company
Insured	Self
Primary Health Plan	Anthem BCBS Traditional
Insurance ID Number	YHA224360478
Group Number	G30017
Copayment/Deductible Amt.	$250 deductible; paid
Secondary Health Plan	Aetna Choice
Secondary Insured's Name	Mark Ruff
Birth Date	09/16/1945
Insurance ID Number	349620118A
Group Number	SE1409
Employer	The Allergy Center
Assignment of Benefits	Y
Signature on File	10/06/2008
Condition unrelated to Employment, Auto Accident, or Other Accident	
Physician	Christopher Connolly, M.D.

Encounter Date: 10/06/2008

Diagnoses

The patient complains of a spiking fever and chills for three days.

Procedures

Saw this new patient in the office. Performed an expanded problem-focused history and exam, with low-complexity decision making. Following the finding of a bulls-eye rash on the patient's left shoulder, ordered a Borellia test tomorrow for suspected Lyme disease.

Claim Case Study 17.19

Patient: Mary Anne Kopelman

From the Patient Information Form

Name	Mary Anne Kopelman
Sex	F
Birth Date	08/24/1975
Marital Status	Married
SSN	230-69-0404
Address	POB 10934 Fort Tyrone Alliance, OH 44601
Telephone	555-427-6019
Employer	Not employed
Insured	Arnold Kopelman – husband
Address	Same
Employer	U.S. Army – Fort Tyrone
Primary Health Plan	TRICARE
Insurance ID Number	230569874
Copayment/Deductible Amt.	$10 copay
Assignment of Benefits	Y
Signature on File	10/06/2008
Condition unrelated to Employment, Auto Accident, or Other Accident	
Physician	Nancy Ronkowski, M.D.

Encounter Date: 10/06/2008

Diagnoses

The patient presents with fatigue.

Procedures

Saw this new patient in the office. Detailed history and exam, with low-complexity decision making; urinalysis.

Claim Case Study 17.20

Patient: Otto Kaar

From the Patient Information Form

Name	Otto Kaar
Sex	M
Birth Date	07/01/1985
Marital Status	Single
SSN	310-66-9248
Address	2467 State Hwy 12
	Toledo, OH 43601
Telephone	555-229-3642
Employer	Not employed
Insured	Self
Health Plan	Medicaid
Insurance ID Number	310669248MC
Copayment/Deductible Amt.	$15 copay
Assignment of Benefits	Y
Signature on File	10/07/2008

Condition unrelated to Employment, Auto Accident, or Other Accident

Physician	David Rosenberg, M.D.

Encounter Date: 10/07/2008

Diagnoses

The patient presents with a carbuncle on the left thumb.

Procedures

Saw this new patient in the office; incised and drained this single abscess.

Chapter 18

RA/EOB/Secondary Case Studies

CHAPTER OUTLINE

Method of Claim Completion of Secondary Claims

Handling Denied Claims

Processing Medicare RAs/EOBs and Preparing Secondary Claims

Processing Commerical Payer RAs/EOBs and Preparing Secondary Claims

Calculating Patients' Balances

Learning Outcomes

This chapter provides an opportunity to demonstrate the ability to work with RAs/EOBs and complete correct secondary claims. There are four sections:

1. **Revising denied claims**
2. **Processing Medicare RAs/EOBs and preparing secondary claims**
3. **Processing commercial payer RAs/EOBs and preparing secondary claims**
4. **Calculating patient balances after primary and secondary payments**

Method of Claim Completion of Secondary Claims

To create secondary claims in Medisoft, you must know how to enter and apply insurance carrier payments in Medisoft, which is beyond the scope of topics covered in the Guide to Medisoft for this text. Therefore, to gain experience in completing the secondary claims in this chapter, you will complete paper CMS-1500 forms. A blank claim form is supplied to you (from the back of the book or printed from the Student Data Template CD-ROM). Complete the secondary claims following the instructions in the text chapter that is appropriate for the particular payer. As in Chapter 17, enter patient copayments as required in the Amount Paid box of the CMS-1500 claim form.

Handling Denied Claims

Claim Case Study 18.1

Patients: Wendy Walker and Andrea Spinelli

An RA/EOB is received from the Medicare HMO plan, as shown in Figure 18.1.

Locate the claim for Wendy Walker in the RA/EOB. Notice that the claim has been denied.

1. What reason is given for the rejected claim? What procedure has been billed in the claim?
2. Refer back to the encounter form for Wendy Walker in Claim Case Study 17.1 (page 551). Does the encounter form contain the same procedure code that is listed in the RA/EOB?
3. Refer next to the patient information form for Wendy Walker in the same case. What is the date of her signature on the patient information form? Do you think she is a new or an established patient?
4. On checking your files, you confirm that Wendy's visit on October 6 was her first visit to the practice. What procedure code will you use to correct the claim you created for her on 10/06/08?
5. In addition to the procedure code, what other item on the claim will you need to change? (Hint: You may need to refer to Table 17.1 on page 546.)

Date prepared: 10/20/2008 **Claim number: 00941108**

Patient's name	Dates of service From – thru	POS	Proc	Qty	Charge amount	Eligible amount	Patient liability	Amt paid provider
Kataline, David	10/03/08 - 10/03/08	11	99202	1	$50.00	$50.00	$10.00	$40.00
Kataline, David	10/03/08 - 10/03/08	11	81000	1	$17.00	$17.00	$ 0.00	$17.00
Walker, Wendy	10/06/08 - 10/06/08	11	99214	1	$59.00	*	*	-0-
Diaz, Samual	10/09/08 - 10/09/08	11	99396	1	$106	$106.00	$10.00	$96.00
Spinelli, Andrea	10/09/08 - 10/09/08	11	69210	1	$34.00	**	**	-0-

* **Incorrect procedure code.**
****The diagnosis is inconsistent with the procedure.**

FIGURE 18.1 RA/EOB from Medicare HMO Plan

6. Assume that you have corrected the claim and resubmitted it. How much do you think Medicare will pay her provider for the visit? Note that Wendy has already paid her copayment for the visit, and that her Medicare HMO pays for 100 percent of covered services.

Locate the claim for Andrea Spinelli in the same RA/EOB (Figure 18.1). Notice that her claim has also been denied.

1. What reason is given for the rejected claim? Look up the diagnosis code connected with the claim (Dx 394.0) in a list of ICD codes. What diagnosis does it stand for?
2. Refer back to the patient information form and encounter form for Andrea Spinelli in Claim Case Study 17.7 (pages 562–563). Based on the patient information form, what is the patient's reason for the visit?
3. Refer to the Dx box on the encounter form. Notice that the description is correct but the code is not. What diagnosis code is required to correct the claim you created for Andrea Spinelli on 10/09/08?
4. Assume that you correct the diagnosis code on the claim and resubmit it. How much do you think Medicare will pay her provider for the visit? Note that Andrea has already paid her copayment for the visit, and that her Medicare HMO pays for 100 percent of covered services.

Claim Case Study 18.2

Patient: Lakshmi Prasad

An RA/EOB is sent by Medicare Nationwide on October 17, 2008. An extract from it, containing three procedures for Lakshmi Prasad, is shown in Figure 18.2.
Notice that, of the three procedures listed, one has been denied.

1. What reason is given in the RA/EOB for the rejected procedure? What is the description of the procedure?
2. Refer back to the encounter form for Lakshmi Prasad in Claim Case Study 17.4 (page 557). Does the encounter form contain the same procedure code that is listed in the RA/EOB?
3. Refer next to Lakshmi Prasad's patient information form. Confirm that Lakshmi is an established patient. Also verify the reason for the visit as described on the patient information form.
4. Next, check the patient information form for Lakshmi's date of birth. Based on her age on the patient information form, what correction should be made to the encounter form and claim information?
5. Since the other two procedures in the claim have already been paid, use a blank CMS-1500 claim form to submit a new claim for the corrected

Date prepared: 10/17/2008 | **Claim number: 10156668**

Patientís name	Dates of service From – thru	POS	Proc	Qty	Charge amount	Eligible amount	Patient liability	Amt paid provider
Prasad, Lakshmi	10/09/08 - 10/09/08	11	88150	1	$ 29.00	$ 29.00	$ 5.80	$ 23.20
Prasad, Lakshmi	10/09/08 - 10/09/08	11	90659	1	$ 68.00	$ 68.00	$ 13.60	$ 54.40
Prasad, Lakshmi	10/09/08 - 10/09/08	11	99397	1	$118.00	*	*	-0-

*Incorrect procedure code.

FIGURE 18.2 Extract from Medicare Nationwide RA/EOB

procedure only. (Note: Even if you created the original claim in Medisoft, you should submit the subsequent claim on a paper CMS-1500 form.)

6. How much do you think Medicare will pay for the corrected procedure? Note that Lakshmi has paid her $100 Medicare deductible for the year, and that the plan plays for 80 percent of covered services (she has a Medicare traditional plan).

Processing Medicare RAs/EOBs and Preparing Secondary Claims

Claim Case Study 18.3

Medicare RA/EOB Analysis

Whenever an RA/EOB is received from a carrier, the payment received for each procedure is posted to each patient's account. If any patients on the RA/EOB have secondary coverage, secondary claims are then prepared. Before doing so, however, the RA/EOB is analyzed to make sure the payments received are in keeping with what is expected, given the office's fee schedule, the patient's insurance plan, and any deductibles or copayments that may be required from the patient.

In Claim Case Study 18.3, an RA/EOB is received from Medicare Nationwide. The first page of the RA/EOB, shown in Figure 18.3 on page 584, contains claim information for four patients who have secondary insurance plans. (The primary claim for each of these patients was created in Chapter 17.) Answer the following questions based on the information in the RA/EOB before preparing the patients' secondary claims.

1. As of October 17, 2008, how many patients on the EOB have paid their Medicare Part B deductible for 2008 in full?
2. Have any of the patients been denied payment for a claim?
3. How do the fees charged by Valley Associates, P.C., compare with the Medicare approved amounts on the claim?
4. How much of the allowed amount for procedure 99204 is Joseph Zylerberg responsible for? What percentage of this will his secondary plan pay, assuming he pays the $15 copay for the visit?
5. How much of the allowed amount for procedure 36415 is Donald Aiken responsible for? How much of this will his secondary plan pay?
6. Notice that the PT RESP amount is shown for each person on the claim. Should you bill the patients for these amounts now?
7. Notice that Wilma Estephan's PT RESP amount is $8.40 for a $14.00 procedure. How much of this amount represents her coinsurance responsibility? Does any of it represent her deductible?
8. The allowed amount for procedure 99211 on Wilma Estephan's claim is $14.00. Normally, Medicare pays 80 percent of the allowed amount, which, in this case, would be $11.20. Why has Medicare paid only $5.60?
9. Given the following figures, taken from the PT RESP field on the RA/EOB, estimate how much you think each secondary payer will pay. Note the following:
   - Joseph Zylerberg's Medicaid plan has a $15 copay.
   - Wilma Estephan's AARP plan does not cover her Medicare Part B deductible.

MEDICARE NATIONWIDE
1000 HIGH ST.
TOLEDO, OH 43601

PROVIDER REMITTANCE
THIS IS NOT A BILL
A PAYMENT SUMMARY AND AN EXPLANATION
OF CODES ARE AT THE END OF THIS STATEMENT

VALLEY ASSOCIATES, P.C.
1400 WEST CENTER STREET
TOLEDO, OH 43601

PAGE: 1 OF 3
DATE: 10/17/08
ID NO.: 6666222

PROVIDER: CHRISTOPHER CONNOLLY, M.D.

PATIENT: ZYLERBERG JOSEPH CLAIM: 900722411
PT RESP: 26.40

FROM DATE	THRU DATE	POS	PROC CODE	UNITS	AMOUNT BILLED	AMOUNT ALLOWED	DEDUCT	COPAY COINS	PROV PAID	REASON CODE
1009	100908	11	99204	1	103.00	103.00	.00	.00	82.40	
1009	100908	11	93000	1	29.00	29.00	.00	.00	23.20	
CLAIM TOTALS:					132.00	132.00	.00	.00	105.60	

CLAIM INFORMATION FORWARDED TO: MEDICAID

PATIENT: LANKHAAR NANCY CLAIM: 900722413
PT RESP: 5.60

FROM DATE	THRU DATE	POS	PROC CODE	UNITS	AMOUNT BILLED	AMOUNT ALLOWED	DEDUCT	COPAY COINS	PROV PAID	REASON CODE
1007	100708	11	99212	1	28.00	28.00	.00	.00	22.40	
CLAIM TOTALS:					28.00	28.00	.00	.00	22.40	

CLAIM INFORMATION FORWARDED TO: AARP

PATIENT: AIKEN DONALD CLAIM: 900722416
PT RESP: 17.20

FROM DATE	THRU DATE	POS	PROC CODE	UNITS	AMOUNT BILLED	AMOUNT ALLOWED	DEDUCT	COPAY COINS	PROV PAID	REASON CODE
1010	101008	11	99203	1	69.00	69.00	.00	.00	55.20	
1010	101008	11	36415	1	17.00	17.00	.00	.00	13.60	
CLAIM TOTALS:					86.00	86.00	.00	.00	68.80	

CLAIM INFORMATION FORWARDED TO: AARP

PATIENT: ESTEPHAN WILMA CLAIM: 900722411
PT RESP: 8.40

FROM DATE	THRU DATE	POS	PROC CODE	UNITS	AMOUNT BILLED	AMOUNT ALLOWED	DEDUCT	COPAY COINS	PROV PAID	REASON CODE
1006	100608	11	99211	1	14.00	14.00*	7.00	.00	5.60	
CLAIM TOTALS:					14.00	14.00	7.00	.00	5.60	

*$7.00 OF THIS ALLOWED AMOUNT HAS BEEN APPLIED TOWARD PATIENT'S DEDUCTIBLE.

CLAIM INFORMATION FORWARDED TO: AARP

FIGURE 18.3 RA/EOB from Medicare Nationwide

Patient	Patient resp. on primary claim	Estimated amount from secondary payer
Zylerberg, J.	26.40	_____ Medicaid
Lankhaar, N.	5.60	_____ AARP
Aiken, D.	17.20	_____ AARP
Estephan, W.	8.40	_____ AARP

Preparing Secondary Claims

Using the information shown in the Medicare Nationwide RA/EOB (Figure 18.3), prepare secondary claims for the following Medicare patients. You will need to base the secondary claims on the primary claims you created for each patient in Chapter 17. Remember to use paper CMS-1500 claim forms rather than the Medisoft program to prepare the claims.

Secondary Claim	Patient	Primary Claim
Claim Case Study 18.3A	Zylerberg, J.	Claim Case Study 17.5 (p. 558)
Claim Case Study 18.3B	Lankhaar, N.	Claim Case Study 17.8 (p. 564)
Claim Case Study 18.3C	Aiken, D.	Claim Case Study 17.9 (p. 566)
Claim Case Study 18.3D	Estephan, W.	Claim Case Study 17.14 (p. 573)

Processing Commerical Payer RAs/EOBs and Preparing Secondary Claims

Claim Case Study 18.4

Commercial RA/EOB Analysis

As with a Medicare RA/EOB, when a commercial RA/EOB is received, before posting payments and preparing secondary claims that may be required, the RA/EOB must be carefully reviewed. When analyzing an RA/EOB from a commercial carrier, you must be familiar with the guidelines of that carrier's particular plan. The type of services covered and the percentage of the coverage will vary, depending on whether the plan is a fee-for-service plan, a managed care plan, a consumer-driven health plan, or some other type. The allowed amounts for each procedure will also vary with different plans, depending on the fee schedule decided upon in the contract between the payer and the provider. The contract will also specify whether there is a discount on the fees.

In Claim Case Study 18.4, an RA/EOB is received from Anthem BCBS Traditional, which is a fee-for-service plan with an 80/20 coinsurance and a $250 deductible. The first page of the RA/EOB, shown in Figure 18.4 on page 586, contains claim information for two patients who have secondary insurance plans through their spouses. (The primary claim for both patients was created in Chapter 17.) Answer the following questions based on the information in the RA/EOB before preparing the patients' secondary claims.

1. What is the name of Karen Giroux's secondary insurance plan?
2. Based on the RA/EOB, how much has Karen Giroux paid up to now toward her 2008 deductible? How much of her deductible is due with this claim? Once she pays this amount, what percentage of her claims will be covered by Aetna?
3. What amount does Karen Giroux owe for procedure 99386?

ANTHEM BCBS TRADITIONAL
900 West Market Street
Cleveland, OH 44101

PROVIDER REMITTANCE

VALLEY ASSOCIATES, P.C.
1400 West Center Street
Toledo, OH 43601

Page: 1 of 2
Date: 10/15/2008
ID # 23AAY20

Dates of service From – thru	POS	Proc	Qty	Charge amount	Eligible amount	Deduct/ Copay	Patient liability	Amt paid provider
PROVIDER: Nancy Ronkowski, M.D.								
CLAIM: 2988876								
Patient's name: Giroux, Karen								
10/07/08 - 10/07/08	11	99386	1	$ 180.00	$ 180.00	$ 50.00	$ 26.00	$104.00
CLAIM INFORMATION FORWARDED TO: MEDICARE NATIONWIDE								
PROVIDER: Christopher Connolly, M.D.								
CLAIM: 2988882								
Patient's name: Ruff, Jean								
10/05/08 - 10/05/08	11	99202	1	$ 75.00	$ 75.00	- 0 -	$ 15.00	$ 60.00
CLAIM INFORMATION FORWARDED TO: AETNA CHOICE								

FIGURE 18.4 RA/EOB from Anthem BCBS Traditional

4. Anthem has paid Dr. Ronkowski $104 for Karen Giroux's claim. How was this amount calculated?
5. What percentage of the eligible charge has Anthem paid for Jean Ruff's claim? Based on the RA/EOB, has she met her $250 deductible?
6. What amount does Jean Ruff owe for procedure 99202? What percentage of the eligible charge does this equal?
7. Suppose Jean Ruff had not met any portion of her deductible and was responsible for the full eligible amount of procedure 99202, $75. Would it still be necessary to send a secondary claim?
8. Based on the RA/EOB, calculate how much each patient is responsible for on the primary claim. Then estimate how much you think each secondary payer will pay. Note the following:
   - The guarantor for Karen Giroux's secondary coverage, her husband Jack, has met his Medicare Part B deductible.
   - Jean Ruff's secondary coverage, provided through her husband's plan, pays for 100 percent of covered services and has a $15 copay.

Patient	*Patient resp. on primary claim*	*Estimated amount from secondary payer*
Giroux, K.	________	_____ Medicare Nationwide
Ruff, J.	________	_____ Aetna Choice

Preparing Secondary Claims

Using the information shown in the Anthem BCBS Traditional RA/EOB (Figure 18.4), prepare secondary claims for both Anthem BCBS Traditional patients. You will need to base the secondary claims on the primary claims you created for each patient in Chapter 17. Remember to use paper CMS-1500 claim forms rather than the Medisoft program to prepare the claims.

Secondary Claim	*Patient*	*Primary Claim*
Claim Case Study 18.4A	Giroux, K.	Claim Case Study 17.17 (p. 576)
Claim Case Study 18.4B	Ruff, J.	Claim Case Study 17.18 (p. 577)

Calculating Patients' Balances

After the insurance carrier makes a decision on a claim and the payment is received and posted, the patient's balance must be calculated. The claim case studies in this section provide practice in calculating balances by providing the latest payment information obtained from RAs/EOBs for each patient in Chapter 17, Claim Cases 17.1 through 17.20. Based on the payment information from the RA/EOB, you must calculate each patient's balance.

Claim Case Study 18.5

Patient: Wendy Walker

The following information is received on an RA/EOB from the Medicare HMO plan. The patient made a $10 copay at the time of the visit.

POS	*PROC*	*BILLED*	*ALLOWED*	*DEDUCT*	*COINS/COPAY*	*PROV PD*
11	**99204**	**103.00**	**103.00**	**0.00**	**10.00**	**93.00**

Patient balance: _____

Claim Case Study 18.6

Patient: Walter Williams

The following information is received on an RA/EOB from Aetna Choice. The patient made a $15 copay at the time of the visit.

POS	*PROC*	*BILLED*	*ALLOWED*	*DEDUCT*	*COINS/COPAY*	*PROV PD*
11	**36415**	**17.00**	**16.00**	**0.00**	**15.00**	**1.00**

Patient balance: _____

Claim Case Study 18.7

Patient: Donna Gaeta

The following information is received from Medicare Nationwide, who pays for the preventive visit as a one-time payment for a new Medicare patient.

POS	*PROC*	*BILLED*	*ALLOWED*	*DEDUCT*	*COINS/COPAY*	*PROV PD*
11	**99387**	**142.00**	**142.00**	**100.00**	**8.40**	**33.60**
11	**93000**	**29.00**	**29.00**	**0.00**	**5.80**	**23.20**
11	**88150**	**29.00**	**29.00**	**0.00**	**5.80**	**23.20**
11	**81000**	**17.00**	**17.00**	**0.00**	**3.40**	**13.60**
11	**36415**	**17.00**	**17.00**	**0.00**	**3.40**	**13.60**

Patient balance: _____

Claim Case Study 18.8

Patient: Lakshmi Prasad

The following information is received on an RA/EOB from Medicare Nationwide. The patient has met the deductible for 2008. (*Note:* The patient was made aware at the time of the visit that preventive visits are not covered by Medicare Nationwide.)

POS	*PROC*	*BILLED*	*ALLOWED*	*DEDUCT*	*COINS/COPAY*	*PROV PD*
11	**99396**	**106.00**	**106.00**	**0.00**	**0.00**	**0.00***

* This procedure is not covered by Medicare Nationwide.

Patient balance:_____

Claim Case Study 18.9

Patient: Joseph Zylerberg

The following information is taken from two RAs/EOBs. The first RA/EOB is from Medicare Nationwide, the primary payer. Note that the patient has met the deductible for the primary payer. The second RA/EOB is from Medicaid, the secondary carrier. The patient's Medicaid copay has not yet been paid for the secondary plan.

PRIMARY CARRIER

POS	*PROC*	*BILLED*	*ALLOWED*	*DEDUCT*	*COINS/COPAY*	*PROV PD*
11	**99204**	**103.00**	**103.00**	**0.00**	**20.60**	**82.40**
11	**93000**	**29.00**	**29.00**	**0.00**	**5.80**	**23.20**

SECONDARY CARRIER

POS	*PROC*	*BILLED*	*ALLOWED*	*DEDUCT*	*COINS/COPAY*	*PROV PD*
11	**99204**	**103.00**	**103.00**	**0.00**	**15.00**	**5.60**
11	**93000**	**29.00**	**29.00**	**0.00**	**0.00**	**5.80**

Patient balance: _____

Claim Case Study 18.10

Patient: Shih-Chi Yang

The following information is received on an RA/EOB from CarePlus Workers' Compensation.

POS	*PROC*	*BILLED*	*ALLOWED*	*DEDUCT*	*COINS/COPAY*	*PROV PD*
11	**26600**	**315.00**	**315.00**	**0.00**	**0.00**	**315.00**
11	**73130**	**91.00**	**91.00**	**0.00**	**0.00**	**91.00**

Patient balance: _____

Claim Case Study 18.11

Patient: Andrea Spinelli

The following information is received on an RA/EOB from the Medicare HMO plan. The patient made a $10 copay at the time of the visit.

POS	PROC	BILLED	ALLOWED	DEDUCT	COINS/COPAY	PROV PD
11	**69210**	**34.00**	**34.00**	**0.00**	**10.00**	**24.00**

Patient balance: _____

Claim Case Study 18.12

Patient: Nancy Lankhaar

The following information is received on two different RAs/EOBs. The first payment is from Medicare, the primary payer. The patient has met the Medicare deductible. The second payment is from AARP, the secondary carrier.

PRIMARY CARRIER

POS	PROC	BILLED	ALLOWED	DEDUCT	COINS/COPAY	PROV PD
11	**99212**	**28.00**	**28.00**	**0.00**	**5.60**	**22.40**

SECONDARY CARRIER

POS	PROC	BILLED	ALLOWED	DEDUCT	COINS/COPAY	PROV PD
11	**99212**	**28.00**	**28.00**	**0.00**	**0.00**	**5.60**

Patient balance: _____

Claim Case Study 18.13

Patient: Donald Aiken

The following information is received on two different RAs/EOBs. The first RA/EOB is from Medicare, the primary payer. The patient has met the Medicare deductible. The second RA/EOB is from the secondary carrier, AARP.

PRIMARY CARRIER

POS	PROC	BILLED	ALLOWED	DEDUCT	COINS/COPAY	PROV PD
11	**99203**	**69.00**	**69.00**	**0.00**	**13.80**	**55.20**
11	**36415**	**17.00**	**17.00**	**0.00**	**3.40**	**13.60**

SECONDARY CARRIER

POS	PROC	BILLED	ALLOWED	DEDUCT	COINS/COPAY	PROV PD
11	**99203**	**69.00**	**69.00**	**0.00**	**0.00**	**13.80**
11	**36415**	**17.00**	**17.00**	**0.00**	**0.00**	**3.40**

Patient balance: _____

Claim Case Study 18.14

Patient: Eric Huang

The following information is received on an RA/EOB from Medicare Nationwide. The patient has not yet met the deductible for 2008.

POS	*PROC*	*BILLED*	*ALLOWED*	*DEDUCT*	*COINS/COPAY*	*PROV PD*
11	**99243**	**97.00**	**97.00**	**26.00**	**14.20**	**56.80**

Patient balance: _____

For the remaining case studies, the RA/EOB information is more limited. The details of each procedure are not given. Based on the information provided, however, you should still be able to calculate each patient's balance. Note that claims for the remaining cases were originally created in Case Studies 17.11 through 17.20 (pages 570–579).

Claim Case Study 18.15

Patient: Isabella Neufeld

Payer	Medicaid
Charge amount	$32.00
Allowed amount	$32.00
Copayment	$15.00, paid at the time of visit
Payment to provider	$17.00
Patient balance:	$______

Claim Case Study 18.16

Patient: Alan Harcar

Payer	Medicare Nationwide
Charge amount	$50.00
Allowed amount	$50.00
Deductible	$50.00
Coinsurance	$ 0.00
Payment to provider	$ 0.00
Patient balance:	$______

Claim Case Study 18.17

Patient: Jose Velaquez

Payer	Anthem BCBS PPO
Charge amount	$193.00
Allowed amount	$135.10 (70% of charge amount)
Copay	$ 20.00, paid at the time of visit
Payment to provider	$ 115.10
Patient balance:	$______

Claim Case Study 18.18

Patient: Wilma Estephan

Primary Payer	Medicare Nationwide
Charge amount	$14.00
Allowed amount	$14.00
Deductible	$ 7.00 ($93 out of $100 already paid)
Coinsurance	$ 1.40
Payment to provider	$ 5.60
Secondary Payer	AARP
Payment to provider	$ 1.40
Patient balance:	$______

Claim Case Study 18.19

Patient: John O'Rourke

Payer	Anthem BCBS PPO
Charge amount	$150.00
Allowed amount	$105.00 (70% of charge amount)
Copay	$ 20.00, paid at the time of visit
Payment to provider	$ 85.00
Patient balance:	$______

Claim Case Study 18.20

Patient: Sylvia Evans

Payer	TRICARE
Charge amount	$46.00 (10/17/2008 claim only)
Allowed amount	$34.50 (75% of charge amount)
Copay	$10.00, paid at the time of visit
Payment to provider	$24.50
Patient balance:	$______

Claim Case Study 18.21

Patient: Karen Giroux

Primary Payer	Anthem BCBC Traditional (80/20 coinsurance; $250 deduct.)
Charge amount	$180.00
Allowed amount	$180.00
Deductible	$ 0.00
Coinsurance	$ 36.00
Payment to provider	$144.00
Secondary Payer	Medicare Nationwide
Payment to provider	$ 0.00 (not a covered service)
Patient balance:	$______

Claim Case Study 18.22

Patient: Jean Ruff

Primary Payer	Anthem BCBC Traditional (80/20 coinsurance; $250 deduct.)
Charge amount	$ 75.00
Allowed amount	$ 75.00
Deductible	$ 0.00
Coinsurance	$ 15.00
Payment to provider	$ 60.00

Secondary Payer	Aetna Choice
Copay	$15.00, not yet paid
Payment to provider	$ 0.00

Patient balance: $______

Claim Case Study 18.23

Patient: Mary Anne Kopelman

Payer	TRICARE
Charge amount	$120.00
Allowed amount	$ 90.00 (75% of charge amount)
Copay	$ 10.00, paid at the time of visit
Payment to provider	$ 80.00

Patient balance: $______

Claim Case Study 18.24

Patient: Otto Kaar

Payer	Medicaid
Charge amount	$57.00
Allowed amount	$57.00
Copay	$15.00, paid at the time of visit
Payment to provider	$42.00

Patient balance: $______

Guide to Medisoft

This Guide contains two parts. Part 1: *Getting Started with Medisoft* provides instructions for starting the Medisoft program and setting up the database files that you will use with Medisoft in the claim case studies in this text. The required files for setting up the database are stored on a backup file on the Student Data Template CD-ROM located inside the back cover of this text. Part 2: *Overview and Practice* provides an introduction to the Medisoft program as well as practice in creating claims in Medisoft.

After you have gone through Parts 1 and 2, you will be able to use Medisoft to create claims if you elect to do so, rather than filling out paper claims. Medisoft can be used to create the claims that appear in the Applying Your Knowledge section at the end of Chapters 9 through 13, as well as for the twenty claim cases in "Chapter 17: Primary Case Studies."

Computer Supplies and Equipment

To use Medisoft with this text, the following items are required:

- Student Data Template CD-ROM, located inside the back cover of this text
- PC with 500 MHz or greater processor speed
- 256 MB RAM
- 500 MB available hard disk space (if saving data to hard drive)
- CD-ROM 2x or faster disk drive
- Mouse or compatible pointing device
- Windows 2000 or Windows XP operating system
- Medisoft Advanced Patient Accounting, Version 11
- External storage device for storing backup copies of the working database
- Printer

Medisoft Advanced Patient Accounting, Version 11, is available to schools adopting *Medical Insurance: A Guide to Coding and Reimbursement*. Information on ordering and installing the software is located in the Instructor's Manual that accompanies the text. Student-at-Home Software Medisoft Advanced Version 11 is available as an option for distance education or for students who want to practice with the software at home.

PART 1: *Getting Started with Medisoft*

Before a medical office begins to create claims using Medisoft, basic information about the practice and its patients must be entered in the program. This preliminary work has been done for you. The medical practice with which you will work is called Valley Associates, P.C. (VAPC). Follow the instructions below to copy the data (currently in the form of a backup file called "VAPC.mbk") from the Student Data Template CD-ROM to your hard drive. Then you will start Medisoft and restore the backup file into the appropriate directory on your hard drive for use with the Medisoft program.

Note that the instructions here assume the use of hard drive C: for setting up the data files from the Student Data Template CD-ROM. If you are working with a different drive, such as a network drive, ask your instructor for guidance in substituting C: with the drive name specific to your computer's setup.

Copying the Required File from the Student Data Template CD-ROM to the Hard Drive

1. Turn on the computer. Insert the Student Data Template CD-ROM in the CD drive.
2. A readme text file appears on the screen. After viewing the information, exit the file.
3. View a directory of files in the CD-ROM drive to locate the backup file labeled "VAPC.mbk."
4. Copy the VAPC.mbk file from the CD-ROM to the folder on the hard drive where you will be saving your work during this course (ask your instructor if you are not sure where to copy the file).
5. When the copying is finished, remove the Student Data Template CD-ROM from the CD drive and store it in a safe place.

Starting Medisoft and Restoring the VAPC Backup File

Follow these instructions to start Medisoft and restore the VAPC backup file for use with Medisoft. First you will create a directory for the data set; then you will restore the data to the new directory. You will only need to follow these instructions once. Thereafter, the data will be available inside the Medisoft program.

1. While holding down the F7 key, use the Start menu on the Windows desktop to open the Medisoft program as follows: Click Start, All Programs, Medisoft, Medisoft Advanced Patient Accounting. When the Find NDCMedisoft Database dialog box appears, release the F7 key. This box asks you to enter the Medisoft data directory.

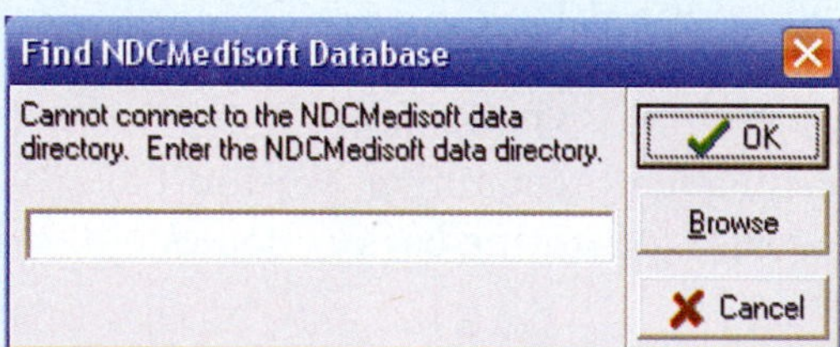

Note: If the Open Practice dialog box appears at this point, see if Valley Associates PC is already displayed in the list of practices. If so, click on it and then click the OK button and skip to step 9 below.

If Valley Associates PC is not displayed in the list of practices, click the New button to create a new data set and continue with step 5 below.

2. Click inside the Find NDCMedisoft Database box to activate it, and then enter *C:\Medidata* (where C is the letter that represents the hard drive you will be using).

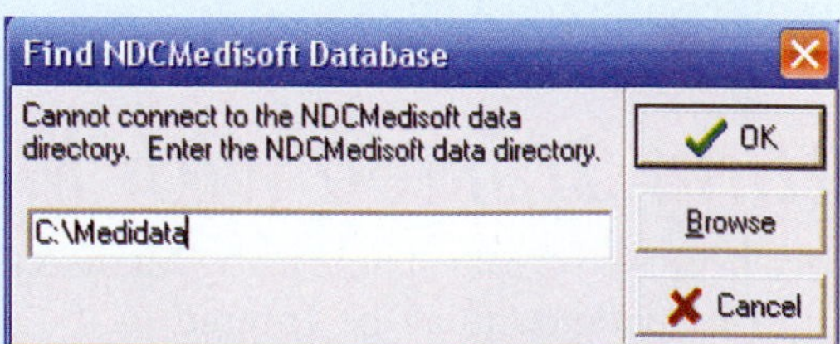

3. Click the OK button. If an Information dialog box appears with the following message, "This is not an existing root data directory. Do you want to create a new one?" appears, click Yes.

4. The Create Data dialog box is displayed. Click the Create a New Set of Data option.

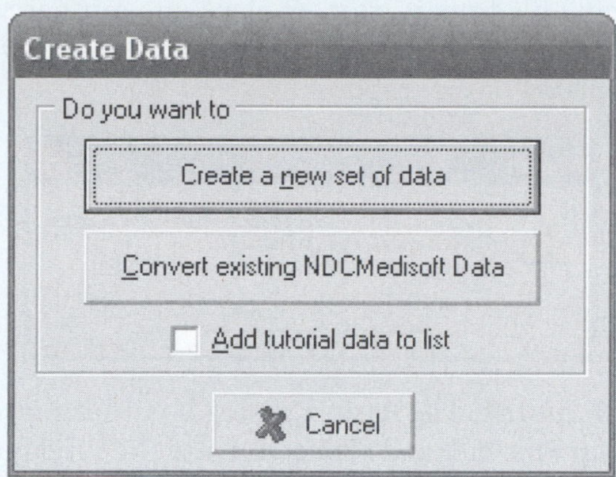

5. The Create a New Set of Data dialog box appears. In the upper box, key *Valley Associates PC*. In the lower box, key *VAPC*. The dialog box should now look like this:

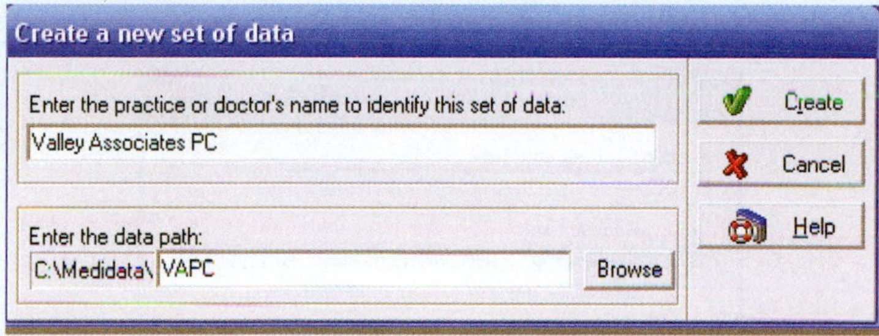

6. Click the Create button. A Confirm dialog box is displayed. Click the Yes button to confirm that you want to create the new directory.
7. After several moments, the Practice Information box appears. In the Practice Name box, key *Valley Associates, P.C.* The remaining boxes can remain blank.

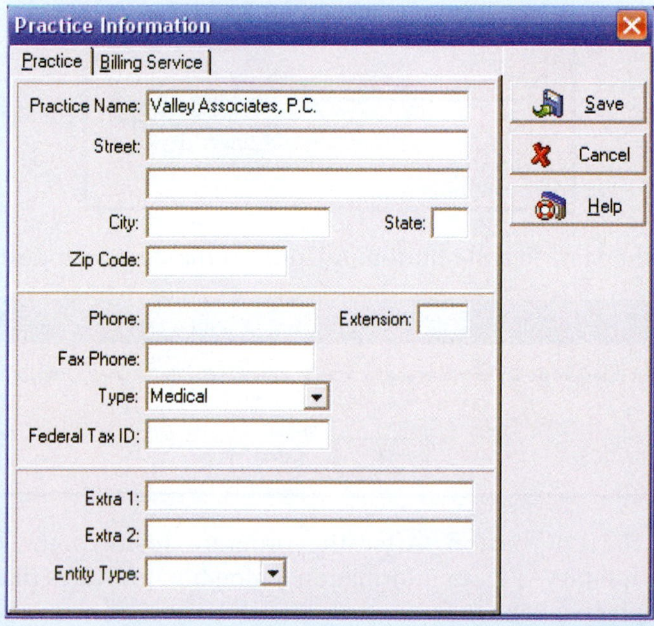

8. Click the Save button.

9. The main window of the Medisoft program is displayed with the name of the new data set, Valley Associates PC, listed on the title bar. To restore the VAPC.mbk file from its storage place on your hard drive to the new directory, first open the File menu and select Restore Data.
10. A Warning dialog box is displayed.

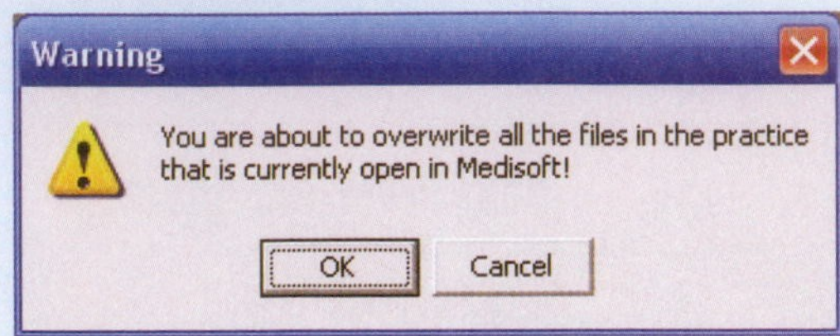

11. Click the OK button. The Restore dialog box is displayed.
12. In the Backup File Path and Name box, use the Find button if necessary to locate the folder on the hard drive where you copied the VAPC.mbk file. With the appropriate folder selected, click the OK button.
13. When you click OK, the VAPC.mbk file is displayed in the Existing Backup Files box on your screen. Click on the VAPC.mbk file to select it. The dialog box should now look like this:

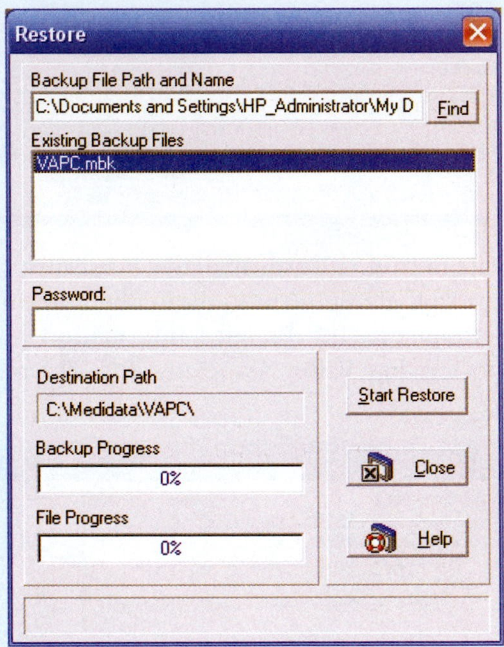

14. Click the Start Restore button. A Confirm dialog box appears.

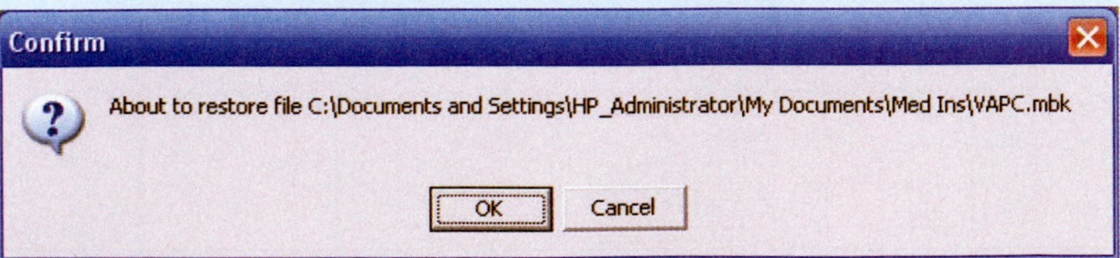

15. Click the OK button. After the program restores the database to C:\Medidata\VAPC, an information dialog box indicates that the restore is complete. Click OK.
16. You are returned to the main Medisoft window. (*Hint:* If the main Medisoft window does not fill the screen, click the Maximize button to expand it.)

17. By default, Medisoft may display a sidebar with four options on the left side of the main window. As the sidebar is not required for this text, open the Window menu and click the Show Side Bar option to toggle it off.
18. The Valley Associates, P.C., database is ready for use.
19. To continue with Part 2: *Overview and Practice,* leave the program open. To exit at this time, open the File menu and click Exit (or click the X in the top right corner of the screen). When the Backup Reminder dialog box appears, click the Exit Program button.

Part 2: *Overview and Practice*

Part 2 of this Guide contains an overview of the Medisoft Advanced Patient Accounting program, including an introduction to the program's databases, an explanation of how claims are created in Medisoft, and illustrations of the major dialog boxes that are used for data entry. Part 2 also provides hands-on practice in using the software to create insurance claims. You will need to be familiar with this information if you decide to use Medisoft to complete the claims in the end-of-chapter material and in "Chapter 17: Primary Case Studies."

Overview

Medisoft, a computerized patient billing system that runs on Microsoft's Windows operating system, is used in this textbook as an example of the type of program with which medical insurance specialists often work. Processing information to complete insurance claim forms is one of the main functions of the Medisoft program.

Medisoft's Database Design

The Medisoft program is designed to collect information and store it in databases. A database is a collection of related facts. For example, a provider database contains information about a practice's physicians while a patient database contains each patient's unique chart number and personal information, including address, phone, employer, assigned provider, and so on. The major databases in the Medisoft program are:

- *Provider:* The provider database has information about the physician(s) as well as the practice, such as the practice's name, address, phone number, and tax and medical identifier numbers.
- *Patient/Guarantor:* Each patient information form is stored in the computer system's patient/guarantor database. The database includes the patient's unique chart number and personal information: name, address, phone number, birth date, Social Security number, gender, marital status, employer, and guarantor (the insured person if other than the patient).
- *Insurance Carriers:* The insurance carrier database contains the names, addresses, plan types, and other data about all insurance carriers used by the practice's patients. This database also stores information about each carrier's electronic claim submission.
- *Diagnosis Codes:* The diagnosis code database contains the most frequently used ICD codes that indicate the reason a service is provided. The practice's encounter form serves as a source document in setting up this database.
- *Procedure Codes:* The procedure code database contains the data needed to create charges. The CPT codes most often used by the practice are selected

for this database. The practice's encounter form is a good source document for these codes also. Other claim data, such as place of service (POS) codes and the charge for each procedure, are stored in this database as well.

- *Transactions:* The transaction database stores information about each patient's visits, diagnoses, and procedures, as well as received and outstanding payments.

How Insurance Claims Are Created in Medisoft

Three major steps are followed to create insurance claims using Medisoft: (1) setting up the practice, (2) entering patient and transaction information, and (3) creating insurance claims.

Setting Up the Practice Before Medisoft can be used to store information about patients and their visits, basic facts about the practice itself are entered into several of the databases mentioned above. Information about the providers in the practice is recorded in the provider database, including provider identification numbers for different carriers. In addition, frequently used diagnosis and procedure codes are entered in their own databases with code descriptions. Finally, insurance carrier data is entered. The insurance carrier database contains information about the carriers that most patients use, as well as options for electronic claim submission and paper claim printing. These databases are created once during the setup of the practice. However, they may be updated as often as necessary.

Entering Patient and Transaction Information Entering patient and transaction information in the database is an ongoing process. After a patient visits a physician in the practice, the medical insurance specialist organizes the information gathered on the patient information form and the encounter form. After analyzing and checking the data, each element is entered in Medisoft. A new record must be created for a new patient, and information on established patients may need to be updated. Next, the appropriate insurance carrier for the visit is selected. Usually, this is the patient's primary insurance carrier, but in workers' compensation cases, for example, the carrier will be different. After that, the purposes of the visit, the diagnosis codes, and the procedure codes are entered, with the appropriate charges.

Creating Insurance Claims When all patient and transaction information has been entered and checked, the medical insurance specialist issues the command to Medisoft to create an insurance claim form. Medisoft then organizes the necessary databases. Within Medisoft, each database is linked, or related, to each of the others by having at least one fact in common. For example, the patient's chart number appears both in the patient/guarantor database and the transaction database, thereby linking the two. Medisoft selects data from each database as needed. The program follows the instructions for printing the form or transmitting the information electronically to the designated receiver, which is often a clearinghouse.

Data Entry in Medisoft

The following section provides illustrations and descriptions of the main areas in which data are entered in Medisoft.

Patient/Guarantor Information The Patient/Guarantor dialog box is where basic information about patients is entered. The dialog box has three "pages," or tabs, used to enter information about patients. Tabs are so named because

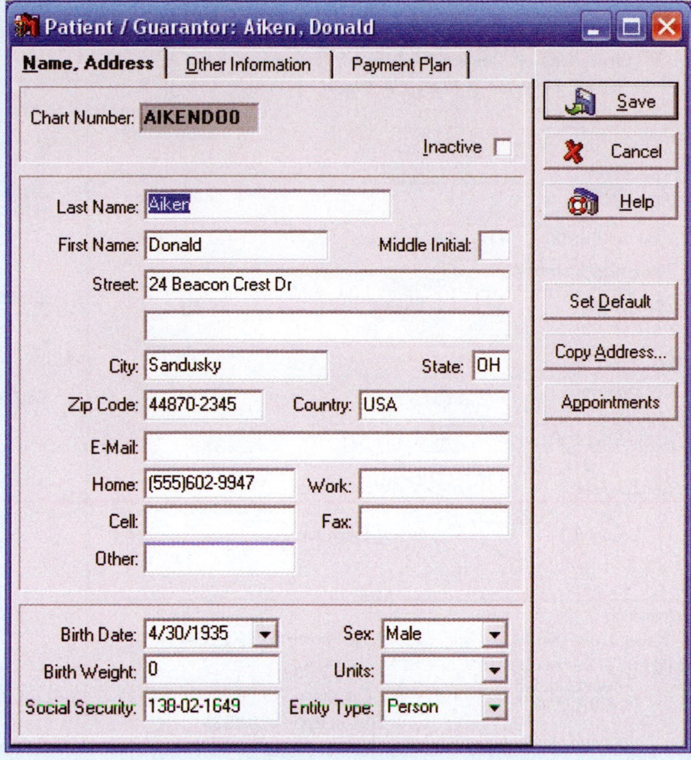

FIGURE 1 Name, Address Tab in the Patient/Guarantor Dialog Box

they resemble the tab on a file folder. When a tab name is clicked, the entire contents of that tab is displayed. Each tab contains fields in which data is keyed. The patient's unique chart number, which can be created by the user or assigned by Medisoft, is entered in the first field in the Name, Address tab of the Patient/Guarantor dialog box (see Figure 1). Then, the patient's personal information (name, address, contact numbers, birth date, Social Security number, and so on) is entered.

Many Medisoft dialog boxes include default entries to save time when various types of data are entered. For example, in the Country field in the Name, Address tab, the entry "USA" automatically appears. If this entry is correct, the user moves on to the next entry, accepting the default. This information is stored when the user clicks the Save button. If the default entry is not correct, other data may be entered and stored in its place.

The second tab in the Patient/Guarantor dialog box, called the Other Information tab, contains information about the patient's employment and other miscellaneous data. The third tab, Payment Plan, is used to enter the terms for the patient's payment plan, provided the practice offers a payment plan and the patient requests one. For the purposes of the Medisoft work in this text, patient information has already been entered in the tabs of the Patient/Guarantor dialog box for you.

Case Information Once a patient's personal information is entered, then a new case can be created each time the patient visits the medical office with a different complaint. A new case is also set up if the insurance carrier differs from the patient's primary carrier, such as in a workers' compensation case, in order to keep the information separate from other office visits. A patient's case information is stored in the Case dialog box (see Figure 2 on page 600).

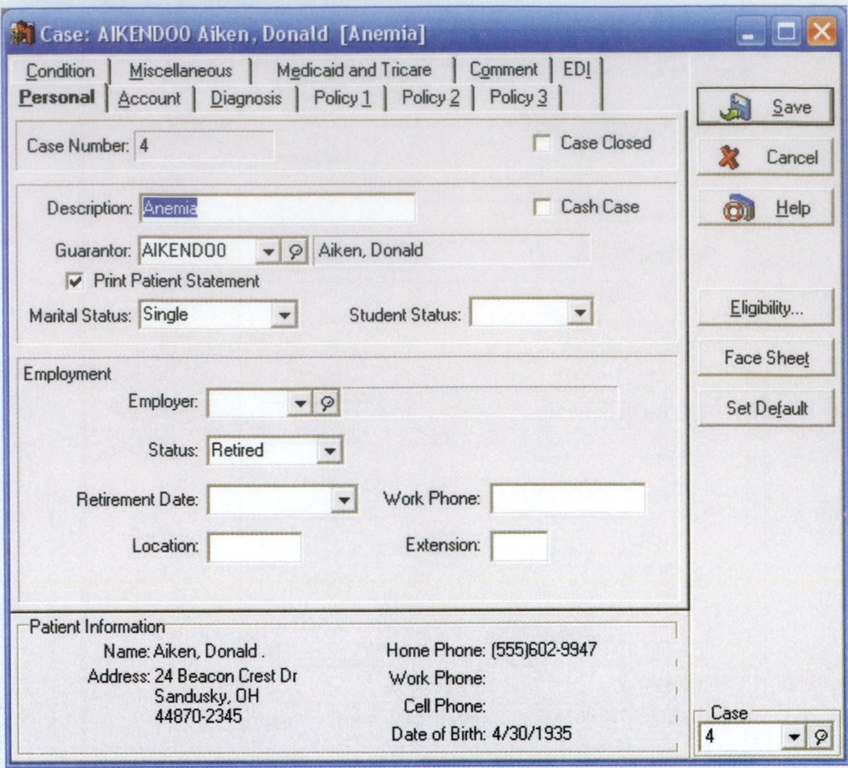

FIGURE 2 Case Dialog Box with the Personal Tab Active

The Case dialog box contains eleven tabs for entering a patient's case information: Personal, Account, Diagnosis, Policy 1, Policy 2, Policy 3, Condition, Miscellaneous, Medicaid and Tricare, Comment, and EDI. These tabs contain information about the patients' billing account, insurance coverage, medical condition, and other miscellaneous information that may be required to create an insurance claim.

As with the tabs in the Patient/Guarantor dialog box, the tabs in the Case dialog box have been filled in for you in the Valley Associates, P.C., database, using information that would have been obtained from each patient's patient information form. Information on the patient's diagnosis, which is obtained from the patient's encounter form for a given visit, has yet to be entered in the Diagnosis tab.

Transaction Entry Transactions—patients' visits and charges, as well as payments and adjustments—are entered in the Transaction Entry dialog box (see Figure 3). When the patient's chart number and case number are selected in the Transaction Entry dialog box, Medisoft displays information previously entered in other dialog boxes, such as the patient's name and birth date, case name, insurance carrier information, and estimated charges, in the top portion of the Transaction Entry dialog box for easy reference.

Charge transactions are created by clicking the New button in the middle portion of the Transaction Entry dialog box, labeled the Charges section. This section is used for entering procedure codes and charges. Procedures are selected in the Procedure field from a drop-down list of procedure codes. The list shows the CPT codes and descriptions that are frequently used by the practice. If the correct procedure has not already been included in Medisoft, a dialog box can be accessed to add it.

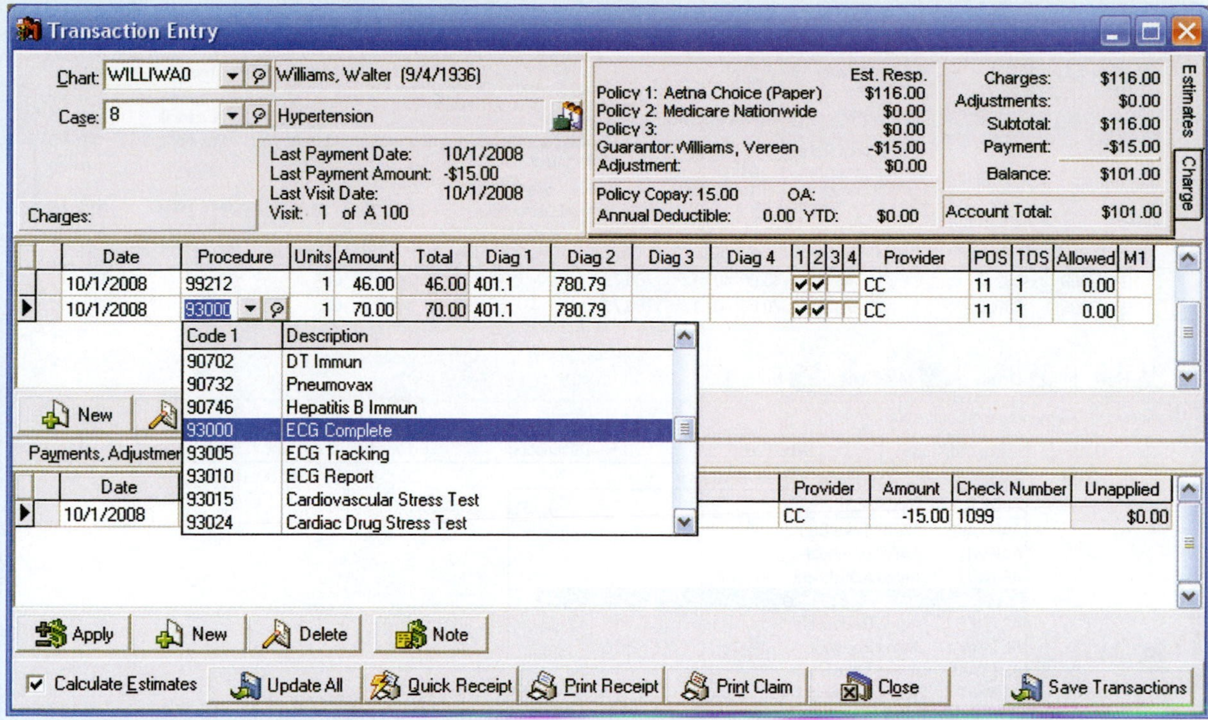

FIGURE 3 Transaction Entry Dialog Box with the Procedure Code Drop-Down List

Patient copayments are entered by clicking the New button in the lower third of the Transaction Entry dialog box, the Payments, Adjustments, and Comments section. This section is used for recording payments received from patients and insurance carriers. The type of payment is selected in the Pay/Adj Code field from a drop-down list of codes (see Figure 4 on page 602). Transaction entries must be saved by clicking the Save Transactions button in the bottom right corner of the dialog box. Any transaction can be edited by clicking in the field to be edited and making the change.

When the transaction entry is complete, a receipt, called a walkout receipt, can be printed for the patient by clicking the Print Receipt button at the bottom of the Transaction Entry dialog box. The walkout receipt is a printed statement showing what the patient paid that day and what is owed. Patients who file their own insurance claims use this information to complete the claim form.

Claim Management

Once a patient's transaction entries have been completed for a visit, a claim can be created. The Claim Management dialog box is used to (1) create batches of claims for transmission, (2) transmit claims electronically or print them on paper forms, and (3), if necessary, make corrections to existing claims. Medisoft creates a list of claims that have been sent by either mode (print or electronic) in the Claim Management dialog box so that each claim can be marked with its status when RA reports arrive from carriers (see Figure 5 on page 602).

If you use Medisoft to complete the claim case studies in this text, you will enter diagnosis and transaction data for patients with a variety of insurance plans in the Valley Associates, P.C., database and then create claims for them in the Claim Management dialog box.

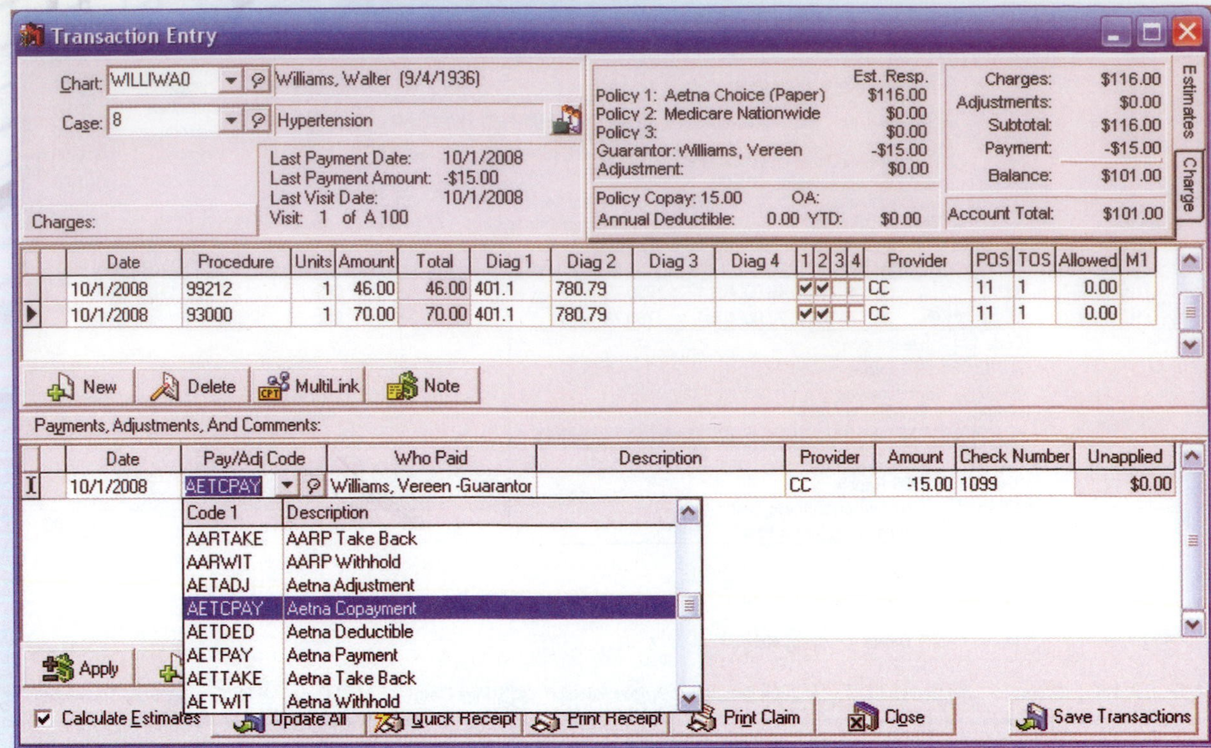

FIGURE 4 Transaction Entry Dialog Box with the Pay/Adj Code Drop-Down List

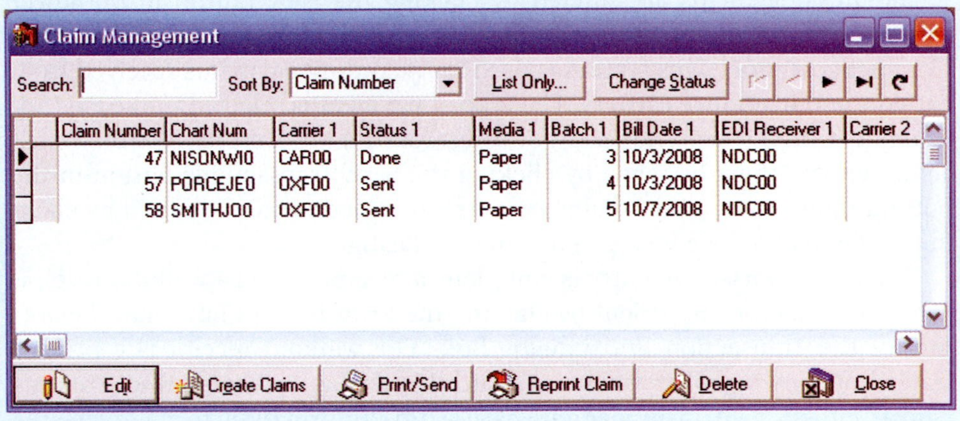

FIGURE 5 Claim Management Dialog Box

> **Important**
> If you have not carried out the instructions in Part 1 of this Guide, including "Starting Medisoft and Restoring the VAPC Backup File," please do so now. You will need the Valley Associates, P.C., data from the restored backup file for this practice session (and for all the Medisoft work in the text).

Practice Session

If you plan to use Medisoft to complete the claim case studies in this text, it is recommended that you complete the hands-on practice session that follows. In this practice session, you will:

- Practice selecting menu options in Medisoft
- Enter the diagnosis and transaction data for a sample patient
- Create and print out an insurance claim for a sample patient
- Learn how to use the Medisoft backup and restore features to save your work.

FIGURE 6 The Medisoft Menu Bar

Practice Selecting Menu Options

The following practice session assumes that you have started the Medisoft program and that the Valley Associates, P.C., database is active. If the database is active, the title bar at the top of the screen will say Valley Associates PC.

The first step in becoming acquainted with Medisoft is to use the program's menu system. Medisoft offers program choices through a group of eight menus. The Medisoft menu bar at the top of the main Medisoft window lists the name of each menu: File, Edit, Activities, Lists, Reports, Tools, Window, and Help (see Figure 6). A Services menu may also be available if the practice is sending electronic prescriptions.

The two menus used the most in the Medisoft activities in *Medical Insurance* are the Lists menu and the Activities menu.

The Lists Menu Most of the data already entered for Valley Associates, P.C., is accessed through the Lists menu. Use the following steps to practice selecting some of the options on the Lists menu.

1. Click the menu name, Lists, to display the Lists menu.

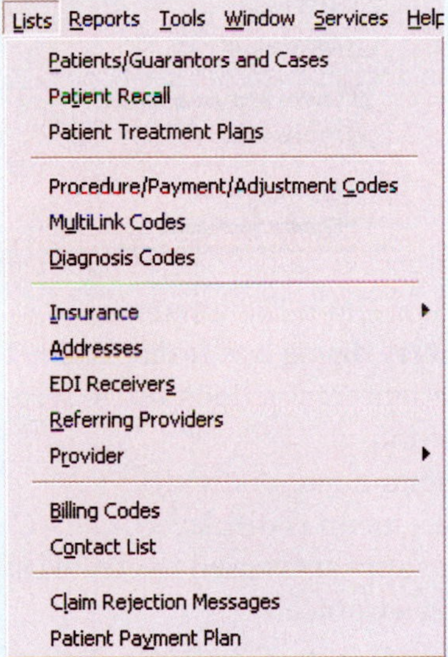

2. Click the first option, Patients/Guarantors and Cases.
3. The Patient List dialog box is displayed. This dialog box contains the names and chart numbers of all the established patients for the medical office.
4. Click the Close button to return to the main Medisoft window.
5. Again, click the menu name, Lists.
6. When the Lists menu is displayed, click Procedure/Payment/Adjustment Codes.
7. The list that appears contains the CPT codes and descriptions for the procedures that are most frequently used by this medical office. Scroll to the bottom of the list. Notice the list also contains a number of codes for accounting purposes, such as take back, withhold, adjustment, copayment, deductible, and payment codes.

8. Click the Close button to return to the main Medisoft window.
9. Using the skills you practiced in the steps above, access two more options from the Lists menu, Diagnosis Codes and Insurance Carriers. The Diagnosis List dialog box lists the ICD codes and descriptions of the diagnoses that are most frequently used by this medical office. The Insurance Carrier List dialog box displays a list of the carriers where most of this office's claims are filed.
10. When you are finished viewing the lists, return to the main Medisoft window.

The Activities Menu Other than the patients' personal and case information, much of the data necessary to create claims is entered through the Activities menu. Follow the steps below to view two options on the Activities menu:

1. Click Activities on the menu bar to display the Activities menu.

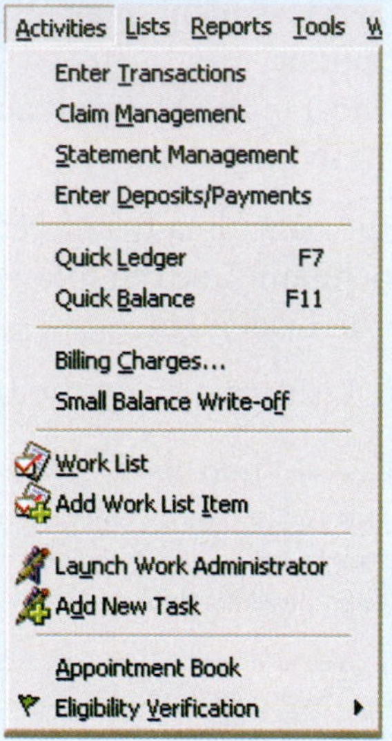

2. Click the first option, Enter Transactions.
3. The Transaction Entry dialog box is displayed. This dialog box is used to enter data about patient transactions and to record charges and payments.
4. Click the Close button.
5. Again, click the menu name, Activities.
6. When the Activities menu is displayed, click Claim Management.
7. The dialog box that appears is used to create claims and then print them or transmit them electronically.
8. Click the Close button.
9. You are returned to the main Medisoft window.

Entering Diagnosis and Transaction Data

This section provides practice in entering a sample patient's diagnosis and transaction information. The sample patient is Robin Caruthers, who has come to the office for a routine visit. Since Mrs. Caruthers is an established patient of the practice, the information on her patient information form has already been entered in the VAPC database. However, as the medical insurance specialist, you will need to enter the diagnosis and transactions for today's visit. After entering this information, you will create a claim.

Entering the Patient's Diagnosis After Mrs. Caruthers finishes her appointment with the doctor, she hands you the encounter form from the visit. Before you enter the transactions on the encounter form, you need to enter the diagnosis code listed on the form. In Medisoft, transactions must be linked to at least one diagnosis code. If they are not, the claim created for the transactions will be rejected by the insurance company.

The encounter form lists her diagnosis for today's visit as 427.41–Ventricular Fibrillation. Follow the steps below to enter this information in her Case dialog box in Medisoft.

1. To display Robin Caruthers' Case dialog box, click Patients/Guarantors and Cases on the Lists menu.
2. When the Patient List dialog box appears, click Caruthers, Robin to highlight the entry. Then click the line that reads Ventricular Fibrillation on the right side of the dialog box to select this case.
3. Click the Edit Case button. The nine tabs for this case appear.
4. Click the Diagnosis tab.
5. In the Default Diagnosis 1 box, key the first two numbers of the diagnosis code 427.41 to highlight the diagnosis code for Ventricular Fibrillation.

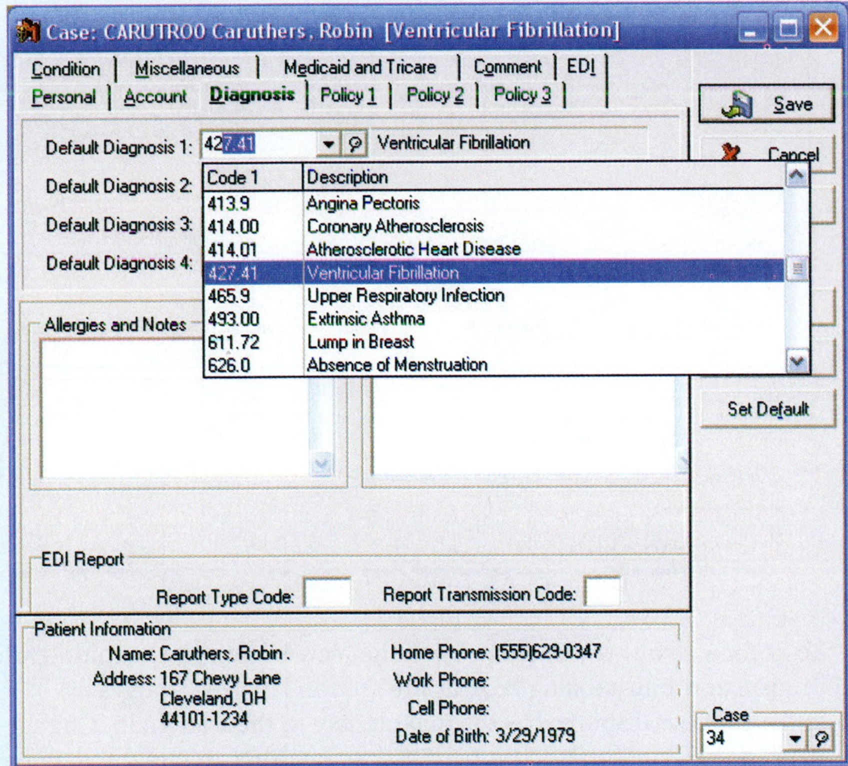

6. Press Enter to select this diagnosis.
7. If an encounter form had more than one diagnosis code indicated, the remaining codes would be entered in the Default Diagnosis 2, 3, and 4 boxes. Since this is the only diagnosis code indicated on the encounter form, click the Save button to save your work.
8. Click the Close button to exit the Patient List dialog box and return to the main Medisoft window.

Entering Transactions Now that Robin Caruthers' diagnosis code has been recorded, follow the steps below to enter the transactions for the visit. In looking at her encounter form, you find that procedure 99212 (Level II, Problem

Focused, established patient) is indicated. In addition to the encounter form, Mrs. Caruthers hands you a check for $20 because her PPO requires a $20 copay per visit. Therefore, you determine that there are two transactions to be recorded for Mrs. Caruthers' visit today—a procedural charge for the office visit and a check copayment.

1. On the Activities menu, select Enter Transactions to display the Transaction Entry dialog box.
2. Key "C" in the Chart box to locate the entry for Robin Caruthers, and then press the Enter key.
3. Notice that Robin Caruthers' current case (Ventricular Fibrillation) and insurance information, including her policy copayment requirement, are displayed in the top section of the Transaction Entry dialog box.

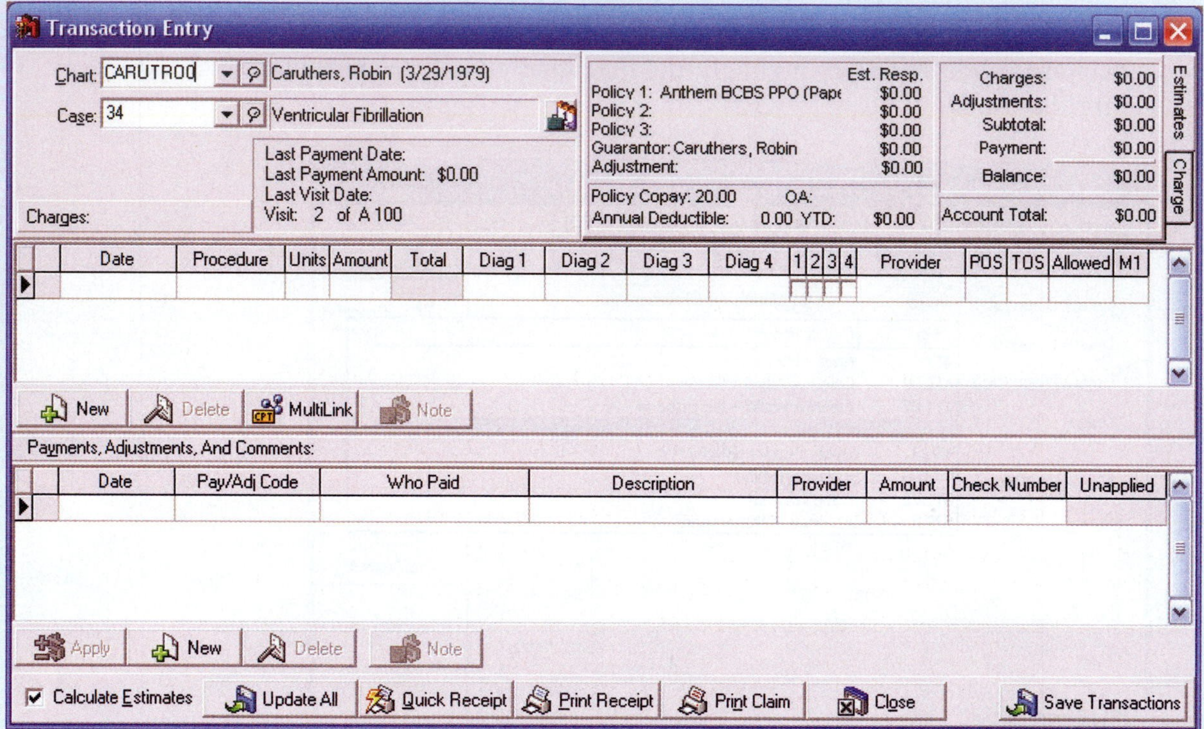

4. To enter a charge transaction, click the New button in the middle of the Transaction Entry dialog box, in the section labeled Charges.
5. Today's date is displayed as the default date in the Date field. Change the date in the Date box to 10/06/2008 (assume that this is the date of the visit on the encounter form) by clicking inside the Date box and then keying 10062008 over the current entry.
6. Press the Tab key to move to the Procedure field.
7. Click the Triangle button in the Procedure field. A drop-down list of procedure codes and descriptions is displayed.
8. To enter procedure code 99212, first key "9" in the Procedure box. Notice that the first code beginning with 9 is highlighted.
9. Key another 9, and then key the rest of the procedure code—212—and press the Tab key. Medisoft inserts the code in the Procedure box and displays the default unit of 1 in the Units box and the default amount of $46.00 in the Amount box. Notice that the diagnosis code entered earlier in the Case dialog box, 427.41, is also displayed.

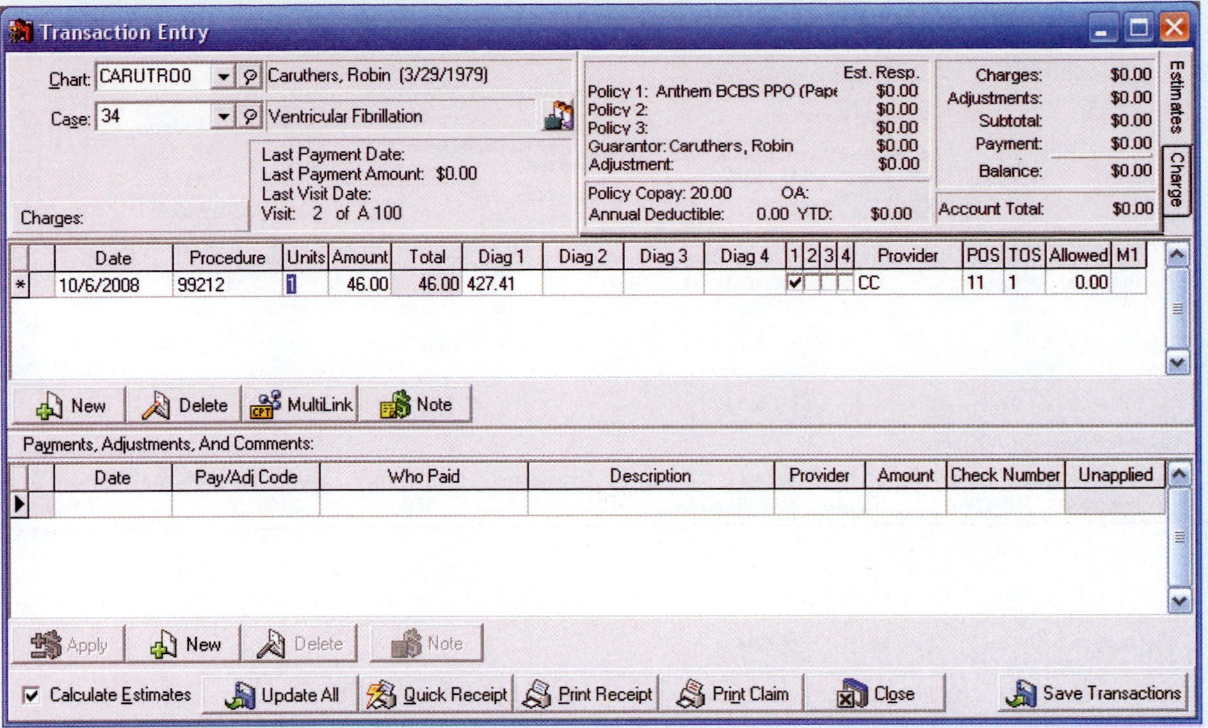

10. Now we will enter Mrs. Caruthers' payment. Payments are entered in the bottom section of the Transaction Entry dialog box. Click the New button in the Payments, Adjustments, and Comments section at the bottom of the dialog box. (An Information box is displayed to remind you that Robin Caruthers' insurance requires a $20.00 copayment for each visit. Click the OK button to continue.)
11. Click the New button again. Make sure the date in the Date box is still 10/06/2008. Press the Tab key twice to save the date entry and move to the Pay/Adj Code box.
12. Click the Triangle button in this box to display the list of payment codes and descriptions. Scroll through the list to locate the code for Mrs. Caruthers' copayment. (Notice, at the top of the Transaction Entry dialog box, that her insurance carrier is Anthem BCBS PPO. Therefore, you are looking for the copayment code for this carrier.) Click the code ANPCPAY for "Anthem BCBS PPO Copayment" to insert it in the Pay/Adj Code box, and then press the Tab key.
13. Medisoft inserts the code in the Pay/Adj Code box and displays the name of the guarantor in the Who Paid box, and the default amount of "–20.00" in the Amount box for this transaction. The minus sign indicates a payment rather than a charge. Notice the Unapplied box at the end of the transaction line also displays the amount of the payment.
14. Click inside the Check Number box, and then key 339 to record the number on Mrs. Caruthers' check (this step is optional). The dialog box should now look like this:

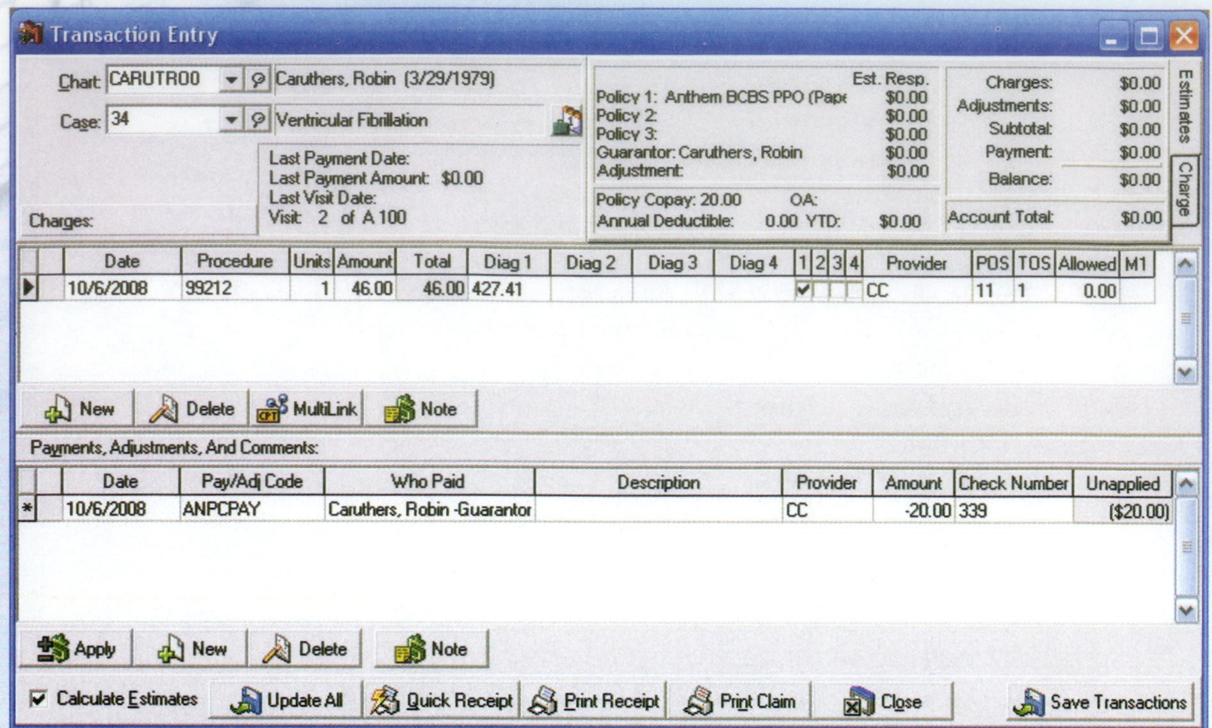

15. The last step in recording the payment is to apply the payment just entered to its corresponding charge. To do this, click the Apply button at the bottom of the Payments, Adjustments, and Comments section of the dialog box. (An Information box appears reminding you that the payment must be applied. Click the OK button to continue.)
16. Click the Apply button again. The Apply Payment to Charges dialog box appears. Click the white background of the This Payment box on the line with the office visit procedure charge (the only procedure charge in this case).
17. Key *20* and press Tab. The payment appears in the This Payment column and the Unapplied box in the upper right corner displays a zero amount. (If the box does not yet display zero, click anywhere in the white space underneath the This Payment column to update it.) The copayment has now been applied to the corresponding office visit charge. (*Note*: It is the standard procedure at Valley Associates, P.C., to apply a patient's copayment to the office visit charge ahead of any other charges.)

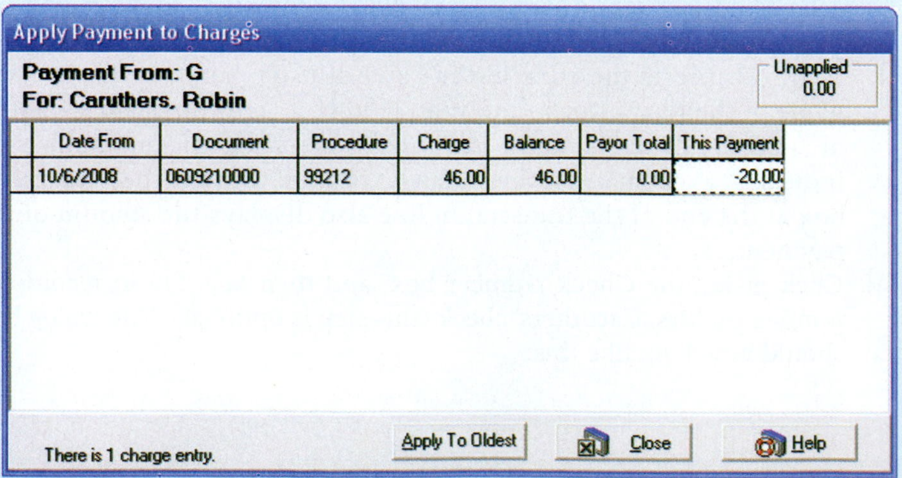

18. Click the Close button to close the Apply Payment to Charges dialog box and return to the Transaction Entry dialog box.
19. Notice the amount in the Unapplied box at the end of the transaction line is now $0.00. Click the Save Transactions button in the lower right corner of the Transaction Entry dialog box to save the information you have entered in the Transaction Entry dialog box.
20. Medisoft displays a Date of Service Validation box for each new transaction before it saves the transaction if the date of the transactions you are saving (10/06/2008) is later than the current date on your computer system. This box asks you to confirm that you want to save the transaction, even though it has a future date.

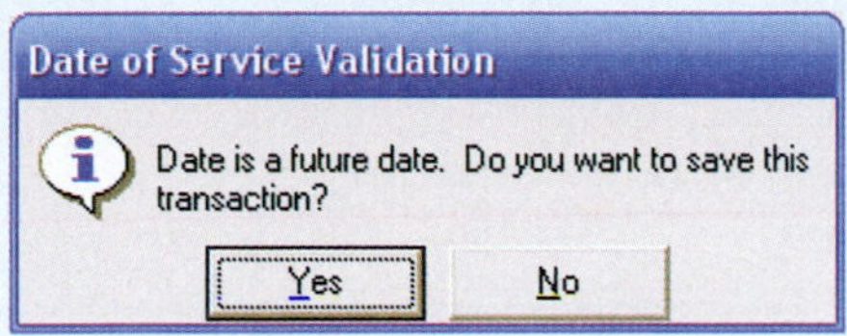

21. For the purposes of the claim cases in *Medical Insurance,* click Yes each time this box appears. In the present Transaction Entry screen, you will need to click Yes two times, as there are two new transactions.
22. Now that the transactions are saved, click the Close button to exit the Transaction Entry dialog box.

You have successfully recorded one charge and one payment for Mrs. Caruthers in the Transaction Entry dialog box.

TIP

Depending on a patient's insurance plan, it may not be necessary to enter a copayment for each visit. If a patient's insurance plan does not require a copayment, simply enter the procedure code(s) for the visit, and then save the transactions.

If you are unsure whether a copayment is required, check the patient's insurance information displayed in the top portion of the Transaction Entry dialog box.

Creating a Claim

Now that Mrs. Caruthers' diagnosis and transaction information for today's visit have been entered in the database, a claim can be created for them.

1. Open the Activities menu, and click Claim Management to display the Claim Management dialog box.
2. Claims that have already been created are listed in this dialog box.
3. Depending on the setting in the Sort By box at the top of the dialog box, the claims will be listed either according to the date they were created, by batch number, or by claim number. For the claim cases in this text, the Sort By box at the top of the dialog box should be set to Claim Number. If it is not, click the triangle button inside the Sort By box to display the list of sorting options, and then click Claim Number.
4. To create a new claim, click the Create Claims button.
5. The Create Claims dialog box appears. This dialog box is used to set the range of claims you want to create. You may create claims for a certain date or range of dates, for a particular chart number or range of chart numbers, and so on.
6. In this instance, you are creating a claim for one chart number. Therefore, in the first Chart Numbers range box, to select Robin Caruthers' chart number, key "C" and then press Enter.
7. Press Tab to get to the second Chart Numbers box. Key "C" again and press Enter. Leave the other boxes blank. (*Note:* If you were creating claims for all the patients' transactions during the day, you would enter today's date in the Transaction Dates boxes and leave the Chart Numbers boxes blank to select all chart numbers for that day.)

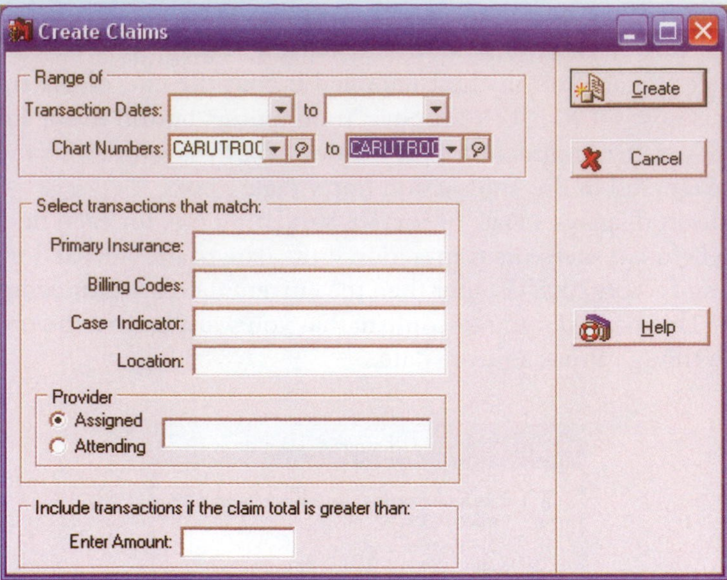

8. To create the claim for the transactions indicated, click the Create button.
9. The Create Claim dialog box closes, and you are returned to the Claim Management dialog box.

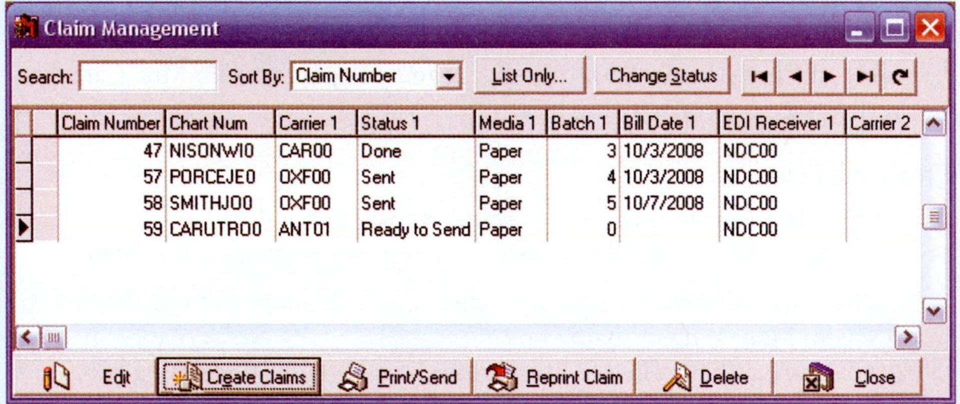

10. Notice that the claim for Robin Caruthers is added to the list of created claims in the Claim Management dialog box (Claim Number 59 in this case). The Status 1 column in the Claim Management dialog box indicates that the claim is "Ready to Send," and the Media 1 column indicates that the claim will be sent as a paper claim. Note that Medisoft assigns numbers to claims based on the order in which the claims are created. Claim numbers will therefore vary with each user.
11. Leave the Claim Management dialog box open for now, as you will use it to print Robin Caruthers' claim in the next section.

Printing a Claim

In Medisoft, claims can be transmitted to insurance carriers electronically or on paper. In most medical offices today, claims are transmitted electronically rather than printed out and mailed, since electronic claims are faster and more cost efficient to process. When a claim is sent electronically, there is no paper claim to refer to. The claim itself is in the form of an electronic file that is sent (for example, over a high-speed cable line) from your computer to a computer at the clearinghouse or office of the payer. The only paper produced is an optional claim verification report that contains the main details of the claim.

Although it is more efficient to send claims electronically in an office setting, for the purposes of the claims created in this text, the program has been set up to prepare claims on paper. (Each insurance carrier's default billing method has been set to Paper rather than Electronic.) With the program set up to produce paper claims, you will be able to check the results of each claim you create. The following instructions take you through the steps of printing Robin Caruthers' claim as an example.

1. Click Robin Caruthers' claim in the Claim Management dialog box to highlight it if it is not already highlighted.

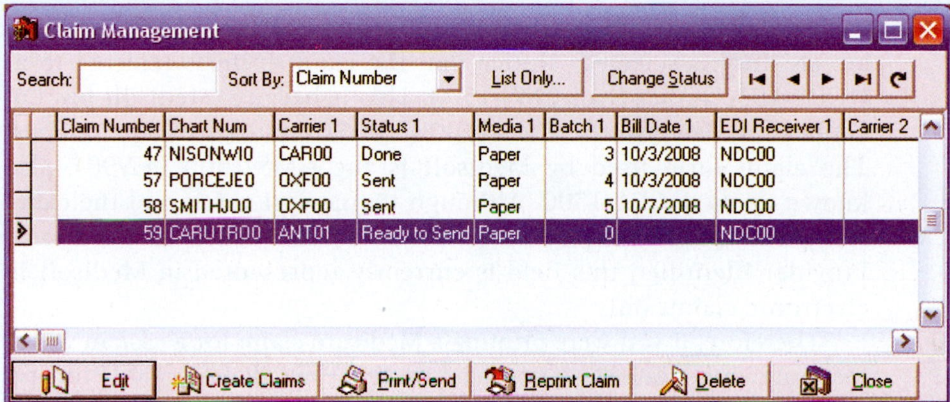

2. To print the claim, click the Print/Send button.
3. The Print/Send Claims dialog box appears.

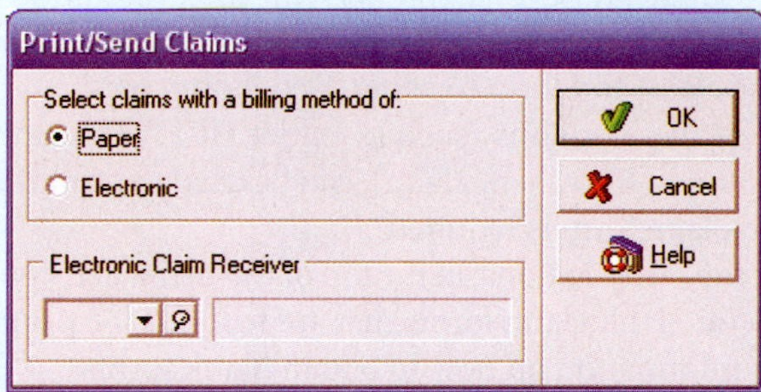

4. Notice the Paper radio button is already selected. (If Robin Caruthers' insurance carrier was set up in the database to receive claims electronically, the Electronic radio button would be selected at this point, and a series of dialog boxes would display leading up to an electronic transmission. In this case, the Paper radio button is used, and a series of dialog boxes will display leading up to the Print dialog box.) Click the OK button to continue.
5. After a moment, the Open Report dialog box appears.

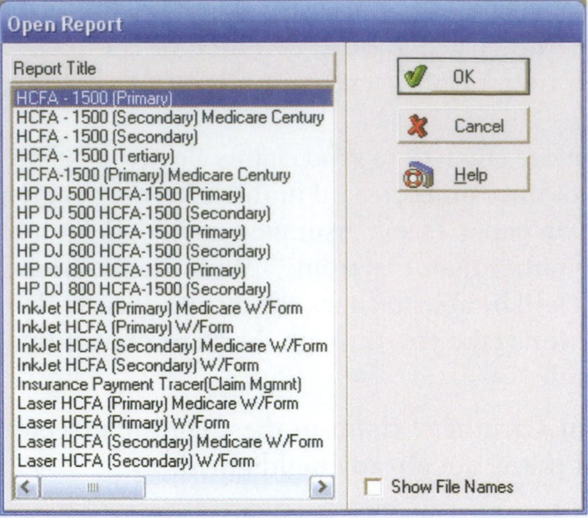
Open Report

Report Title
HCFA - 1500 (Primary)
HCFA - 1500 (Secondary) Medicare Century
HCFA - 1500 (Secondary)
HCFA - 1500 (Tertiary)
HCFA-1500 (Primary) Medicare Century
HP DJ 500 HCFA-1500 (Primary)
HP DJ 500 HCFA-1500 (Secondary)
HP DJ 600 HCFA-1500 (Primary)
HP DJ 600 HCFA-1500 (Secondary)
HP DJ 800 HCFA-1500 (Primary)
HP DJ 800 HCFA-1500 (Secondary)
InkJet HCFA (Primary) Medicare W/Form
InkJet HCFA (Primary) W/Form
InkJet HCFA (Secondary) Medicare W/Form
InkJet HCFA (Secondary) W/Form
Insurance Payment Tracer(Claim Mgmnt)
Laser HCFA (Primary) Medicare W/Form
Laser HCFA (Primary) W/Form
Laser HCFA (Secondary) Medicare W/Form
Laser HCFA (Secondary) W/Form

OK
Cancel
Help
Show File Names

TIP
Blank claim forms for use with Medisoft can be printed out from the Student Data Template CD-ROM. Be sure to select the file "Medisoft claim form.pdf."
When printing the form in Adobe Reader, select the Page Scaling option in the Print menu that produces the largest form—in this case, usually the option "None"—so that the form fills the full page when printed. This is the size the Medisoft program uses.

6. In this dialog box, the appropriate claim form for the type of claim you are creating is selected. Notice that the claim form is referred to as HCFA-1500 rather than CMS-1500. This is because Medisoft has not yet been updated to the CMS-1500 (08/05) version for paper claims. The claim form used by Medisoft is the CMS-1500 (12/90), also known as the HCFA-1500. Although the newest version of the claim form, the CMS-1500 (08/05), allows for the use of the National Provider Identifier, this field is currently represented in Medisoft in electronic claims only.

   Therefore, if you were printing a Medicare claim for a case in which Medicare is the primary carrier, you would select HCFA-1500 (Primary) Medicare Century to select the correct printing format for a Medicare primary claim in Medisoft. In our example, Robin Caruthers' primary insurance carrier is Anthem BCBS PPO, so the HCFA-1500 (Primary) option at the top of the list would be selected—the form used for a commercial claim.

   Note also, at the bottom of the list of claim formats in the Open Report dialog box, there are several options with the description "W/Form." The InkJet HCFA W/Form and the Laser HCFA W/Form options are designed to print the claim and form together. Depending on the type of printer you have, one of these options (such as InkJet HCFA Primary W/Form in the case of the Robin Caruthers' claim), can be used to print the claim on blank paper—no claim form is required.

   Select the other options, at the top of the list, when you are printing the claim data on blank claim forms that are fed into the printer (see the margin tip for information on how to obtain blank forms).

   Now that you are familiar with the options in the Open Report dialog box, click the option that is most suitable for your printer and the type of claim you are creating, and then click the OK button.
7. The Print Report Where? dialog box appears, asking if you want to preview the report, or if you want the claim sent directly to the printer or exported to a file. Click the preview option, and then click Start.
8. After a few seconds, the Data Selection Questions dialog box is displayed. To select Robin Caruthers' claim, key "C" in the first Chart Number Range box, and press Enter. Then tab once to get to the second Chart Number Range box. Key "C" again, and press Enter. Then click the OK button.

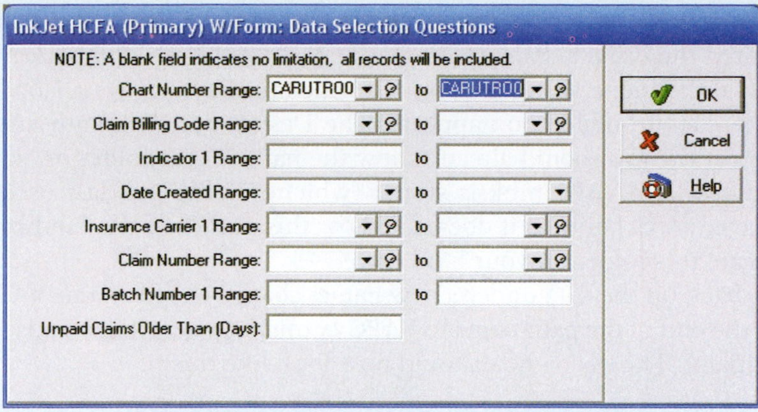

9. The claim is displayed in the Preview Report window. Click the printer icon at the top of the window to send the claim to the printer.
10. A Print dialog box displays. Click OK to continue.
11. After a few seconds, the claim is printed. Click the Close button when you are finished to exit the Print Preview window.
12. If you printed the claim, notice that the Status column for Robin Caruthers' claim in the Claim Management dialog box now reads Sent instead of Ready to Send. (If you previewed the claim but never printed it, the Status column will still read Ready to Send because the claim has not actually been printed yet.)
13. Click the Close button to exit the Claim Management dialog box. You have successfully printed the claim form for Robin Caruthers.

Backing Up Data While Exiting Medisoft

When entering data in Medisoft, it is important to back up your work regularly for safekeeping. A backup copy of the database files prevents you from losing your work if the hard drive fails, or if you accidentally delete data while working. If you are working in an instructional environment where you share computers, it is essential that you back up your work on exiting the program and then restore it at the beginning of the next session to be sure you are working with your own data. For practice in backing up, follow these steps to backup the data entered during this practice session.

1. In Medisoft, you can back up your data at any time using the Backup option on the File menu. However, by default, Medisoft also gives you the option to back up your data each time you exit the program. Click the Exit option on the File menu to exit Medisoft.
2. The Backup Reminder dialog box appears.

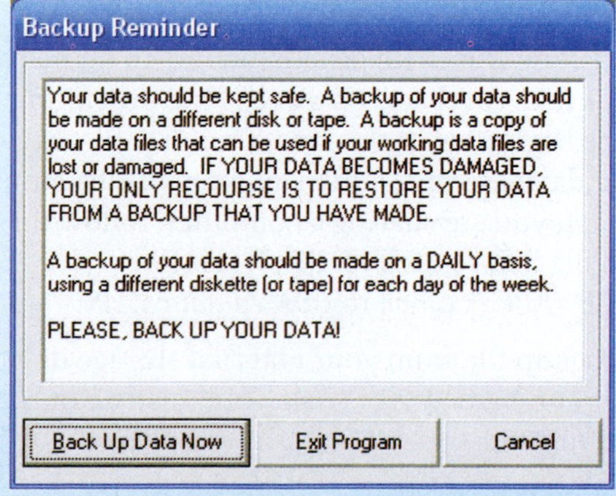

3. You will back up your data to the folder on your hard drive where you stored the original backup file, VAPC.mbk, only you will back it up under a new name, using your initials. Click the Back Up Data Now button.
4. The Backup dialog box appears. The Destination File Path and Name box at the top should already show the name of the folder on your hard drive where VAPC.mbk is stored (whichever file was last used is displayed by default). If it does not show this path, use the Find button to locate this folder on your hard drive.
5. To back up the data under a new name, change the file name VAPC.mbk at the end of the path name to ***VAPCxxx.mbk*** (where xxx stands for your initials). The dialog box should now look like this:

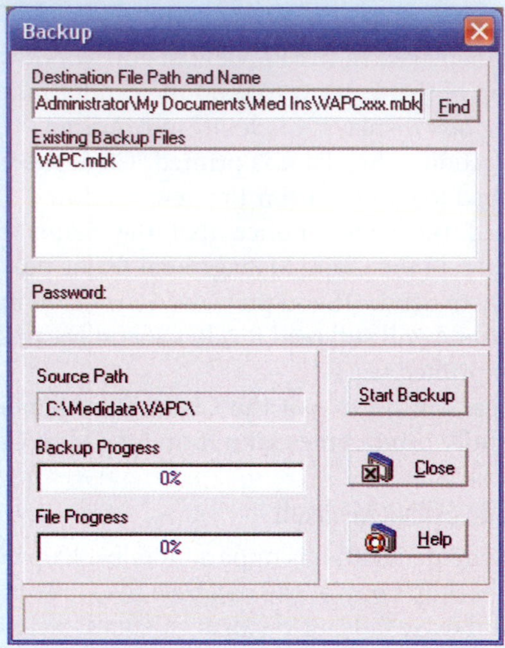

6. Click the Start Backup button.
7. Medisoft backs up the data under the new name and displays an Information box indicating that the backup is complete.
8. Click the OK button to close the Information dialog box and exit the Medisoft program.
9. For safekeeping, copy your new backup file from your hard drive to an external storage device, such as a flash drive or a CD-ROM. A separate backup copy prevents you from losing your work if the hard drive fails or if you or someone else accidentally deletes data on the computer.

Restoring a Backup File

If you are sharing a computer with other students in an instructional environment, it is essential that you back up your work on exiting the program and then restore it at the beginning of the next session. This way if another user alters the data in the database in the interim, you will be sure you are working with your own data. If you are sharing a computer, follow these steps to restore your latest backup file before each Medisoft session.

To restore the file *VAPCxxx.mbk* to *C:\Medidata\VAPC:*

1. Copy your backup file from your external storage device to the assigned location on your hard drive. (Ask your instructor if you are not sure which folder this is.)

2. Hold down the F7 key, and start Medisoft by clicking Start, All Programs, Medisoft, and Medisoft Advanced Patient Accounting. When the Find NDCMedisoft Database box appears, release the F7 key.
3. Enter ***C:\Medidata*** (where *C* is the letter that represents the hard drive you will be using), and click the OK button.
4. When the Open Practice dialog box appears, click on Valley Associates PC to select it (if it is not already selected), and then click OK.
5. Open the File menu, and click Restore Data.
6. When the Warning box appears, click OK. The Restore dialog box appears.
7. Use the Find button if necessary to locate your assigned storage folder on the hard drive (the folder used in step 1 above). Locate VAPCxxx.mbk in the list of existing backup files displayed for that folder, and click on it to attach it to the Backup File Path and Name at the top of the dialog box. The end of the path name should read \ . . . \VAPCxxx.mbk.
8. The Destination Path at the bottom of the box should already be C:\Medidata\VAPC. Leave this as it is. The dialog box should now look like this:

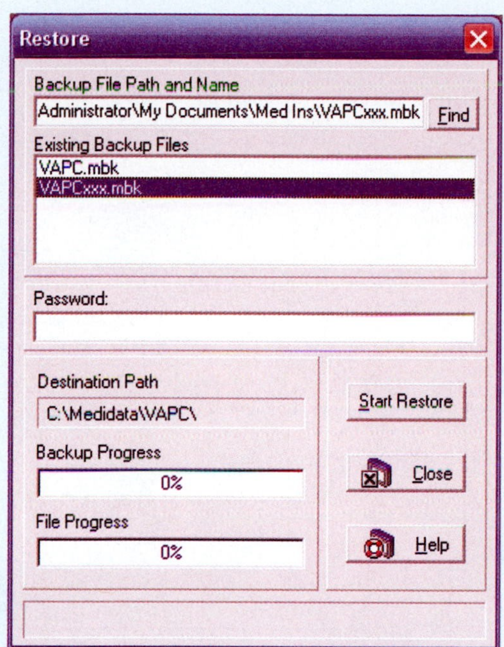

9. Click the Start Restore button.
10. When the Confirm box appears, click OK.
11. An Information box appears indicating that the restore is complete. Click OK to continue.
12. The Restore dialog box disappears. You are ready to begin the new session.

APPENDIX A

Medical Specialties and Taxonomy Codes

This table lists the medical specialties and taxonomy codes for allopathic and osteopathic physicians. The *Health Care Provider Taxonomy* (Washington Publishing Company/NUCC) contains codes for many other categories of providers, such as behavioral, chiropractic providers, and facilities. The Provider Taxonomy Code List is published (released) twice a year on July 1st and January 1st. The July publication is effective for use on October 1st and the January publication is effective for use on April 1st.

Code	*Definition.*
193200000X	Multi-Specialty: A business group of one or more individual practitioners, who practice with different areas of specialization.
193400000X	Single Specialty: A business group of one or more individual practitioners, all of whom practice with the same area of specialization.
207K00000X	Allergy & Immunology
207KA0200X	Allergy
207K10005X	Clinical & Laboratory Immunology
207L00000X	Anesthesiology
207LA0401X	Addiction Medicine
207LC0200X	Critical Care Medicine
207LP2900X	Pain Medicine
207LP3000X	Pediatric Anesthesiology
208U00000X	Clinical Pharmacology
208C00000X	Colon & Rectal Surgery
207N00000X	Dermatology
207NI0002X	Clinical & Laboratory Dermatological Immunology
207NS0135X	Dermatological Surgery
207ND0900X	Dermatopathology
207ND0101X	MOHS-Micrographic Surgery
207NP0225X	Pediatric Dermatology
207P00000X	Emergency Medicine
207PE0004X	Emergency Medical Services
207PT0002X	Medical Toxicology
207PP0204X	Pediatric Emergency Medicine
207PS0010X	Sports Medicine
207PE0005X	Undersea & Hyperbaric Medicine
207Q00000X	Family Practice
207QA0401X	Addiction Medicine
207QA0000X	Adolescent Medicine
207QA0505X	Adult Medicine
207QG0300X	Geriatric Medicine
207QS0010X	Sports Medicine

Code	*Definition.*
208D00000X	General Practice
208M00000X	Hospitalist
207R00000X	Internal Medicine
207RA0401X	Addiction Medicine
207RA0000X	Adolescent Medicine
207RA0201X	Allergy & Immunology
207RC0000X	Cardiovascular Disease
207RI0001X	Clinical & Laboratory Immunology
207RC0001X	Clinical Cardiac Electrophysiology
207RC0200X	Critical Care Medicine
207RE0101X	Endocrinology, Diabetes, & Metabolism
207RG0100X	Gastroenterology
207RG0300X	Geriatric Medicine
207RH0000X	Hematology
207RH0003X	Hematology & Oncology
207RI0008X	Hepatology
207RI0200X	Infectious Disease
207RI0011X	Interventional Cardiology
207RM1200X	Magnetic Resonance Imaging (MRI)
207RX0202X	Medical Oncology
207RN0300X	Nephrology
207RP1001X	Pulmonary Disease
207RR0500X	Rheumatology
207RS0012X	Sleep Medicine
207RS0010X	Sports Medicine
209800000X	Legal Medicine
	Medical Genetics
207SG0202X	Clinical Biochemical Genetics
207SC0300X	Clinical Cytogenetics
207SG0201X	Clinical Genetics (MD)
207SG0203X	Clinical Molecular Genetics
207SM0001X	Molecular Genetic Pathology
207SG0205X	Ph.D. Medical Genetics
207T00000X	Neurological Surgery
204D00000X	Neuromusculoskeletal Medicine & OMM
204C00000X	Neuromusculoskeletal Medicine, Sports Medicine
207U00000X	Nuclear Medicine
207UN0903X	In Vivo & In Vitro Nuclear Medicine
207UN0901X	Nuclear Cardiology
207UN0902X	Nuclear Imaging & Therapy
207V00000X	Obstetrics & Gynecology
207VC0200X	Critical Care Medicine
207VX0201X	Gynecological Oncology
207VG0400X	Gynecology
207VM0101X	Maternal & Fetal Medicine
207VX0000X	Obstetrics
207VE0102X	Reproductive Endocrinology
207W00000X	Ophthalmology
204E00000X	Oral & Maxillofacial Surgery
207X00000X	Orthopaedic Surgery
207XS0114X	Adult Reconstructive Orthopaedic Surgery

Code	*Definition.*
207XX0004X	Foot & Ankle Orthopaedics
207XS0106X	Hand Surgery
207XS0117X	Orthopaedic Surgery of the Spine
207XX0801X	Orthopaedic Trauma
207XP3100X	Pediatric Orthopaedic Surgery
207XX0005X	Sports Medicine
207Y00000X	Otolaryngology
207YS0123X	Facial Plastic Surgery
207YX0602X	Otolaryngic Allergy
207YX0905X	Otolaryngology/Facial Plastic Surgery
207YX0901X	Otology & Neurotology
207YP0228X	Pediatric Otolaryngology
207YX0007X	Plastic Surgery within the Head & Neck
207YS00112X	Sleep Medicine
	Pain Medicine
208VP0014X	Interventional Pain Medicine
208VP0000X	Pain Management
	Pathology
207ZP0101X	Anatomic Pathology
207ZP0102X	Anatomic Pathology & Clinical Pathology
207ZB0001X	Blood Banking & Transfusion Medicine
207ZP0104X	Chemical Pathology
207ZP0105X	Clinical Pathology/Laboratory Medicine
207ZC0500X	Cytopathology
207ZD0900X	Dermatopathology
207ZF0201X	Forensic Pathology
207ZH0000X	Hematology
207ZI0100X	Immunopathology
207ZM0300X	Medical Microbiology
207ZP0007X	Molecular Genetic Pathology
207ZN0500X	Neuropathology
207ZP0213X	Pediatric Pathology
208000000X	Pediatrics
2080A0000X	Adolescent Medicine
2080I0007X	Clinical & Laboratory Immunology
2080P0006X	Developmental—Behavioral Pediatrics
2080T0002X	Medical Toxicology
2080N001X	Neonatal—Perinatal Medicine
2080P0008X	Neurodevelopmental Disabilities
2080P0201X	Pediatric Allergy & Immunology
2080P0202X	Pediatric Cardiology
2080P0203X	Pediatric Critical Care Medicine
2080P0204X	Pediatric Emergency Medicine
2080P0205X	Pediatric Endocrinology
2080P0206X	Pediatric Gastroenterology
2080P0207X	Pediatric Hematology—Oncology
2080P0208X	Pediatric Infectious Diseases
2080P0210X	Pediatric Nephrology
2080P0214X	Pediatric Pulmonology
2080P0216X	Pediatric Rheumatology
2080S0012X	Sleep Medicine
2080S0010X	Sports Medicine

Code	*Definition.*
208100000X	Physical Medicine & Rehabilitation
2081P2900X	Pain Medicine
2081P0010X	Pediatric Rehabilitation Medicine
2081P0004X	Spinal Cord Injury Medicine
2081S0010X	Sports Medicine
208200000X	Plastic Surgery
2082S0099X	Plastic Surgery Within the Head & Neck
2082S0105X	Surgery of the Hand
	Preventive Medicine
2083A0100X	Aerospace Medicine
2083T0002X	Medical Toxicology
2083X0100X	Occupational Medicine
2083P0500X	Preventive Medicine/Occupational Environmental-Medicine
2083P0901X	Public Health & General Preventive Medicine
2083S0010X	Sports Medicine
2083P0011X	Undersea and Hyperbaric Medicine
	Psychiatry & Neurology
2084A0401X	Addiction Medicine
2084P0802X	Addiction Psychiatry
2084P0804X	Child & Adolescent Psychiatry
2084N0600X	Clinical Neurophysiology
2084F0202X	Forensic Psychiatry
2084P0805X	Geriatric Psychiatry
2084P0005X	Neurodevelopmental Disabilities
2084N0400X	Neurology
2084N0402X	Neurology with Special Qualifications in Child Neurology
2084P2900X	Pain Medicine
2084P0800X	Psychiatry
2084S0012X	Sleep Medicine
2084S0010X	Sports Medicine
2084V0102X	Vascular Neurology
	Radiology
2085B0100X	Body Imaging
2085R0202X	Diagnostic Radiology
2085U0001X	Diagnostic Ultrasound
2085N0700X	Neuroradiology
2085N0904X	Nuclear Radiology
2085P0229X	Pediatric Radiology
2085R0001X	Radiation Oncology
2085R0205X	Radiological Physics
2085R0203X	Therapeutic Radiology
2085R0204X	Vascular & Interventional Radiology
208600000X	Surgery
2086S0120X	Pediatric Surgery
2086S0122X	Plastic & Reconstructive Surgery
2086S0105X	Surgery of the Hand
2086S0102X	Surgical Critical Care
2086X0206X	Surgical Oncology

Code	*Definition.*
2086S0127X	Trauma Surgery
2086S0129X	Vascular Surgery
208G00000X	Thoracic Surgery (Cardiothoracic Vascular Surgery)
204F00000X	Transplant Surgery
208800000X	Urology
2088PO231X	Pediatric Urology

APPENDIX B

Place of Service Codes

Codes designated as F are facility codes; those with NF are nonfacility physician practice codes. The rate calculations for nonfacility locations take into account the higher overhead expenses such as the cost of clinical staff, supplies, and equipment, collectively called practice expense, generally borne by providers in these settings. The facility rates paid to providers usually are lower because the hospital/facility is reimbursed separately for overhead costs associated with patient care.

01	pharmacy	NF
03	school	NF
04	homeless shelter	NF
05	Indian Health Service freestanding facility	
06	Indian Health Service provider-based facility	
07	Tribal 638 freestanding facility	
08	Tribal 638 provider-based facility	
09	prison/correctional facility	NF
11	office	NF
12	home	NF
13	assisted living facility	NF
14	group home	NF
15	mobile unit	NF
20	urgent care facility	NF
21	inpatient hospital	F
22	outpatient hospital	F
23	emergency room, hospital	F
24	ambulatory surgical center F, or NF for payable procedures not on ASC list	
25	birthing center	NF
26	military treatment facility	F
31	skilled nursing facility	F
32	nursing facility	NF
33	custodial care facility	NF
34	hospice	F
41	ambulance, land	F
42	ambulance, air or water	F
49	independent clinic	NF
50	federally qualified health center	NF
51	inpatient psychiatric facility	F
52	psychiatric facility, partial hospitalization	F
53	community mental health center	F
54	intermediate care facility/mentally retarded	NF
55	residential substance abuse treatment facility	NF
56	psychiatric residential treatment center	F
57	nonresidential substance abuse treatment facility	NF

60	mass immunization center	NF
61	comprehensive inpatient rehabilitation facility	F
62	comprehensive outpatient rehabilitation facility	NF
65	end-stage renal disease treatment facility	NF
71	state or local public health clinic	NF
72	rural health clinic	NF
81	independent laboratory	NF
99	other place of service	NF

Appendix C

Professional Websites

Government Sites and Resources

CCI

The Medicare Correct Coding Initiative automated edits are online at
cms.hhs.gov/physicians/cciedits/default.asp

CMS

Coverage of the Centers for Medicare and Medicaid Services: Medicare, Medicaid, SCHIP, HIPAA, CLIA topics
www.cms.hhs.gov
Medicare Learning Network: cms.hhs.gov/mlngeninfo
Online Medicare manuals: cms.hhs.gov/manuals/IOM/list.asp
Medicare Physician Fee Schedule: cms.hhs.gov/PhysicianFeeSched

HCPCS

General information on HCPCS
www.cms.hhs.gov/MedHCPCSGenInfo
Annual alphanumeric Healthcare Common Procedure Coding System file
www.cms.hhs.gov/MedHCPCSReleaseCodeSets
SADMERC
www.palmettogba.com
Health Information Technology
The U.S. Department of Health & Human Services (HHS) website for health IT Initiatives.
hhs.gov/healthinformationtechnology

HIPAA

Home page
www.cms.hhs.gov/HIPAAGenInfo
Questions and Answers on HIPAA Privacy Policies
answers.hhs.gov
HIPAA Privacy Rule
"Standards for Privacy of Individually Identifiable Health Information; Final Rule." 45 CFR Parts 160 and 164. *Federal Register 65*, no. 250 (2000).
www.hss.gov/ocr/hipaa/finalreg.html

ICD

NCHS (National Center for Health Statistics) posts the ICD-9-CM addenda and guidelines
www.cdc.gov/nchs/icd9.htm

WHO The International Statistical Classification of Diseases and Related Health Problems, tenth revision. is posted on the World Health Organization site
www.who.int/whosis/icd10

NUBC

The National Uniform Billing Committee develops and maintains a standardized data set for use by institutional providers to transmit claim and encounter information. This group is in charge of the 837I and the CMS-1450 (UB 04) claim formats.
www.nubc.org

NUCC

The National Uniform Claim Committee develops and maintains a standardized data set for use by the non-institutional health care community to transmit claim and encounter information. This group is in charge of the 837P and the CMS-1500 claim formats.
www.nucc.org

OCR

The Office of Civil Rights of the HHS enforces the HIPAA Privacy Rule; Privacy Fact Sheets are online at
www.hhs.gov/ocr/hipaa

OIG

The Office of Inspector General of the HHA home page links to fraud and abuse, advisory opinions, exclusion list, and other topics
www.oig.hhs.gov
Model compliance programs are found at
oig.hhs.gov/fraud/complianceguidance.html

TRICARE and CHAMPVA

General TRICARE information
www.tricare.osd.mil
CHAMPVA Overview
www.va.gov/hac

WPC

Washington Publishing Company is the link for HIPAA Transaction and Code Sets implementation guides. It also assists in the maintenance and distribution of these HIPAA-related code lists:

- Provider Taxonomy Codes
- Claim Adjustment Reason Codes
- Claim Status Codes
- Claim Status Category Codes
- Health Care Services Decision Reason Codes
- Insurance Business Process Application Error Codes
- Remittance Remark Codes

www.wpc-edi.com

Billing and Insurance

BlueCross BlueShield Association
www.bluecares.com
The Kaiser Family Foundation Web site provides in-depth information on key health policy issues such as Medicaid, Medicare, and prescription drugs.
www.kff.org
Various sites, such as www.benefitnews.com, www.erisaclaim.com and www.erisa.com, cover EMTALA, ERISA regulations and updates concerning provider and patient appeals of managed care organizations.
State insurance commissioners
www.omc.state.ct.us

Electronic Medical Records

AHIMA Coverage of Related Topics Located Under the Practice Brief tab on the AHIMA Home Page:
www.ahima.org
Maintaining a Legally Sound Health Record
The Legal Process and Electronic Health Records
Implementing Electronic Signatures
HIM Practice Transformation/EHR's Impact on HIM Functions
Core Data Sets for the Physician Practice Electronic Health Record

Computer-based Patient Record Institute (CPRI)
www.cpri.org
Medical Record Institute
www.medrecinst.com

Associations

AAFP American Academy of Family Physicians
www.aafp.org
AAHAM American Association of Healthcare Administrative Management
www.aaham.org
AAMA American Association of Medical Assistants
www.aama-ntl.org
AAMT American Association for Medical Transcription (changing to Association for Integrity of Healthcare Documentation)
www.aamt.org
AAPC American Academy of Professional Coders
www.aapc.com
ACA International (formerly American Collectors Association)
www.acainternational.org
AHIP America's Health Plans
Links to Member Health Plans
www.ahip.org
ACHE American College of Healthcare Executives
www.ache.org
AHIMA American Health Information Management Association
www.ahima.org

AMB Association of Medical Billers
www.billers.com
AHLA American Health Lawyers Association
www.healthlawyers.org
AHA American Hospital Association
www.aha.org
AMA American Medical Association
www.ama-assn.org
AMT American Medical Technologists
www.amt1.com
ANA American Nursing Association
www.ana.org
HBMA Healthcare Billing and Management Association
www.hbma.com
HFMA Healthcare Financial Management Association
www.hfma.org
MGMA Medical Group Management Association
www.mgma.org
PAHCOM Professional Association of Health Care Office Management
www.pahcom.com

Selected Professional Coding Resources

Note that many commercial vendors of the annual coding books offer package prices for the year's CPT, ICD-9-CM, and HCPCS references. Professional organizations may also offer discounts.

American Academy of Professional Coders (AAPC)
309 West 700 South
Salt Lake City, UT 84101
800 626 CODE
www.aapc.com
Certification courses/examinations and coding-related publications

AHA Coding Clinic for ICD-9-CM
AHA Order Services
PO Box 92683
Chicago, IL 60675-2683
800 242 2626
www.ahaonlinestore.com
Official Coding Guidelines for ICD-9-CM

American Association of Health Information Management (AHIMA)
233 North Michigan Avenue, Suite 2150
Chicago, IL 60601-5800
312 233 1100
www.ahima.org
Certification courses/examinations and coding-related publications

AMA Press
PO Box 930884
Atlanta, GA 31193-0884
800 621 8335
www.amapress.com

Annual Editions of CPT, ICD, and HCPCS
www.ama-assn.org/go/CPT
CPT Assistant and CPT Clinical Examples

The Coding Institute
2272 Airport Road South
Naples, FL 34112
800 508 2582
www.codinginstitute.com
Coding resources in medical specialties; seminars

Coding Strategies, Inc.
5401 Dallas Hwy, Suite 606
Powder Springs, GA 30132
877 6 CODING
www.codingstrategies.com
Medical coding education and specialty publications

Conomikes Reports, Inc.
12233 W. Olympic Blvd., Suite 116
Los Angeles, CA 90064
800 421 6512
www.conomikes.com
Newsletters and handbooks

hcPro
200 Hoods Lane
Marblehead, MA 01945
800 650 6787
www.hcpro.com
Training materials and E-newsletters

Ingenix, Inc.
St. Anthony Publishing/Medicode
2525 Lake Park Blvd.
Salt Lake City, UT 84120
800 INGENIX
www.ingenix.com
Annual editions of ICD-9-CM, CPT, and HCPCS books; newsletters, and electronic reference manuals

MMHSI/Coders Central
800 253 4945
Online resource for coding reference books
www.coderscentral.com

Medical Management Institute
Campus Bookstore
11405 Old Roswell Road
Alpharetta, GA 30004
800 334 5725
www.CodingCourse.com
Annual editions of ICD-9-CM, CPT, and HCPCS books; seminars

NCHS
National Center for Health Statistics
3311 Toledo Road
Hyattsville, MD 20782-2064

301 458 4000
ICD-9-CM code set, addenda, and coding guidelines available for downloading
www.cdc.gov/nchs/icd9.htm

Practice Management Information Corp. (PMIC)
4727 Wilshire Boulevard
Los Angeles, CA 90010
800 MEDSHOP
www.medicalcodingbooks.com
Annual Editions of CPT, ICD-9-CM, and HCPCS Code Books; publications on practice management and coding reimbursement

www.icd9coding.com
Online Web site for ICD and DRG codes

UCG/DecisionHealth
11300 Rockville Pike, Suite 1100
Rockville, MD 20852
301 287 2700
www.decisionhealth.com
Newsletters, especially ICD-9/CPT Coding Pro and Specialty Coders' Pink Sheets; publications

United States Government Printing Office:
Federal Register
www.access.gpo.gov

APPENDIX D

Forms

CMS-1500 (08/05)

1500

HEALTH INSURANCE CLAIM FORM

APPROVED BY NATIONAL UNIFORM CLAIM COMMITTEE 08/05

PICA | PICA

CARRIER

1. MEDICARE (Medicare #) | MEDICAID (Medicaid #) | TRICARE CHAMPUS (Sponsor's SSN) | CHAMPVA (Member ID#) | GROUP HEALTH PLAN (SSN or ID) | FECA BLK LUNG (SSN) | OTHER (ID)

1a. INSURED'S I.D. NUMBER (For Program in Item 1)

2. PATIENT'S NAME (Last Name, First Name, Middle Initial)

3. PATIENT'S BIRTH DATE MM DD YY SEX M F

4. INSURED'S NAME (Last Name, First Name, Middle Initial)

5. PATIENT'S ADDRESS (No., Street)

6. PATIENT RELATIONSHIP TO INSURED Self Spouse Child Other

7. INSURED'S ADDRESS (No., Street)

CITY | STATE

8. PATIENT STATUS Single Married Other

CITY | STATE

ZIP CODE | TELEPHONE (Include Area Code) ( )

Employed | Full-Time Student | Part-Time Student

ZIP CODE | TELEPHONE (INCLUDE AREA CODE) ( )

9. OTHER INSURED'S NAME (Last Name, First Name, Middle Initial)

10. IS PATIENT'S CONDITION RELATED TO:

11. INSURED'S POLICY GROUP OR FECA NUMBER

a. OTHER INSURED'S POLICY OR GROUP NUMBER

a. EMPLOYMENT? (CURRENT OR PREVIOUS) YES NO

a. INSURED'S DATE OF BIRTH MM DD YY SEX M F

b. OTHER INSURED'S DATE OF BIRTH MM DD YY SEX M F

b. AUTO ACCIDENT? YES NO PLACE (State)

b. EMPLOYER'S NAME OR SCHOOL NAME

c. EMPLOYER'S NAME OR SCHOOL NAME

c. OTHER ACCIDENT? YES NO

c. INSURANCE PLAN NAME OR PROGRAM NAME

d. INSURANCE PLAN NAME OR PROGRAM NAME

10d. RESERVED FOR LOCAL USE

d. IS THERE ANOTHER HEALTH BENEFIT PLAN? YES NO *If yes*, return to and complete item 9 a-d.

PATIENT AND INSURED INFORMATION

READ BACK OF FORM BEFORE COMPLETING & SIGNING THIS FORM.

12. PATIENT'S OR AUTHORIZED PERSON'S SIGNATURE I authorize the release of any medical or other information necessary to process this claim. I also request payment of government benefits either to myself or to the party who accepts assignment below.

SIGNED ____________ DATE ____________

13. INSURED'S OR AUTHORIZED PERSON'S SIGNATURE I authorize payment of medical benefits to the undersigned physician or supplier for services described below.

SIGNED ____________

14. DATE OF CURRENT: MM DD YY ◀ ILLNESS (First symptom) OR INJURY (Accident) OR PREGNANCY(LMP)

15. IF PATIENT HAS HAD SAME OR SIMILAR ILLNESS. GIVE FIRST DATE MM DD YY

16. DATES PATIENT UNABLE TO WORK IN CURRENT OCCUPATION FROM MM DD YY TO MM DD YY

17. NAME OF REFERRING PHYSICIAN OR OTHER SOURCE

17a.

17b. NPI

18. HOSPITALIZATION DATES RELATED TO CURRENT SERVICES FROM MM DD YY TO MM DD YY

19. RESERVED FOR LOCAL USE

20. OUTSIDE LAB? YES NO $ CHARGES

21. DIAGNOSIS OR NATURE OF ILLNESS OR INJURY. (Relate Items 1,2,3 or 4 to Item 24e by Line)

1. ___ . ___ 3. ___ . ___

2. ___ . ___ 4. ___ . ___

22. MEDICAID RESUBMISSION CODE | ORIGINAL REF. NO.

23. PRIOR AUTHORIZATION NUMBER

	24. A. DATE(S) OF SERVICE From MM DD YY	To MM DD YY	B. PLACE OF SERVICE	C. EMG	D. PROCEDURES, SERVICES, OR SUPPLIES (Explain Unusual Circumstances) CPT/HCPCS MODIFIER	E. DIAGNOSIS POINTER	F. $ CHARGES	G. DAYS OR UNITS	H. EPSDT Family Plan	I. ID. QUAL.	J. RENDERING PROVIDER ID. #
1										NPI	
2										NPI	
3										NPI	
4										NPI	
5										NPI	
6										NPI	

25. FEDERAL TAX I.D. NUMBER SSN EIN

26. PATIENT'S ACCOUNT NO.

27. ACCEPT ASSIGNMENT? (For govt. claims, see back) YES NO

28. TOTAL CHARGE $

29. AMOUNT PAID $

30. BALANCE DUE $

31. SIGNATURE OF PHYSICIAN OR SUPPLIER INCLUDING DEGREES OR CREDENTIALS (I certify that the statements on the reverse apply to this bill and are made a part thereof.)

SIGNED DATE

32. SERVICE FACILITY LOCATION INFORMATION

a. NPI b.

33. BILLING PROVIDER INFO & PHONE # ( )

a. NPI b.

PHYSICIAN OR SUPPLIER INFORMATION

NUCC Instruction Manual available at: www.nucc.org

UB-04

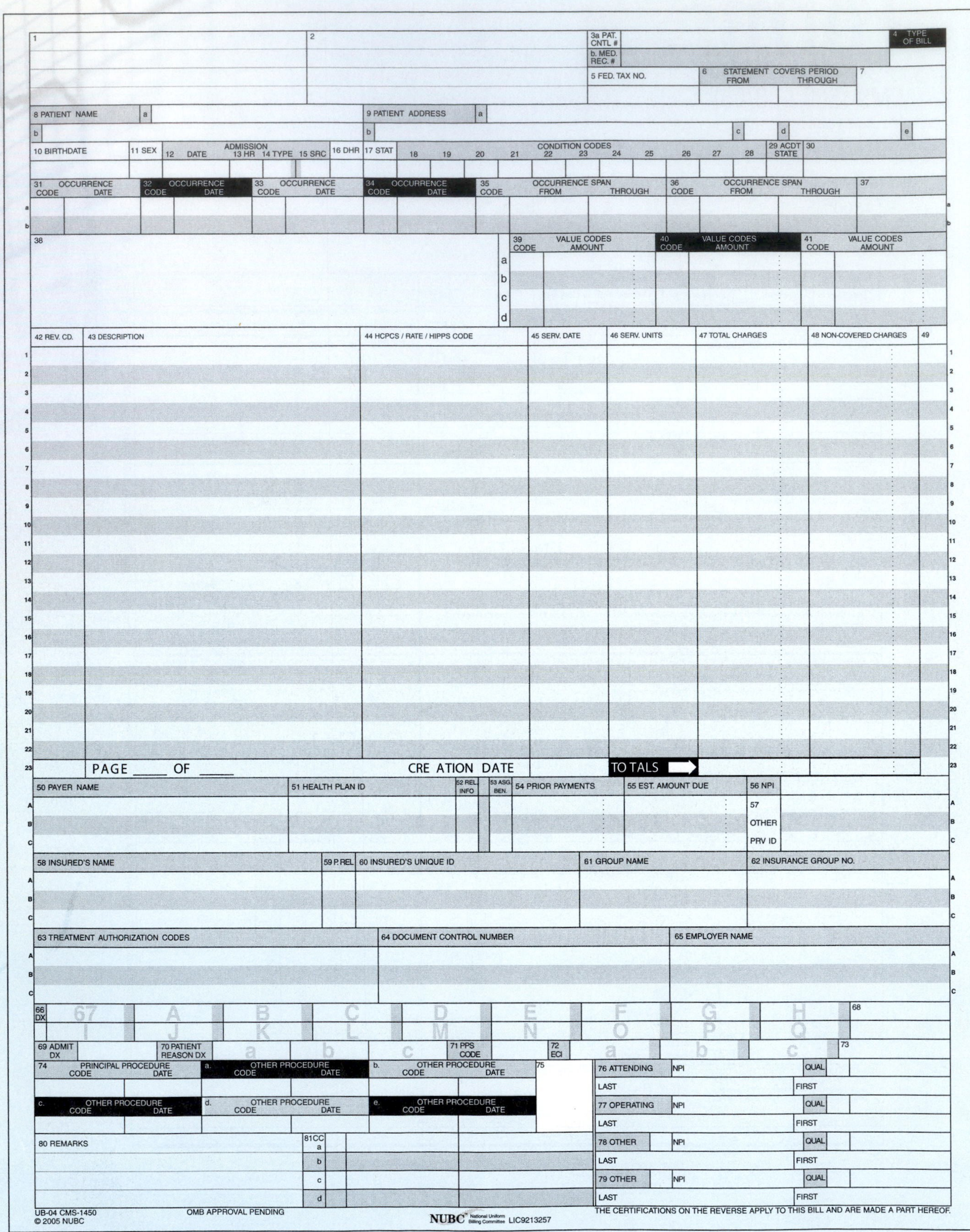

1
2
3a PAT. CNTL #
4 TYPE OF BILL
b. MED. REC. #
5 FED. TAX NO.
6 STATEMENT COVERS PERIOD FROM THROUGH
7
8 PATIENT NAME a
9 PATIENT ADDRESS a
b
b c d e
10 BIRTHDATE
11 SEX
ADMISSION 12 DATE 13 HR 14 TYPE 15 SRC
16 DHR
17 STAT
CONDITION CODES 18 19 20 21 22 23 24 25 26 27 28
29 ACDT STATE
30
31 OCCURRENCE CODE DATE
32 OCCURRENCE CODE DATE
33 OCCURRENCE CODE DATE
34 OCCURRENCE CODE DATE
35 OCCURRENCE SPAN CODE FROM THROUGH
36 OCCURRENCE SPAN CODE FROM THROUGH
37
a
b
38
39 VALUE CODES CODE AMOUNT
40 VALUE CODES CODE AMOUNT
41 VALUE CODES CODE AMOUNT
a
b
c
d
42 REV. CD.
43 DESCRIPTION
44 HCPCS / RATE / HIPPS CODE
45 SERV. DATE
46 SERV. UNITS
47 TOTAL CHARGES
48 NON-COVERED CHARGES
49
1 2 3 4 5 6 7 8 9 10 11 12 13 14 15 16 17 18 19 20 21 22
23 PAGE ____ OF ____ CREATION DATE TOTALS
50 PAYER NAME
51 HEALTH PLAN ID
52 REL. INFO
53 ASG. BEN.
54 PRIOR PAYMENTS
55 EST. AMOUNT DUE
56 NPI
57 OTHER PRV ID
A B C
58 INSURED'S NAME
59 P. REL
60 INSURED'S UNIQUE ID
61 GROUP NAME
62 INSURANCE GROUP NO.
A B C
63 TREATMENT AUTHORIZATION CODES
64 DOCUMENT CONTROL NUMBER
65 EMPLOYER NAME
A B C
66 DX
67 A B C D E F G H
I J K L M N O P Q
68
69 ADMIT DX
70 PATIENT REASON DX a b c
71 PPS CODE
72 ECI a b c
73
74 PRINCIPAL PROCEDURE CODE DATE
a. OTHER PROCEDURE CODE DATE
b. OTHER PROCEDURE CODE DATE
75
76 ATTENDING NPI QUAL
LAST FIRST
c. OTHER PROCEDURE CODE DATE
d. OTHER PROCEDURE CODE DATE
e. OTHER PROCEDURE CODE DATE
77 OPERATING NPI QUAL
LAST FIRST
80 REMARKS
81CC a b c d
78 OTHER NPI QUAL
LAST FIRST
79 OTHER NPI QUAL
LAST FIRST
UB-04 CMS-1450
© 2005 NUBC
OMB APPROVAL PENDING
NUBC National Uniform Billing Committee LIC9213257
THE CERTIFICATIONS ON THE REVERSE APPLY TO THIS BILL AND ARE MADE A PART HEREOF.

Abbreviations

AAMA	American Association of Medical Assistants
AAMT	American Association for Medical Transcription
AAPC	American Academy of Professional Coders
ABN	advance beneficiary notice
a.c.	before meals
adm	admitted
AHIMA	American Health Information Management Association
AMA	American Medical Association
AMT	American Medical Technologists
ANSI	American National Standards Institute
AP	anterior-posterior
APC	ambulatory patient classification
A/R	accounts receivable
ASC	ambulatory surgical center
ASU	ambulatory surgical unit
BCBS	Blue Cross and Blue Shield
b.i.d.	twice a day
BLK Lung	black lung
BMI	body mass index
BP	blood pressure
BUN	blood urea nitrogen
bx	biopsy
ca	cancer
C&S	culture and sensitivity
cc	cubic centimeter
CC	(1) physicians' records: chief complaint, (2) hospital documentation: comorbidities and complications
CCA	Certified Coding Associate
CCI	Correct Coding Initiative (national; Medicare)
CCS	Certified Coding Specialist
CCS-P	Certified Coding Specialist-Physician-Based
CCYY	year, indicates entry of four digits for the century (CC) and year (YY)
CE	covered entity
CHAMPUS	Civilian Health and Medical Program of the Uniformed Services, now TRICARE
CHAMPVA	Civilian Health and Medical Program of the Department of Veterans Affairs
CLIA	Clinical Laboratory Improvement Amendment
cm	centimeter
CMA	Certified Medical Assistant
CMS	Centers for Medicare and Medicaid Services
CNS	central nervous system
COB	coordination of benefits
COBRA	Consolidated Omnibus Budget Reconciliation Act of 1985
COP	conditions of participation
CPC	Certified Professional Coder
CPC-H	Certified Professional Coder-Hospital Outpatient Facility
CPE	complete physical exam
CPT	*Current Procedural Terminology*
CSRS	Civil Service Retirement System
CV	cardiovascular
D&C	dilation and curettage
DD	day, indicates entry of two digits for the day
DEERS	Defense Enrollment Eligibility Reporting System
DME	durable medical equipment
DOB	date of birth
DOS	date of service
DPT	diphtheria, pertussis, and tetanus
DRG	diagnosis-related group
DRS	designated record set
dx	diagnosis
EDI	electronic data interchange
EEG	electroencephalogram
EENT	eyes, ears, nose, and throat
EFT	electronic funds transfer
EIN	Employee Identification Number
EKG	electrocardiogram
EMC	electronic media claim
E/M code	Evaluation and Management code
EMG	emergency
EMR	electronic medical record
ENMT	ears, nose, mouth, and throat
ENT	ears, nose, and throat
EOB	explanation of benefits
EOC	episode of care
EP	established patient
EPSDT	Early and Periodic Screening, Diagnosis, and Treatment
ER	emergency room
ERISA	Employee Retirement Income Security Act of 1974
ETOH	alcohol
F	female
FECA	Federal Employee Compensation Act
FEHBP	Federal Employees Health Benefits Program
FERS	Federal Employees Retirement System
FH	family history
FI	fiscal intermediary
FICA	Federal Insurance Contribution Act
FMAP	Federal Medicaid Assistance Percentage
F/U	follow-up
FUO	fever, unknown origin
Fx	fracture
g, gm	gram
GI	gastrointestinal
GPCI	geographic practice cost index
gr	grain
GTIN	Global Trade Item Number
GU	genitourinary
GYN	gynecologic, gynecologist
h	hour
H&P	history and physical
HBA	health benefits adviser
HCFA	Health Care Financing Administration, currently CMS
HCPCS	Healthcare Common Procedure Coding System
HEDIS	Health Employer Data and Information Set
HEENT	head, eyes, ears, nose, and throat
HGB	hemoglobin

HHA	home health agency
HHS	Department of Health and Human Services
HiB	hemophilus influenza type B vaccine
HIM	health information management
HIPAA	Health Insurance Portability and Accountability Act
HMO	health maintenance organization
HPI	history of present illness
HS	hour of sleep
hx	history
I&D	incision and drainage
ID, I.D.	identification
ID #, I.D. #	identification number
ICD-9-CM	*International Classification of Diseases*, Ninth Revision, *Clinical Modification*
ICU	intensive care unit
IM	intramuscular
INFO	information
IPA	individual practice association
IV	intravenous
JCAHO	Joint Commission on Accreditation of Healthcare Organizations
kg	kilogram
L	liter
LCD	local coverage determination
LLQ	left lower quadrant
LMP	last menstrual period
LPN	licensed practical nurse
LUQ	left upper quadrant
m	meter
M	male
MA	medical assistant
mcg	microgram
MCM	Medicare Carriers Manual
MCO	managed care organization
MD	medical doctor
mEq	milliequivalent
MFS	Medicare Fee Schedule
mg	milligram
mL	milliliter
mm	millimeter
MM	month, indicates entry of two digits for the month
MMA	Medicare Modernization Act
MMR	measles, mumps, and rubella
MRN	Medicare Remittance Notice, Medicare Redetermination Notice
MS	musculoskeletal
MSA	Medicare Savings Account
MSN	Medicare Summary Notice
MTF	Military Treatment Facility
MTS	Medicare Transaction System
NCCI	National Correct Coding Initiative
NCQA	National Committee for Quality Assurance
NDC	National Drug Codes
NEC	not elsewhere classified
NEMB	notice of exclusion from Medicare benefits
Neuro	neurologic, neurological
NO.	number
nonPAR	nonparticipating
NOS	not otherwise specified
NP	(1) new patient, (2) nurse-practitioner
NPI	National Provider Identifier
n.p.o.	nothing per os (by mouth)
NPP	Notice of Privacy Practices
NUCC	National Uniform Claim Committee
OB	obstetrics
OCR	Office of Civil Rights
OIG	Office of the Inspector General
OMB	Office of Management and Budget
op	operative
opt	optional
OSHA	Occupational Safety and Health Administration
OV	office visit
OWCP	Office of Workers' Compensation Programs
OZ	product number, Health Care Uniform Code Council
PA	physician's assistant
P&A	percussion and auscultation
p.c.	after meals
PCM	Primary Care Manager (TRICARE)
PCP	primary care physician/provider
PE	physical exam
PECOS	Provider Enrollment Chain and Ownership System
PH #	phone number
PHI	protected health information
PIN	provider identifier number
PMH	past medical history
PMPM	per member per month
po	postoperative
p.o.	per os (by mouth)
POS	place of service
PPD	purified protein derivative of tuberculin test
PPO	preferred provider organization
PPS	Prospective Payment System
p.r.n.	as desired or as needed
PSA	prostate-specific antigen
PSO	provider-sponsored organization
psych	psychiatric
pt	patient
q.	every
q.d.	every day
q.h.	every hour
q.i.d.	four times a day
q.o.d.	every other day
QIO	quality improvement organization
q.2h.	every two hours
QUAL.	qualifier
RA	remittance advice
RBRVS	Resource-Based Relative Value Scale (Medicare)
REF.	reference
Resp	respiratory
RHIA	Registered Health Information Administration
RHIT	Registered Health Information Technology
RLQ	right lower quadrant
RMA	Registered Medical Assistant
RN	registered nurse
R/O	rule out
ROS	review of systems
RTC	return to clinic
RUG	Resource Utilization Group
RUQ	right upper quadrant
RVS	relative value scale
RVU	relative value unit
Rx	prescription
SCHIP	State Children's Health Insurance Program
SDA	same-day appointment

SDI	state disability insurance
SH	social history
SNF	skilled nursing facility
SOAP	subjective/objective/assessment/plan
SOF	signature on file
S/P	status post
SSDI	Social Security Disability Insurance
SSI	Supplemental Security Income
SSN	Social Security number
stat, STAT	immediately
STD	sexually transmitted disease
subq, subcu	subcutaneous
T&A	tonsillectomy and adenoidectomy
TANF	Temporary Assistance for Needy Families
TCS	(HIPAA Electronic) Transaction and Code Sets
temp	temperature
t.i.d.	three times a day
TM	tympanic membrane
TPA	third-party claims administrator
TPO	treatment, payment, and operations
TPR	temperature, pulse, and respirations
UA	urinalysis
UC	urine culture
UCR	usual, customary, and reasonable
UHDDS	Uniform Hospital Discharge Data Set
UPC	Universal Product Code
UPIN	Unique Physician Identification Number
URI	upper respiratory infection
USIN	Unique Supplier Identification Number
UTI	urinary tract infection
VD	venereal disease
VIS	vaccine information sheet
VP	Vendor Product Number
VS	vital signs
wbc	white blood cells
WBC	white blood count
yo	year old
YY	year, indicates entry of two digits for the year; may also be noted as CCYY, which allows for entry of four digits for the century (CC) and year (YY)

Glossary

A

abuse Actions that improperly use another person's resources.

accept assignment (acceptance of assignment) A participating physician's agreement to accept the allowed charge as payment in full.

access The ability or means necessary to read, write, modify, or communicate information or otherwise use a system resource.

accounts receivable (A/R) Monies owed to a medical practice by its patients and third-party payers.

Accredited Standards Committee X12, Insurance Subcommittee (ASC X12N) The ANSI-accredited standards development organization that maintains the administrative and financial electronic transactions standards adopted under HIPAA.

Acknowledgment of Receipt of Notice of Privacy Practices Form accompanying a covered entity's Notice of Privacy Practices; covered entities must make a good-faith effort to have patients sign the acknowledgment.

acute Describes an illness or condition having severe symptoms and a short duration; can also refer to a sudden exacerbation of a chronic condition.

addenda Updates to the ICD-9-CM diagnostic coding system.

Additional Documentation Request Carrier request for information during a Medicare Medical Review.

add-on code Procedure that is performed and reported only in addition to a primary procedure; indicated in CPT by a plus sign (+).

adjudication The process followed by health plans to examine claims and determine benefits.

adjustment An amount (positive or negative) entered in a patient billing program to change a patient's account balance.

administrative code set Under HIPAA, required codes for various data elements, such as taxonomy codes and place of service (POS) codes.

administrative services only (ASO) Contract under which a third-party administrator or an insurer agrees to provide administrative services to an employer in exchange for a fixed fee per employee.

Admission of Liability Carrier's determination that an employer is responsible for an employee's claim under workers' compensation.

admitting diagnosis (ADX) The patient's condition determined by a physician at admission to an inpatient facility.

advance beneficiary notice (ABN) Medicare form used to inform a patient that a service to be provided is not likely to be reimbursed by the program.

adverse effect Condition caused by a drug that has been used correctly.

advisory opinion An opinion issued by CMS or the OIG that becomes legal advice for the requesting party; a requesting party who acts according to the advice is immune from investigation on the matter; the advisory opinion provides guidance for others in similar matters.

aging Classification of accounts receivable by the length of time an account is due.

allowed charge The maximum charge that a health plan pays for a specific service or procedure; also called allowable charge, maximum fee, and other terms.

Alphabetic Index The section of the ICD-9-CM in which diseases and injuries with corresponding diagnosis codes are presented in alphabetical order.

ambulatory care Outpatient care.

ambulatory patient classification (APC) A Medicare payment classification for outpatient services.

ambulatory surgical center (ASC) A clinic that provides outpatient surgery.

ambulatory surgical unit (ASU) A hospital department that provides outpatient surgery.

American Academy of Professional Coders (AAPC) National association that fosters the establishment and maintenance of professional, ethical, educational, and certification standards for medical coding.

American Association of Medical Assistants National association that fosters the profession of medical assisting.

American Association for Medical Transcription National association fostering the profession of medical transcription.

American Health Information Management Association (AHIMA) National association of health information management professionals that promotes valid, accessible, yet confidential health information and advocates quality health care.

American Medical Association (AMA) Member organization for physicians that aims to promote the art and science of medicine, improve public health, and promote ethical, educational, and clinical standards for the medical profession.

American National Standards Institute (ANSI) Organization that sets standards for electronic data interchange on a national level.

ancillary services Supplemental medical services such as diagnostic services and occupational therapy that support the diagnosis and treatment of patients' conditions.

appeal A request sent to a payer for reconsideration of a claim adjudication.

appellant One who appeals a claim decision.

assignment of benefits Authorization by a policyholder that allows a health plan to pay benefits directly to a provider.

assumption coding Reporting undocumented services that the coder assumes have been provided because of the nature of the case or condition.

at-home recovery care Assistance with the activities of daily living provided for a patient in the home.

attending physician The clinician primarily responsible for the care of the patient from the beginning of a hospitalization.

audit Methodical review; in medical insurance, a formal examination of a physician's accounting or patient medical records.

authorization (1) Document signed by a patient to permit release of particular medical information under the stated specific conditions. (2) A health plan's system of approving payment of benefits for services that satisfy the plan's requirements for coverage; see *preauthorization*.

autoposting Software feature that enables automatic entry of payments on a remittance advice to credit an individual's account.

B

bad debt An account deemed uncollectible.

balance billing Collecting the difference between a provider's usual fee and a payer's lower allowed charge from the insured.

bankruptcy Legal declaration that a person is unable to pay his or her debts.

benefits The amount of money a health plan pays for services covered in an insurance policy.

billing provider The person or organization (often a clearinghouse or billing service) sending a HIPAA claim, as distinct from the pay-to provider who receives payment.

billing service Company that provides billing and claim processing services.

birthday rule The guideline that determines which of two parents with medical coverage has the primary insurance for a child; the parent whose day of birth is earlier in the calendar year is considered primary.

BlueCard A Blue Cross and Blue Shield program that provides benefits for plan subscribers who are away from their local areas.

Blue Cross A primarily nonprofit corporation that offers prepaid medical benefits for hospital services and some outpatient, home care, and other institutional services.

Blue Cross and Blue Shield Association (BCBS) The national licensing agency of Blue Cross and Blue Shield plans.

Blue Shield A primarily nonprofit corporation that offers prepaid medical benefits for physician, dental, and vision services and other outpatient care.

bundling A single procedure code that covers a group of related procedures.

business associate A person or organization that performs a function or activity for a covered entity but is not part of its workforce.

C

capitation Payment method in which a prepayment covers the provider's services to a plan member for a specified period of time.

capitation rate (cap rate) The contractually set periodic prepayment to a provider for specified services to each enrolled plan member.

carrier Health plan; also known as insurance company, payer, or third-party payer.

carve out A part of a standard health plan that is changed under a negotiated employer-sponsored plan; also refers to subcontracting of coverage by a health plan.

case mix index A measure of the clinical severity or resource requirements of the patients in a particular hospital or treated by a particular clinician during a specific time period.

cash flow The inflow of payments from patients and payers to a medical practice and the outflow from the practice of payments to suppliers and staff; based on the actual movement of money rather than amounts that are receivable or payable.

catastrophic cap The maximum annual amount a TRICARE beneficiary must pay for deductible and cost share.

catchment area A geographic area usually within approximately forty miles of military inpatient treatment facilities; under TRICARE, the facility in a patient's area must issue a nonavailability statement before the patient can be treated at a nonmilitary facility.

categorically needy A person who receives assistance from government programs such as Temporary Assistance for Needy Families (TANF).

category In the ICD-9-CM, a three-digit code used to classify a particular disease or injury.

Category I codes Procedure codes found in the main body of CPT (Evaluation and Management, Anesthesia, Surgery, Pathology and Laboratory, Radiology, and Medicine).

Category II codes Optional CPT codes that track performance measures for a medical goal such as reducing tobacco use.

Category III codes Temporary codes for emerging technology, services, and procedures that are used instead of unlisted codes when available.

CCI column 1/column 2 code pair edit A Medicare code edit under which CPT codes in column 2 will not be paid if reported for the same patient on the same day of service by the same provider as the column 1 code.

CCI modifier indicator A number that shows whether the use of a modifier can bypass a CCI edit.

CCI mutually exclusive code (MEC) edit Under the CCI edits, both services represented by MEC codes could not have reasonably been done during a single patient encounter, so they will not both be paid by Medicare; only the lower-paid code is reimbursed.

Centers for Medicare and Medicaid Services (CMS) Federal agency within the Department of Health and Human Services (HHS) that runs Medicare, Medicaid, clinical laboratories (under the CLIA program), and other government health programs.

certificate Term for a Blue Cross and Blue Shield medical insurance policy.

certification number Number returned electronically by a health plan when approving a referral authorization request.

CHAMPUS Now the TRICARE program; formerly the Civilian Health and Medical Program of the Uniformed Services (Army, Navy, Air Force, Marine Corps, Coast Guard, Public Health Service, and National Oceanic and Atmospheric Administration) that serves spouses and children of active-duty service members, military retirees and their families, some former spouses, and survivors of deceased military members.

CHAMPVA The Civilian Health and Medical Program of the Department of Veterans Affairs (previously know as the Veterans Administration) that shares health care costs for families of veterans with 100 percent service-connected disabilities and the surviving spouses and children of veterans who die from service-connected disabilities.

charge-based fee structure Fees based on the amounts typically charged for similar services.

charge capture Office procedures that ensure that billable services are recorded and reported for payment.

charge master A hospital's list of the codes and charges for its services.

chart number A unique number that identifies a patient.

chief complaint (CC) A patient's description of the symptoms or other reasons for seeking medical care from a provider.

chronic An illness or condition with a long duration.

Civilian Health and Medical Program of the Department of Veterans Affairs See *CHAMPVA*.

claim adjustment group codes (GRP) Codes used by a payer on an RA/EOB to indicate the general type of reason code for an adjustment.

claim adjustment reason code (RC) Code used by a payer on an RA/EOB to explain why a payment does not match the amount billed.

claimant Person or entity exercising the right to receive benefits.

claim attachment Documentation that a provider sends to a payer in support of a health care claim.

claim control number Unique number assigned to a health care claim by the sender.

claim filing indicator code Administrative code used to identify the type of health plan.

claim frequency code (claim submission reason code) Administrative code that identifies the claim as original, replacement, or void/cancel action.

claim scrubber Software that checks claims to permit error correction for clean claims.

claim status category codes Codes used by payers on a HIPAA 277 to report the status group for a claim, such as received or pending.

claim status codes Codes used by payers on a HIPAA 277 to provide a detailed answer to a claim status inquiry.

claim turnaround time The time period in which a health plan is obligated to process a claim.

clean claim A claim that is accepted by a health plan for adjudication.

clearinghouse A company (billing service, repricing company, or network) that converts nonstandard transactions into standard transactions and transmits the data to health plans; also handles the reverse process, changing standard transactions from health plans into nonstandard formats for providers.

Clinical Laboratory Improvement Amendments (CLIA) federal law establishing standards for laboratory testing performed in hospital-based facilities, physicians' office laboratories, and other locations; administered by CMS.

CMS See *Centers for Medicare and Medicaid Services*.

CMS-1450 Paper claim for hospital services; also known as the UB-92.

CMS-1500 Paper claim for physician services.

CMS-1500 (08/05) Current paper claim approved by the NUCC.

CMS HCPCS Workgroup Federal government committee that maintains the Level II HCPCS code set.

code edits Computerized screening system used to identify improperly or incorrectly reported codes.

code linkage The connection between a service and a patient's condition or illness; establishes the medical necessity of the procedure.

code set Alphabetic and/or numeric representations for data. Medical code sets are systems of medical terms that are required for HIPAA transactions. Administrative (nonmedical) code sets, such as taxonomy codes and ZIP codes, are also used in HIPAA transactions.

coding The process of assigning numerical codes to diagnoses and procedures/services.

coexisting condition Additional illness that either has an effect on the patient's primary illness or is also treated during the encounter.

coinsurance The portion of charges that an insured person must pay for health care services after payment of the deductible amount; usually stated as a percentage.

collection agency Outside firm hired by a practice or facility to collect overdue accounts from patients.

collections The process of following up on overdue accounts.

collections specialist Administrative staff member with training in proper collections techniques.

combination code A single code that classifies both the etiology and the manifestation of an illness or injury.

Common Working File (CWF) Medicare's master patient/procedural database.

comorbidity Admitted patient's coexisting condition that affects the length of the hospital stay or the course of treatment.

compliance Actions that satisfy official guidelines and requirements.

compliance plan A medical practice's written plan for the following: the appointment of a compliance officer and committee; a code of conduct for physicians' business arrangements and employees' compliance; training plans; properly prepared and updated coding tools such as job reference aids, encounter forms, and documentation templates; rules for prompt identification and refunding of overpayments; and ongoing monitoring and auditing of claim preparation.

complication Condition an admitted patient develops after surgery or treatment that affects the length of hospital stay or the course of further treatment.

concurrent care Medical situation in which a patient receives extensive, independent care from two or more attending physicians on the same date of service.

conditions of participation (Medicare) (COP) Regulations concerning provider participation in the Medicare program.

Consolidated Omnibus Budget Reconciliation Act (COBRA) Federal law requiring employers with more than twenty employees to allow employees who have been terminated for reasons other than gross misconduct to pay for coverage under the employer's group health plan for eighteen months after termination.

consultation Service performed by a physician to advise a requesting physician about a patient's condition and care; the consultant does not assume responsibility for the patient's care and must send a written report back to the requestor.

consumer-driven health plan (CDHP) Type of medical insurance that combines a high-deductible health plan with a medical savings plan that covers some out-of-pocket expenses.

contract An enforceable voluntary agreement in which specific promises are made by one party in exchange for some consideration by the other party.

convention Typographic techniques or standard practices that provide visual guidelines for understanding printed material.

conversion factor Dollar amount used to multiply a relative value unit to arrive at a charge.

coordination of benefits (COB) A clause in an insurance policy that explains how the policy will pay if more than one insurance policy applies to the claim.

copayment An amount that a health plan requires a beneficiary to pay at the time of service for each health care encounter.

corporate integrity agreement A compliance action under which a provider's Medicare billing is monitored by the Office of the Inspector General.

Correct Coding Initiative (CCI) Computerized Medicare system to prevent overpayment for procedures.

Correct Coding Initiative edits Pairs of CPT or HCPCS Level II codes that are not separately payable by Medicare except under certain circumstances; the edits apply to services by the same provider for the same beneficiary on the same date of service.

cost share Coinsurance for a TRICARE or CHAMPVA beneficiary.

Coverage Issues Manual (CIM) Information about Medicare-qualified clinical trials, treatments, therapeutic interventions, diagnostic testing, durable medical equipment, therapies, and services referenced in the HCPCS code manual.

covered entity (CE) Under HIPAA, a health plan, clearinghouse, or provider that transmits any health information in electronic form in connection with a HIPAA transaction; does not specifically include workers' compensation programs, property and casualty programs, or disability insurance programs.

covered services Medical procedures and treatments that are included as benefits under an insured's health plan.

counseling Physician's discussion with a patient and/or family about diagnostic results, prognosis, treatment options, and/or instructions.

CPT *Current Procedural Terminology*, a publication of the American Medical Association.

credentialing Periodic verification that a provider or facility meets the professional standards of a certifying organization; physician credentialing involves screening and evaluating qualifications and other credentials, including licensure, required education, relevant training and experience, and current competence.

creditable coverage History of health insurance coverage for calculation of COBRA benefits.

credit bureaus Organizations that supply information about consumers' credit history and relative standing.

credit reporting Analysis of a person's credit standing during the collections process.

crossover claim Claim for a Medicare or Medicaid beneficiary; Medicare is the primary payer and automatically transmits claim information to Medicaid as the secondary payer.

cross-reference Directions in printed material that tell a reader where to look for additional information.

crosswalk A comparison or map of the codes for the same or similar classifications under two coding systems; it serves as a guide for selecting the closest match.

***Current Procedural Terminology* (CPT)** Publication of the American Medical Association containing the HIPAA-mandated standardized classification system for reporting medical procedures and services performed by physicians.

cycle billing Type of billing in which patients with current balances are divided into groups to even out statement printing and mailing throughout a month, rather than mailing all statements once a month.

D

database An organized collection of related data items having a specific structure.

data element The smallest unit of information in a HIPAA transaction.

data format An arrangement of electronic data for transmission.

date of service The date of a patient encounter for medical services.

day sheet In a medical office, a report that summarizes the business day's charges and payments, drawn from all the patient ledgers for the day.

deductible An amount that an insured person must pay, usually on an annual basis, for health care services before a health plan's payment begins.

Defense Enrollment Eligibility Reporting System (DEERS) The worldwide database of TRICARE and CHAMPVA beneficiaries.

de-identified health information Medical data from which individual identifiers have been removed; also known as a redacted or blinded record.

dependent A person other than the insured, such as a spouse or child, who is covered under a health plan.

descriptor The narrative part of a CPT code that identifies the procedure or service.

designated record set (DRS) A covered entity's records that contain protected health information (PHI); for providers, the designated record set is the medical/financial patient record.

destination payer In HIPAA claims, the health plan receiving the claim.

determination A payer's decision about the benefits due for a claim.

development Payer process of gathering information in order to adjudicate a claim.

diagnosis A physician's opinion of the nature of a patient's illness or injury.

diagnosis code The number assigned to a diagnosis in the *International Classification of Diseases.*

diagnosis-related groups (DRG) A system of analyzing conditions and treatments for similar groups of patients used to establish Medicare fees for hospital inpatient services.

diagnostic statement A physician's description of the main reason for a patient's encounter; may also describe related conditions or symptoms.

direct provider Clinician who treats the patient face-to-face, in contrast to an indirect provider such as a laboratory.

disability compensation program A plan that reimburses the insured for lost income when the insured cannot work because of an illness or injury, whether or not it is work-related.

disallowed charge An item on a remittance advice that identifies the difference between the allowable charge and the amount the physician charged for a service.

disclosure The release, transfer, provision of, access to, or divulging in any other manner of information outside the entity that holds it.

discounted fee-for-service A negotiated payment schedule for health care services based on a reduced percentage of a provider's usual charges.

documentation The systematic, logical, and consistent recording of a patient's health status—history, examinations, tests, results of treatments, and observations—in chronological order in a patient medical record.

documentation template Physician practice form used to prompt the physician to document a complete review of systems (ROS) when done and the medical necessity for the planned treatment.

domiciliary care Care provided in the home; or providing care and living space, such as a home for disabled veterans.

downcoding A payer's review and reduction of a procedure code (often an E/M code) to a lower level than reported by the provider.

dual-eligible A Medicare-Medicaid beneficiary.

durable medical equipment (DME) Medicare term for reusable physical supplies such as wheelchairs and hospital beds that are ordered by the provider for use in the home; reported with HCPCS Level II codes.

durable medical equipment, prosthetics, orthotics, and supplies (DMEPOS) Category of HCPCS services.

Durable Medical Equipment Regional Carrier (DMERC) Medicare contractor that processes claims for durable medical equipment, prosthetics, orthotics, and supplies.

E

Early and Periodic Screening, Diagnosis, and Treatment (EPSDT) Medicaid's prevention,, early detection, and treatment program for eligible children under the age of twenty-one.

E code Alphanumeric ICD code for an external cause of injury or poisoning.

edits Computerized screening system used to identify improperly or incorrectly reported codes.

8371 HIPAA-mandated electronic transaction for hospital claims.

elective surgery Nonemergency surgical procedure that can be scheduled in advance.

electronic claim A health care claim that is transmitted electronically; also known as an electronic media claim (EMC).

electronic data interchange (EDI) The system-to-system exchange of data in a standardized format.

electronic funds transfer (EFT) Electronic routing of funds between banks.

electronic media Electronic storage media, such as hard drives and removable media, and transmission media used to exchange information already in electronic storage media, such as the Internet. Paper transmission via fax and voice transmission via telephone are not electronic transmissions.

electronic medical record (EMR) A running collection of health information that provides immediate electronic access by authorized users.

electronic remittance Payment made through electronic funds transfer.

electronic remittance advice See *remittance advice.*

E/M See *evaluation and management code.*

emancipated minor A person who has reached the legal age for an emancipated minor under state law.

embezzlement Stealing of funds by an employee or contractor.

emergency A situation in which a delay in the treatment of the patient would lead to a significant increase in the threat to life or body part.

Employee Retirement Income Security Act of 1974 (ERISA) A federal law that provides incentives and protection against litigation for companies that set up employee health and pension plans.

encounter An office visit between a patient and a medical professional.

encounter form A listing of the diagnoses, procedures, and charges for a patient's visit; also called the superbill.

encryption A method of scrambling transmitted data so it cannot be deciphered without the use of a confidential process or key.

episode-of-care (EOC) option A flat payment by a health plan to a provider for a defined set of services, such as care provided for a normal pregnancy, or for services for a certain period of time, such as a hospital stay.

eponym A name or phrase that is formed from or based on a person's name; usually describes a condition or procedure associated with that person.

established patient Patient who has received professional services from a provider (or another provider with the same specialty in the same practice) within the past three years.

ethics Standards of conduct based on moral principles.

etiology The cause or origin of a disease.

etiquette Standards of professional behavior.

evaluation and management (E/M) codes Procedure codes that cover physicians' services performed to determine the optimum course for patient care; listed in the Evaluation and Management section of CPT.

excluded parties Individuals or companies that, because of reasons bearing on professional competence, professional performance, or financial integrity, are not permitted by the OIG to participate in any federal health care programs.

excluded service A service specified in a medical insurance contract as not covered.

explanation of benefits (EOB) Document sent by a payer to a patient that shows how the amount of a benefit was determined.

explanation of Medicare benefits (EOMB) See *Medicare Summary Notice.*

external audit Audit conducted by an organization outside of the practice, such as a federal agency.

F

Fair and Accurate Credit Transaction Act (FACTA) Laws designed to modify the Fair Credit Reporting Act to protect the accuracy and privacy of credit reports.

Fair Credit Reporting Act (FCRA) Law requiring consumer reporting agencies to have reasonable and fair procedures to protect both consumers and business users of the reports.

Fair Debt Collection Practices Act of 1977 (FDCPA) Laws regulating collection practices.

family deductible Fixed, periodic amount that must be met by the combination of payments for covered services to each individual of an insured/dependent group before benefits from a payer begin.

Federal Employee Compensation Act (FECA) A federal law that provides workers' compensation insurance for civilian employees of the federal government.

Federal Employees Health Benefits Program (FEHBP) The health insurance program that covers employees of the federal program.

Federal Employees Retirement System (FERS) Disability program for employees of the federal government.

Federal Insurance Contribution Act (FICA) The federal law that authorizes payroll deductions for the Social Security Disability Program.

Federal Medicaid Assistance Percentage (FMAP) Basis for federal government Medicaid allocations to individual states.

fee-for-service Method of charging under which a provider's payment is based on each service performed.

fee schedule List of charges for services performed.

final report A report filed by the physician in a state workers' compensation case when the patient is discharged.

financial policy A practice's rules governing payment for medical services from patients.

firewall A software system designed to block unauthorized entry to a computer's data.

first report of injury A report filed in state workers' compensation cases that contains the employer's name and address, employee's supervisor, date and time of accident, geographic location of injury, and patient's description of what happened.

fiscal intermediary Government contractor that processes claims for government programs; for Medicare, the fiscal intermediary (FI) processes Part A claims.

Flexible Blue The Blue Cross and Blue Shield consumer-driven health plan.

flexible savings account (FSA) Type of consumer-driven health funding plan option that has employer and employee contributions; funds left over revert to the employer.

formulary A list of a health plan's selected drugs and their proper dosages; often a plan pays only for the drugs it lists.

fragmented billing Incorrect billing practice in which procedures covered under a single bundled code are unbundled and separately reported.

fraud Intentional deceptive act to obtain a benefit.

G

gatekeeper See *primary care physician.*

gender rule Coordination of benefits rule for a child insured under both parents' plans under which the father's insurance is primary

geographic practice cost index (GPCI) Medicare factor used to adjust providers' fees to reflect the cost of providing services in a particular geographic area relative to national averages.

global period The number of days surrounding a surgical procedure during which all services relating to the procedure—preoperative, during the surgery, and postoperative—are considered part of the surgical package and are not additionally reimbursed.

global surgical rule See *surgical package.*

grievance Right of a medical practice to file a complaint with the state insurance commission if it has been treated unfairly by a payer.

grouper Software used to assign DRGs based on patients' diagnoses during hospitalization.

group health plan Under HIPAA, a plan (including a self-insured plan) of an employer or employee organization to provide health care to the employees, former employees, or their families. Plans that are self-administered and have fewer than fifty participants are not group health plans.

guarantor A person who is the insurance policyholder for a patient of the practice.

guarantor billing Grouping patient billing under the insurance policyholder; the guarantor receives statements for all patients covered under the policy.

guardian An adult legally responsible for care and custody of a minor.

H

HCFA See *Centers for Medicare and Medicaid Services.*

HCFA-1450 See *CMS-1450.*

HCFA-1500 See *CMS-1500 (08/05).*

Health and Human Services (HHS) The U.S. Department of Health and Human Services, whose agencies have authority to create and enforce HIPAA regulations.

health care claim An electronic transaction or a paper document filed with a health plan to receive benefits.

Healthcare Common Procedure Coding System (HCPCS) Procedure codes for Medicare claims, made up of CPT codes (Level I) and national codes (Level II).

Health Care Financing Administration See *Centers for Medicare and Medicaid Services.*

Health Care Fraud and Abuse Control Program Government program to uncover misuse of funds in federal health care programs; run by the Office of the Inspector General.

Health Employer Data and Information Set (HEDIS) Set of standard performance measures on the quality of a health care plan collected and disseminated by the National Committee for Quality Assurance (NCQA).

health information management (HIM) Hospital department that organizes and maintains patient medical records; also profession devoted to managing, analyzing, and utilizing data vital for patient care, making the data accessible to health care providers.

Health Insurance Portability and Accountability Act (HIPAA) of 1996 Federal act that set forth guidelines for standardizing the electronic data interchange of administrative and financial transactions, exposing fraud and abuse in government programs, and protecting the security and privacy of health information.

health maintenance organization (HMO) A managed health care system in which providers agree to offer health care to the organization's members for fixed periodic payments from the plan; usually members must receive medical services only from the plan's providers.

health plan Under HIPAA, an individual or group plan that either provides or pays for the cost of medical care; includes group health plans, health insurance issuers, health maintenance organizations, Medicare Part A or B, Medicaid, TRICARE, and other government and nongovernment plans.

Health Professional Shortage Area (HPSA) Medicare-defined geographical area offering participation bonuses to physicians.

health reimbursement account (HRA) Type of consumer-driven health plan funding option under which an employer sets aside an annual amount an employee can use to pay for certain types of health care costs.

health savings account (HSA) Type of consumer-drive health plan funding option under which employers, employees, both employers and employees, or individuals set aside funds that can be used to pay for certain types of health care costs.

high-deductible health plan (HDHP) Type of health plan combining high-deductible insurance, usually a PPO with a relatively low premium, and a funding option to pay for patients' out-of-pocket expenses up to the deductible.

HIPAA claim Generic term for the HIPAA X12N 837 professional health care claim transaction.

HIPAA Claim Status—Inquiry/Response The HIPAA X12N 276/277 transaction in which a provider asks a health plan for information on a claim's status and receives an answer from the plan.

HIPAA Coordination of Benefits The HIPAA ASCX12N 837 transaction that is sent to a secondary or tertiary payer on a cliam with the primary payer's remittance advice.

HIPAA Electronic Health Care Transactions and Code Sets (TCS) The HIPAA rule governing the electronic exchange of health information.

HIPAA Eligibility for a Health Plan The HIPAA X12N 270/217 transaction in which a provider asks a health plan for information on a patient's eligibility for benefits and receives an answer from the plan.

HIPAA Health Care Claims or Equivalent Encounter Information/Coordination of Benefits The HIPAA X12N 837 transaction that a provider uses to report professional, institutional, or dental claims and that is also used to send a secondary or tertiary payer claim with the primary payer's RA/EOB data.

HIPAA Health Care Payment and Remittance Advice The HIPAA X12N 835 transaction used by a health plan to describe a payment in response to a health care claim.

HIPAA National Identifier HIPPA-mandated identification systems for employers, health care providers, health plans, and patients; the NPI, National Provider System, and employer system are in place; health plan and patient systems are yet to be created.

HIPAA Privacy Rule Law that regulates the use and disclosure of patients' protected health information (PHI).

HIPAA Referral Certification and Authorization The HIPAA X12N 278 transaction in which a provider asks a health plan for approval of a service and the health plan responds, providing a certification number for an approved request.

HIPAA Security Rule Law that requires covered entities to establish administrative, physical, and technical safeguards to protect the confidentiality, integrity, and availability of health information.

HIPPA transaction General term for the electronic transactions, such as claim status inquiries, health care claim transmittal, and coordination of benefits regulated under the HIPAA Health Care Transactions and Code Sets standards.

home health agency (HHA) Organization that provides home care services to patients.

home health care Care given to patients in their homes, such as skilled nursing care.

home plan Blue Cross and Blue Shield plan in the community where the subscriber has contracted for coverage.

hospice Public or private organization that provides services for terminally ill people and their families.

hospice care Palliative care for people with terminal illnesses.

host plan Participating provider's local Blue Cross and Blue Shield plan.

I

ICD code System of diagnosis codes based on the *International Classification of Diseases*.

ICD-9-CM Abbreviated title of *International Classification of Diseases*, Ninth Revision, *Clinical Modification*.

ICD-9-CM Official Guidelines for Coding and Reporting American Hospital Association publication that provides rules for selecting and sequencing diagnosis codes correctly in both the inpatient and outpatient environments.

incident-to Term for services of allied health professionals, such as nurses, technicians, and therapists, provided under the physician's direct supervision that may be billed under Medicare.

indemnify A health plan's agreement to reimburse a policyholder for covered losses.

indemnity Protection from loss.

indemnity plan Type of medical insurance that reimburses a policyholder for medical services under the terms of its schedule of benefits.

independent medical examination (IME) Examination by a physician to confirm that an individual is permanently disabled that is conducted at the request of a state workers' compensation office or an insurance carrier.

independent (or individual) practice association (IPA) Type of health maintenance organization in which physicians are self-employed and provide services to both HMO members and nonmembers.

indirect provider Clinician who does not interact face-to-face with the patient, such as a laboratory.

individual deductible Fixed amount that must be met periodically by each individual of an insured/dependent group before benefits from a payer begin.

individual health plan (IHP) Medical insurance plan purchased by an individual, rather than through a group affiliation.

individual relationship code Administrative code that specifies the patient's relationship to the subscriber (insured).

information technology (IT) The development, management, and support of computer-based hardware and software systems.

informed consent The process by which a patient authorizes medical treatment after discussion about the nature, indications, benefits, and risks of a treatment a physician recommends.

initial preventive physical examination (IPPE) Medicare benefit of a preventive visit for new beneficiaries.

inpatient A person admitted to a medical facility for services that require an overnight stay.

Inpatient Prospective Payment System (IPPS) Medicare payment system for hospital services; based on diagnosis-related groups (DRGs).

insurance aging report A report grouping unpaid claims transmitted to payers by the length of time that they remain due, such as 30, 60, 90, or 120 days.

insurance commission State's regulatory agency for the insurance industry that serves as liaison between patient and payer and between provider and payer.

insured The policyholder or subscriber to a health plan or medical insurance policy; also known as guarantor.

intermediary See *fiscal intermediary*.

internal audit Self-audit conducted by a staff member or consultant as a routine check of compliance with reporting regulations.

***International Classification of Diseases*, Ninth Revision, *Clinical Modification*(ICD-9-CM)** Publication containing the HIPAA-mandated standardized classification system for diseases and injuries developed by the World Health Organization and modified for use in the United States.

J

job reference aid List of a medical practice's frequently reported procedures and diagnoses.

Joint Commission on Accreditation of Healthcare Organizations (JCAHO) Organization that reviews accreditation of hospitals and other organizations/programs.

K

key component Factor required to be documented for various levels of evaluation and management services.

L

late effect Condition that remains after an acute illness or injury has completed its course.

late enrollee Category of enrollment in a commercial health plan that may have different eligibility requirements.

LCD Local coverage determination.

Level II HCPCS national codes.

Level II modifiers HCPCS national code set modifiers.

liable Legally responsible.

lifetime limit See *maximum benefit limit*.

limiting charge In Medicare, the highest fee (115 percent of the Medicare Fee Schedule) that nonparticipating physicians may charge for a particular service.

line item control number On a HIPAA claim, the unique number assigned by the sender to each service line item reported.

local coverage determination (LCD) Notices sent to physicians that contain detailed and updated information about the coding and medical necessity of a specific Medicare service.

Local Medicare Review Policy (LMRP) See *local coverage determination*.

M

main number The five-digit procedure code listed in the CPT.

main term The word in boldface type that identifies a disease or condition in the ICD-9-CM Alphabetic Index.

malpractice Failure to use an acceptable level of professional skill when giving medical services that results in injury or harm to a patient.

managed care System that combines the financing and the delivery of appropriate, cost-effective health care services to its members.

managed care organization (MCO) Organization offering some type of managed health care plan.

manifestation Characteristic sign or symptom of a disease.

master patient index Hospital's main patient database.

maximum benefit limit The amount an insurer agrees to pay for an insured's covered expenses over the course of the insured person's lifetime.

M code Classification number that identifies the morphology of neoplasms.

means test Process of fairly determining a patient's ability to pay.

Medicaid A federal and state assistance program that pays for health care services for people who cannot afford them.

MediCal California's Medicaid program.

medical coder Medical office staff member with specialized training who handles the diagnostic and procedural coding of medical records.

medical error Failure of a planned action to be completed as intended or the use of a wrong plan to achieve an aim.

medical insurance Financial plan that covers the cost of hospital and medical care.

medical insurance specialist Medical office administrative staff member who handles billing, checks insurance, and processes payments.

medically indigent Medically needy.

medically needy Medicaid classification for people with high medical expenses and low financial resources, although not sufficiently low to receive cash assistance.

medical necessity Payment criterion of payers that requires medical treatments to be appropriate and provided in accordance with generally accepted standards of medical practice. To be medically necessary, the reported procedure or service must match the diagnosis, be provided at the appropriate level, not be elective, not be experimental, and not be performed for the convenience of the patient or the patient's family.

medical necessity denial Refusal by a health plan to pay for a reported procedure that does not meet its medical necessity criteria.

medical record A file that contains the documentation of a patient's medical history, record of care, progress notes, correspondence, and related billing/financial information.

Medical Review (MR) Program A payer's procedures for ensuring that providers give patients the most appropriate care in the most cost-effective manner.

Medical Savings Account (MSA) The Medicare health savings account program.

medical standards of care State-specified performance measures for the delivery of health care by medical professionals.

medical terminology The terms used to describe diagnoses and procedures; based on anatomy.

Medicare The federal health insurance program for people sixty-five or older and some people with disabilities.

Medicare Advantage Medicare plans other than the Original Medicare Plan.

Medicare beneficiary A person covered by Medicare.

Medicare card Insurance identification card issued to Medicare beneficiaries.

Medicare carrier A private organization under contract with CMS to administer Medicare Part B claims in an assigned region.

Medicare Carriers Manual (MCM) Guidelines established by Medicare about coverage for HCPCS Level II services; references to the MCM appear in the HCPCS code book.

Medicare health insurance claim number (HICN) Medicare beneficiary's identification number; appears on the Medicare card.

Medicare Modernization Act (MMA) Short name for the Medicare Prescription Drug, Improvement, and Modernization Act of 2003, which included a prescription drug benefit.

Medicare Outpatient Adjudication remark codes (MOA) Remittance advice codes that explain Medicare payment decisions.

Medicare Part A (Hospital Insurance [HI]) The part of the Medicare program that pays for hospitalization, care in a skilled nursing facility, home health care, and hospice care.

Medicare Part B (Supplementary Medical Insurance [SMI]) The part of the Medicare program that pays for physician services, outpatient hospital services, durable medical equipment, and other services and supplies.

Medicare Part C Managed care health plans offered to Medicare beneficiaries under the Medicare Advantage program.

Medicare Part D Prescription drug reimbursement plans offered to Medicare beneficiaries.

Medicare-participating agreement Describes physicians and other providers of medical services who have signed agreements with Medicare to accept assignment on all Medicare claims.

Medicare Physician Fee Schedule (MPFS) The RBRVS-based allowed fees that are the basis for Medicare reimbursement.

Medicare Redetermination Notice (MRN) Resolution of a first appeal for Medicare fee-for-service claims; a written decision notification letter is due within sixty days of the appeal.

Medicare Secondary Payer (MSP) Federal law requiring private payers who provide general health insurance to Medicare beneficiaries to be the primary payers for beneficiaries' claims.

Medicare Summary Notice (MSN) Type of remittance advice from Medicare to beneficiaries to explain how benefits were determined.

Medigap Insurance plan offered by a private insurance carrier to supplement Medicare Original Plan coverage.

Medi-Medi beneficiary Person who is eligible for both Medicare and Medicaid benefits.

Military Treatment Facility (MTF) Government facility providing medical services for members and dependents of the uniformed services.

minimum necessary standard Principle that individually identifiable health information should be disclosed only to the extent needed to support the purpose of the disclosure.

modifier A number that is appended to a code to report particular facts. CPT modifiers report special circumstances involved with a procedure or service. HCPCS modifiers are often used to designate a body part, such as left side or right side.

monthly enrollment list Document of eligible members of a capitated plan registered with a particular PCP for a monthly period.

moribund Approaching death.

multiple modifiers Two or more modifiers used to augment a procedure code.

N

National Committee for Quality Assurance (NCQA) Organization that collects and disseminates the HEDIS information rating the quality of health maintenance organizations.

national coverage determination (NCD) Medicare policy stating whether and under what circumstances a service is covered by the Medicare program.

National Patient ID (Individual Identifier) Unique individual identification system to be created under HIPAA National Identifiers.

National Payer ID (Health Plan ID) Unique health plan identification system to be created under HIPAA National Identifiers.

National Provider Identifier (NPI) Under HIPAA, unique ten-digit identifier assigned to each provider by the National Provider System.

National Uniform Claim Committee (NUCC) Organization responsible for the content of health care claims.

negligence In the medical profession, failure to perform duties properly according to the state-required standard of care.

network A group of providers having participation agreements with a health plan. Using in-network providers is less expensive for the plan's enrollees.

network model HMO A type of health maintenance organization in which physicians remain self-employed and provide services to both HMO members and nonmembers.

new patient A patient who has not received professional services from a provider (or another provider with the same specialty in the same practice) within the past three years.

nonavailability statement A form required for preauthorization when a TRICARE member seeks medical services in other than military treatment facilities.

noncovered services Medical procedures that are not included in a plan's benefits.

nonparticipating (nonPAR) provider A provider who chooses not to join a particular government or other health plan.

nontraumatic injury A condition caused by the work environment over a period longer than one work day or shift; also known as occupational disease or illness.

not elsewhere classified (NEC) An ICD-9-CM abbreviation indicating the code to be used when an illness or condition cannot be placed in any other category.

Notice of Contest Carrier's determination to deny liability for an employee's workers' compensation claim.

Notice of Exclusions from Medicare Benefits (NEMB) CMS form given by a participating provider to a Medicare patient before providing a noncovered service; provides written notification that Medicare will not pay and states the estimated charge for which the patient will be responsible.

Notice of Privacy Practices (NPP) A HIPAA-mandated description of a covered entity's principles and procedures related to the protection of patients' health information.

not otherwise specified (NOS) An ICD-9-CM abbreviation indicating the code to be used when no information is available for assigning the illness or condition a more specific code.

O

observation services Medical service furnished in a hospital to evaluate an outpatient's condition or determine the need for admission as an inpatient.

occupational diseases or illnesses Conditions caused by the work environment over a period longer than one workday or shift; also known as nontraumatic injuries.

Occupational Safety and Health Administration (OSHA) Federal agency that regulates workers' health and safety risks in the workplace.

Office for Civil Rights (OCR) Government agency that enforces the HIPAA Privacy Act.

Office of the Inspector General (OIG) Government agency that investigates and prosecutes fraud against government health care programs such as Medicare.

Office of Workers' Compensation Programs (OWCP) The office of the U.S. Department of Labor that administers the Federal Employees' Compensation Act.

OIG Compliance Program Guidance for Individual and Small Group Physician Practices OIG publication that explains the recommended features of compliance plans for small providers.

OIG Fraud Alert Notices issued by the OIG to advise providers about potentially fraudulent or noncompliant actions regarding billing and reporting practices.

OIG Work Plan The OIG's annual list of planned projects under the Medicare Fraud and Abuse Initiative.

open-access plans Type of health maintenance organization in which a member can visit any specialist in the plan's network without a referral.

open enrollment period Span of time during which a policyholder selects from an employer's offered benefits; often used to describe the fourth quarter of the year for employees in employer-sponsored health plans or the designated period for enrollment in a Medicare or Medigap plan.

operations (health care) Activities such as conducting quality assessment and improvement, developing protocol, and reviewing the competence or qualifications of health care professionals and actions to implement compliance with regulations.

Original Medicare Plan The Medicare fee-for-service plan.

other ID number Additional provider identification number supplied on a health care claim.

out-of-network A provider that does not have a participation agreement with a plan. Using out-of-network providers is more expensive for the plan's enrollees.

out-of-pocket Expenses the insured must pay before benefits begin.

outpatient A patient who receives health care in a hospital setting without admission; the length of stay is generally less than twenty-three hours.

Outpatient Prospective Payment System (OPPS) The payment system for Medicare Part B services that facilities provide on an outpatient basis.

outside laboratory Purchased laboratory services.

overpayment An improper or excessive payment to a provider as a result of billing or claims processing errors for which a refund is owed by the provider.

P

panel In CPT, a single code grouping laboratory tests that are frequently done together.

participating physician/provider (PAR) A provider who agrees to provide medical services to a payer's policyholders according to the terms of the plan's contract.

participation Contractual agreement by a provider to provide medical services to a payer's policyholders.

password Confidential authentication information composed of a string of characters.

patient aging report A report grouping unpaid patients' bills by the length of time that they remain due, such as 30, 60, 90, or 120 days.

patient information form Form that includes a patient's personal, employment, and insurance company data needed to complete a health care claim; also known as a registration form.

patient ledger Record of all charges, payments, and adjustments made on a particular patient's account.

patient ledger card Card used to record charges, payments, and adjustments for a patient's account.

patient refunds Monies that are owed to patients.

patient statement A report that shows the services provided to a patient, total payments made, total charges, adjustments, and balance due.

payer Health plan or program.

payer of last resort Regulation that Medicaid pays last on a claim when a patient has other insurance coverage.

pay-for-performance (P4P) Health plan financial incentives program to encourage providers to follow recommended care management protocols.

payment plans Patients' agreements to pay medical bills over time according to an established schedule.

pay-to provider The person or organization that is to receive payment for services reported on a HIPAA claim; may be the same as or different from the billing provider.

PECOS See *Provider Enrollment Chain and Ownership System.*

pending Claim status during adjudication when the payer is waiting for information from the submitter.

permanent disability Condition that prevents a person in a disability compensation program from doing any job.

permanent national codes HCPCS Level II codes.

per member per month (PMPM) Periodic capitated prospective payment to a provider that covers only services listed on the schedule of benefits.

pharmacy Facility or location where drugs and other medically related items and services are sold, dispensed, or otherwise provided directly to patients.

pharmacy benefit manager Company that operates an employer's pharmacy benefits program, buying drugs, setting up the formulary, and pricing the prescriptions for the insured.

physical status modifier Code used in the Anesthesia Section of CPT with procedure codes to indicate the patient's health status.

physician of record Provider under a workers' compensation claim who first treats the patient and assesses the level of disability.

place of service (POS) code HIPAA administrative code that indicates where medical services were provided.

plan summary grid Quick-reference table for frequently billed health plans.

point-of-service (POS) option In HMOs, plan that permits patients to receive medical services from non-network providers; this choice requires a larger patient payment than visits with network providers.

policyholder Person who buys an insurance plan; the insured, subscriber, or guarantor.

practice management program (PMP) Business software designed to organize and store a medical practice's financial information; often includes scheduling, billing, and electronic medical records features.

preauthorization Prior authorization from a payer for services to be provided; if preauthorization is not received, the charge is usually not covered.

precertification Generally, preauthorization for hospital admission or outpatient procedure; see *preauthorization*.

preexisting condition Illness or disorder of a beneficiary that existed before the effective date of insurance coverage.

preferred provider organization (PPO) Managed care organization structured as a network of health care providers who agree to perform services for plan members at discounted fees; usually, plan members can receive services from non-network providers for a higher charge.

premium Money the insured pays to a health plan for a health care policy.

prepayment plan Payment before medical services are provided.

preventive medical services Care that is provided to keep patients healthy or to prevent illness, such as routine checkups and screening tests.

Primary Care Manager (PCM) Provider who coordinates and manages the care of TRICARE beneficiaries.

primary care physician (PCP) A physician in a health maintenance organization who directs all aspects of a patient's care, including routine services, referrals to specialists within the system, and supervision of hospital admissions; also known as a gatekeeper.

primary diagnosis Diagnosis that represents the patient's major illness or condition for an encounter.

primary insurance (payer) Health plan that pays benefits first when a patient is covered by more than one plan.

primary procedure The most resource-intensive (highest paid) CPT procedure done during a patient's encounter.

principal diagnosis (PDX) The condition that after study is established as chiefly responsible for a patient's admission to a hospital.

principal procedure The main service performed for the condition listed as the principal diagnosis for a hospital inpatient.

prior authorization number Identifying code assigned by a government program or health insurance plan when preauthorization is required; also called the certification number.

private disability insurance Insurance plan that can be purchased to provide benefits when illness or injury prevents employment.

privileging The process of determining a health care professional's skills and competence to perform specific procedures as a participant in, or an affiliate of, a health care facility or system. Once a facility privileges a practitioner, the practitioner may perform those specific procedures.

procedure code Code that identifies medical treatment or diagnostic services.

professional component (PC) The part of the relative value associated with a procedure code that represents a physician's skill, time, and expertise used in performing it; contrast with the *technical component*.

professional courtesy Providing free medical services to other physicians.

prognosis The physician's prediction of outcome of disease and likelihood of recovery.

progress report A report filed by the physician in state workers' compensation cases when a patient's medical condition or disability changes; also known as a supplemental report.

prompt-pay laws Regulations that obligate payers to pay clean claims within a certain time period.

prospective audit Internal audit of particular claims conducted before they are transmitted to payers.

prospective payment Payment for health care made before the services are provided.

Prospective Payment System (PPS) Medicare system for payment for institutional services.

protected health information (PHI) Individually identifiable health information that is transmitted or maintained by electronic media.

provider Person or entity that supplies medical or health services and bills for or is paid for the services in the normal course of business. A provider may be a professional member of the health care team, such as a physician, or a facility, such as a hospital or skilled nursing home.

Provider Enrollment Chain and Ownership System (PECOS CMS national database of participating providers.

provider-sponsored organization (PSO) Capitated Medicare managed care plan in which the physicians and hospitals that provide treatment also own and operate the plan.

provider withhold Amount withheld from a provider's payment by an MCO under contractual terms; may be paid if stated financial requirements are met.

Q

qualifier Two-digit code for a type of provider identification number other than the National Provider Identifier (NPI).

quality improvement organization (QIO) State-based group of physicians who are paid by the government to review aspects of the Medicare program, including the quality and appropriateness of services provided and fees charged.

qui tam "Whistle-blower" cases in which a relator accuses another party of fraud or abuse against the federal government.

R

RA/EOB Remittance advice/explanation of benefits. Payer document detailing the results of claim adjudication and payment.

real-time Information technology term for computer systems that update information the same time they receive it; the sender and receiver "converse" by inquiring and responding to data while remaining connected.

reasonable fee The lower of either the fee the physician bills or the usual fee, unless special circumstances apply.

reconciliation Comparison of two numbers to determine whether they differ.

redetermination First level of Medicare appeal processing.

referral Transfer of patient care from one physician to another.

referral number Authorization number given by a referring physician to the referred physician.

referral waiver Document a patient is asked to sign guaranteeing payment when a required referral authorization is pending.

referring physician The physician who refers the patient to another physician for treatment.

registration Process of gathering personal and insurance information about a patient during admission to a hospital.

relative value scale (RVS) System of assigning unit values to medical services based on an analysis of the skill and time required of the physician to perform them.

relative value unit (RVU) A factor assigned to a medical service based on the relative skill and time required to perform it.

relator Person who makes an accusation of fraud or abuse in a *qui tam* case.

remittance The statement of the results of the health plan's adjudication of a claim.

remittance advice (RA) Health plan document describing a payment resulting from a claim adjudication; also called an explanation of benefits (EOB).

remittance advice remark codes (REM) Codes that explain payers' payment decisions.

rendering provider Term used to identify the physician or other medical professional who provides the procedure reported on a health care claim if other than the pay-to provider.

reprice Contractual reduction of a physician's fee schedule.

repricer Vendor that processes out-of-network claims for payers.

required data element Information that must be supplied on an electronic claim.

resource-based fee structure Setting fees based on the relative skill and time required to provide similar services.

resource-based relative value scale (RBRVS) Federally mandated relative value scale for establishing Medicare charges.

respondeat superior Doctrine making the employer responsible for employees' actions.

responsible party Person or entity other than the insured or the patient who will pay a patient's charges.

restricted status A category of Medicaid beneficiary.

retention schedule A practice policy that governs which information from patients' medical records is to be stored, for how long it is to be retained, and the storage medium to be used.

retroactive payment Payer's payment for health care after the services are provided

retrospective audit An internal audit conducted after claims are processed by payers and after RAs have been received for comparison with submitted charges.

rider Document that modifies an insurance contract.

roster billing Under Medicare, simplified billing for pneumococcal, influenza virus, and hepatitis B vaccines.

S

schedule of benefits List of the medical expenses that a health plan covers.

screening services Tests or procedures performed for a patient who does not have symptoms, abnormal findings, or any past history of the disease; used to detect an undiagnosed disease so that medical treatment can begin.

secondary condition Additional diagnosis that occurs at the same time as a primary diagnosis and that affects its treatment.

secondary insurance (payer) The health plan that pays benefits after the primary plan pays when a patient is covered by more than one plan.

secondary procedure Procedure performed in addition to the primary procedure.

secondary provider identifier On HIPAA claims, identifiers that may be required by various plans in addition to the NPI, such as a plan identification number.

section guidelines Usage notes provided at the beginnings of CPT sections.

Section 125 cafeteria plan Employers' health plans that are structured under income tax laws to permit funding of premiums with pretax payroll deductions.

self-funded (insured) employer A company that creates its own insurance plan for its employees, rather than using a carrier; the plan assumes payment risk, contracts with physicians, and pays for claims from its fund.

self-pay patient A patient who does not have insurance coverage.

separate procedure Descriptor used in the Surgery Section of CPT for a procedure that is usually part of a surgical package but may also be performed separately or for a different purpose, in which case it may be billed.

service line information On a HIPAA claim, information about the services being reported.

silent PPOs Managed care organization that purchases a list of a PPO's participating providers and pays those providers' claims for its enrollees according the contract's fee schedule even though the providers do not have contracts with the silent PPO. A provider can avoid having to work with a silent PPO by making sure his or her contract includes language prohibiting the PPO from selling his or her name to another party.

situational data element Information that must be supplied on a claim when certain other data elements are provided.

skilled nursing facility (SNF) Health care facility in which licensed nurses provide nursing and/or rehabilitation services under a physician's direction.

skip trace The process of locating a patient who has not paid on an outstanding balance.

small group health plan Under HIPAA, generally a health plan sponsored by an employer with fewer than fifty employees.

SNODENT Systemized nomenclature of dentistry.

SNOMED Systemized nomenclature of medicine.

SOAP (subjective/objective/assessment/plan) Documentation format in which encounter information is grouped into four sections containing the patient's subjective descriptions of signs and symptoms; the physician's notes on the objective information regarding the condition and examination/test results; the physician's assessment, or diagnosis, of the condition; and the plan of treatment.

Social Security Disability Insurance (SSDI) The federal disability compensation program for salaried and hourly wage earners, self-employed people who pay a special tax, and widows, widowers, and minor children with disabilities whose deceased spouse/parent would qualify for Social Security benefits if alive.

special report Note explaining the reasons for a new, variable, or unlisted procedure or service; describes the patient's condition and justifies the procedure's medical necessity.

spend-down State-based Medicaid program requiring beneficiaries to pay part of their monthly medical expenses.

sponsor The uniformed service member in a family qualified for TRICARE or CHAMPVA.

staff model HMO A type of HMO in which member providers are employees of the organization and provide services for HMO-member patients only.

standards of care (medical) State-specified performance measures for the delivery of health care by medical professionals.

State Children's Health Insurance Program (SCHIP) Program offering health insurance coverage for uninsured children under Medicaid.

statistical analysis durable medical equipment regional carrier (SADMERC) CMS contractors who provide assistance in determining which HCPCS codes describe DMEPOS items for Medicare billing purposes.

stop-loss provision Protection against the risk of large losses or severely adverse claims experience; may be included in a participating provider's contract with a plan or bought by a self-funded plan.

subcapitation Arrangement under which a capitated provider prepays an ancillary provider for specified medical services for plan members.

subcategory In ICD-9-CM, a four-digit code number.

subclassification In ICD-9-CM, a five-digit code number.

subpoena A order of a court for a party to appear and testify in a court of law.

subpoena *duces tecum* An order of a court directing a party to appear, to testify, and to bring specified documents or items.

subscriber The insured.

subterm Word or phrase that describes a main term in the ICD-9-CM Alphabetic Index.

Summary Plan Description (SPD) Legally required document for self-funded plans that states beneficiaries' benefits and legal rights.

superbill Listing of the diagnoses, procedures, and charges for a patient's visit; also called the encounter form.

supplemental insurance Insurance plan, such as Medigap, that provides benefits for services that are not normally covered by a primary plan.

supplemental report Report filed by the physician in state workers' compensation cases when a patient's medical condition or disability changes; also known as progress report.

Supplemental Security Income (SSI) Government program that helps pay living expenses for low-income older people and those who are blind or have disabilities.

supplementary term Nonessential word or phrase that helps define a code in the ICD-9-CM; usually enclosed in parentheses or brackets.

surgical package Combination of services included in a single procedure code for some surgical procedures inCPT.

suspended Claim status during adjudication when the payer is developing the claim.

T

Table of Drugs and Chemicals Reference listing of drugs and chemicals in the ICD-9-CM Alphabetic Index.

Tabular List Section of the ICD-9-CM in which diagnosis codes are presented in numerical order.

taxonomy code Administrative code set under HIPAA used to report a physician's specialty when it affects payment.

technical component The part of the relative value associated with a procedure code that reflects the technician's work and the equipment and supplies used in performing it; in contrast to the *professional component*.

Telephone Consumer Protection Act of 1991 Federal law that regulates consumer collections to ensure fair and ethical treatment of debtors; governs calling hours and methods.

Temporary Assistance for Needy Families (TANF) Government program that provides cash assistance for low-income families.

temporary disability Condition that keeps a person with a private disability compensation program from working at the usual job for a short time, but from which the worker is expected to recover completely and return to work.

temporary national codes HCPCS Level II codes available for use but not part of the standard code set.

tertiary insurance The third payer on a claim.

third-party claims administrator (TPA) Company that provides administrative services for health plans but is not a contractual party.

third-party payer Private or government organization that insures or pays for health care on the behalf of beneficiaries; the insured person is the first party, the provider the second party, and the payer the third party.

tiered network Plan feature that pays more to providers that the plan rates as providing the highest-quality, most cost-effective medical services.

TPO See *treatment, payment, and operations.*

trace number A number assigned to a HIPAA 270 electronic transaction sent to a health plan to inquire about patient eligibility for benefits.

transaction Under HIPAA, structured set of data transmitted between two parties to carry out financial or administrative activities related to health care; in a medical billing program, financial exchange that is recorded, such as a patient's copayment or deposit of funds into the provider's bank account.

traumatic injury Injury caused by a specific event or series of events within a single workday or shift.

treatment, payment, and health care operations (TPO) Under HIPAA, patients' protected health information may be shared without authorization for the purposes of treatment, payment, and operations.

TRICARE Government health program that serves dependents of active-duty service members, military retirees and their families, some former spouses, and survivors of deceased military members; formerly called CHAMPUS.

TRICARE Extra TRICARE'S managed care health plan that offers a network of civilian providers.

TRICARE for Life Program for beneficiaries who are both Medicare and TRICARE eligible.

TRICARE Prime The basic managed care health plan offered by TRICARE.

TRICARE Reserve Select (TRS) TRICARE coverage for reservists.

TRICARE Standard The fee-for-service health plan offered by TRICARE.

truncated coding Diagnoses that are not coded at the highest level of specificity available.

Truth in Lending Act Federal law requiring disclosure of finance charges and late fees for payment plans.

U

UB-04 Currently mandated paper claim for hospital billing.

UB-92 Former paper hospital claim; also known as the CMS-1450.

unbundling The incorrect billing practice of breaking a panel or package of services/procedures into component parts and reporting them separately.

uncollectible accounts Monies that cannot be collected from the practice's payers or patients and must be written off.

Uniform Hospital Discharge Data Set (UHDDS) Classification system for inpatient health data.

unlisted procedure A service that is not listed in CPT; it is reported with an unlisted procedure code and requires a special report when used.

unspecified An incompletely described condition that must be coded with an unspecified ICD code.

upcoding Use of a procedure code that provides a higher payment than the code for the service actually provided.

urgently needed care In Medicare, a beneficiary's unexpected illness or injury requiring immediate treatment; Medicare plans pay for this service even if it is provided outside the plan's service area.

usual, customary, and reasonable (UCR) Setting fees by comparing the usual fee the provider charges for the service, the customary fee charged by most providers in the community, and the fee that is reasonable considering the circumstances.

usual fee Fee for a service or procedure that is charged by a provider for most patients under typical circumstances.

utilization Pattern of usage for a medical service or procedure.

utilization review Payer's process to determine the appropriateness of hospital-based health care services delivered to a member of a plan.

utilization review organization (URO) Organization hired by a payer to evaluate the medical necessity of procedures before they are provided to a member of a plan.

V

V code Alphanumeric code in the ICD-9-CM that identifies factors that influence health status and encounters that are not due to illness or injury.

verification report Report created by a medical billing program to permit double-checking of basic claim content before transmission.

vocational rehabilitation Retraining program covered by workers' compensation to prepare a patient for reentry into the workforce.

W

waiting period Time period between an insured's date of enrollment and the date insurance coverage is effective.

waived tests Particular low-risk laboratory tests that Medicare permits physicians to perform in their offices.

walkout receipt Medical billing program report given to a patient that lists the diagnoses, services provided, fees, and payments received and due after an encounter.

Welfare Reform Act law that established the Temporary Assistance for Needy Families program in place of the Aid to Families with Dependent Children program and that tightened Medicaid eligibility requirements.

workers' compensation insurance State or federal plan that covers medical care and other benefits for employees who suffer accidental injury or become ill as a result of employment.

write off (noun: write-off) To deduct an amount from a patient's account because of a contractual agreement to accept a payer's allowed charge or for other reasons.

Index

Abbreviations, ICD-9-CM, 116, 120–121
Abuse. *See* Fraud and abuse detection and investigation
Acceptance of assignment, 96, 97, 344
Access control, 56
Accident claims, 266
Accidents, E codes (ICD-9-CM), 123
Accounts receivable (A/R), 20
Accreditation Association for Ambulatory Health Care, Inc. (AAHC), 301
Accrediting organizations, 301, 518–521
Acknowledgment of Receipt of Notice of Privacy Practices, 81–82
Acute conditions, 128–129
Add-on codes (CPT), 152, 155, 171
Addenda, ICD-9-CM codes, 112
Additional Documentation Request (ADR), Medicare, 352–353
Adjudication, 20, 449–452
  automated review, 450
  defined, 449
  determination, 451–452
  initial processing, 449–450
  manual review, 450–451
  payment of claim, 452
Adjustments, 95
  claim, 458–460
  RA/EOB, 458–460
Administrative code sets (NUCC), 258
Administrative services only (ASO) contracts, 289
Admission of Liability, 429
Admitting diagnosis (ADX), 524
Advance beneficiary notice (ABN), Medicare, 341–344
  blank or blanket, 343
  modifiers, 342–343
Advance Notice for Elective Surgery Form, 344
Adverse effects, E codes (ICD-9-CM), 123
Advisory opinions (OIG), 209
Aetna, 14, 300
Aging population, 3, 377, 380, 514
Aging reports
  insurance, 453, 454
  patient, 495
Agreement for Patient Payment of Noncovered Services, 88
Aid to Families with Dependent Children (AFDC), 377
AIDS/HIV, statutory reports, 53–55
Allowed charges, 225–227
Alphabetic Index. *See* ICD-9-CM codes, Alphabetic Index
Ambulatory care, 514
Ambulatory patient classification (APC) system, 529
Ambulatory surgical center (ASC), 514
Ambulatory surgical unit (ASU), 514
American Academy of Professional Coders (AAPC), 27–28
American Association for Medical Transcription (AAMT), 55
American Association of Medical Assistants (AAMA), 26
American Health Information Management Association (AHIMA), 26, 27–28, 55, 125, 147, 505, 524
American Hospital Association (AHA), 125, 147, 524
American Medical Accreditation Program (AMAP), 301
American Medical Association (AMA), 144, 146, 157, 189
  CPT Assistant, 156
  Documentation Guidelines for Evaluation and Management Services, 165, 216–219
  National Uniform Claim Committee (NUCC), 239, 258, 316
American Medical Technologist (AMT), 26
Ancillary services, 179
Anesthesia codes (CPT), 169–171
  add-on codes, 171
  modifiers, 170–171
  reporting, 171
  structure, 170
Answering machines, confidentiality and, 55
Anti-kickback statute, 60–61
Appeals, 464–466
  basic steps, 464–465
  Medicare, 465, 466
  options after rejection of, 465
  worker's compensation, 433
Appellant, 464
Appendixes (CPT), 155–156
Arteriosclerotic cardiovascular disease, ICD-9-CM coding for, 133–134
Arteriosclerotic heart disease, ICD-9-CM coding for, 133–134
Assignment of Benefits form, 81
Assignment of benefits statement, 81
  acceptance of assignment, 96, 97, 344
  secondary insurance coverage, 89–90
Assumption coding, 211
At-home recovery care, 514
Attachments
  HCPCS claims, 192
  HIPAA 837 claims, 266–267
Attending physician, 515
Audits
  compliance, 215–219, 320
  Medicare, 352–353
  postpayment, 466–467
Authorization to release information, 52–56
  hospital consent, 517
  preauthorizations and, 88
  requests other than TPO, 53–55
  Signature on File (SOF), 246, 257
  treatment, payment, and health care operations (TPO), 48–52, 81
Authorization to Use or Disclose Health Information, 54
Automated editing
  in adjudication, 450
  manual review of, 450–451
  Medicare National Correct Coding Initiative (CCI), 207–209, 339, 351, 450
Automobile insurance, 472
Away From Home Care®, 302

Backups, 57
Bad debt, 503–505
Balance billing, 226–227, 458
Balanced Budget Act (1997), 375
Bankruptcy, 504
Base unit, in relative value scale, 222–223
Benefits. *See also* Medical insurance
  defined, 5
  providers of. *See* Providers
  schedule of health care, 5
Bilateral modifiers (CPT), 176
Billing/collections manager, 493
Billing process, 485–492. *See also* Claims preparation and processing; Compliant billing
  aging report, 453
  check-in, 18, 86–92, 316
  check-out, 18–19, 98–100, 316
  communication in, 21, 23–24
  cycle billing, 491
  errors relating to
    code linkage, 210–211
    downcoding, 211, 463
    Medicare Medical Review (MR) Program, 352–353
    overpayment, 468
    unbundling, 172–173, 175, 211, 212
    upcoding, 211
  establishing financial responsibility, 17, 86–88, 315–316
  financial policies and procedures, 96–98, 405–406, 487, 488
  follow-up and collections, 21, 453–455
  hospitalization, 521–524, 529–536
  individual patient billing versus guarantor billing, 491–492
  information technology in, 22, 24
  management of fee schedule, 221–222, 307–312
  Medicaid, 194–196, 388
  Medicare
    Clinical Laboratory Improvement Amendments (CLIA), 178, 354
    duplicate claims, 353
    electronic billing, 351
    HCPCS, 194–196
    incident-to billing, 354
    Medical Review (MR) Program, 352–353
    Medicare as secondary payer, 351, 468–477, 516
    preauthorization, 354
    roster billing, 354
    split billing, 353
    timely filing, 352
  patient billing program. *See* MediSoft
  patients' statements, 20–21, 486–491
  payer adjudication, 20, 449–452, 458
  payment methods of patients, 98–99, 499–500
  payment over time, 98, 99, 499–500
  preregistration of patient, 16–17, 75–85, 315
  private payer, 196, 312–320
  procedures in, 21
  review of billing compliance, 19, 316
  review of coding compliance, 19, 316
  steps in, 16–21, 315–320
  workers' compensation, 433–434
Billing provider, 247
Birthday rule, 91
Blood and blood-forming organ diseases, ICD-9-CM coding for, 133
Blue Cross and Blue Shield Association (BCBS), 14, 147, 300–303
  BlueCard program, 303
  Flexible Blue Plan, 303
  subscriber identification card, 301, 302
  types of plans, 302–303
BlueCard program, 303
Bookkeeper, 493
Braces (ICD-9-CM), 120
Brackets (ICD-9-CM), 120
Bundled codes, 171–172, 175, 212
Burns, ICD-9-CM coding for, 136
Business associates, 47–48

Cafeteria plans, 290
California Relative Value Studies, 222–223
Capitation and capitation management, 320–321
  billing for capitated visits, 254
  billing for excluded services, 321
  claim write-offs, 321
  described, 9–10, 228–229
  parties in, 5
  patient eligibility, 320
  referral requirements, 321
Capitation rate (cap rate), 228–229
Career opportunities
  billing/collections manager, 493
  collections specialists, 493
  health information technician, 4
  medical administrative support, 4
  medical assistant, 4, 25–26
  medical coders, 27–28
  medical insurance specialist. *See* Medical insurance specialists
Cash payments, 98
Catastrophic cap
  CHAMPVA, 411
  TRICARE Standard, 401–402
Catchment area, 403
Categorically needy persons, 375
Categories (ICD-9-CM), 117
Category I codes (CPT), 145–147
Category II codes (CPT), 145–147, 180
Category III codes (CPT), 145–147, 180
CCI column 1/column 2 code pair edits, 207–208
CCI modifier indicators, 209
CCI mutually exclusive code (MED) edits, 208
Centers for Medicare and Medicaid Services (CMS), 45–46, 112, 144, 157, 189, 190–192, 333
  Documentation Guidelines for Evaluation and Management Services, 165, 216–219
  HCPCS codes. *See* HCPCS codes
  ICD-9-CM codes. *See* ICD-9-CM codes

Medicaid. *See* Medicaid
Medical Provider Analysis and Review (MedPar), 530
Medicare. *See* Medicare
Certification number, 88
Certified Coding Specialist (CCS), 28
Certified Coding Specialist—Physician-based (CCS-P), 28
Certified Medical Assistant (CMA), 25–26
Certified Professional Coder (CPC; CPC-H), 28
CHAMPUS (Civilian Health and Medical Program of the Uniformed Services), 399. *See also* TRICARE
CHAMPVA (Civilian Health and Medical Program of the Veterans Administration), 409–412
administration of, 16
authorization card, 409
claims processing, 411–412
costs, 411
covered medical services, 409–410
eligibility requirements, 409
excluded services, 410
preauthorization, 410
providers, 410–411
third-party liability, 411
CHAMPVA for Life, 411
CHAMPVA Maximum Allowable Charge (CMAC), 411
Charge-based fee structures, 222
Charge master, 522
Charge slips. *See* Encounter forms
Chart numbers, 83
Charts. *See* Patient medical records
Cheat sheets (job reference aids), 214–215
Check, payment by, 98
Check-in process, patient, 18, 86–92, 316
Check-out process, patient, 18–19, 98–100, 316
Chief complaint (CC), 38–39, 124
Childbirth complications, ICD-9-CM coding for, 134
Children. *See* Minors
Chronic conditions, 128–129
Cigna Health Care, 300
Circulatory disease, ICD-9-CM coding for, 133–134
Civil Service Retirement System (CSRS), 333, 434, 435–436
Claim adjustment group codes, 458
Claim adjustment reason codes, 458, 459–460
Claim control number, 265
Claim filing indicator codes, 261
Claim frequency code, 266
Claim monitoring and follow-up, 21, 453–455
Claim note, 266
HIPAA 837 claims, 355
ICD-9-CM claims, 115, 119–120
Claim scrubbers, 271
Claim status category codes, 453
Claim status codes, 453–454
Claim submission reason codes, 266
Claim turnaround time, 433, 453
Claimant, 464
Claims preparation and processing, 20, 36–65, 95–101, 238–273, 316–318. *See also* MediSoft
background, 239
calculations of patient charges, 95–101
charges billed, 96, 98
charges due at time of service, 95–96, 98–101
communication with patients about, 98–100
insured's financial responsibilities, 95–96
limits on patient charges and possible reimbursements, 95–96
walkout receipts, 99–101
CHAMPVA, 411–412
claim content, 239
CMS-1500. *See* CMS-1500 (08/05)
compliant billing, 19, 205–215, 316
errors in, 210–211
knowledge of billing rules, 205–210
strategies for compliance, 212–215
disability compensation, 436–437
electronic claims. *See* Electronic claims
fee-for-service, 315–320
determining additional coverage, 315
internal review of claims before submission, 316
verifying patient eligibility under primary insurance, 315–316
fee structures, 220–223
providers' usual fees, 220–221
relative value scale (RVS), 222–223, 425
resource-based relative value scale (RBRVS), 223–224, 341
usual, customary, and reasonable (UCR) fees, 222
fraudulent. *See* Fraud and abuse detection and investigation
HIPAA 837 electronic claims. *See* HIPAA 837 claims
hospital care, 514–524, 529–536
admission, 312, 515–516
coding, 524–526
discharge and billing, 521–524, 529–536
records of treatments and charges, 518–521
remittance advice processing, 530
introduction, 238–239
Medicaid. *See* Medicaid, claims processing
Medicare. *See* Medicare, claims processing
patient medical records, 36–45
defined, 36
electronic, 43–45
paper-based, 43
standards, 36–45
payment methods, 225–229
allowed charges, 225–227
capitation, 9–10, 228–229
contracted fee schedule, 228–229
procedures in, 315–320
remittance advice/explanation of benefits (RA/EOB), 452, 456–463
secondary payers, 468–477
steps in
claim status determination, 453–455
claims processing, 316–318
claims transmission, 20, 87, 267–271, 316–318, 351
coding, 18–19, 124, 387
encounter form preparation, 321
gathering of patient information, 16–17, 75–85
insurance verification, 86–92, 315–316
linkage and compliance review, 339
record retention, 505
third-party payer adjudication, 20, 449–452
TRICARE, 405–406
secondary claims, 474
timely filing requirement, 406
TRICARE regions, 405
workers' compensation, 429–433, 433–434
Clean claims, 271, 289
Clean Claims Act and/or Prompt Payment Act, 289
Clearinghouses, 47, 269
Clinical Laboratory Improvement Amendments (CLIA), 178, 354
Closed-panel plans, 293
CMS-1450, 530
CMS-1500 (08/05), 408
claims processing, 238, 239–259
CHAMPVA claims, 411–412
form locators, 356–361
Medicaid claims, 387–390
Medicare claims, 351–354, 356–361, 472–474
patient information, 239–246
physician or supplier information, 247–257
private payers, 316–318
secondary insurance claims, 470
summary of claim information, 258–259
taxonomy codes, 257, 258, 320
TRICARE claims, 406, 407, 408
Medicare, 238, 239–259, 356–361, 472–474
sample form, 240, 319, 322
workers' compensation, 433–434
CMS HCPCS Workgroup, 190–192
COB (coordination of benefits). *See* Coordination of benefits (COB)
COBRA (Consolidated Omnibus Budget Reconciliation Act of 1985), 291
Code edits. *See also* Automated editing
code linkage, 205, 210–211
medical necessity, 205
Medicare National Correct Coding Initiative (CCI), 207–209, 339, 351, 450
private payer, 210
Code linkage, 205, 206, 210–211, 266, 339
Code sets
list of. *See also* CPT codes; HCPCS codes; ICD-9-CM codes
standards, 58
Codes. *See also* Coding compliance
coding certification, 27–28
diagnosis. *See also* Diagnosis codes; ICD-9-CM codes
errors relating to coding process, 211
procedure. *See also* CPT codes; HCPCS codes; Procedure codes
updating, 112, 146–147, 192–193, 196
Coding certification, 27–28
Coding compliance
audits, 215–219
external, 215–216
internal, 216, 316
compliance errors, 210–211
defined, 19
Medicare, Correct Coding Initiative (CCI), 207–209, 339, 351, 450
preparation of job reference aids (cheat sheets), 214–215
refunds of overpayments, 468
regulations and requirements, 247–257
disability and workers compensation, 429, 433–434
hospitalization, 524–526
Medicaid, 385, 387, 388–390
Medicare, 194–196, 355–361
private payers, 210
review of, 19, 316
Coexisting conditions, 124
Coinsurance, 7
insured financial responsibility for, 227
Medicare, 472
Collection agencies, 500–501
selecting, 501
when to use, 500–501
Collections from patients, 21, 95–101, 492–505
billing before or after insurance payments, 96
copayment, 87, 95, 97, 309–310
deciding when to bill, 96
deductible, 96
financial arrangements for large bills, 98, 99
financial policy and procedures, 96–98, 213–214, 485–486, 487, 488
fraud prevention, 493
pretreatment, 516–517
process and methods, 494–498
collection agencies, 500–501
collections calls, 496–498, 503
collections letters, 496, 497
credit arrangements and payment plans, 98–99, 499–500
credit reporting, 501–502
organization, 492–493
payment methods, 98–99
prepayment plans, 500
record retention, 505
skip tracing, 502–503
writing off uncollectible accounts, 503–505
at time of service, 95–96
Collections specialists, 493
Colons (ICD-9-CM), 120
Combination codes, 117
Common Working File (CWF), Medicare, 336
Communications skills, 21, 23–24
with patients, 84, 98–101
with providers, 94
with third-party payers, 92, 320, 454–455
Comorbidities, 525
Complaints, patient privacy, 50
Compliance audits, 215–219
external, 216, 320
internal, 215–216
Compliance plan, 63–65. *See also* Coding compliance; Compliant billing
code of conduct, 64
compliance, defined, 19
compliance officer and committee, 64
ongoing training, 65
parts of, 64
refunds of overpayments, 468
Compliance Program Guidance for Individual and Small Group Physician Practices, 213–214
Compliance review. *See* Linkage and compliance review
Compliant billing, 205–215, 316
defined, 19
documentation in, 36–45
errors in, 210–211
hospital, 530
knowledge of billing rules, 205–210
review of billing compliance, 19, 316
strategies for compliance, 212–215

Complications, 525
Computer technology
in claims processing. *See also* MediSoft
database of patients, 83–84
database of payers, 92
patient billing program. *See also* MediSoft
scheduling systems, 75–76
Concurrent care, 450
Confidential information
electronic medical records, 43–45
exceptions to confidentiality requirements, 53–55
court order, 53–55
de-identified health information, 55
research data, 55
statutory reports, 53–55
workers' compensation cases, 53
guidelines for release, 48–56, 88–89
HIPAA Privacy Rule, 47, 48–56
protected health information (PHI), 48–56
psychotherapy notes, 55
state statutes, 48, 55–56
Congenital anomalies, ICD-9-CM coding for, 134
Consent, 39, 516, 517
Consolidated Omnibus Budget Reconciliation Act (COBRA; 1985), 291
Consultations
defined, 160
E/M codes, 160, 168
referrals versus, 314
Consumer-driven health plans (CDHPs), 292, 296–299
billing under, 298–299
comparison with other options, 13
described, 12–13
funding options, 296–298
types of plans, 296–298
Contract provisions
managed care organization, 304–307
parties in, 5
Contracted fee schedule, 228–229
Contrast material, 177
Conversion factor, 223–224
Coordinated care plans, Medicare, 348–349
Coordination of benefits (COB), 90–91, 264, 315
billing secondary payers, 468–477
Medicare, 470–477
Coordination of care, 164–165, 348–349
Copayment
collection of, 87, 95, 97, 309–310
health maintenance organization (HMO), 10
in managed care participation contract, 309–310
Coronary atherosclerosis, ICD-9-CM coding for, 133–134
Correct Coding Initiative (CCI), 207–209, 339, 351, 450
Cost containment, health maintenance organization (HMO), 10–11, 13
Cost-sharing
health maintenance organization (HMO), 10
TRICARE, 401–403
Counseling (E/M code), 164
Court order, release of information under, 53–55
Coventry Health Care, 300
Coverage Issues Manual (CIM), 196, 207
Covered entities, HIPAA, 47
Covered medical services
CHAMPVA, 409–410
defined, 5
in managed care participation contracts, 305
Medicaid, 384
TRICARE Standard, 402
Covered services, 87, 308
CPT Assistant, 156
CPT codes
add-on codes, 152, 155, 171
Anesthesia section, 169–171
add-on codes, 171
modifiers, 170–171
reporting, 171
structure, 170
annual revisions, 146–147
appendixes, 155–156
code edits, 210
coding steps, 156–157
current code requirement, 145, 147
defined, 18
descriptors, 145
Evaluation and Management section (E/M codes), 157–168
auditing codes, 215–219
code selection, 161–165
consultations, 160
development of, 157–158
modifiers, 160–161
new and established patients, 159–160
referrals, 160
reporting, 165–168
structure of codes, 158–159
format of, 146
index, 147–149
code ranges, 149
cross-references and convention, 149, 151–152
main terms, 147–148
modifying terms, 147–148
sample entries, 148
job reference aids (cheat sheets), 214–215
linkage between ICD-9-CM codes and, 205, 206, 210–211, 266, 339
main text, 149–152
format, 151–152
guidelines, 150–151
symbol for add-on codes, 152
symbol for conscious sedation, 152
symbol for FDA approval pending, 152
symbols for changed codes, 152
Medicine section, 179–180
reporting, 179–180
structure and modifiers, 179
modifiers, 152–155, 212–213
Anesthesia section, 170–171
bilateral, 176
determining need for, 157
Evaluation and Management section, 160–161
listing of, 154
Medicine section, 179
Pathology and Laboratory section, 177–178
Radiology section, 177
Surgical section, 173–175
use of, 152–155
organization of, 146
origins of, 144–145
Pathology and Laboratory section, 177–178
panels, 177–178
reporting, 178
special reports, 178
structure and modifiers, 178
unlisted procedures, 178
Radiology section, 176–177
contrast material, 177
reporting, 177
special reports, 176–177
structure and modifiers, 177
unlisted procedures, 176–177
Surgery section, 171–176
modifiers, 173–175
reporting, 175–176
separate procedures, 172–173
structure, 173
surgical package, 171–172
types of, 145, 180
updating, 146–147
Credentialing, 301
Credit arrangements, 98–99, 499–500
Credit bureaus, 501
Credit card payments, 98–99, 100, 486, 489
Credit counseling, 499
Credit-debit information, 267
Credit reporting, 501–502
Creditable coverage, 291
Cross-references
CPT, 149, 151–152
ICD-9-CM, 115
Crosswalk, 113, 261–262
Current Procedural Terminology, Fourth Edition (CPT), 18, 144. *See also* CPT codes; Procedure codes
Cycle billing, 491

Data elements, HIPAA 837 claims, 260–263, 272–273, 355–356
Day sheet, 487
De-identified health information, 55
Death benefits, workers' compensation, 427
Debit card payments, 98–99
Deductible, 7
CHAMPVA, 411
collection of, 96
family, 290
high-deductible health plan (HDHP), 296, 297
individual, 290
insured financial responsibility for, 290
Medicare, 472
TRICARE Standard, 402
Defense Enrollment Eligibility Reporting System (DEERS), 399
Denial of claims
medical necessity, 451–452
reasons for, 463
Department of Health and Human Services (HHS), 45, 333, 376. *See also* Centers for Medicare and Medicaid Services (CMS); Office of the Inspector General (OIG)
Medicaid claims, 385
New Freedom Initiative, 376
Department of Labor, Pension and Welfare Benefits Administration (EBSA), 289
Descriptors, 145
Designated record set (DRS), 49
Destination payer, 264
Determination, 451–452
Development of claims, 450–451
Diagnosis codes, 111–136. *See also* ICD-9-CM codes
defined, 18, 111
HIPAA 837 claims, 355
hospital, 524–525
introduction to, 111–112
linkage between procedure codes and, 205, 206, 210–211, 266, 339
source of, 111
updating, 112
Diagnosis-related groups (DRGs), 527, 528
Diagnostic and Statistical Manual of Mental Disorders (DSM), 133
Diagnostic statement, 114
Digestive system diseases, ICD-9-CM coding for, 134
Direct data entry (DDE), 270
Direct provider, 82
Disability compensation programs, 6, 434–437. *See also* Workers' compensation
Civil Service Retirement System (CSRS), 434
claims processing, 436–437
Federal Employees Retirement System (FERS), 435–436
New Freedom Initiative, 376
Social Security Disability Insurance (SSDI), 434
Supplemental Security Income (SSI), 435
Veteran's Pension Program, 434
veterans' programs, 436
workers' compensation, 423–434
Disability terminology, 428
Disabled persons
Medicaid eligibility, 379
Medicare eligibility, 333, 470–471
Discharge summaries, documentation of, 40–41
Disclosure of patient information. *See also* Confidential information
by e-mail, 87
by fax, 87
HIPAA Privacy Rule and, 48–56
by telephone, 55, 87
Discounted fee-for-service payment, 292
Discounts
for out-of-network visits, 316
professional courtesy, 213
for prompt payment, 309
uninsured/low-income patient, 214
Documentation, 36–45. *See also* Claims preparation and processing; Patient information; Patient medical records
Additional Documentation Request (ADR), Medicare, 352–353
collection process, 498
defined, 36
Documentation Guidelines for Evaluation and Management Services, 165, 216–219
electronic, 43–45
legal status, 36–37
Medical Review (MR) Program, Medicare, 352–353
paper-based, 43
standards, 36–45
AMA/CMS, 165, 216–219
contents of medical records, 37
discharge summaries, 40–41
Documentation Guidelines for Evaluation and Management Services, 165, 216–219
evaluation and management (E/M), 38–40
medical record formats, 37–38. *See also* Patient medical records
National Committee for Quality Assurance (NCQA), 301
patient encounters, 36–43
patient examinations, 38–39
patient-related issues, 36–37
procedural services, 41–42
progress reports, 39, 41
termination of provider-patient relationship, 42–43

Documentation templates, 215
Downcoding, 211, 463
Dropping to paper, 271
Drug reactions, E codes (ICD-9-CM), 123
Dual-eligibles, 387
Duplicate claims, Medicare, 353
Durable medical equipment (DME), 189

E codes (ICD-9-CM), 122, 123–124
E-mail, disclosure of patient information by, 87
Early and Periodic Screening, Diagnosis, and Treatment (EPSDT), 255, 376
Elective surgery, 310–311, 344
Electronic claims, 87. *See also* HIPAA 837 claims
  billing secondary payers, 469
  clearinghouses, 47, 269
  Medicare, 351
Electronic data interchange (EDI), 46–47, 269, 529–530
Electronic funds transfer (EFT), 462
Electronic Medicaid Eligibility Verification System (EMEVS), 380
Electronic medical records (EMR), 22, 518
Electronic patient record systems, 43–45
Electronic transactions, standards for, 47, 57–59
Embezzlement, 493
Emergency care, 14
  codes for, 252–253
  CPT codes, 168
  defined, 514
Emergency Medical Treatment and Active Labor Act (EMTALA), 14
Emergency room treatment, 14
Employee Retirement Income Security Act (ERISA; 1974), 289
Employer identification number (EIN), 59
Employment opportunities. *See* Career opportunities
Encounter forms, 92–94
  computer technology and, 94
  defined, 92
  estimating charges and reimbursement from, 98
  prenumbered, 94
Encryption, 56
End-stage renal disease (ESRD), Medicare eligibility, 333, 471–472
Endocrine diseases, ICD-9-CM coding for, 133
Energy Employees Occupational Illness Compensation Program, 424
Episode of care (EOC) option, 295
Eponyms, 117
EPSDT (Early and Periodic Screening, Diagnosis, and Treatment), 255, 376
Equal Employment Opportunity (EEO) regulations, 64
Errors, in billing process
  code linkage, 210–211
  downcoding, 211, 463
  Medicare Medical Review (MR) Program, 352–353
  overpayment, 468
  unbundling, 175, 211, 212
  upcoding, 211
Errors and omissions (E&O) insurance, 64
Essential hypertension, ICD-9-CM coding for, 134
Established patients
  database of patients, 83
  defined, 74
  Evaluation and Management section (E/M codes), 159–160
  patient information form, 82
  updating information on, 82, 83
Estimated length of stay (ELOS), 529
Ethics, 25
Etiology of disease, 114, 116
Etiquette, 25
Evaluation and Management Code Assignment Audit form, 217–218
Evaluation and Management (E/M) codes (CPT), 38–40, 157–168
  auditing codes, 215–219
  auditing tools to verify code selection, 216–218
  benchmarking with national averages, 212
  code selection, 161–165
  consultations, 160
  development of, 157–158
  modifiers, 160–161
  new and established patients, 159–160
  referrals, 160
  reporting, 165–168
  structure, 158–159
Excluded parties, 209–210
Excluded services. *See also* Noncovered/overlimit services
  billing for, 321
  CHAMPVA, 410
  collection for, 95–96
  defined, 5
  Medicaid, 384
  Medicare, 338–339, 341, 342
  procedures for, 87–88
  TRICARE Standard, 403
Explanation of benefits (EOB). *See* Remittance advice/explanation of benefits (RA/EOB)
  Explanation of Medicare Benefits (EOMB), 346
  flexible savings accounts, 298
External audits, 215–216

Fair and Accurate Credit Transaction Act (FACTA), 501
Fair Credit Reporting Act (FCRA), 501
Fair Debt Collection Practices Act (FDCPA; 1977), 494
False Claims Act (FCA), 60, 63, 353, 383
Family deductible, 290
Family history (FH), 162–163
Fax, disclosure of patient information by, 87
FECA (Federal Employees' Compensation Act) number, 245, 423, 424
Federal Black Lung Program, 424, 472
Federal Coal Mine Health and Safety Act, 424
Federal Employees' Compensation Act (FECA), 245, 423, 424
Federal Employees Health Benefits Program (FEHBP), 288
Federal Employees Retirement System (FERS), 435–436
Federal Insurance Contribution Act (FICA), 435
Federal Medicaid Assistance Percentage (FMAP) program, 374
Federal poverty level (FPL), 377
Federal regulation of medical insurance, 15–16
Federal workers' compensation plans, 423–424
Fee-for-service plans, 7, 8
  claims processing, 315–320
    internal review of claims before submission, 316
    verifying patient eligibility under primary insurance, 315–316
  for indemnity plans, 6–7, 315–320
  Medicaid, 385
  Medicare, 350
  Medicare private fee-for-service (PFFS), 349
  TRICARE Standard, 401–403
Fee schedules, 220–223
  comparing physician and payer fees, 220–222
  management of, 221–222, 307–312
  payer, 222–224
    contracted, 228–229
    Medicare, 222–224, 226, 308–312, 341, 351–352
    relative value scale (RVS), 222–223, 425
    resource-based relative value scale (RBRVS), 223–224, 341
    usual, customary, and reasonable (UCR) fees, 222
  provider
    providers' usual fees, 220–221
    sources of physician, 220–221
1500 Health Insurance Claim Form Reference Instruction Manual for 08/05 Version, 239
Fifth-digit requirement (ICD-9-CM), 119
Financial policies and procedures, 96–98, 213–214, 485–486, 487, 488
First-dollar coverage, 293
First-party payers, 5, 9–10
First report of injury, 429, 432
Fiscal intermediaries, 336
Flexible Blue Plan, 303
Flexible savings accounts (FSAs), 298
Form samples. *See also* Letter samples
  Acknowledgment of Receipt of Notice of Privacy Practices, 82
  Advance Notice for Elective Surgery Form, 344
  Agreement for Patient Payment of Noncovered Services, 88
  Assignment of Benefits, 81
  Authorization to Use or Disclose Health Information, 54
  CMS-1500 (08/05), 240, 319, 322, 408
  Encounter Form, 93
  Evaluation and Management Code Assignment Audit form, 217–218
  Financial Arrangements for Services, 99
  Financial Policy, 97
  Hospital Consent Form, 517
  Insurance Aging Report, 454
  Medicaid
    Eligibility Verification Log, 383
    Identification Coupon, 382
  Medical History, 77–78
  Medicare
    Advance Beneficiary Notice (ABN), Medicare, 341
    Notice of Exclusions from Medicare Benefits (NEMB), 342
    Request for Redetermination, 466
    Secondary Payer Determination Form, 519–520, 519–523
    Secondary Payer Screening Questionnaire, 471
    Summary Notice (MSN), 347
  Notice of Privacy Practices, 50–51
  Patient Information Form, 79
  Patient Referral Form, 89
  Patient Request for Accounting of Disclosures, 52
  Physician's Progress Report, 431
  Preauthorized Credit Card Payment, 100
  Precertification Form for Hospital Admission and Surgery, 312
  Private Pay Agreement, 386
  Referral Waiver, 90
  Self-Referral, 90
  UB-04, 531–535
  Walkout Receipt, 101
  workers' compensation
    First Report of Injury Form, 432
    Physician's Progress Report Form, 431
    Workers' Compensation Physician Report, 430
Formulary, 291
Fractures, ICD-9-CM coding for, 135
Fragmented billing, 175
Fraud and abuse detection and investigation
  abuse, defined, 61
  collections process, 493
  compliance plan, 63–65
  enforcement and penalties, 62–63
  examples of fraud, 60–62
  federal government, 59–62
    OIG Work Plan, 209–210, 530
  fraud, defined, 61
  Medicaid, 60, 62–63, 380, 382–383
  Medicare, 60, 62–63, 346, 530
    audits, 352–353
    Quality Improvement Organizations (QIOs), 527–528
  prevention, 60, 63–65, 380
  qui tam cases, 60
  TRICARE, 406–409

Gender rule, 91
Genitourinary system, ICD-9-CM coding for, 134
Geographic practice cost index (GPCI), 223
Global periods, 172, 212, 352, 429
Global surgery concept, 172
Global Trade item Number (GTIN), 250
Government-sponsored health care programs, 15–16
  CHAMPVA, 16. *See also* CHAMPVA
  Medicaid, 15. *See also* Medicaid
  Medicare, 15. *See also* Medicare
  TRICARE, 15. *See also* TRICARE
  workers' compensation. *See* Workers' compensation
Grievances, 468
Group health plans (GHP), 6, 290–292
  eligibility for benefits, 290–291
  employer-sponsored medical insurance, 287–288

Group health plans (GHP)—*Cont.*
Federal Employees Health Benefits (FEHB) program, 288
portability and required coverage, 291–292
Group/network HMO, 294–295
GRP (group codes), 458
Guarantor, 76
Guarantor billing, 491–492

HCFA-1500. See CMS-1500 (08/05)
HCPCS codes, 145, 189–196
billing procedures, 194–196
coding steps, 193
Level I Current Procedural Terminology, 189
Level II National Codes, 189, 191, 192–193
Level III codes (phased out), 189
Medicare requirement, 192, 351
modifiers, 194, 195
origins of, 189–192
reporting quantities, 194
sections, 190
temporary versus permanent codes, 190–192
updates, 192–193, 196
Health care benefits. *See* Benefits
Health care claims. *See also entries beginning with* "claim"
conditions for payment, 6–7
defined, 6
indemnity plan, 6–7
Health Care Financing Administration (HCFA). *See* Centers for Medicare and Medicaid Services (CMS)
Health Care Fraud and Abuse Control Program, 60
Health care industry, 3–6
aging population, 3, 377, 380, 514
cost increases in, 3–4
employment opportunities in, 4. *See also* Career opportunities
Health Industry Business Communications Council (HIBCC), 250
Health information management (HIM), 515
Health information technicians, 4
Health insurance. *See* Medical insurance
Health Insurance Association of America (HIAA), 147
Health Insurance Portability and Accountability Act (HIPAA; 1996), 46–59, 112, 189, 291
Administrative Simplification provision, 46–47
complying with, 47–48
Electronic Transaction and Code Sets Standards, 47, 57–59
Privacy Rule, 47, 48–56, 81–82, 84
Security Rule, 47, 56–57, 84, 99, 505
Health maintenance organizations (HMOs), 8–11, 293–295
Blue Cross and Blue Shield coverage, 302
business models
group/network HMO, 294–295
independent practice association HMO, 295
point-of-service plan, 11, 13, 292
staff HMO, 293
comparison with other options, 13
examples of benefits, 14
hospital care, 529
Medicaid coverage, 385
medical management practices, 10–11
cost containment, 10–11, 13
quality improvement, 11
Medicare, 348
Medicare coordinated care plans, 348
Health Net, 300
Health plans, 4–5, 47. *See also* Medical insurance
Health Professional Shortage Areas (HPSAs), 340
Health reimbursement accounts (HRAs), 297
Health savings accounts (HSAs), 297–298
Healthcare Common Procedure Coding System (HCPCS). *See* HCPCS codes
High-deductible health plan (HDHP), 296, 297
HIPAA 270/271 Eligibility for a Health Plan, 315
HIPAA 276, 267, 453
HIPAA 277, 267, 453
HIPAA 278 Referral and Authorization, 314
HIPAA 837 claims
claims preparation and processing, 238–239, 260–267, 388
billing secondary payers, 469
claim attachments, 266–267
claim information, 265–266
claim organization, 260–263, 272–273
credit-debit information, 267
Medicare, 355–356
payer information, 264–265
private payers, 316–318
provider information, 261
service line information, 266
subscriber information, 261
Medicaid, 388
Medicare
assumed care date/relinquished care date, 356
diagnosis codes, 355
insurance type code, 356
Medicare assignment code, 355
Notes (NTE) segment, 355
TRICARE, 406
workers' compensation, 433–434
HIPAA 837I, 529, 530
HIPAA 837P, 260, 529
HIPAA Electronic Transaction and Code Sets Standards, 47, 57–59
HIPAA Eligibility for a Health Plan, 87
HIPAA Privacy Rule, 47
Acknowledgment of Receipt of Notice of Privacy Practices, 81–82
authorizations to release, 52–56
disclosures, 48–56, 84
examples of compliance, 49–52
exemptions, 49
workers' compensation and, 428–429
HIPAA Referral Certification and Authorization, 88
HIPAA Security Rule, 47, 56–57, 84
disposition of electronic protected health information, 505
identity theft and, 99
HIPAA X12 276/277 Health Care Claim Status Inquiry/Response, 267, 453–454
HIPAA X12 837 Health Care Claim or Equivalent Encounter Information, 238–239, 260–267, 388
claim attachments, 266–267
claim information, 265–266
claim organization, 260–263, 272–273
credit-debit information, 267
payer information, 264–265
provider information, 261
service line information, 266
subscriber information, 261
History of present illness (HPI), 39, 162, 218–219
HIV/AIDS, statutory reports, 53–55
HMOs. *See* Health maintenance organizations (HMOs)
Home health agency (HHA), 514
Home health care, 514
Home plans, Blue Cross/Blue Shield, 303
Hospice care, 514
Hospital care, 513–536. *See also* Surgical procedures
claims processing, 514–524, 529–536
admission, 312, 515–516
coding, 524–526
discharge and billing, 521–524, 529–536
records of treatments and charges, 518–521
remittance advice processing, 530
encounter forms for, 94
ICD-9-CM for, 113
inpatient, 513–514, 524–528
integrated delivery systems, 514
outpatient or ambulatory, 168, 514
payers and payment methods, 526–529
Medicare, 526–529
private payers, 529
regulation by Joint Commission on Accreditation of Healthcare Organizations (JCAHO), 518–521
TRICARE Standard, 403
Hospital Consent Form, 517
Hospital Insurance (HI; Medicare, Part A), 334
Host plans, Blue Cross/Blue Shield, 303
Humana Inc., 300
Hypertension, ICD-9-CM coding for, 134
Hypertensive heart disease, ICD-9-CM coding for, 134

ICD-9-CM codes, 111–136
addenda, 112
Alphabetic Index, 113, 114–117, 525
abbreviations, 116
common terms, 117
cross-references, 115
eponyms, 117
locating primary diagnosis in, 124
M (morphology) codes, 132
main terms, 114
multiple codes and connecting words, 116–117
Neoplasm Table, 131–132
notes, 115
sample entries, 114
subterms, 114
supplementary terms, 115
Table of Drugs and Chemicals, 123
turnover lines, 115
in claims processing, 249–250
code edits, 210
coding steps, 124
defined, 18
described, 111–112
fifth-digit requirement, 119
HIPAA 837 claims, 355
hospital, 525–526
hospitalization, 524–525
job reference aids (cheat sheets), 214–215
linkage between CPT codes and, 205, 206, 210–211, 266, 339
nature of, 111–112
new revision, ICD-10-CM, 112–113
Official Guidelines for Coding and Reporting, 125–130
coexisting conditions, 124
highest level of certainty, 129
highest level of specificity, 130
primary diagnosis, 128
specific diagnoses, 130–136
organization of, 113
origins of, 111–112
Tabular List, 113, 117–122, 525–526, 526
abbreviations, 120–121
categories, 117
multiple codes, 121–122
notes, 119
punctuation, 120
sample entries, 119
subcategories, 117–118
subclassification, 118
supplementary classifications, 122–124
symbols, 119–120, 121
verifying code in, 124
updates, 112
Volume 3, 525–526
ICD-10-CM codes, 112–113
Identification cards. *See* Insurance cards
Identity theft, 99
Identity verification
for patient, 78–80
for person requesting information, 82
Ill-defined conditions, ICD-9-CM coding for, 135
Immunity disorders, ICD-9-CM coding for, 133
Immunizations, CPT codes, 152, 179–180
In-network providers, 401
Incident-to billing, 354
Indemnity plans, 6–7, 295–296, 315–320
commercial insurance carriers, 14
comparison with other options, 13
group policies, 6
individual policies, 6
Indentions (CPT), 151
Independent medical examination (IME), 427
Independent practice associations (IPAs)
health maintenance organizations, 295
Medicare coordinated care plans, 348
Indirect provider, 82
Individual deductible, 290
Individual health plans (IHP), 289
Individual policies, 6
Individual relationship code, 261
Infectious diseases, ICD-9-CM coding for, 130
Information technology, 47–48. *See also* MediSoft; Practice management programs (PMPs)
importance of, 22, 518
limitations of, 22
Informed consent, 39
Initial preventive physical examination (IPPE), 338
Injury, ICD-9-CM coding for, 135–136
Inpatient care, 513–514, 524–528
Inpatient principal diagnosis, 526
Inpatient principal procedure, 526
Inpatient Prospective Payment System (IPPS), 527
Insurance
disability, 6
liability, 472
medical. *See* Medical insurance

Insurance aging report, 453, 454
Insurance cards, 78–80, 86
  Blue Cross/Blue Shield, 301, 302
  CHAMPVA, 409
  Medicaid, 380, 381, 382
  Medicare, 335, 336
  POS plan, 307
  precertification requirement on, 311
  TRICARE, 400
Insurance verification, 86–92
  communications with third-party payers, 92
  eligibility of new patients, 86–92, 315
  insurance card, 78–80, 86. *See also* Insurance cards
  preauthorizations for services, 88
  primary versus secondary insurance, 89–91
  referrals to specialists, 88–89
Insured, 76
Integrated delivery systems, 514
Internal audits, 216, 316, 320
International Classification of Diseases, Ninth Revision, *Clinical Modification* (ICD-9-CM), 18, 111–112. *See also* Diagnosis codes; ICD-9-CM codes
Internet
  portals, 86
  as research tool, 24
  security symbol for information, 56
Ischemic heart disease, ICD-9-CM coding for, 133

Job reference aids (cheat sheets), 214–215
Joint Commission on Accreditation of Healthcare Organizations (JCAHO), 301, 518–521

Kaiser Permanente, 300
Key components (E/M code), 164

Laboratory requirements, 86, 178, 213, 315
  Clinical Laboratory Improvement Amendments (CLIA), 354
Late effects, 129
Late enrollees, 290
Legal environment. *See also* Fraud and abuse detection and investigation
  legal status of medical records, 36–37
  medical professional liability
  physician-patient relationship, 36–37
Letter samples. *See also* Form samples
  termination letter, 43
  utilization review organization, 313
Level I codes. *See* CPT codes
Level II codes. *See* HCPCS codes
Level II modifiers (HCPCS), 194, 195
Level III codes, 189
Liability insurance, 472
Lifetime limit, 290
Lifetime reserve (LTR), Medicare, 516–517
Limiting charge, 345
Line item control number, 266
Linkage and compliance review, 205, 206, 210–211, 266, 339
List of Excluded Individuals/Entities (LEIE), 209–210
Local coverage determinations (LCDs), Medicare, 341
Local Medicare Review Policies (LMRP), 341
Log files, 56
Long-term care
  described, 514
  spend-down programs, 380
  spousal impoverishment protection, 377
Longshore and Harbor Workers' Compensation Act (LHWCA), 423
Low-income patients, discounts for, 214
Lozenge (ICD-9-CM), 120

M (morphology) codes, 132
Main term (ICD-9-CM), 114
Managed care, 7–8
Managed care organizations (MCOs), 7–8
  appointment scheduling, 76
  Blue Cross/Blue Shield plans, 302–303
  growth of, 8
  hospital care, 529
  laboratory requirements, 86
  Medicaid coverage, 385
  origins of, 8
  participation contracts, 304–312
  plan types, 8–16
    consumer-driven health plans, 12–13
    health maintenance organization (HMO), 8–11
    preferred provider organization (PPO), 11–12
    provider-sponsored organization (PSO), 348
  TRICARE Extra, 404
  TRICARE Prime, 403–404
Manifestation, 116–117
Manual review, 450–451
Master patient index, 515
Maximum benefit limit
  CHAMPVA, 411
  defined, 290
  TRICARE, 401
Means tests, 504
Medi-Medi beneficiaries, 387, 474–476
Mediation, 433
Medicaid, 15, 374–390
  administration of, 15, 374
  billing procedures, 194–196, 388
  claims processing, 387–390
    coding, 387
    fee-for-service plans, 385
    managed care, 385
    payment for services, 385–386
    submission of claims, 387
    unacceptable billing practices, 388
  covered services, 384
  eligibility requirements
    enrollment verification, 380–383
    federal, 375–377
    state, 374, 377–380
  enrollment verification, 380–383
  establishment of, 374
  excluded services, 384
  fraud detection and investigation, 60, 62–63, 380, 382–383
  hospital care, 526
  insurance card, 380, 381, 382
  Medi-Medi beneficiaries, 387, 474–476
  payment for services, 385–386
  preauthorization, 384
  resubmission code, 250
  spend-down programs, 380
  third-party liability, 386–387
  types of plans
    fee-for-service, 385
    managed care, 385
MediCal, 377, 387
Medical administrative support, 4
Medical assistants, 4, 25–26
Medical coders, 27–28
Medical history, 76, 77–78, 162–163
Medical insurance. *See also* Medical insurance specialists; *specific programs*
  accrediting organizations, 301, 518–521
  career opportunities. *See* Career opportunities
  contract, 5
  cost increases, 3–4
  defined, 4
  extent of coverage, 14, 315
  group or individual policies, 6
  payers, 14–16
    determining financial responsibility, 17
    government-sponsored, 15–16
    private-sector, 14
    self-funded (self-insured) plans, 15
  plan types, 6–14
    indemnity, 6–7
    managed care, 7–14
  policy types, 6
  regulation
    federal, 45–46
    state, 46
  reimbursement, capitation, 9–10
  terminology, 4–5
  verifying coverage, 515
Medical insurance specialists, 16–21, 22–28
  attributes, 24–25
  certification, 25–28
    Certified Coding Specialist (CCS), 28
    Certified Medical Assistant (CMA), 25–26
    Certified Professional Coder (CPC; CPC-H), 28
    Registered Health Information Technician (RHIT), 26
    Registered Medical Assistant (RMA), 25–26
  characteristics for success, 23–25
  communications skills of. *See* Communications skills
  computer technology and. *See* Computer technology
  described, 22–23
  diagnosis codes and, 111–112
  education, 25–26
  job functions, 16
  medical billing process and, 16–21
  medical ethics and etiquette, 25
  roles and responsibilities, 23
  securing and advancing on job, 25–28
Medical necessity, defined, 5, 37
Medical necessity review, 86
  code edit, 205
  coding errors relating to, 211
  medical necessity denial of claim, 451–452
  Medicare, 338–339
  postpayment audit, 466–467
Medical professional liability, 37, 64
Medical Provider Analysis and Review (MedPar), 530
Medical records. *See* Patient medical records
Medical Review (MR) Program, Medicare, 352–353
Medical Savings Account (MSA) plans, 349
Medical standards of care, 36–37
Medically needy persons, 377
Medicare, 15, 333–362
  administration of, 15, 333–334
  appeals, 465, 466
  audit types, 352–353
  billing procedures, 194–196, 351–354, 516
  claims processing, 336–339, 351–354
    Clinical Laboratory Improvement Amendments (CLIA), 354
    CMS-1500, 238, 239–259, 356–361, 472–474
    Correct Coding Initiative (CCI), 207–209, 339, 351
    duplicate claims, 353
    electronic billing, 351
    electronic transmission, 351
    exclusions, 338–339, 341
    Explanation of Medical Benefits (EOMB), 346
    fiscal intermediaries, 336
    global surgical package, 352
    HCPCS codes required for, 192, 351
    HIPAA 837 claims, 355–356
    HIPAA 837 form locators, 355–356
    hospitalization, 516–517, 518–521
    ICD-9 codes required for, 111–112
    incident-to billing, 354
    Local Medicare Review Policies (LMRP), 341
    Medicare as secondary payer, 351, 356, 468–477, 516
    RA/EOB, 470
    regulation of, 194–196
    release of information statements, 81–82
    roster billing, 354
    split billing, 353
    timely filing requirement, 352
  Clinical Laboratory Improvement Amendments (CLIA), 178, 354
  Common Working File (CWF), 336
  coordinated care plans, 348–349
  coverage and benefits, 335–339
  eligibility requirements, 333–335, 470–471
  establishment of, 333
  fee-for-service plans, 350
  fee schedules, 222–224, 226, 308–312, 341, 351–352
  fraud detection and investigation, 60, 62–63, 346, 352–353, 530
    audits, 352–353
    Quality Improvement Organizations (QIOs), 527–528
  hospital care, 526–529
    diagnosis-related groups (DRGs), 527, 528
    inpatient payment system, 527–528
    outpatient payment systems, 529
  incident-to billing, 354
  insurance card, 335, 336
  Medi-Medi beneficiaries, 387, 474–476
  Medical Review (MR) Program, 352–353
  Medicare Advantage plans, 335, 348–349
  medigap insurance, 349–351
    described, 350
    Medicare Summary Notice (MSN), 346, 347
  nonparticipating providers, 344–345
    payment for acceptance of assignment, 344
    payment for unassigned claims, 345
  Notice of Exclusions from Medicare Benefits (NEMB), 341, 342

Medicare—*Cont.*
Original Medicare Plan, 346
overpayments, 468
participating providers, 340–344
advance beneficiary notice (ABN), 341–344
incentives, 340
payments, 341–344
patient rights under, 466, 518
preauthorization, 354
private fee-for-service (PFFS) plans, 349
programs, 334–335
excluded services, 338–339, 341, 342
not medically necessary services, 338–339
Part A, 334
Part B, 334–335, 337–338
Part C, 335
Part D, 335
roster billing, 354
as secondary payer, 346, 351, 468–477, 516
supplemental insurance, described, 351
surgical procedures, 351–354
Medicare, Medicaid, and SCHIP Benefits and Improvement Act (BIPA; 2000), 465
Medicare Advantage, 335, 348–349
Medicare carriers, 355
Medicare Carriers Manual (MCM), 196, 207
Medicare Catastrophic Coverage Act (1988), 112
Medicare Comprehensive Limiting Charge Compliance Program (CLCCP), 345
Medicare Fee Schedule (MFS), 341–342
Medicare health insurance claim number (HICN), 335–339
Medicare Modernization Act (MMA), 297–298, 335, 349
Medicare Outpatient Adjudication remark codes (MOA), 458
Medicare Physician Fee Schedule (MPFS), 224, 226, 308–312, 341, 351–352
Medicare Prescription Drug, Improvement, and Modernization Act (2003), 297–298, 335, 349
Medicare Redetermination Notice (MRN), 465, 467
Medicare Secondary Payer (MSP), 470–477, 516
Medicare Summary Notice (MSN), 346, 347
Medigap insurance, 349–351
CMS-1500 claim completion, 360–362
coverage, 350
described, 350
Medicare Summary Notice (MSN), 346, 347
Medisoft, Guide to, 593-615
Medisoft, as example of practice management program, 22
claim transmission, 269
data entry
patient information, 242
payer information, 241
Service Line Information, 251
tips for, 267
EMC verification report, 270
Patient/Guarantor Dialog box, 83
Patient List, 83
security setup, 57
Mental disorders, ICD-9-CM coding for, 133
Mental Health Parity Act, 292
Metabolic diseases, ICD-9-CM coding for, 133
Microsoft Windows, 24
Military Health System (MHS), 406
Military Treatment Facility (MTF), 401
Minimum necessary standard, 49, 50, 210
Minors
birthday rule to determine primary insurance, 91
Early and Periodic Screening, Diagnosis, and Treatment (EPSDT), 376
gender rule to determine primary insurance, 91
Medicaid eligibility, 374, 375
Medicare eligibility, 333
release of information statement, 83
State Children's Health Insurance Program (SCHIP), 375
state programs for, 377–379
Temporary Assistance for Needy Families (TANF), 375, 377
MOA (Medicare outpatient adjudication remark codes), 458
Modifiers
advance beneficiary notice (ABN), Medicare, 341, 344
CPT, 152–155, 212–213
Anesthesia section, 170–171
assigning, 155
bilateral, 176
determining need for, 157
Evaluation and Management section, 160–161
listing of, 154
meaning of, 155
Medicine section, 179
Pathology and Laboratory section, 178
Radiology section, 177
Surgical section, 173–175
use of, 152–155
HCPCS, 194, 195
Monthly enrollment list, 320
Multiple codes (ICD-9-CM)
code also, 122
code first underlying disease, 121
use additional code, 122
use additional code, if desired, 122
Musculoskeletal and connective tissue diseases, ICD-9-CM coding for, 134

Name of patient, 80
National Association of Insurance Commissioners, 300
National Center for Health Statistics (NCHS), 111, 112, 125
National Committee for Quality Assurance (NCQA), 301
National coverage determinations (NCDs), Medicare, 341
National Drug Codes (NDC), 250
National Health Care Anti-Fraud Association, 59
National identifiers, 58–59
National Medicaid EDI HIPAA Workgroup (NMEH), 387
National Provider identifier (NPI), 59, 239, 248, 307, 320
National Uniform Claim Committee (NUCC), 239, 258, 316
NEC (not elsewhere classified), 116, 120–121, 192
Neoplasms, ICD-9-CM coding for, 131–132
Nervous system disorders, ICD-9-CM coding for, 133
Network of providers, 8, 10
New Freedom Initiative, 376
New patients
defined, 74
Evaluation and Management section (E/M codes), 159–160
patient information, 74–82
assignment of benefits, 81
database of patients, 83–84
patient information form, 76–78, 79
verifying insurance eligibility of, 86–92, 315
New procedures, payment for, 309
Newborns' and Mothers' Health Protection Act, 291–292
No-fault insurance, 472
No-shows, billing for, 309
Nonavailability statements (NAS), 403
Noncovered/overlimit services, 5, 87–88, 95–96, 403. *See also* Excluded services
Nonparticipating (nonPAR) providers, 87
allowed charges, 226
collection for services, 96
defined, 76
discounts for out-of-network visits, 316
Medicare
payment for acceptance of assignment, 344
payment for unassigned claims, 345
TRICARE, 400–401
NOS (not otherwise specified), 120–121
Not elsewhere classified (NEC), 116, 120–121, 192
Not medically necessary services, Medicare, 338–339
Not Otherwise Classified (NOC) drugs, 358
Not otherwise specified (NOS), 120–121
Not required (NR) elements, 261
Notes segment, 266
HIPAA 837 claims, 355
ICD-9-CM, 115, 119–120
Notice of Contest, 429
Notice of Exclusions from Medicare Benefits (NEMB), 341, 342
Notice of Privacy Practices (NPP), 49, 501
Notice of Workers' Compensation Coverage, 424
NTE segment, HIPAA 837 claims, 355
Nutritional diseases, ICD-9-CM coding for, 133

Occupational diseases or illnesses, 425
Occupational Safety and Health Administration (OSHA), 64, 178, 423
Office for Civil Rights (OCR), 62–63
Office of Personnel Management (OPM), 288
Office of the Inspector General (OIG), 60–63
Compliance Program Guidance for Individual and Small Group Physician Practices, 213–214
False Claims Act, 60, 63, 353, 383
OIG Work Plan, 209–210, 530
price-fixing avoidance, 309
Office of Workers' Compensation Programs (OWCP), 423–424
OIG Work Plan, 209–210, 530
Open-access/open-panel plans, 11, 293
Open enrollment periods, 288
Original Medicare Plan, 346
Other health insurance (OHI), 405
Other id number, 248
Out-of-network providers, 10, 87, 96, 311, 316, 401
Out-of-pocket expense, 7
Outpatient Prospective Payment System (OPPS), 529
Outpatient services, 168, 514
Outside laboratory, 249
Overpayments
Medicare, 468
refunding, 468, 504–505
Oxford Health Plans, 300

Pain terminology, 427–428
Panels, 177–178
Paper-based medical records, 43
parasitic diseases, ICD-9-CM coding for, 130
Parentheses (ICD-9-CM), 120
Part A, Medicare, 334
Part B, Medicare, 334–335, 337–338
Part C, Medicare, 335
Part D, Medicare, 335
Participating (PAR) providers
allowed charges, 225–227
CHAMPVA, 410–411
defined, 76
Medicare, 340–344
incentives, 340
payments, 341–342
TRICARE, 400
Participation, 8
Participation contracts, 304–312
Passwords, 56
Past medical history (PMH), 162
Pathology and Laboratory codes (CPT), 177–178
panels, 177–178
reporting, 178
special reports, 178
structure and modifiers, 178
unlisted procedures, 178
Patient aging reports, 495
Patient billing program
names of programs. *See also* MediSoft
write-off of capitated accounts, 321
Patient examinations, documentation of, 38–39
Patient Financial Agreement, 88
Patient information, 74–85. *See also* Patient medical records
CMS-1500 form locators, 239–246
communications with patients, 84, 98–101
computer technology and, 83–84. *See also* MediSoft
confidentiality of
exceptions to confidentiality requirements, 53–55
guidelines for release, 88–89
established patients, 82
new patients, 74–82
patient rights to, 466
preregistration process, 16–17
release of. *See* Authorization to release information
updating, 83, 263
Patient information form (PIF)
CMS-1500 claims, 239–246
for established patients, 82
for new patients, 76–78
sample form, 79
in verifying eligibility for insurance benefits, 86–88
Patient ledger, 18–19
Patient medical records, 36–45. *See also* Patient information
Acknowledgment of Receipt of Notice of Privacy Practices, 81–82
billing for copies of, 52, 95
chart numbers, 83
database of patients, 83–84
defined, 36
disability compensation and, 428–429

documentation standards, 36–45
discharge summaries, 40–41
medical record formats, 37–38
office procedure note, 41–42
patient encounters, 37–38
patient examinations, 38–39
progress reports, 39, 41
termination of provider-patient relationship, 42–43
electronic, 43–45
formats
problem-oriented medical record (POMR) format, 37–38
SOAP format, 37–38, 39
during hospitalization, 518–521
legal status, 36–37
paper-based, 43
patient rights to information in, 466
Patients, established. *See* Established patients
Patients, new. *See* New patients
Patients' statements, 20–21, 486–491
content of, 489
relating to practice management program, 489–491
Pay-for-performance (P4P), 11, 300
Pay-to provider, 247
Payer of last resort, 387
Payers, 14–16. *See also* Claims preparation and processing; Third-party payers
adjudication, 20, 449–452, 458
defined, 5
government-sponsored plans, 15–16
private plans, 14
self-funded plans, 15
Payment methods of patients
cash, 98
check, 98
credit arrangements, 98–99, 499–500
credit/debit card, 98–99
Payment per member per month (PMPM), 229, 294–295
Peer review organizations (PROs), 354, 527–528
Pending claims, 453
Per member per month (PMPM) fee, 9–10
Perinatal conditions, ICD-9-CM coding for, 135
Permanent national codes (HCPCS), 192
Personal Responsibility and Work Opportunity Reconciliation Act (1996), 377
Photo identification, 80
Physical status modifier, 170–171
Physician information, CMS-1500 claims, 247–257. *See also* Providers
Physician of record, workers' compensation, 429
Physician practice manager. *See also* Practice manager
Place of service (POS) code, 252
Plan summary grids, 313–314
Point-of-service (POS) plans, 11, 292, 295
Blue Cross/Blue Shield coverage, 302
comparison with other options, 13
Poisoning, ICD-9-CM coding for, 135–136
Policies
group insurance, 6
individual insurance, 6
Policyholder, 4–5, 76
Portals, 86
Postpayment audits, 466–467
Practice management programs (PMP). *See also* MediSoft
Practice management programs (PMPs), 22
entering insurance information, 92
entering patient information, 83–84
entering payer information, 241
relating patients' statements to, 489–491
Practice manager
management of fee schedule, 221–222
payments over time, 98, 99, 499–500
Preauthorization, 88, 310
CHAMPVA, 410
health maintenance organization (HMO), 10
Medicaid, 384
Medicare, 354
meeting requirements for, 315–316
of surgical procedures, 310–312
TRICARE Standard, 403
Precertification. *See* Preauthorization
Preexisting condition exclusions, 5, 291
Preferred provider organizations (PPOs), 11–12, 292–293, 294
Blue Cross/Blue Shield coverage, 303
comparison with other options, 13
contracted fee schedules, 224
hospital care, 529
Medicare, 348
silent, avoiding, 310
Pregnancy and childbirth coverage, 291
Pregnancy complications, ICD-9-CM coding for, 134
Premium, 7, 290
Prepayment plans, 500
Preregistration of patients, 16–17, 75–85, 315
Prescription drugs
cost controls of HMOs, 10
Medicare Prescription Drug, Improvement, and Modernization Act (2003), 297–298, 335, 349
Presenting problem (E/M code), 164
Pretreatment patient payment collection, 516–517
Preventive medical services, 295
CPT codes, 168
defined, 5
health maintenance organization (HMO), 11
Medicare
covered procedures, 338, 339
exclusion, 338–339
Price fixing, avoiding, 309
Primary Care Manager (PCM), 403–404
Primary care physician (PCP), 10
patient eligibility for insurance benefits, 86–92, 315
referrals from, 385
termination of patient relationship, 42–43
verifying, 86
Primary diagnosis, 124, 128
Primary insurance
coordination of benefits, 89–91
defined, 89
determining primary coverage, 315–316
Medicare, 357–359
for minors, 91
verifying patient eligibility under, 315–316
Primary procedures, 152
Principal diagnosis (PDX), 524
Principal procedure, 526
Prior authorization. *See* Preauthorization
Prior authorization number, 88
Privacy officers, 48
Privacy policy, 49–51. *See also* Confidential information; Patient medical records
Private fee-for-service (PFFS), Medicare, 349
Private payers, 14, 287–322. *See also* Blue Cross and Blue Shield Association (BCBS); Indemnity plans; Managed care organizations (MCOs)
billing, 196, 312–320
Blue Cross and Blue Shield Associations, 300–303
capitation management, 320–321
CCI edits, 210
CMS-1500 claims, 316–318
compensation and billing guidelines, 307–312
group health plans (GHP), 287–288, 290–292
hospital care, 529
individual plans, 289
list of major payers and accrediting groups, 300, 301
participation contracts, 304–312
sample private pay agreement, 386
self-funded plans, 289
services provided, 299
third-party claims administrators, 289
types of plans, 292–299
Problem-oriented medical record (POMR) format, 37–38
Procedural services, 41–42
Procedure codes. *See also* CPT codes; HCPCS codes
defined, 18
hospital, 525–526
introduction to, 144–145
linkage between diagnosis codes and, 205, 206, 210–211, 266, 339
Professional component, CPT code, 155
Professional courtesy discounts, 213
Progress reports
documentation of, 39, 41
workers' compensation, 429, 431
Prompt payment
discounts for, 309
prompt-pay laws, 453
Prospective audits, 216
Prospective Payment System (PPS), 527, 529
Protected health information (PHI), 48–56
authorizations for release of, 52–56
in claims transmission, 266, 268
in collection process, 501, 503
disclosure for treatment, payment, and health care operations (TPO), 48–52, 81
dual-eligible status and, 387
group health plans and, 289
on RA/EOB, 470
Provider-sponsored organizations (PSOs), Medicare coordinated care plans, 348
Provider withhold, 229
Providers
CMS-1500 (08/05) claim information, 247–257
communication with, 94
as covered entities under HIPAA, 47
defined, 5
direct versus indirect, 82
documenting encounters with, 37–43
establishing financial responsibility, 17, 86–88, 315–316
information for CMS-1500 claims, 247–257
information for HIPAA 837 claims, 261
Medicare, 340–345
National Provider identifier (NPI), 59, 239, 248, 307, 320
network of, 8, 10
nonparticipating. *See* Nonparticipating (nonPAR) providers
participating. *See* Participating (PAR) providers
primary care. *See* Primary care physician (PCP)
TRICARE, 399–401
usual fees, 220–221
Psychotherapy notes, release of, 55
Puerperium complications, ICD-9-CM coding for, 134

Qualified independent contractor (QIC), 406
Qualifier, 248
Quality improvement, health maintenance organization (HMO), 11
Quality Improvement Organization (QIO), 354, 527–528
Qui tam cases, 60

RA/EOB. See Remittance advice/explanation of benefits (RA/EOB)
Radiology codes, CPT, 176–177
contrast material, 177
reporting, 177
special reports, 176–177
structure and modifiers, 177
unlisted procedures, 176–177
Railroad Retirement Board, 333
Reconciliation, 462–463
Record retention, 505
Redetermination, 465–467
Referral numbers, 88–89
Referral waivers, 89, 90
Referrals
in capitation management, 321
consultations versus, 314
determining requirements for, 88–89
E/M codes, 160
in health maintenance organizations (HMOs), 10, 11
insurance verification by specialist's office, 88–89
meeting requirements for, 315–316
referral numbers, 88–89
self-referrals
patient, 11, 89
physician, 60–61
Referring physician, 75
Refunds, 468, 504–505
Registered Health Information Administrator (RHIA), 26
Registered Health Information Technician (RHIT), 26
Registered Medical Assistant (RMA), 25–26
Registration, hospital, 515–516
Regulation of medical insurance
accrediting organizations, 301
federal, 45–46
state, 46
Reimbursement
capitation, 9–10
fee-for-service, 6–7
Relative value scale (RVS), 222–223, 425
Relative value unit (RVU), 223

Release of information. *See* Authorization to release information
REM (remark codes), 458, 461
Remittance advice/explanation of benefits (RA/EOB), 452
adjustments, 458–460
contents of, 456–457
denial management, 463
hospital, 530
procedures for posting, 462–463
remark codes, 458, 461
reviewing, 462
Rendering provider, 247
Repricer, 316
Required data elements, 261
Required if applicable (RIA) elements, 261
Research data, release of information for, 55
Resource-based fee structures, 222
Resource-based relative value scale (RBRVS), 223–224, 341
Respiratory system diseases, ICD-9-CM coding for, 134
Respondeat superior, 63
Responsible party, 261
Restricted status, 380–381
Retention schedule, 505
Retrospective audits, 216
Return service requested, 489
Review of systems (ROS), 39, 162, 215
Roster billing, 354
Routing slips. *See* Encounter forms

SADMERC (statistical analysis durable medical equipment carrier), 192
Sarbanes-Oxley Act of 2002, 60–61
Schedule of benefits, 5
Scheduling systems, 75–76
Screening service, 338
Second-party payers, 5, 9–10
Secondary insurance
billing secondary payers, 468–477
claims processing, 468–477
coordination of benefits, 89–91
defined, 89
Medicare as, 351, 356, 470–474
TRICARE claims processing, 474
Secondary procedures, 152
Section 125 cafeteria plans, 290
Section guidelines (CPT), 150–151
Security policy, 57
Self-funded (self-insured) plans, 15, 289, 424
Self-pay patients, 96
Self-Referral form, 90
Self-referrals
patient, 11, 89
physician, 60–61
Semicolons (CPT), 151
Sense organ disorders, ICD-9-CM coding for, 133
Separate procedures (CPT), 172–173
Service line information
CMS-1500 claims, 250, 251
HIPAA 837 claims, 266
Signature on File (SOF), 246, 257
Signs, coding, 129–130
Silent PPOs, 310
Situational data elements, 261
Skilled nursing facilities (SNF), 513
Skin and subcutaneous diseases, ICD-9-CM coding for, 134
Skip tracing, 502–503
SOAP format, 37–38, 39
Social history (SH), 163
Social Security Act, 333, 374, 385
Social Security Disability Insurance (SSDI), 434
Special needs plans (SNPs), Medicare coordinated care plans, 348–349
Special reports (CPT), 151
Pathology and Laboratory section, 178
Radiology section, 176–177
Spend-down programs, 380
Split billing, Medicare, 353
Spousal Impoverishment Protection, 377
Staff HMO, 293
Stark rules, 60–61
State Children's Health Insurance Program (SCHIP), 375
States
assignment of benefits and, 81
implementation of Welfare Reform Act, 377
Medicaid benefits, 377–380
Medicaid eligibility requirements, 374
privacy regulations of, 48, 55–56
prohibition of silent PPOs, 310
prompt-pay laws, 453
regulation of medical insurance, 46
workers' compensation plans, 424–426
Statistical analysis durable medical equipment carrier (SADMERC), 192
Statutory reports, HIV/AIDS information, 53–55
Stop-loss provision, 306
Subcapitation, 295
Subcategories (ICD-9-CM), 117–118
Subclassification (ICD-9-CM), 118
Subpoena, 53
Subpoena *duces tecum*, 53
Subscribers, 76
HIPAA 837 claim information, 261
Subterms (ICD-9-CM), 114
Summary Plan Description (SPD), 289
Superbills, 93. *See also* Encounter forms
Supplemental insurance
coordination of benefits, 89–91
defined, 89
Medicare, described, 351
Supplemental Security Income (SSI), 377, 379, 435
Supplementary Medical Insurance (SMI; Medicare Part B), 334–335
Supplementary terms (ICD-9-CM), 115
Surgery codes
CPT, 171–176
modifiers, 173–175
reporting, 175–176
separate procedures, 172–173
structure, 173
surgical package, 171–172
ICD-9-CM, 130
Surgical procedures
elective surgery, 310–311, 344
health care facilities providing, 514
in managed care participation contract, 310–311
Medicare, 351–352, 353, 354
preauthorization of, 310–312
surgical package, 171–172, 352
Suspected diagnosis, 524–525
Suspended claims, 450–451
Symbols
CPT, 152
ICD-9-CM, 119–120, 121
Symptoms, coding, 129–130

Table of Drugs and Chemicals, 123
Tabular List. *See* ICD-9-CM codes, Tabular List
Taxonomy codes, 257, 258, 320
Technical component, CPT code, 155
Telephone
collections calls using, 496–498, 503
disclosure of patient information by, 55, 87
skip trace calls, 503
Telephone Consumer Protection Act (1991), 494
Temporary Assistance for Needy Families (TANF), 375, 377
Termination
of nonpaying patients, 504
of patient-provider relationship, 42–43
of patients in HMOs and POSs, 295
of workers' compensation and benefits, 432–433
Tertiary insurance
coordination of benefits, 89–91
defined, 89
Third-party claims administrators (TPAs), 289, 305
Third-party payers, 5, 9–10
adjudication, 449–452
CHAMPVA claims and, 411
communication skills with, 92, 320, 454–455
Medicaid claims and, 386–387
Ticket to Work and Work Incentives Improvement Act (TWWIIA; 1999), 376
Tiered networks, 291
Title IX, Social Security Act, 385
Trace number, 87
Training and education
compliance with regulations, 65
medical insurance specialist, 25–26
Transactions, 46–47
Treatment, payment, and health care operations (TPO), 48–52, 81, 515
TRICARE, 399–409
administration of, 15
claims processing, 405–406, 474
defined, 15
eligibility requirements, 399
fraud and abuse, 406–409
identification cards, 400
providers, 399–401
network and non-network, 401
nonparticipating, 400–401
participating, 400
reimbursement, 401
secondary claims, 474
types of plans, 401–405
TRICARE Extra, 404
TRICARE for Life, 404–405
TRICARE Maximum Allowable Charge (TMAC), 401
TRICARE Prime, 403–404
TRICARE Reserve Select (TRS), 404
TRICARE Standard, 401–403
Truncated coding, 211
Truth in Lending Act, 499
Turnover (carryover) lines (ICD-9-CM), 115
UB-04 (uniform billing 2004), 530, 531–536
Unassigned claims, payment for, 97, 345
Unbundling, 172–173, 175, 211, 212
Uncollectible accounts, 503–505
Unconfirmed diagnosis, 524–525
Uniform Hospital Discharge Data Set (UHDDS), 524
Uninsured patients, discounts for, 214
UnitedHealth Group, 14, 300
Universal claim form. *See* CMS-1500 (08/05)
Universal Product Codes (UPC), 250
Unlisted procedures (CPT), 151, 253
Pathology and Laboratory section, 178
Radiology section, 176–177
Unspecified, 120–121
UP-92 (uniform billing 1992), 530
Upcoding, 211
Urgently needed care, 348
Usual, customary, and reasonable (UCR) payment structures, 222
Usual fees, 220–221
Utilization review, 306
Utilization Review Accreditation Commission (URAC), 301
Utilization review organization (URO), 311, 313

V codes (ICD-9-CM), 122
Vaccine coding (CPT), 152, 179–180
Verification. *See* Insurance verification
Veteran's disability compensation, 436
Veterans Health Care Eligibility Reform Act (1996), 409
Vocational rehabilitation, 427

Waiting period, 290
Waiver of patient payment, Medicare, 346
Waiver of tests, 354
Walkout receipts, 99–101
Welfare Reform Act (1996), 377
WellPoint, Inc., 300
Wellpoint, Inc., 14
Whistleblower cases, 60
Women's Health and Cancer Rights Act, 172, 292
Workers' compensation, 6, 423–434
appeals, 433
billing process, 433–434
claims processing, 429–434
classification of injuries, 426–427
eligibility requirements, 424–425
benefits, 425
covered injuries and illnesses, 425–426
establishment of, 423–424
federal plans, 423–424
HIPAA Privacy Rule and, 428–429
Medicare coverage and, 472
Occupational Safety and Health Administration (OSHA), 64, 178, 423
release of information for, 53
state plans, 424–426
termination of compensation and benefits, 432–433
terminology, 427–428
World Health Organization (WHO), 111–112
Write off, 504